AMERICAN ACADEMY
OF OPHTHALMOLOGY®
Protecting Sight. Empowering Lives.

MW01701626

6 | Pediatric Ophthalmology and Strabismus

2022–2023
BCSC
Basic and Clinical Science Course™

EB Published after collaborative review with the European Board of Ophthalmology subcommittee

The American Academy of Ophthalmology is accredited by the Accreditation Council for Continuing Medical Education (ACCME) to provide continuing medical education for physicians.

The American Academy of Ophthalmology designates this enduring material for a maximum of 15 *AMA PRA Category 1 Credits*™. Physicians should claim only the credit commensurate with the extent of their participation in the activity.

CME expiration date: June 1, 2025. *AMA PRA Category 1 Credits*™ may be claimed only once between June 1, 2022, and the expiration date.

BCSC® volumes are designed to increase the physician's ophthalmic knowledge through study and review. Users of this activity are encouraged to read the text and then answer the study questions provided at the back of the book.

To claim *AMA PRA Category 1 Credits*™ upon completion of this activity, learners must demonstrate appropriate knowledge and participation in the activity by taking the posttest for Section 6 and achieving a score of 80% or higher. For further details, please see the instructions for requesting CME credit at the back of the book.

Cover image: From BCSC Section 12, *Retina and Vitreous.* Confocal scanning laser ophthalmoscopy multicolor fundus image (30° field of view) of a healthy eye. *(Courtesy of Lucia Sobrin, MD.)*

FSC www.fsc.org MIX Paper from responsible sources FSC® C001701

Printed in China.

Basic and Clinical Science Course

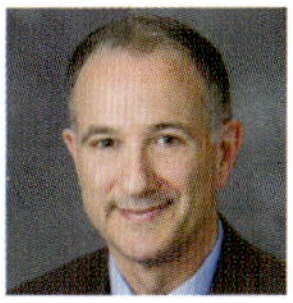

Christopher J. Rapuano, MD, Philadelphia, Pennsylvania
Senior Secretary for Clinical Education

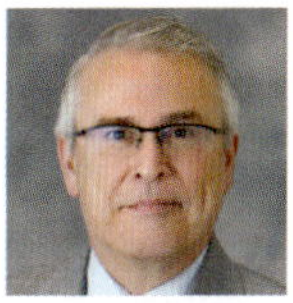

J. Timothy Stout, MD, PhD, MBA, Houston, Texas
Secretary for Lifelong Learning and Assessment

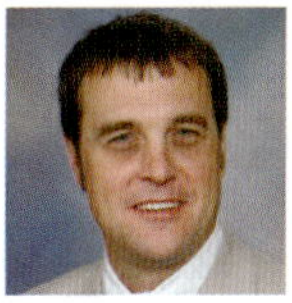

Colin A. McCannel, MD, Los Angeles, California
BCSC Course Chair

Section 6

Faculty for the Major Revision

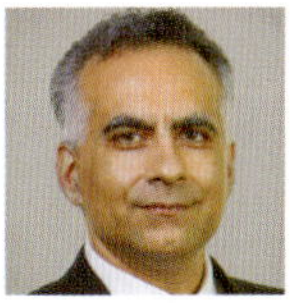

Arif O. Khan, MD
Chair
Abu Dhabi, United Arab Emirates

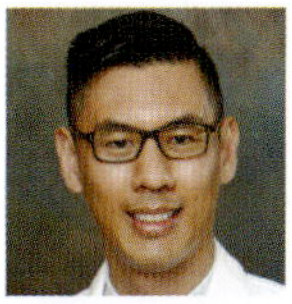

Ta Chen Peter Chang, MD
Miami, Florida

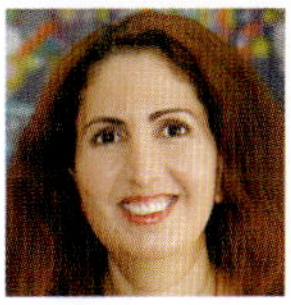

Mays A. El-Dairi, MD
Durham, North Carolina

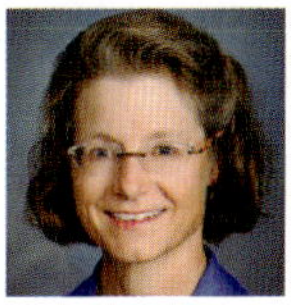

Katherine A. Lee, MD, PhD
Boise, Idaho

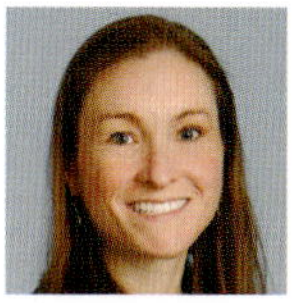

Virginia Miraldi Utz, MD
Cincinnati, Ohio

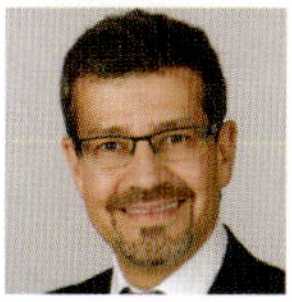

Kamiar Mireskandari, MBChB, PhD
Toronto, Canada

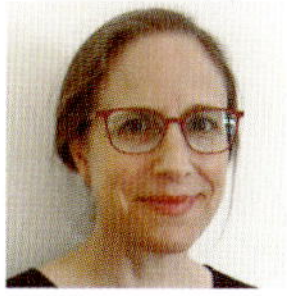

Kristina Tarczy-Hornoch, MD, DPhil
Seattle, Washington

The Academy acknowledges the following committees for review of this edition:

Committee on Aging: Aaron M. Miller, MD, MBA, Houston, Texas

Vision Rehabilitation Committee: Linda M. Lawrence, MD, Salina, Kansas

BCSC Resident/Fellow Reviewers: Sharon L. Jick, MD, *Chair,* St Louis, Missouri; Arpine Barsegian, MD; Stephanie N. Kletke, MD; Archana Nair, MD; Daniel G. Nelson, MD; Alisa Prager, MD; Michael A. Puente Jr, MD; Margaret McDougal Runner, MD; Allison Umfress, MD; Hersh Varma, MD; Ivy Zhu, MD

Practicing Ophthalmologists Advisory Committee for Education: George S. Ellis Jr, MD, *Primary Reviewer*, New Orleans, Louisiana; Cynthia S. Chiu, MD, Oakland, California; Bradley D. Fouraker, MD, Tampa, Florida; Philip R. Rizzuto, MD, Providence, Rhode Island; Gaurav K. Shah, MD, Town and Country, Missouri; Rosa A. Tang, MD, MPH, MBA, Houston, Texas; Troy M. Tanji, MD, Waipahu, Hawaii; Michelle S. Ying, MD, Ladson, South Carolina

The Academy also acknowledges the following committee for assistance in developing Study Questions and Answers for this BCSC Section:

Resident Self-Assessment Committee: Evan L. Waxman, MD, PhD, *Chair,* Pittsburgh, Pennsylvania; Robert A. Beaulieu, MD, Southfield, Michigan; Benjamin W. Botsford, MD, New York, New York; Olga M. Ceron, MD, Grafton, Massachusetts; Kevin Halenda, MD, Cleveland, Ohio; Amanda D. Henderson, MD, Baltimore, Maryland; Andrew M. Hendrick, MD, Atlanta, Georgia; Joshua Hendrix, MD, Dalton, Georgia; Matthew B. Kaufman, MD, Portland, Oregon; Zachary A. Koretz, MD, MPH, Pittsburgh, Pennsylvania; Kevin E. Lai, MD, Indianapolis, Indiana; Kenneth C. Lao, MD, Temple, Texas; Yasha S. Modi, MD, New York, New York; Mark E. Robinson, MD, MPH, Columbia, South Carolina; Jamie B. Rosenberg, MD, New York, New York; Tahira M. Scholle, MD, Houston, Texas; Ann Shue, MD, Sunnyvale, California; Jeong-Hyeon Sohn, MD, Shavano Park, Texas; Misha F. Syed, MD, League City, Texas; Parisa Taravati, MD, Seattle, Washington; Sarah Van Tassel, MD, New York, New York; Matthew S. Wieder, MD, Scarsdale, New York; Jules A. Winokur, MD, Great Neck, New York

In addition, the Academy recognizes the important contributions of E. Mitchel Opremcak, MD, and Sheila Angeles-Han, MD, MSc, in the development of Chapter 25, and Grace Prakalapakorn, MD, Michael Chiang, MD, and Robert Sisk, MD, in the development of Chapter 27.

EB

European Board of Ophthalmology: Lotte Welinder, MD, *Liaison*, Aalborg, Denmark; Anna P. Maino, MBBS, PGCert, Manchester, United Kingdom; Sara F. Syed, MBBChir, MACantab, PGClinEd, Manchester, United Kingdom

Financial Disclosures

Academy staff members who contributed to the development of this product state that within the 24 months prior to their contributions to this CME activity and for the duration of development, they have had no financial interest in or other relationship with any entity that produces, markets, resells, or distributes health care goods or services consumed by or used in patients, or with any competing commercial product or service.

The authors and reviewers state that within the 24 months prior to their contributions to this CME activity and for the duration of development, they have had the following financial relationships:*

Dr El-Dairi: Syneos Health (C)

Dr Fouraker: Addition Technology (C, L), AJL Ophthalmic SA (C, L), Alcon (C, L), OASIS Medical (C, L)

Dr Khan: Alcon (C), Novartis (C)

Dr Lai: Twenty/Twenty Therapeutics (C)

Dr Miller: Leadiant Biosciences (C, L), Luminopia (C)

Dr Miraldi Utz: Retrophin (S), Spark Therapeutics (C)

Dr Mireskandari: Bayer (S), Santen (C)

Dr Modi: Alimera Sciences (C), Allergan (C), Carl Zeiss (C), Genentech (C), Novartis (C), Théa Laboratories (C)

Dr Robinson: Horizon Therapeutics (O)

Dr Shah: Allergan (C, L, S), Bausch + Lomb (L), DORC Dutch Ophthalmic Research Center (International) BV (S), Regeneron Pharmaceuticals (C, L, S)

Dr Tang: EMD Serono (L), Horizon Therapeutics (C, S), Immunovant (S), Novartis (S), Quark Pharmaceuticals (C, S), Regenera Pharma (S), Sanofi (L), ZEISS (L)

Dr Tarczy-Hornoch: Amgen (O)

Dr Van Tassel: AbbVie (C), Aerie Pharmaceuticals (C), Allergan (C), Bausch + Lomb (C), Carl Zeiss Meditec (C), Equinox (C), New World Medical (C, L)

The other authors and reviewers state that within the 24 months prior to their contributions to this CME activity and for the duration of development, they have had no financial interest in or other relationship with any entity that produces, markets, resells, or distributes health care goods or services consumed by or used in patients, or with any competing commercial product or service.

* C = consultant fee, paid advisory boards, or fees for attending a meeting; E = employed by or received a W-2 from a commercial company; L = lecture fees or honoraria, travel fees or reimbursements when speaking at the invitation of a commercial company; O = equity ownership/stock options in publicly or privately traded firms, excluding mutual funds; P = patents and/or royalties for intellectual property; S = grant support or other financial support to the investigator from all sources, including research support from government agencies, foundations, device manufacturers, and/or pharmaceutical companies

Recent Past Faculty

Steven M. Archer, MD
Rebecca Sands Braverman, MD
Robert W. Hered, MD
Gregg T. Lueder, MD
Mary A. O'Hara, MD

In addition, the Academy gratefully acknowledges the contributions of numerous past faculty and advisory committee members who have played an important role in the development of previous editions of the Basic and Clinical Science Course.

American Academy of Ophthalmology Staff

Dale E. Fajardo, EdD, MBA, *Vice President, Education*
Beth Wilson, *Director, Continuing Professional Development*
Denise Evenson, *Director, Brand & Creative*
Susan Malloy, *Acquisitions and Development Manager*
Stephanie Tanaka, *Publications Manager*
Rayna Ungersma, *Manager, Curriculum Development*
Jasmine Chen, *Manager, E-Learning*
Sarah Page, *Online Education & Licensing Manager*
Lana Ip, *Senior Designer*
Beth Collins, *Medical Editor*
Amanda Fernandez, *Publications Editor*
Eric Gerdes, *Interactive Designer*
Lynda Hanwella, *Publications Specialist*
Debra Marchi, *Administrative Assistant*

American Academy of Ophthalmology
655 Beach Street
Box 7424
San Francisco, CA 94120-7424

Contents

Introduction to the BCSC

The Basic and Clinical Science Course (BCSC) is designed to meet the needs of residents and practitioners for a comprehensive yet concise curriculum of the field of ophthalmology. The BCSC has developed from its original brief outline format, which relied heavily on outside readings, to a more convenient and educationally useful self-contained text. The Academy updates and revises the course annually, with the goals of integrating the basic science and clinical practice of ophthalmology and of keeping ophthalmologists current with new developments in the various subspecialties.

The BCSC incorporates the effort and expertise of more than 100 ophthalmologists, organized into 13 Section faculties, working with Academy editorial staff. In addition, the course continues to benefit from many lasting contributions made by the faculties of previous editions. Members of the Academy Practicing Ophthalmologists Advisory Committee for Education, Committee on Aging, and Vision Rehabilitation Committee review every volume before major revisions, as does a group of select residents and fellows. Members of the European Board of Ophthalmology, organized into Section faculties, also review volumes before major revisions, focusing primarily on differences between American and European ophthalmology practice.

Organization of the Course

The Basic and Clinical Science Course comprises 13 volumes, incorporating fundamental ophthalmic knowledge, subspecialty areas, and special topics:

1 Update on General Medicine
2 Fundamentals and Principles of Ophthalmology
3 Clinical Optics and Vision Rehabilitation
4 Ophthalmic Pathology and Intraocular Tumors
5 Neuro-Ophthalmology
6 Pediatric Ophthalmology and Strabismus
7 Oculofacial Plastic and Orbital Surgery
8 External Disease and Cornea
9 Uveitis and Ocular Inflammation
10 Glaucoma
11 Lens and Cataract
12 Retina and Vitreous
13 Refractive Surgery

References

Readers who wish to explore specific topics in greater detail may consult the references cited within each chapter and listed in the Additional Materials and Resources section at the back of the book. These references are intended to be selective rather than exhaustive, chosen by the BCSC faculty as being important, current, and readily available to residents and practitioners.

Multimedia

This edition of Section 6, *Pediatric Ophthalmology and Strabismus*, includes multimedia—videos, interactive content ("activities"), and online case studies—related to topics covered in the book. The multimedia content is available to readers of the print and electronic versions of Section 6 (www.aao.org/bcscvideo_section06, www.aao.org/bcscactivity_section06, and www.aao.org/bcsccasestudy_section06). Mobile-device users can scan the QR codes below (a QR-code reader may need to be installed on the device) to access the multimedia.

Videos   Activities   Case Studies

Self-Assessment and CME Credit

Each volume of the BCSC is designed as an independent study activity for ophthalmology residents and practitioners. The learning objectives for this volume are given on page 1. The text, illustrations, and references provide the information necessary to achieve the objectives; the study questions allow readers to test their understanding of the material and their mastery of the objectives. Physicians who wish to claim CME credit for this educational activity may do so by following the instructions given at the end of the book.*

Conclusion

The Basic and Clinical Science Course has expanded greatly over the years, with the addition of much new text, numerous illustrations, and video content. Recent editions have sought to place greater emphasis on clinical applicability while maintaining a solid foundation in basic science. As with any educational program, it reflects the experience of its authors. As its faculties change and medicine progresses, new viewpoints emerge on controversial subjects and techniques. Not all alternate approaches can be included in this series; as with any educational endeavor, the learner should seek additional sources, including Academy Preferred Practice Pattern Guidelines.

The BCSC faculty and staff continually strive to improve the educational usefulness of the course; you, the reader, can contribute to this ongoing process. If you have any suggestions or questions about the series, please do not hesitate to contact the faculty or the editors.

The authors, editors, and reviewers hope that your study of the BCSC will be of lasting value and that each Section will serve as a practical resource for quality patient care.

*This activity meets the Self-Assessment CME requirements defined by the American Board of Ophthalmology (ABO). Please be advised that the ABO is not an accrediting body for purposes of any CME program. ABO does not sponsor this or any outside activity, and ABO does not endorse any particular CME activity. Complete information regarding the ABO Self-Assessment CME Maintenance of Certification requirements is available at https://abop.org/maintain-certification/cme-self-assessment/.

Objectives

Upon completion of BCSC Section 6, *Pediatric Ophthalmology and Strabismus,* the reader should be able to

- describe techniques for evaluating young children that provide the maximum information gain with the least trauma and frustration
- describe the anatomy and physiology of the extraocular muscles
- explain the classification and diagnosis of amblyopia
- describe the treatment options for amblyopia
- describe the commonly used tests for the diagnosis and measurement of strabismus
- classify the various esodeviations and exodeviations
- describe the management of each type of esodeviation and exodeviation
- identify pattern and vertical strabismus, as well as special forms of strabismus
- select a treatment plan for pattern, vertical, and special forms of strabismus
- list the features of the various forms of nystagmus seen in children, including their significance
- state the possible complications of strabismus surgery, including guidelines to minimize them
- describe an approach to the diagnosis of decreased vision in children
- state various causes of congenital and acquired ocular infections in children, including a logical plan for the diagnosis and management of each type
- list the most common lacrimal drainage system abnormalities found in children

- describe a management plan for the most common lacrimal drainage system abnormalities occurring in children
- list the most common diseases and malformations of the anterior segment occurring in children
- describe the diagnostic findings and treatment options for childhood glaucoma
- identify common types of childhood cataract and other lens disorders
- describe a diagnostic and management plan for childhood cataracts
- identify appropriate diagnostic tests for pediatric uveitis
- identify various vitreoretinal, optic nerve head, and metabolic diseases and disorders that occur in children
- describe the characteristic findings of accidental and nonaccidental ocular trauma in childhood
- list the characteristics of ocular tumors and neuro-oculocutaneous syndromes occurring in children
- describe potential social barriers to treatment of children who require long-term eye care

CHAPTER 1

The Pediatric Eye Evaluation

This chapter includes related videos. Go to www.aao.org/bcscvideo_section06 or scan the QR codes in the text to access this content.

Highlights

- Flexibility, creativity, playfulness, and patience are valuable assets for the pediatric ophthalmologist.
- The use of *crowding bars* is recommended if a child's visual acuity is tested using single optotypes.
- In infants, fixation preference testing is commonly used, but *preferential looking* tests can quantify visual acuity.

General Considerations

Children and their ophthalmic needs can differ greatly from the patients and ocular conditions encountered in adult ophthalmology. Each childhood developmental level requires a different examination approach. With proper preparation and a positive attitude, the ophthalmologist can find the examination of pediatric patients to be both enjoyable and rewarding.

Examinations are typically more successful when patients are relaxed. The outpatient clinic atmosphere should be welcoming, preferably with dedicated waiting area(s) for children and families. Many pediatric practitioners forego the traditional white coat because some children may be afraid of it. The examination begins as the practitioner enters the room and gathers important information via observation about the child's visual behavior, ability to ambulate, any abnormal head position, any dysmorphic features, familial disorders (note parents and siblings), and family social dynamics. A parent's smartphone may contain photos and videos that prove useful in establishing a diagnosis and a condition's progression over time.

Clinicians should introduce themselves to the child and family and establish and maintain eye contact with the child. Being relaxed, open, and playful during the examination helps create a "safe" environment. Gaining the child's trust enables a faster and better examination, easier follow-up visits, and greater parental support. Family members may also need reassurance; parental anxiety may exacerbate the child's anxiety. Asking children easy questions can help them feel confident; a simple joke can relax both child and parent. It is important to work with the child's family, enlisting their help and respecting their concerns.

CLINICAL PEARL

Children enjoy being regarded as "big" as well as correcting adults' mistakes; pretending to grossly overestimate the patient's age or grade level and then asking, "Is that right?" can boost a child's confidence.

In addition to a standard medical history, the pediatric eye assessment includes relevant prenatal/perinatal history (pregnancy or perinatal complications including prematurity), developmental milestones, and family history of strabismus or other childhood eye disorders.

During the examination, the practitioner should sit at the child's eye level; some children prefer sitting in a parent's lap. Describe the examination to children in terms that they can understand. Because cooperation may be fleeting, the examination elements that are most critical for diagnosis and management are best addressed early. The most threatening parts of the examination should be performed last. A long examination lane with different types of distance-fixation targets (including remotely activated videos and mechanical animals 6 meters from the examination chair) is optimal. It is best to have a variety of near-fixation targets with details that stimulate accommodation (a muscle light is not an accommodative target) (Fig 1-1).

CLINICAL PEARL

Explain what is happening in terms familiar to a child, such as "I want to show you something special" instead of "I need to examine you." Use "magic sunglasses" for the stereo glasses, "special flashlight" for the retinoscope, "funny hat" for the indirect ophthalmoscope, and "magnifying glass" for the indirect lens.

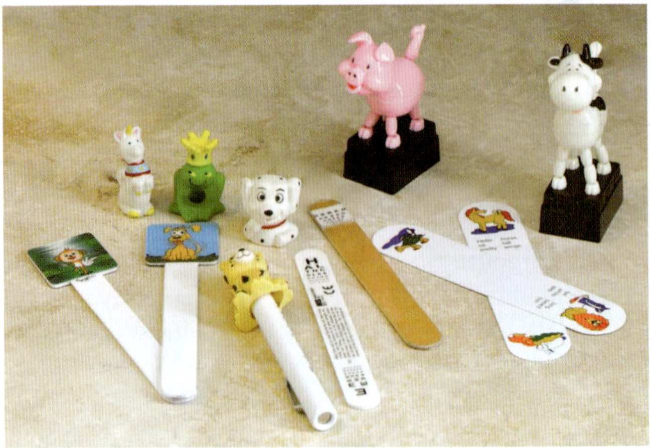

Figure 1-1 Small toys, pictures, and eye charts are used as accommodative near-fixation targets. *(Courtesy of Robert W. Hered, MD.)*

For a child who has difficulty cooperating with the examination, some combination of rest periods, persuasion, persistence, patience, and rewards is usually successful. It is important to engage the child and caregivers in decisions regarding how to proceed. If a child is having a bad day, it may be best to stop the examination and schedule another appointment.

> **CLINICAL PEARL**
>
> If an infant was fussy during the first visit, ask the caregiver to bring the infant to the follow-up visit hungry, and feed him or her during the examination. If dilation in the clinic is a barrier to successful examination, consider having parents give dilating drops at home ahead of time. Review possible adverse effects.

Brief restraint may sometimes be needed, especially for eyedrop administration or fundoscopy in infants and younger children. Provide agency to the older child by offering a choice between helping and being held. Always consider the physical and emotional consequences of restraining a child and apologize to the child afterward if restraint is used. Depending on the nature of the ocular problem, a sedated examination or an examination under anesthesia may be considered.

A pattern of poor adherence to treatment and follow-up recommendations should alert providers to the possibility of neglect, or at least of barriers to care that may benefit from social services (see Chapter 28 in this volume). Pediatric practitioners are obligated to report suspected neglect or abuse to the appropriate social agencies.

Note that the caregiver bringing a child to appointments may not be the child's legal guardian and therefore may not be authorized to provide consent, such as for surgery.

Examination: Specific Elements

A pediatric eye examination requires different techniques and devices than an adult examination. For example, sensorimotor evaluation (which will be discussed in detail in Chapter 6) is often required. Sensorimotor examination should begin with the tests that are least dissociating with respect to binocularity, such as stereoacuity testing, followed by motility testing; monocular visual acuity testing and pupil exams are dissociating and should be performed later in the examination, so as not to affect the sensorimotor exam.

Vision Assessment

The clinician's approach to vision assessment varies depending on the child's age, developmental level, and cooperativeness.

Recognition visual acuity

In older children, recognition visual acuity is tested using linear letter optotypes whenever possible. Sloan letters, consisting of C, D, H, K, N, O, R, S, V and Z, are ideal because they have been shown to be equally recognizable. The optotypes should be spaced so the distance between each optotype is no greater than the width of the optotypes on any given line (see BCSC Section 3, *Clinical Optics and Vision Rehabilitation,* for further discussion of visual acuity charts). Computerized visual acuity test systems allow for randomization of optotype presentation, preventing memorization.

An adhesive patch is the most reliable occluder for monocular testing because it reduces the possibility that the child will "peek" around the occluder. A fogging occluder may be indicated for patients with nystagmus (see Chapter 12). Patients with vision worse than 20/400 may need to move closer to the chart until they can see the 20/400 optotype, in which case, the numerator for the visual acuity is the distance in feet (eg, if the 20/400 optotype is only seen at 5 feet, and the chart is calibrated for 20 feet, visual acuity is noted as 5/400).

Younger and/or preliterate children may need to be tested with alternative optotypes, preferably the LEA symbols (Fig 1-2) or the reduced set of 4 letter optotypes known as the HOTV test. Allen figures, though commonly used, are not as well standardized, and may be culturally biased. Some children are confused by linear arrays and need to be shown single optotypes; in this case, the use of crowding bars (see Fig 1-2B) around each optotype is recommended, because testing with uncrowded optotypes will underestimate the actual visual acuity deficits in patients with amblyopia.

> **CLINICAL PEARL**
>
> Matching cards allow testing in children who can't or won't name optotypes. Handouts with test optotypes may be given to families to practice at home ahead of time.

Because results may vary with different methods, test details (optotype; linear vs single crowded presentation) should always be recorded. When transitioning to a new method during ongoing amblyopia treatment, retesting with the method used at the previous visit helps assess for interval change. Table 1-1 shows normative data for HOTV recognition visual acuity for children at different ages, as measured by an eye care professional (these are not the

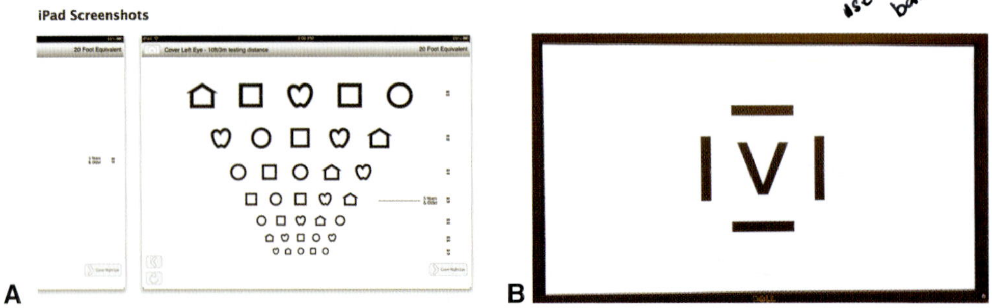

Figure 1-2 Recognition visual acuity testing. **A,** LEA optotypes; screenshot of an American Association for Pediatric Ophthalmology and Strabismus iPad application for visual acuity screening. **B,** Crowding bars around a single-letter optotype displayed on a clinic monitor for distance visual acuity testing. *(Part A courtesy of Mae Millicent W. Peterseim, MD. Childhood Vision Screening.* Focal Points: Clinical Practice Perspectives. *American Academy of Ophthalmology; 2018, Module 4. Part B courtesy of Kristina Tarczy-Hornoch, MD, DPhil.)*

Table 1-1 Monocular HOTV Optotype Recognition Acuity Test Results in Preschool Children

Age (y)	Mean Visual Acuity	Threshold Visual Acuity[a]
2½	20/30	20/63
3	20/30	20/50
4	20/25	20/40
5	20/20	20/32

[a] Over 95% of children with normal vision are expected to achieve this level of visual acuity or better.

Information from Pan Y, Tarczy-Hornoch K, Cotter SA, et al; Multi-Ethnic Pediatric Eye Disease Study Group. Visual acuity norms in preschool children: The Multi-Ethnic Pediatric Eye Disease Study. *Optom Vis Sci.* 2009;86(6):607–612.

same as referral thresholds in the context of primary care vision screening). Further tips for checking visual recognition acuity can be found in BCSC Section 3, *Clinical Optics and Vision Rehabilitation,* in the "Quick-Start Guide to Optics and How to Refract."

CLINICAL PEARL

While checking vision, the practitioner can make the child feel successful by initially presenting optotypes that can be readily discerned and then saying, "That's too easy—let's try this one."

Fixation and following behavior

In infants and toddlers who are too young to undergo optotype testing, fixation and following (tracking) behavior is tested. Each eye is tested while the fellow eye is occluded. Consistent objection to occlusion of 1 eye but not the other suggests a clinically significant difference in visual acuity between the eyes. The size of the smallest target tracked at a given viewing distance (eg, face vs 2-in toy) may be noted for each eye. Normal development of fixation and following behavior is described in Chapter 15.

CLINICAL PEARL

Children can tire quickly of the same toy; have several accommodative near targets available and apply the "1 toy, 1 look" rule. Photos or videos on a phone can also be used as near-fixation targets.

Fixation preference testing may also be performed; this is assessed under binocular viewing conditions. This is not a measure of monocular visual acuity, but it does provide information about how strongly the nondominant eye is suppressed with both eyes open. For a patient with strabismus, the first step in fixation preference testing is determining the preferred, or dominant, eye. The second step is to determine how well the child holds or maintains fixation with the nonpreferred eye. Starting from fixation with the nonpreferred eye, with the preferred eye occluded, the occluder is removed; the examiner notes whether fixation is maintained with the nondominant eye or reverts to the dominant eye (and, if the latter, how quickly) (Video 1-1). The patient's ability to maintain fixation through a blink or smooth pursuit is also noted.

VIDEO 1-1 Fixation preference testing.
Animation developed by Steven M. Archer, MD, and Kristina Tarczy-Hornoch, MD, DPhil.

For children with microstrabismus or no strabismus, the induced tropia test is used to determine the preferred eye (see the Appendix at the back of this volume for strabismus terminology). When a 10 prism diopter (Δ) to 20Δ base-down prism is introduced over the right eye, the child may

1. shift fixation upward (keep using right eye)
2. not shift fixation (keep using left eye)
3. alternate fixation (no preference)

The test is repeated with the prism over the left eye. If the child prefers the same eye on both tests, a fixation preference is present. A child who has no fixation preference *either* alternates fixation *or* consistently prefers the eye with prism or the eye without prism regardless of which eye has the prism.

To determine how well the child holds or maintains fixation with the nonpreferred eye, the examiner occludes the preferred eye, holding a base-down prism under the occluder, so that the child is initially fixating with the nonpreferred eye; when the occluder is removed, with the prism still in place, the examiner notes whether fixation is maintained with the nondominant eye, or if it reverts to the dominant eye (as described above for strabismic patients; see Video 1-1).

Fixation behavior and fixation preference testing can be described using the CSM (Central, Steady, and Maintained) notation. Fixation during monocular viewing is described as *central* (foveal) or *noncentral* (eccentric), and *steady* (stable eye position) or *nonsteady* (roving eye movement or nystagmus). *Maintained* refers to fixation that is held during binocular viewing after the opposite eye is uncovered during fixation preference testing. Table 1-2 describes gradations of fixation preference and their corresponding CSM notation.

A child with a strong fixation preference is more likely to have amblyopia than a child with weak or absent fixation preference, but strong fixation preference does not necessarily indicate amblyopia. Conversely, weak or absent fixation preference does not rule out amblyopia.

Cotter SA, Tarczy-Hornoch K, Song E, et al; Multi-Ethnic Pediatric Eye Disease Study Group. Fixation preference and visual acuity testing in a population-based cohort of preschool children with amblyopia risk factors. *Ophthalmology.* 2009;116(1):145–153. Erratum appears in *Ophthalmology.* 2009;116(2):174.

Preferential looking tests

In infants and children who are too young to do optotype testing, quantitative vision can be assessed using forced-choice preferential looking techniques. The child is shown a card with a black-and-white grating (Teller Acuity Cards II, Precision Vision; Fig 1-3,

Table 1-2 Examples of Fixation Preference Grading, in Order of Increasing Fixation Preference

Fixation Preference	Examination Finding	CSM Notation
None	Child spontaneously alternates fixation or shows no fixation preference (eg, always prefers eye without prism on induced tropia testing)	CSM alternates
Weak preference, holds well with fellow eye	Fixation preference is present, but the child maintains fixation well with the nonpreferred eye during binocular viewing (>3 seconds, through smooth pursuit, through blinks)	CSM prefers right or left CSM through blink
Strong preference, holds briefly with fellow eye	Fixation preference is present; child can maintain fixation only briefly with the nonpreferred eye during binocular viewing (1–3 seconds, not through pursuit or blink)	CSM to blink CSM briefly
Strong preference, does not hold with fellow eye	Fixation preference is present, and the child cannot maintain fixation with the nonpreferred eye during binocular viewing (<1 second) Monocular fixation with the nonpreferred eye may be central and steady, central but unsteady, or eccentric and unsteady	CSnM CnSnM nCnSnM

C = central; nC = noncentral; S = steady; nS = nonsteady; M = maintained; nM = nonmaintained.

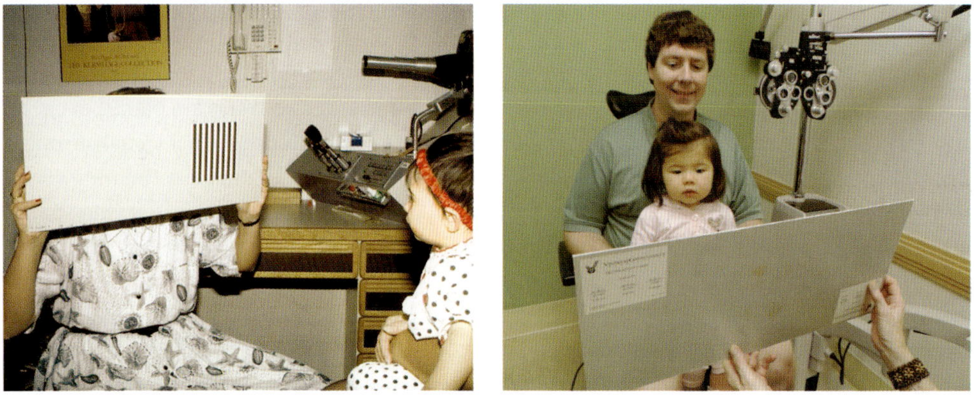

Figure 1-3 Teller Acuity Cards can be used to measure visual acuity in a preverbal child. If the pattern is visible to the child, the child looks toward the grating; otherwise, the stripes blend into the gray background and the child shows no preference for looking toward the side of the card with the grating. *(Left image courtesy of John W. Simon, MD; right image courtesy of Lee R. Hunter, MD.)*

Video 1-2) or vanishing optotype (Cardiff Acuity Test) on one half, and a homogeneous gray area of equal mean luminance on the other. The observer notes where the child looks upon being shown the card, then checks to see whether it was toward the stimulus. As the stripes in the grating or figure outline become finer (higher *spatial frequency*), fixation behavior approaches chance at the child's resolution threshold. Other preferential looking tests of grating acuity include the LEA Grating Acuity Test (LEA Test Intl/Good-Lite Company), and Patti Stripes Square Wave Grating Paddles (Precision Vision). Table 1-3 shows the average grating resolution acuity at different ages.

Table 1-3 Monocular Grating Resolution Acuity Test Results for Forced-Choice Preferential Looking Using Teller Acuity Cards

Age (Mo)	Mean Grating Acuity (Cycles/Degree)[a]	Snellen Fraction Notation of Similar Spatial Frequency[b]
1	0.94	20/640
4	2.68	20/220
6	5.65	20/110
12	6.42	20/93
24	9.57	20/63
36	21.81	20/28

[a] One cycle = 1 pair of black-and-white grating stripes. The number of cycles per degree of visual angle is a measure of spatial frequency.

[b] Even for a similar spatial frequency, grating resolution acuity is not comparable to optotype recognition acuity. Snellen fraction notations are provided only as a familiar indicator of spatial frequency. Snellen fraction notation denominators are rounded to 2 significant figures.

Information from Mayer DL, Beiser AS, Warner AF, Pratt EM, Raye KN, Lang JM. Monocular acuity norms for the Teller Acuity Cards between ages 1 month and 4 years. *Invest Ophthalmol Vis Sci.* 1995;36(3):671–685.

VIDEO 1-2 Teller Acuity Card testing.
Courtesy of Lee R. Hunter, MD.

Visual evoked potential

The visual evoked potential (VEP) is an objective tool for quantifying visual function that does not rely on a child's verbal or motor responses. In this test, electrodes are placed over the occipital lobe to measure cortical electrical signals produced in response to a visual stimulus (see BCSC Section 5, *Neuro-Ophthalmology*). The sweep VEP is a method for estimating visual acuity in preverbal children. The child views a series of bar or grid patterns of varying spatial frequency. The amplitude of the VEP waveform decreases with increasing spatial frequency, yielding a threshold spatial frequency estimate of grating resolution acuity. VEP estimates of monocular grating resolution acuity in infants are higher than estimates based on behavioral (preferential looking) tests; based on visual cortical responses, the infant visual system can resolve a spatial frequency of about 5 cycles per degree at 1 month of age and well over 10 cycles per degree by 6 months of age (compare to Table 1-3 for results from preferential looking tests).

Hamer RD, Norcia AM, Tyler CW, Hsu-Winges C. The development of monocular and binocular VEP acuity. *Vision Res.* 1989;29(4):397–408.

Dynamic Retinoscopy

Noncycloplegic retinoscopy at near is a way to assess accommodation. In an emmetropic child with normal accommodation, the retinoscopic reflex will be close to neutralized if the child is focused appropriately on a near target located at the examiner's working distance. Because the examiner can also assess how quickly the refractive state changes during a switch from far to near fixation, this technique is often termed *dynamic retinoscopy*. A poor accommodative response may indicate the need for hyperopic correction or a near-point add. Hypoaccommodation occurs more frequently in children with Down syndrome or cerebral palsy than in the general pediatric population.

Visual Field Testing

Visual fields can be assessed once visual fixation has developed (usually by 4 months of age). If the introduction of a peripheral target while the child is fixating on an interesting central target induces a saccade toward the peripheral target, this indicates vision in the corresponding hemifield. Confrontation visual fields can be approximated in children old enough to identify or count fingers placed in each peripheral quadrant. School-aged children can often be evaluated with manual or automated perimetry.

Pupil Testing

The pupillary light reflex is not reliably present until approximately 30 weeks' gestational age. Pupils are usually miotic in newborns and gradually increase in size until preadolescence. Accurate pupil testing in young children is complicated by the smaller pupil and difficulty controlling accommodation. Pupil evaluation can be facilitated by careful observation, easily accessible control of room lights to allow continued observation during changes in room illumination, and the use of appropriate distance-fixation targets. Digital photography can also be useful for observing and documenting pupil size and symmetry.

Brückner Test

In the *Brückner test,* the direct ophthalmoscope is used to obtain a red reflex simultaneously in both eyes (Fig 1-4). Foveation of the ophthalmoscope filament dims the red reflex. If strabismus is present, the deviated eye will have a lighter and brighter reflex than the fixating eye; media opacities and refractive errors can also cause unequal red reflexes. The positions of the corneal light reflexes can also be assessed. This test is often used by primary care practitioners to screen for vision disorders.

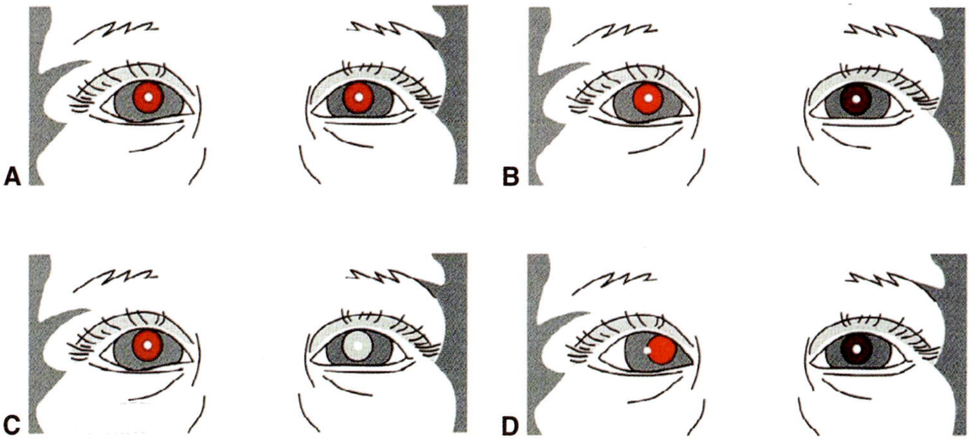

Figure 1-4 Brückner test. **A,** Symmetric red reflex. **B,** Asymmetric red reflex due to anisometropia. **C,** Asymmetric red reflex, absent in the left eye due to cataract. **D,** Asymmetric red reflex, brighter in the deviated right eye due to strabismus. *(Adapted from Mae Millicent W. Peterseim, MD. Childhood Vision Screening.* Focal Points: Clinical Practice Perspectives. *American Academy of Ophthalmology; 2018, Module 4. Courtesy of Alfred G. Smith, MD, ©1991.)*

Anterior Segment Examination

Children old enough to sit by themselves can usually be enticed to hold the "motorcycle handles" of the slit lamp long enough for a brief examination. A younger child may be positioned at the slit lamp while in a parent's lap. Children unable or unwilling to cooperate for standard slit-lamp examination may be examined with a portable slit lamp, surgical loupes, or a 20.00 diopter (D) handheld lens used as a simple magnifier with illumination from an indirect ophthalmoscope.

Intraocular Pressure Measurement

It is not always easy or possible to perform formal tonometry in children. Accurate tonometry requires a relaxed patient. Handheld devices such as the Icare tonometer (Icare Finland Oy) or Tono-Pen (Reichert Technologies) can be very useful for measuring intraocular pressure (IOP) in children. The Tono-Pen or the Perkins Tonometer (Haag-Streit USA) may be used to test infants when they are sleeping or feeding in the supine position.

Digital palpation, though not quantitative, can provide a gross assessment of IOP. Interpretation requires practice and correlation with formal tonometry tests in the same patient.

Cycloplegic Refraction

Because of the relationship between accommodation and ocular convergence, refraction with cycloplegic agents is a particularly important test in the evaluation of any patient who has issues relating to binocular vision and ocular motility.

Cycloplegic and mydriatic agents

Cyclopentolate hydrochloride (1%) is the preferred cycloplegic drug for routine use in children. Use of a weaker concentration of cyclopentolate (0.2% to 0.5%) is suggested in infants. *Tropicamide* (0.5% or 1%) alone is usually not potent enough for complete cycloplegia in children. *Atropine* (1% drops or ointment) is used by some ophthalmologists, particularly in young children with accommodative esotropia or dark irides, but this drug causes prolonged blurring and is more often associated with adverse effects (see the section "Adverse effects of cycloplegic agents"). Although *phenylephrine* (2.5%) has no cycloplegic effect, it is often used in combination with 1 or more cycloplegic agents for maximum dilation.

Table 1-4 describes typical usage of common cycloplegic drugs. The duration of action varies greatly between drugs. Darker irides may be more resistant to dilation and cycloplegia. Mydriasis begins earlier and lasts longer than cycloplegia; thus, a dilated pupil does not

Table 1-4 Common Cycloplegic Agents

Medication	Typical Administration Schedule	Time to Cycloplegia	Duration of Action
Tropicamide	1 drop every 5 min × 2; wait 30 min	20–40 min	4–6 hours
Cyclopentolate hydrochloride	1 drop every 5 min × 2; wait 30 min	30–60 min	1–2 days
Atropine sulfate	1 drop; wait 90 min. Alternatively, 1–3 drops per day × 1–4 days; then 1 drop morning of appointment	45–120 min	7–14 days

necessarily indicate complete cycloplegia. For patients with poorly controlled accommodative esotropia, repeat cycloplegic refraction is important to ensure full correction of hyperopia.

Administering eyedrops in children

Most young children are apprehensive about eyedrops. It may help improve the child's cooperation for the remainder of the examination if someone other than the physician instills the eyedrops. Eyedrops may be described to the child as feeling "like a splash of swimming pool water." Some practitioners administer a topical anesthetic drop first, while others use the cycloplegic drops alone; some use a compounded drop (containing more than 1 mydriatic/cycloplegic agent) or spray.

> **CLINICAL PEARL**
>
> An anesthetic drop may be called a "tickle drop" and the child can be encouraged to laugh when it is administered.

Adverse effects of cycloplegic agents

Local allergic reactions to cycloplegic drugs may include conjunctivitis, edematous eyelids, and dermatitis. Cycloplegic agents may also cause nonallergic systemic symptoms, which may be more common in children with lighter irides; these include fever, dry mouth, flushing, tachycardia, constipation, urinary retention, nausea, dizziness, and delirium. Treatment is discontinuation of the drug, with supportive measures as necessary. A severe reaction should be managed in an emergency care setting. Adverse effects are more common with atropine than other agents. Note that 1 drop of 1% atropine contains 0.5 mg of atropine. See also BCSC Section 2, *Fundamentals and Principles of Ophthalmology,* Part V: Ocular Pharmacology.

Refraction technique

Refraction is generally performed after cycloplegia. Streak retinoscopy is an objective technique that can be used with children of any age; it is described in detail in Chapter 4 of BCSC Section 3, *Clinical Optics and Vision Rehabilitation*. Retinoscopy may be performed with loose trial lenses, or through a phoropter for children who are able to reliably participate. Accurate retinoscopy must be performed in the child's visual axis and at a controlled working distance. Autorefractors may also be used after cycloplegia. Subjective phoropter refraction or refinement is an option for older children.

Fundus Examination

The fundus examination is typically done last and can be challenging in infants and toddlers. It is helpful to reduce the illumination on the indirect ophthalmoscope. It is important to obtain an adequate view of at least the optic nerve and macula. This is facilitated by distracting the child with a distant target or a toy held near the examiner's head (to the examiner's right for the child's right eye). Examination for retinopathy of prematurity (ROP) constitutes a special situation in which it is essential to view the far retinal periphery, which usually requires restraint, topical anesthesia, an eyelid speculum, and scleral depression (see Chapter 24 in this volume for discussion of ROP).

Inpatient Examination of Children at the Bedside

In the inpatient setting, it is important to consult with the family and/or the nursing team regarding examination timing. When testing visual acuity using a near-vision testing card, use the recommended standardized testing distance, with habitual refractive correction if possible, and do not test visual acuity at near after cycloplegia. Dilation may not be appropriate in patients requiring frequent neurologic assessment, including pupil assessment. Dilating eyedrops should be ordered and documented in the medication administration record, and primary care team members should be informed if pupils were pharmacologically dilated. Important findings should be communicated verbally to the primary team, in addition to being documented in the consultation report.

PART I

Strabismus

CHAPTER 2

Anatomy of the Extraocular Muscles

This chapter includes a related activity. Go to www.aao.org/bcscactivity_section06 or scan the QR code in the text to access this content.

Highlights

- The courses of the oblique muscles result in vertical action (depression for the superior oblique and elevation for the inferior oblique).
- The trochlea functions as a pulley to redirect the action of the superior oblique muscle.
- All other extraocular muscles also have pulley-like structures, which are formed by connective tissues of the orbit.
- Anterior ciliary blood vessels are disrupted during strabismus surgery; thus, simultaneous surgery on 3 or more rectus muscles incurs a risk for anterior segment ischemia.

Origin, Course, Insertion, and Innervation of the Extraocular Muscles

There are 7 extraocular muscles (EOMs): the 4 rectus muscles (lateral, medial, superior, and inferior), the 2 oblique muscles, and the levator palpebrae superioris muscle. Figure 2-1 shows an anterior view of the EOMs and their relationships to one another; these relationships can also be explored in Activity 2-1.

ACTIVITY 2-1 Extraocular muscles.
Activity developed by Mary A. O'Hara, MD.

Table 2-1 summarizes the characteristics of the EOMs; Chapter 3 in this volume describes EOM functions. BCSC Section 5, *Neuro-Ophthalmology,* discusses the ocular motor nerves in more detail; Section 2, *Fundamentals and Principles of Ophthalmology,* extensively illustrates the anatomical structures mentioned in this chapter.

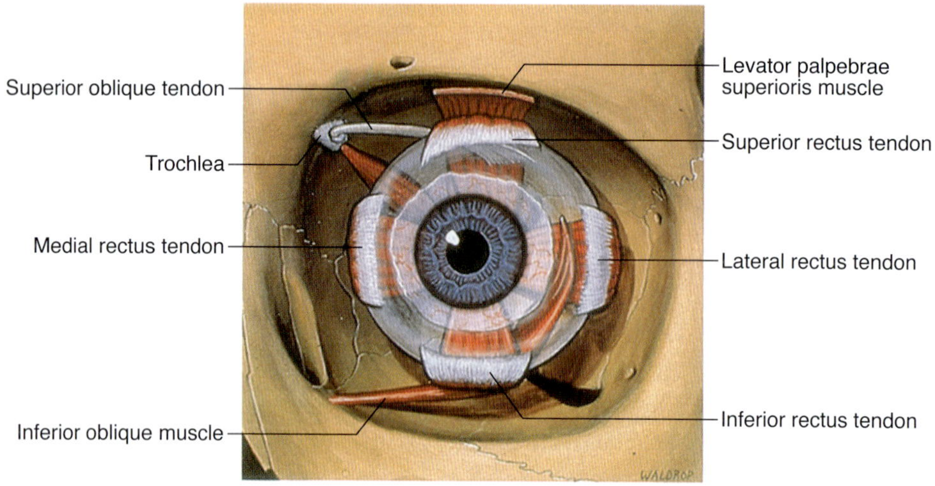

Figure 2-1 Extraocular muscles, frontal composite view, left eye. *(Reproduced with permission from Dutton JJ.* Atlas of Clinical and Surgical Orbital Anatomy. *Saunders; 1994:23.)*

Horizontal and Vertical Rectus Muscles

The horizontal and vertical rectus muscles arise from the annulus of Zinn. The horizontal rectus muscles are

- the *medial rectus muscle,* which courses along the medial orbital wall
- the *lateral rectus muscle,* which courses along the lateral orbital wall

The vertical rectus muscles are

- the *superior rectus muscle,* which courses anteriorly, upward over the eyeball, and laterally, forming an angle of 23° with the visual axis or the midplane of the eye in primary position (Fig 2-2; see also Chapter 3, Fig 3-4)
- the *inferior rectus muscle,* which courses anteriorly, downward, and laterally along the floor of the orbit, forming an angle of 23° with the visual axis or midplane of the eye in primary position (see Chapter 3, Fig 3-4)

The rectus muscles are thin and ribbonlike near their scleral insertions. Although it is often referred to as a tendon, the region of the muscle adjacent to the insertion consists of striated muscle fibers along with tendinous tissue.

Surgical considerations

The sclera is thinnest just posterior to the 4 rectus muscle insertions, increasing the risk of scleral perforation during small rectus muscle recessions.

Oblique Muscles

The *superior oblique muscle* originates from the orbital apex, above the annulus of Zinn, and passes anteriorly and upward along the superomedial wall of the orbit. The muscle becomes tendinous before passing through the trochlea, a cartilaginous saddle attached

Table 2-1 Extraocular Muscles

Muscle	Approx. Length of Active Muscle (mm)	Origin	Anatomical Insertion and Distance From Limbus (mm)	Direction of Pull	Arc of Contact (mm)	Innervation
Medial rectus (MR)	40	Annulus of Zinn	Up to 5.5 mm from medial limbus	90°	7.0	Lower CN III
Lateral rectus (LR)	40	Annulus of Zinn	Up to 6.9 mm from lateral limbus	90°	12.0	CN VI
Superior rectus (SR)	40	Annulus of Zinn	Up to 7.7 mm from superior limbus	23°	6.5	Upper CN III
Inferior rectus (IR)	40	Annulus of Zinn	Up to 6.5 mm from inferior limbus	23°	6.5	Lower CN III
Superior oblique (SO)	32	Orbital apex, above annulus of Zinn (functional origin at the trochlea)	Posterior to equator in superotemporal quadrant	51°	7–8	CN IV
Inferior oblique (IO)	37	Behind inferior orbital rim, lateral to lacrimal fossa	Lateral to area of macula	51°	15.0	Lower CN III
Levator palpebrae superioris (LPS)	40	Orbital apex, above annulus of Zinn	Septa of pretarsal orbicularis and anterior surface of tarsus	—	—	Upper CN III

CN = cranial nerve.
See also Chapter 3, Figures 3-3 through 3-5.

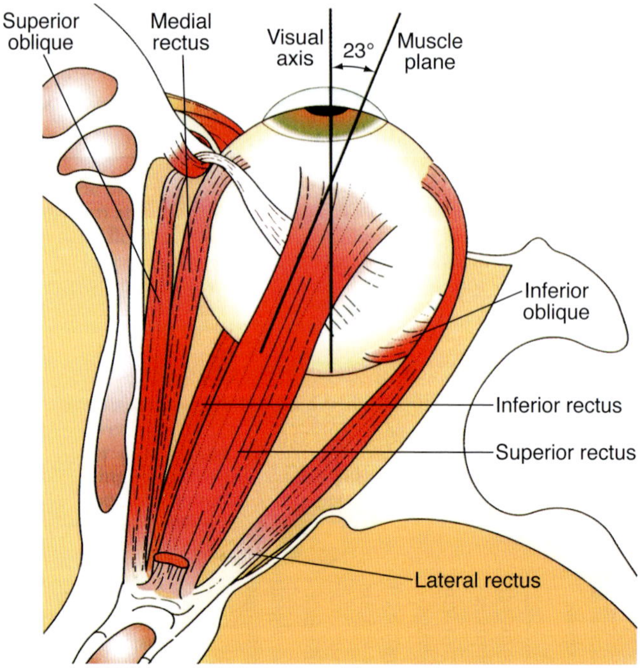

Figure 2-2 The extrinsic muscles of the right eyeball in primary position, seen from above. Note that only the origin and insertion of the inferior oblique muscle are visible in this view. *(Modified with permission from Yanoff M, Duker J, eds.* Ophthalmology. *2nd ed. Mosby; 2004:549.)*

to the frontal bone in the superior nasal orbit. The combination of the trochlea and the superior oblique tendon is known as the *tendon–trochlea complex.*

The trochlea functions as a pulley, redirecting the tendon inferiorly, posteriorly, and laterally; the tendon forms an angle of 51° with the visual axis or midplane of the eye in primary position (see Chapter 3, Fig 3-5). The tendon emerges from the Tenon capsule 2 mm nasally and 5 mm posteriorly to the nasal insertion of the superior rectus muscle. Passing under the superior rectus muscle, the tendon inserts posterior to the equator in the superotemporal quadrant of the eyeball, almost or entirely laterally to the midvertical plane or center of rotation (see Chapter 3, Fig 3-5). With its functional origin anterior to the equator and its insertion posterior to the equator, the superior oblique muscle's contribution to vertical eye movement is to depress the eye by pulling the back of the eye upward.

The *inferior oblique muscle* originates inferonasally from the periosteum of the maxillary bone, just posterior to the orbital rim and lateral to the orifice of the lacrimal fossa. It courses laterally, superiorly, and posteriorly, going inferior to the inferior rectus muscle and inserting under the lateral rectus muscle in the posterolateral portion of the globe, in the area of the macula. Like the superior oblique muscle, the inferior oblique muscle forms an angle of 51° with the visual axis or midplane of the eye in primary position. The vertical action of the inferior oblique muscle is to elevate the eye by pulling the back of the eye downward (see Chapter 3, Fig 3-5). Most inferior oblique muscles have a single belly, but approximately 10% have 2 parallel bellies (or, even more rarely, 3).

Surgical considerations

Surgery on the inferior oblique muscle requires careful inspection … quadrant to ensure that all muscle bellies are identified; otherwise, t… cle may not be sufficiently altered, and additional surgery may be require….

Levator Palpebrae Superioris Muscle

The *levator palpebrae superioris muscle* arises at the orbital apex from the lesser wing of the sphenoid bone, just superior to the annulus of Zinn. At its origin, the muscle blends with the superior rectus muscle inferiorly and with the superior oblique muscle medially. The levator palpebrae superioris passes anteriorly, lying just above the superior rectus muscle; the fascial sheaths of these 2 muscles are connected. The levator palpebrae superioris muscle becomes an aponeurosis in the region of the superior fornix. This muscle has both a cutaneous and a tarsal insertion. See BCSC Section 7, *Oculofacial Plastic and Orbital Surgery,* for additional information.

Relationship of the Rectus Muscle Insertions

Starting at the medial rectus and proceeding to the inferior rectus, lateral rectus, and superior rectus muscles, the rectus muscles insert progressively farther from the limbus. Drawing a continuous curve through these insertions yields a spiral, known as the *spiral of Tillaux* (Fig 2-3). The temporal side of each vertical rectus muscle insertion is farther from the limbus (ie, more posterior) than is the nasal side.

Innervation of Extraocular Muscles

Cranial nerve (CN) VI (abducens) innervates the lateral rectus muscle; CN IV (trochlear), the superior oblique muscle; and CN III (oculomotor), the levator palpebrae superioris, superior rectus, medial rectus, inferior rectus, and inferior oblique muscles. Cranial nerve III

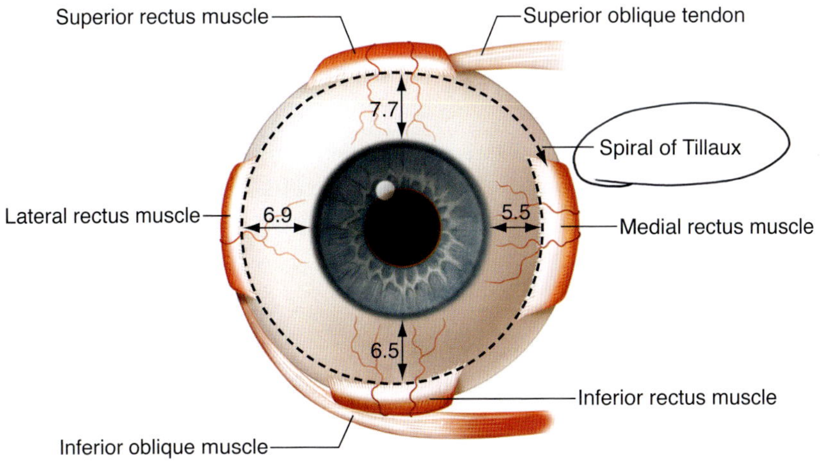

Figure 2-3 Spiral of Tillaux, right eye. *Note:* The insertion distances, given in millimeters, are maximum values. Insertion distances vary among individuals. *(Illustration by Christine Gralapp.)*

as an upper and a lower division: the upper division supplies the levator palpebrae superioris and superior rectus muscles, and the lower division supplies the medial rectus, inferior rectus, and inferior oblique muscles. The parasympathetic innervation of the sphincter pupillae (responsible for pupil constriction) and ciliary muscle (responsible for accommodation) travels with the branch of the lower division of CN III that supplies the inferior oblique muscle.

The nerve supplying the inferior oblique muscle enters the lateral portion of the muscle, where it crosses the inferior rectus muscle. The nerves to the rectus muscles and the superior oblique muscle enter the muscles approximately one-third of the distance from the origin to the insertion (or trochlea, in the case of the superior oblique muscle).

Surgical considerations

Surgery on the inferior oblique muscle can damage its nerve or the accompanying parasympathetic fibers and can result in an enlarged or tonic pupil. Injury to the nerve of a rectus muscle is less likely but may occur if an instrument is thrust more than 26 mm posterior to a rectus muscle's insertion.

Orbital and Fascial Relationships

Within the orbit, a complex musculofibroelastic structure suspends the globe, supports the EOMs, and compartmentalizes the fat pads (Figs 2-4, 2-5).

Surgical Considerations

Connective tissue abnormalities can result in strabismus; examples include connective tissue entrapment in blowout fractures and extraocular muscle pulley heterotopy.

Adipose Tissue

The eye is supported and cushioned within the orbit by a large amount of fatty tissue. External to the muscle cone, fatty tissue ends about 10 mm from the limbus. Fatty tissue is also present inside the muscle cone, separated from the sclera by the Tenon capsule (see Fig 2-5).

Surgical considerations

During strabismus surgery, special care must be taken to avoid violating the integrity of the Tenon capsule 10 mm or more posterior to the limbus. If this occurs, fatty tissue prolapsing through the capsule can form a restrictive adhesion to sclera, muscle, intermuscular septum, or conjunctiva, limiting ocular motility.

Muscle Cone

The muscle cone lies posterior to the equator and consists of the EOMs, their sheaths, and the intermuscular septum. The posterior intermuscular septum separates the intraconal and extraconal fat pads (see Fig 2-5).

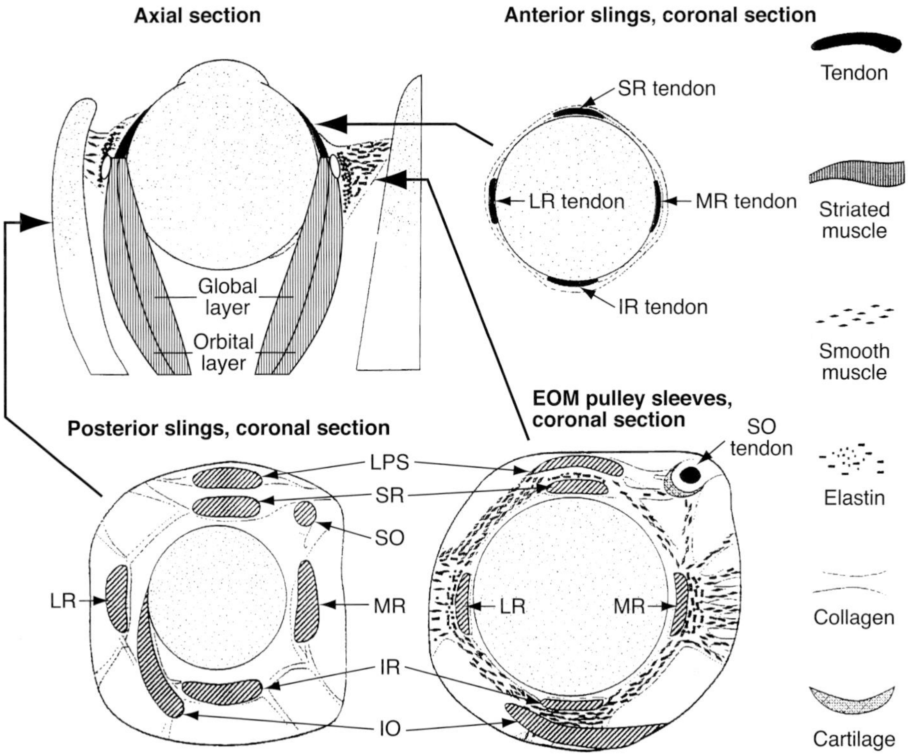

Figure 2-4 Structure of orbital connective tissues. EOM = extraocular muscle; IO = inferior oblique; IR = inferior rectus; LPS = levator palpebrae superioris; LR = lateral rectus; MR = medial rectus; SO = superior oblique; SR = superior rectus. The 3 coronal views represent cross sections at the levels indicated by arrows in axial section. *(Reprinted with permission from SLACK Incorporated. Modified with permission from Demer JL, Miller JM, Poukens V. Surgical implications of the rectus extraocular muscle pulleys.* J Pediatr Ophthalmol Strabismus. *1996;33(4):208–218.)*

Surgical considerations

CN IV is outside the muscle cone and is usually not affected by a retrobulbar block. However, any EOM could be reached by a retrobulbar needle and injured by injection of local anesthetic.

Muscle Capsule

Each rectus muscle has a surrounding fascial capsule that extends with the muscle from its origin to its insertion. These capsules are thin posteriorly, but near the equator they thicken as they pass through the sleeve of the Tenon capsule in the region of the EOM pulleys (see the section The Pulley System), continuing anteriorly with the muscles to their insertions. Anterior to the equator, between the undersurface of the muscle and the sclera, there is almost no fascia, only connective tissue footplates that connect the muscle to the globe. The smooth, avascular surface of the muscle capsule allows the muscles to slide easily over the globe.

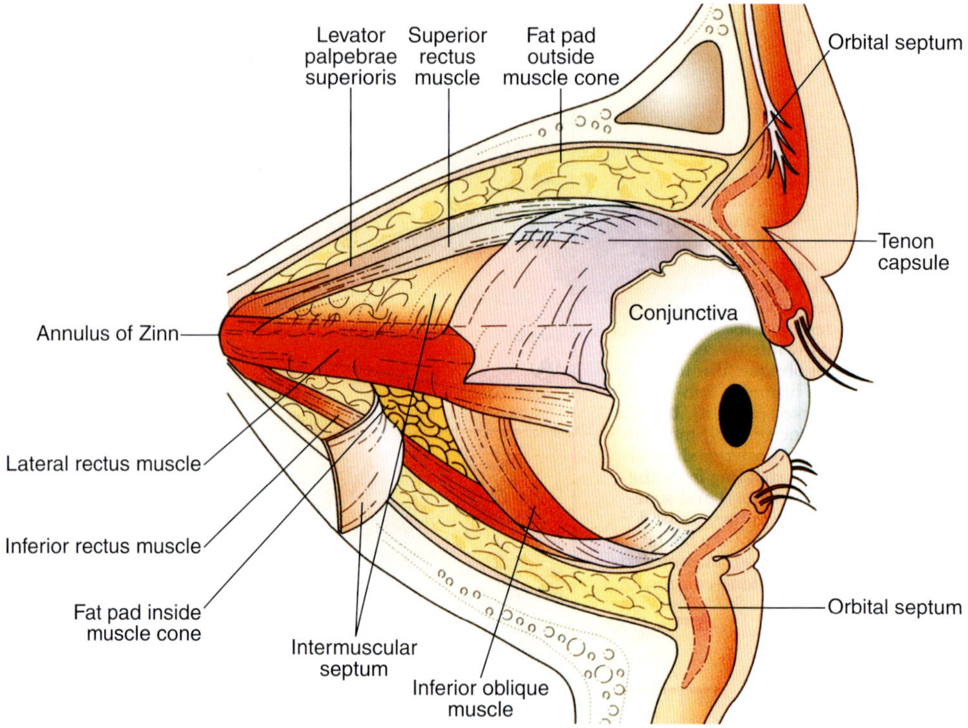

Figure 2-5 The muscle cone contains 1 fat pad and is surrounded by another; these 2 fat pads are separated by the rectus muscles and intermuscular septum. Note that the intermuscular septum does not extend all the way back to the apex of the orbit. *(Modified with permission from Yanoff M, Duker J, eds.* Ophthalmology. *2nd ed. Mosby; 2004:553.)*

Surgical considerations

Maintaining the integrity of the muscle capsules during surgery reduces intraoperative bleeding and provides a smooth muscle surface with less risk of adhesion formation. When suturing a muscle within its capsule, it is important to secure the muscle fibers themselves; if only the muscle capsule is sutured to the globe, the muscle can retract backward, resulting in a slipped muscle.

The Tenon Capsule and Intermuscular Septum

The Tenon capsule *(fascia bulbi)* is the principal orbital fascia and forms the envelope within which the eyeball moves (Fig 2-6). The Tenon capsule fuses posteriorly with the optic nerve sheath and anteriorly with the intermuscular septum, merging with conjunctiva and sclera 3 mm from the limbus. The portion of the Tenon capsule posterior to the globe is thin and flexible, enabling free movement of the optic nerve, ciliary nerves, and ciliary vessels as the globe rotates, while separating the orbital fat inside the muscle cone from the sclera. At and just posterior to the equator, the Tenon capsule is thick and tough, suspending the globe like a trampoline by means of connections to the periorbital tissues. The global layer of the 4 rectus muscles penetrates this thick fibroelastic tissue approximately

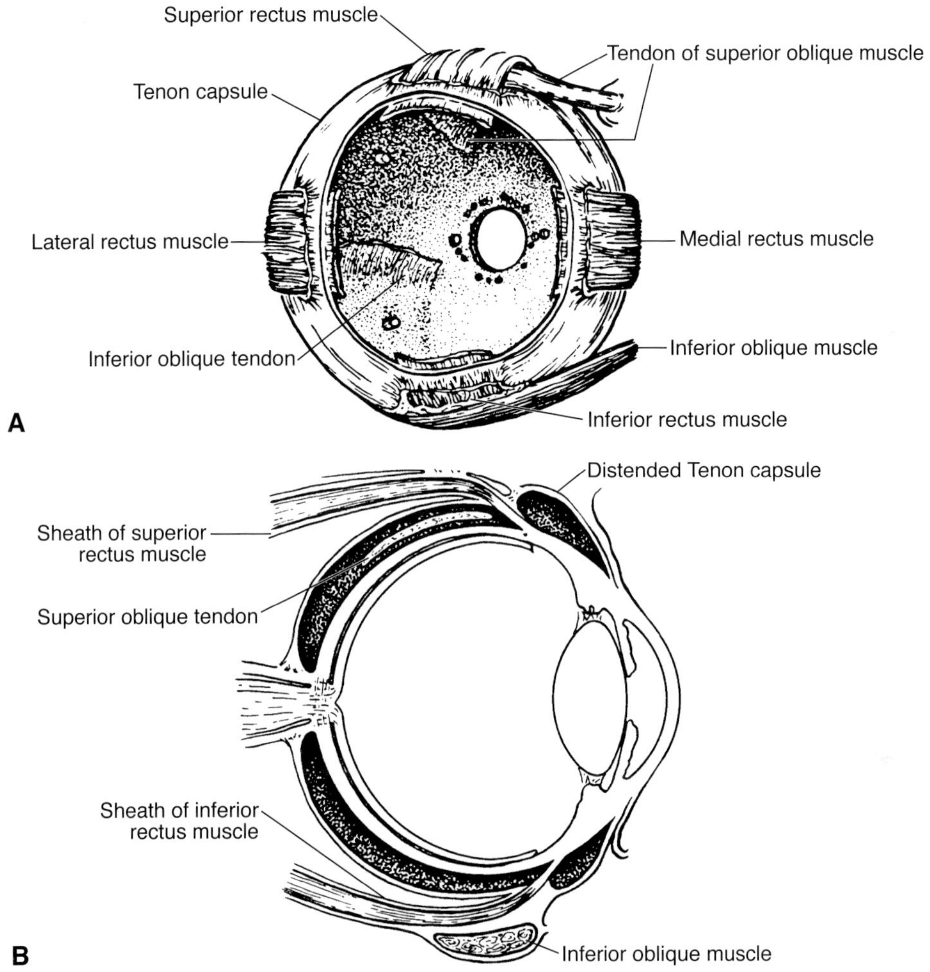

Figure 2-6 The Tenon capsule. **A,** Anterior and posterior orifices of the Tenon capsule shown after enucleation of the globe. **B,** The Tenon space shown by injection with India ink. *(Modified from Charpy A.* Muscles et capsule de Tenon. *In: Poirier P, Charpy A, eds.* Traité d'Anatomie Humaine; *vol 5, no 2. Masson; 1912:539.)*

10 mm posterior to their insertions. The oblique muscles penetrate the Tenon capsule anterior to the equator. The Tenon capsule continues forward over these 6 EOMs and separates them from the orbital fat and structures lying outside the muscle cone.

Surgical considerations

The intermuscular septum (especially between the rectus and oblique muscles) is a useful point of reference when trying to locate a muscle that has been "lost" during surgery or as a result of trauma. Extensive dissection of the intermuscular septum is not necessary for rectus muscle recession surgery, but during resection surgery, dissection helps prevent excessive advancement of connective tissue with the muscle. The connective tissues of the Tenon capsule and intermuscular septum thin with age; as a result, less dissection is required during strabismus surgery in adults than in children.

The Pulley System

The superior oblique muscle is the EOM whose mechanical action is most obviously redirected through an anatomical pulley at the trochlea; however, orbital connective tissues form fibroelastic pulley-like structures around all other EOMs as well. These pulleys, which consist of collagen, elastin, and smooth muscle, are located near the equator, where the muscles pass through connective tissue sleeves to penetrate the Tenon capsule. Dynamic magnetic resonance imaging (MRI) studies show that, in some cases, the pulleys act mechanically as the rectus muscle origins. The pulleys may also serve to stabilize the path of the posterior EOMs relative to the orbit, preventing sideslipping or movement perpendicular to the muscle axis (see Fig 2-4). Numerous extensions from the EOM sheaths attach to the orbit and help support the muscles and the globe.

The inferior oblique muscle originates near the orbital rim and enters its connective tissue pulley inferior to the inferior rectus muscle, where the oblique muscle penetrates the Tenon capsule. The inferior oblique pulley and inferior rectus pulley join to form the Lockwood ligament (Fig 2-7), to which a dense neurofibrovascular bundle running along the lateral border of the inferior rectus muscle is attached; this bundle contains the inferior oblique motor nerve (see Chapter 13, Fig 13-1). This complex acts mechanically as the functional origin of the inferior oblique muscle.

EOMs (other than the levator palpebrae superioris) exhibit a distinct 2-layer organization: an outer *orbital layer,* which acts only on connective tissue pulleys, and an inner *global layer,* which inserts on the sclera to move the globe (see Fig 2-4). The *active pulley hypothesis* proposes that a pulley's position can be shifted by contraction of the orbital layer. This concept remains controversial; whether there is actual innervational control of the pulleys is still debated. Normal pulleys shift only slightly in the coronal plane, even during large eye movements; however, high-resolution MRI scans indicate that the pulleys are located only a short distance from the globe center, so that even small shifts in pulley position could have a large impact on EOM pulling direction.

Heterotopy (malpositioning) of the rectus pulleys may cause some cases of incomitant strabismus and A or V patterns (see Chapter 9); these anomalies can mimic oblique muscle dysfunction by misdirecting the forces of the rectus muscles. Bony abnormalities, such as those seen in association with craniosynostosis, can also alter the direction of pull of rectus muscles by causing malpositioning of the pulleys. Age-related connective tissue laxity may result in acquired pulley heterotopy and associated strabismus, such as sagging eye syndrome and adult-onset distance esotropia.

Peragallo JH, Pineles SL, Demer JL. Recent advances clarifying the etiologies of strabismus. *J Neuroophthalmol.* 2015;35(2):185–193.

Other Connective Tissue Attachments of Rectus Muscles

The inferior rectus muscle is bound to the lower eyelid by the fascial extension from its sheath (see Fig 2-7). The superior rectus muscle is more loosely bound to the levator palpebrae superioris muscle.

Surgical considerations

Resection of the inferior rectus muscle tends to narrow the fissure by elevating the lower eyelid. *Recession* of the inferior rectus muscle tends to widen the palpebral fissure,

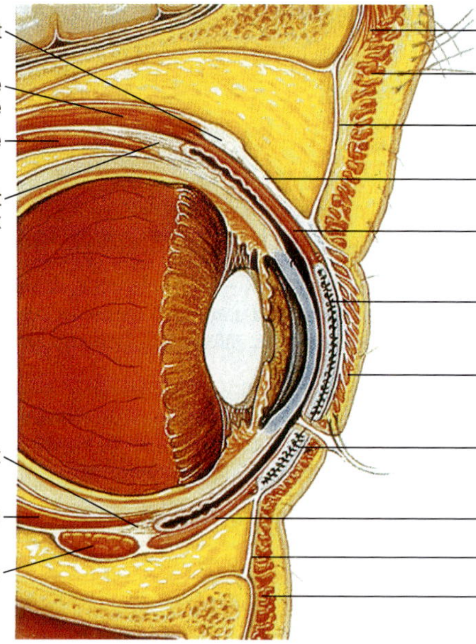

Figure 2-7 Attachments of the upper and lower eyelids to the vertical rectus muscles *(Modified with permission from Buckley EG, Freedman S, Shields MB, eds.* Atlas of Ophthalmic Surgery, *vol III:* Strabismus and Glaucoma. *Mosby Year Book; 1995:15.)*

resulting in lower eyelid retraction. Resection of the superior rectus muscle may pull the eyelid downward, narrowing the palpebral fissure, but moderate recession of this muscle does not usually cause upper eyelid retraction. In hypotropia, a pseudoptosis may be present because the upper eyelid tends to follow the superior rectus muscle.

There is a connective tissue frenulum connecting the lateral rectus muscle to the underlying inferior oblique at its insertion, and a similar one connecting the superior rectus to the underlying superior oblique tendon. During recession or resection of the lateral rectus muscle or superior rectus muscle, severing the connective tissue attachments to the adjacent oblique muscle helps prevent unintended consequences, such as the inferior oblique muscle being advanced with the lateral rectus muscle.

The medial rectus is the only rectus muscle that does not have an oblique muscle running tangential to it. This makes surgery on the medial rectus less complicated but means that there is neither a point of reference if the surgeon becomes disoriented nor a point of attachment if the muscle is lost.

Blood Supply of the Extraocular Muscles

Arterial System

Branches of the ophthalmic artery provide the most important blood supply to the EOMs. The *lateral muscular branch* supplies the lateral rectus, superior rectus, and superior oblique muscles; the *medial muscular branch,* the larger of the 2 muscular branches, supplies the inferior rectus, medial rectus, and inferior oblique muscles. The *lacrimal artery* partially supplies the lateral rectus muscle. Various branches of the ophthalmic artery supply the levator palpebrae superioris muscle. In addition, a branch of the maxillary artery, the *infraorbital artery,* also partially supplies the inferior oblique and inferior rectus muscles.

The muscular branches give rise to the *anterior ciliary arteries* accompanying the rectus muscles; each rectus muscle has 1–4 anterior ciliary arteries. These arteries pass through the episclera of the globe and supply blood to the anterior segment (almost all of the temporal half of the anterior segment circulation and most of the nasal half of the anterior segment circulation). Through anastomoses in the perilimbal region, conjunctival vessels may also contribute to the blood supply of the anterior segment. The commonly held notion that the lateral rectus has fewer ciliary vessels than the other rectus muscles has been challenged by anatomical studies showing that the number of ciliary vessels is similar for the lateral rectus and other rectus muscles.

Johnson MS, Christiansen SP, Rath PP, et al. Anterior ciliary circulation from the horizontal rectus muscles. *Strabismus.* 2009;17(1):45–48.

Surgical considerations

Simultaneous surgery on 3 rectus muscles may induce anterior segment ischemia, particularly in older or vasculopathic patients.

Venous System

The venous system parallels the arterial system, emptying into the *superior* and *inferior orbital veins.* Generally, 4 or more *vortex veins* are located posterior to the equator; these are often found near the nasal and temporal margins of the superior rectus and inferior rectus muscles. Although the number and position of the vortex veins vary, the location of 2 of them in the orbit is consistent: the inferotemporal quadrant, just posterior to the inferior oblique muscle; and the superotemporal quadrant, just posterior to the superior oblique tendon.

Surgical considerations

When surgery is performed near the vortex veins, accidental severing of a vein is possible, especially during recession or resection of the inferior rectus or superior rectus muscle, weakening of the inferior oblique muscle, or exposure of the superior oblique muscle tendon. Hemostasis can be achieved with cautery or with an absorbable hemostatic sponge.

Structure of the Extraocular Muscles

The important functional characteristics of muscle fibers are contraction speed and fatigue resistance. The eye muscles participate in motor acts that are among the fastest in the human body (saccadic eye movements) and also among the most sustained (gaze fixation and vergence movements). Like skeletal muscle, EOM is voluntary striated muscle. However, EOM differs from typical skeletal muscle. In the EOMs, the ratio of nerve fibers to muscle fibers is very high (1:3–1:5)—up to 10 times higher than the ratio of nerve axons to muscle fibers in skeletal muscle. This high ratio may enable accurate eye movements that are controlled by an array of systems ranging from the primitive vestibular-ocular reflex to highly evolved vergence movements.

The muscle fibers can be either singly or multiply innervated. Singly innervated fibers are fast-twitch generating. Approximately 90% and 80% of the fibers are singly innervated in the global and orbital layers, respectively. The global singly innervated muscle fibers include 3 types (red, intermediate, and white), defined by mitochondrial content. The red fibers are the most fatigue resistant and the white fibers are the least. The orbital singly innervated fibers all have high mitochondrial content and high fatigue resistance; they are considered the major contributor to sustained EOM force in primary and deviated positions. This muscle fiber type is the most affected by denervation from damage to the motor nerves or the end plates, as occurs after botulinum toxin injection.

The function of the multiply innervated fibers of the orbital and global layers is not clear. These fibers are not seen in the levator palpebrae superioris. They are thought to be involved in the finer control of fixation and in smooth and finely graded eye movements, particularly vergence control.

Compartmentalization of Extraocular Muscles

There is evidence for compartmentalization of rectus muscle innervation. Studies in primates and humans have shown distinct superior and inferior zones of innervation within horizontal rectus muscles. Segregation of innervational input may explain why some abducens nerve injuries affect the superior portion of the muscle more than the inferior portion, with associated small vertical deviations.

Demer JL. Compartmentalization of extraocular muscle function. *Eye (Lond)*. 2015;29(2): 157–162.

CHAPTER 3

Motor Physiology

This chapter includes a related video. Go to www.aao.org/bcscvideo_section06 or scan the QR code in the text to access this content.

Highlights

- Sherrington's law, which states that when an agonist muscle contracts, its antagonist relaxes, refers to the innervation controlling a duction or a *monocular* movement.
- Strabismus that increases in a particular gaze direction may be caused by a weakness of the agonist, a restriction of its antagonist, or a combination of these 2 factors.
- Having a patient look to each of the 6 cardinal positions of gaze helps isolate the primary movement of each extraocular muscle.
- Hering's law, which states that yoked eye muscles receive a similar amount of innervation when making conjugate change in eye position, refers to innervation controlling a version or a *binocular* movement.

Basic Principles and Terms

Ocular Rotations

Ocular rotations can be clinically considered as

- *horizontal rotations* about a vertical axis, corresponding to medial and lateral gaze
- *vertical rotations* about a horizontal axis, corresponding to upward and downward gaze
- *torsional rotations* about the line of sight or *visual axis*

Positions of Gaze

Positions of gaze include

- *primary position:* the position of the eyes when they are fixating straight ahead
- *secondary diagnostic positions:* straight up, straight down, right gaze, and left gaze

- *tertiary diagnostic positions:* the 4 oblique positions of gaze: up and right, up and left, down and right, down and left, as well as the right and left head-tilt positions
- *cardinal positions:* up and right, up and left, right, left, down and right, down and left (Fig 3-1); these correspond to the primary fields of action of the extraocular muscles (EOMs) (see the section "Field of action")

See Chapter 6 for additional discussion of the positions of gaze.

Extraocular Muscle Action

The breadth of the insertion of each EOM stabilizes the eye and mitigates changes in action that would otherwise occur in different eye positions. For example, when the eye looks upward, the insertion of the medial rectus muscle moves upward accordingly. Concurrently, the inferior fibers tighten and the superior fibers slacken, in effect shifting the net vector from the muscle downward toward its original position. See also Activity 2-1 in Chapter 2.

Muscle pulleys

Regardless of eye position or whether the insertion points have been moved surgically, the rectus muscles are still constrained to pass through the same openings in the Tenon capsule as they course from the orbital apex to the eye. The orbital connective tissue sheaths surrounding these openings have been described as muscle pulleys. See Chapter 2 for further discussion of the pulley system.

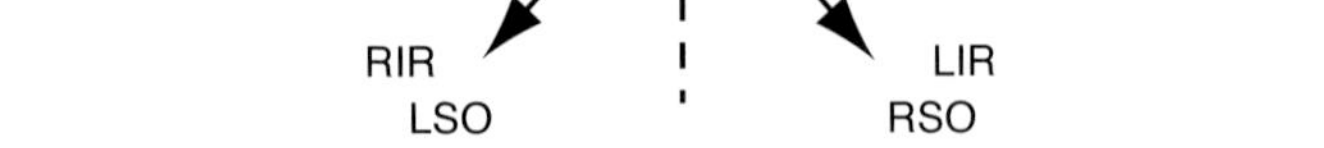

Gaze position	Yoke muscles
Eyes up and right	RSR and LIO
Eyes up and left	LSR and RIO
Eyes right	RLR and LMR
Eyes left	LLR and RMR
Eyes down and right	RIR and LSO
Eyes down and left	LIR and RSO

Figure 3-1 The 6 cardinal positions of gaze, which correspond to the primary fields of action of the extraocular muscles. RSR = right superior rectus; LIO = left inferior oblique; LSR = left superior rectus; RIO = right inferior oblique; RLR = right lateral rectus; LMR = left medial rectus; LLR = left lateral rectus; RMR = right medial rectus; RIR = right inferior rectus; LSO = left superior oblique; LIR = left inferior rectus; RSO = right superior oblique.

Arc of contact

In primary position, each muscle wraps around the globe for several millimeters before reaching its insertion on the sclera. The length of muscle in contact with the globe is called the *arc of contact* (Table 2-1 in Chapter 2 gives the arc of contact for each of the oculorotatory EOMs). The point where the muscle first contacts the globe is the effective insertion of the muscle. As the muscle contracts and the eye rotates toward the muscle, the effective insertion moves forward on the globe, toward the scleral insertion point, and the arc of contact decreases. The muscle remains tangential to the globe at its effective insertion, maintaining the same torque through much of the eye movement.

Eye Movements

Motor Units

A motor unit comprises an individual motor nerve fiber and several muscle fibers. *Electromyography (EMG),* which can be used to record the electrical activity of motor units, is a useful research tool in the investigation of normal and abnormal innervation of eye muscles.

> **CLINICAL PEARL**
>
> A portable EMG device connected to an insulated needle can be used during injection of botulinum toxin into eye muscles to help the surgeon localize the appropriate muscle within the orbit, especially when the muscle has been operated on previously.

Recruitment during fixation or following movement

Recruitment is the orderly increase in the number of activated motor units, which increases the strength of muscle contraction. For example, as the eye moves farther into abduction, the brain activates more and more lateral rectus motor units to help pull the eye temporally. In addition, as the eye fixates farther into abduction, the firing frequency of each motor unit increases until it reaches a peak (several hundred per second, for some motor units).

Monocular Eye Movements

Ductions

Ductions are monocular rotations of the eye:

- *adduction* is movement of the eye nasally
- *abduction* is movement of the eye temporally
- *elevation* (*supraduction* or *sursumduction*) is an upward rotation of the eye
- *depression* (*infraduction* or *deorsumduction*) is a downward rotation of the eye
- *intorsion (incycloduction)* is a nasal rotation of the superior pole of the vertical meridian
- *extorsion (excycloduction)* is a temporal rotation of the superior pole of the vertical meridian

The following important terms relate to the muscles used in monocular eye movements:

- *agonist:* the primary muscle moving the eye in a given direction
- *synergist:* the muscle in the same eye as the agonist that acts with the agonist to produce a given movement (eg, the inferior oblique muscle is a synergist with the agonist superior rectus muscle for elevation of the eye)
- *antagonist:* the muscle in the same eye as the agonist that acts in the direction opposite to that of the agonist (eg, the medial rectus and lateral rectus muscles are antagonists)

Sherrington's law of reciprocal innervation states that increased innervation of a given EOM is accompanied by a reciprocal decrease in innervation of its antagonist. For example, as the right eye adducts, innervation of the right medial rectus muscle increases and innervation of the right lateral rectus muscle decreases (Fig 3-2).

Field of action

Field of action refers to the position of gaze (1 of the cardinal positions) in which the effect of the specific EOM is most readily observed. For the lateral rectus muscle, the direction of rotation and field of action are both abduction; for the medial rectus muscle, they are both adduction. However, for the vertically acting muscles, the direction of rotation and the field of action are not the same. For example, the inferior oblique muscle is an abductor and elevator, pulling the eye up and out, but its field of action (where the elevating action is best observed) is with the eye elevated in adduction. Similarly, the superior oblique muscle is an abductor and depressor, pulling the eye down and out, but its field of action (where the depression action is best observed) is in adduction and depression.

The clinical significance of fields of action is that a deviation (eg, strabismus) that increases with gaze in a given direction may result from weakness of the muscle that normally pulls the eye in that direction, from restriction of its antagonist muscle, or from a combination of these 2 factors.

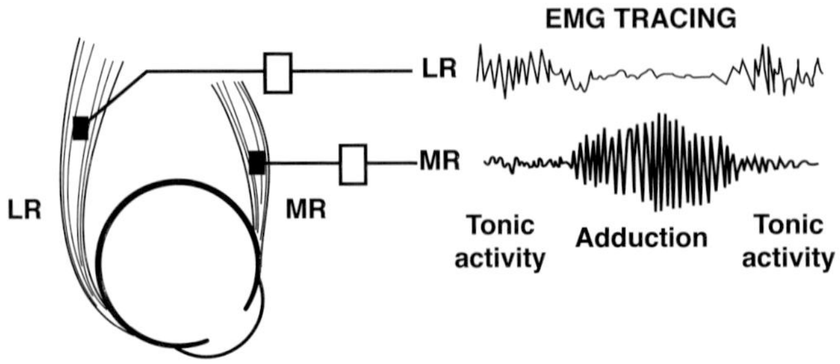

Figure 3-2 Electromyography (EMG) tracing from lateral and medial rectus muscles (right eye viewed from above) demonstrating Sherrington's law. As the eye adducts, there is a strong EMG signal from the medial rectus muscle, while its antagonist, the lateral rectus muscle, relaxes, showing a weak EMG signal. *(Reprinted from Wright KW, Spiegel PH, Thompson LS (eds).* Handbook of Pediatric Strabismus and Amblyopia. *Springer-Verlag; 2006:63.)*

Primary, secondary, and tertiary actions

When the eye is in primary position, the medial and lateral rectus muscles move the eye only horizontally and therefore have a primary horizontal action. Anatomic studies have shown that the innervation to the horizontal rectus muscles is compartmentalized in some patients, which may explain the finding of small vertical actions of these muscles in these cases (see Chapter 2). Table 3-1 summarizes the EOM actions.

The vertical rectus muscles have a direction of pull that is mostly vertical as their primary action, but in primary position, the angle of pull from origin to insertion is inclined 23° to the visual axis (or midplane of the eye), giving rise to a secondary *torsional* action (intorsion for the superior rectus, extorsion for the inferior rectus). Both muscles have tertiary adduction effect. The oblique muscles are inclined 51° to the vertical axis, resulting in a primary action of torsion and a secondary action of vertical rotation (depression for the superior oblique, elevation for the inferior oblique). The sole action of the levator palpebrae superioris is elevation of the upper eyelid.

Changing muscle action with different gaze positions

Gaze position can alter the effect of EOM contractions on the rotation of the eye. In each of the cardinal positions (see Fig 3-1), each of the EOMs has a different effect on the eye's rotation, based on the orientation of the muscle plane to the visual axis. In each cardinal position, the angle between the visual axis and the direction of pull of the muscle being tested is minimized, thus maximizing the horizontal effect of the medial or lateral rectus muscle or the vertical effect of the superior rectus, inferior rectus, superior oblique, or inferior oblique muscle.

By having the patient move the eyes to the 6 cardinal positions, the clinician can isolate and evaluate the ability of each of the EOMs to move the eye. See also the section Binocular Eye Movements.

When the eye is in primary position, the *horizontal rectus muscles* share a common horizontal plane that contains the visual axis (Fig 3-3). The clinician can assess the relative strength of the horizontal rectus muscles by observing the horizontal excursion of the eye as it moves medially from primary position to test the medial rectus and laterally to test the lateral rectus.

Table 3-1 Action of the Extraocular Muscles Referenced to Primary Position

Muscle[a]	Primary	Secondary	Tertiary
Medial rectus	Adduction	—	—
Lateral rectus	Abduction	—	—
Inferior rectus	Depression	Extorsion	Adduction
Superior rectus	Elevation	Intorsion	Adduction
Inferior oblique	Extorsion	Elevation	Abduction
Superior oblique	Intorsion	Depression	Abduction
Levator palpebrae superioris[b]	Elevation of upper eyelid	—	—

[a] The superior muscles are intortors; the inferior muscles, extortors. The vertical rectus muscles are adductors; the oblique muscles, abductors.

[b] *Note:* The levator palpebrae superioris is not oculorotatory.

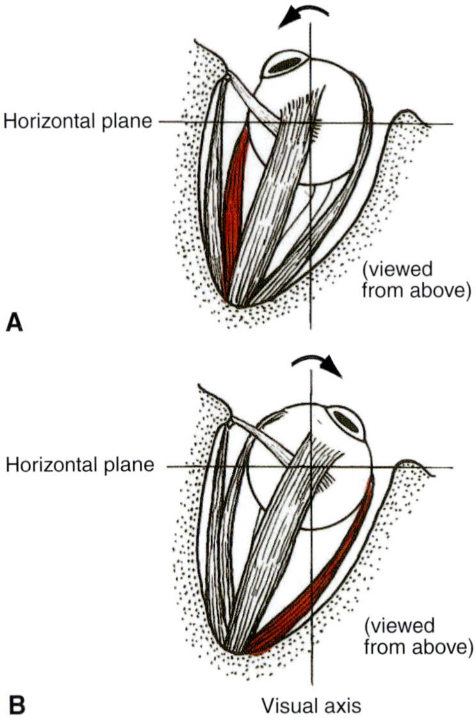

Figure 3-3 The horizontal rectus muscle actions viewed from above. **A,** Right medial rectus muscle. **B,** Right lateral rectus muscle. *(Modified with permission from von Noorden GK.* Atlas of Strabismus. *4th ed. Mosby;1983:3.)*

The actions of the vertical rectus and oblique muscles are more complex. With insertions anterior to the center of rotation of the globe and, in primary position, the 23° angle between the muscle planes and the visual axis (Fig 3-4), the *superior* and *inferior rectus muscles* have 3 actions: primary vertical, secondary torsion, and tertiary adduction.

The relative vertical strength of the vertical rectus muscles can be most readily observed by aligning the visual axis parallel to the muscle plane axis—that is, when the eye is rotated 23° into abduction. In this position, the superior rectus becomes a pure elevator and the inferior rectus a pure depressor. To minimize the vertical action of these muscles, the visual axis should be perpendicular to the muscle axis at a position of 67° of adduction. In this position, the superior rectus action would be pure intorsion, and the inferior rectus action would be pure extorsion. Because the globe cannot adduct this far, the vertical rectus muscles maintain significant elevating and depressing action even in maximal voluntary adduction.

With insertions posterior to the center of rotation of the globe and, in primary position, the 51° angle between the muscle planes and the visual axis (Fig 3-5), the *superior* and *inferior oblique muscles* have 3 actions: primary torsion, secondary vertical, and tertiary abduction. In 51° adduction, the muscle plane is aligned with the visual axis, and the vertical action of the oblique muscle can be most readily observed. When the eye abducts 39°, the visual axis becomes perpendicular to the muscle plane, and the muscle action is mainly torsion.

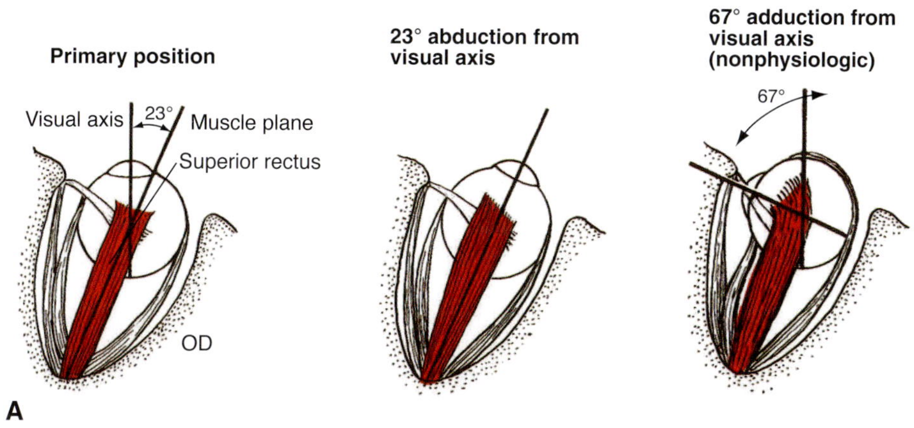

Right superior rectus muscle action(s)		
Elevation Intorsion Adduction	Elevation	Intorsion Adduction (minor)

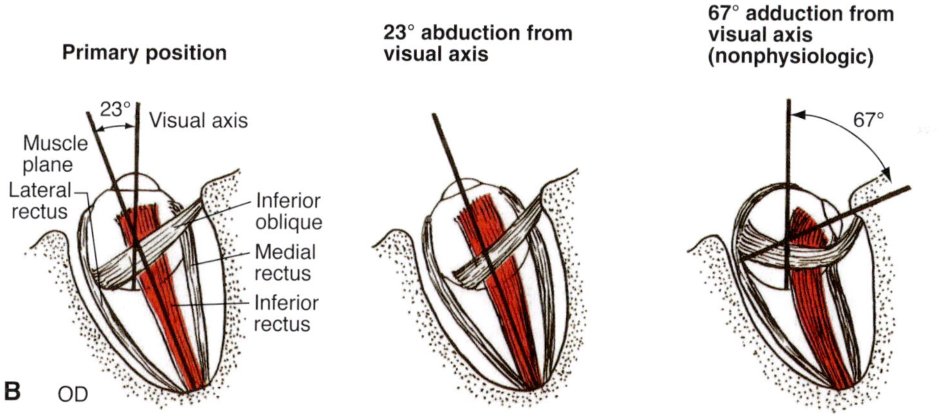

Right inferior rectus muscle action(s)		
Depression Extorsion Adduction	Depression	Extorsion Adduction (minor)

Figure 3-4 Vertical rectus muscle actions change with change in gaze position. **A,** Right superior rectus, viewed from above. **B,** Right inferior rectus, viewed from below. *(Modified with permission from von Noorden GK.* Atlas of Strabismus. *4th ed. Mosby;1983:7.)*

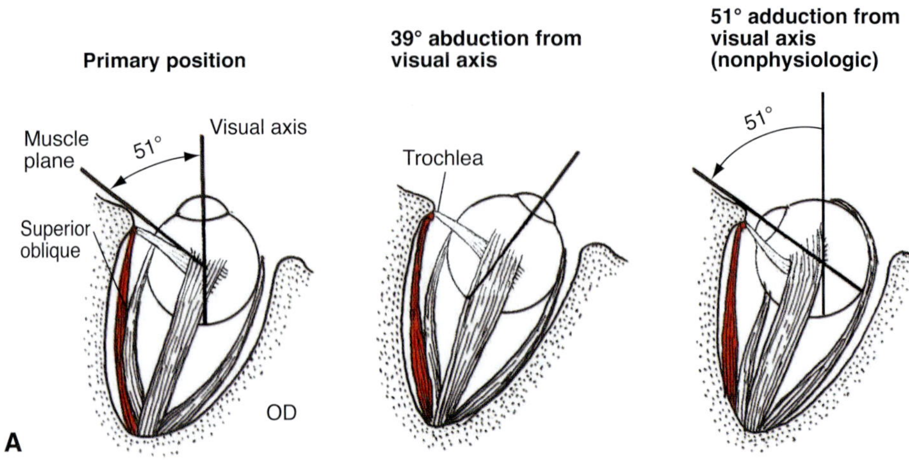

Right superior oblique muscle action(s)		
Intorsion Depression Abduction	Intorsion Abduction	Depression Intorsion

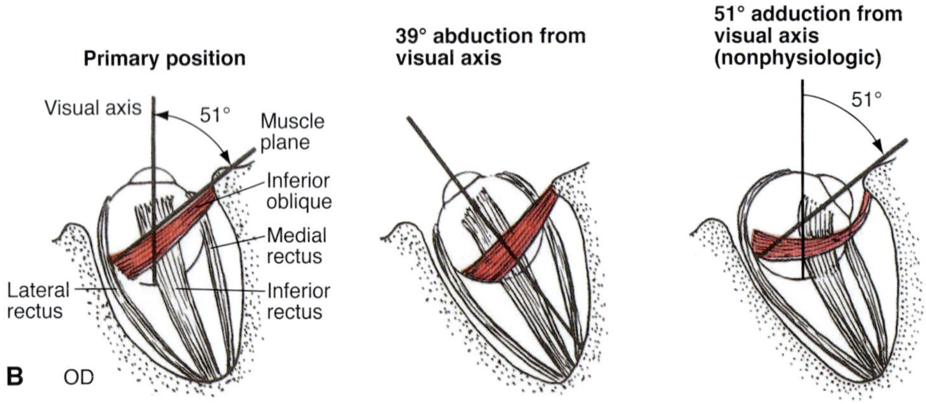

Right inferior oblique muscle action(s)		
Extorsion Elevation Abduction	Extorsion Abduction	Elevation Extorsion

Figure 3-5 Oblique muscle actions change with change in gaze position. **A,** Right superior oblique, viewed from above. **B,** Right inferior oblique, viewed from below. *(Modified with permission from von Noorden GK.* Atlas of Strabismus. *4th ed. Mosby; 1983:7.)*

Binocular Eye Movements

Versions

When binocular eye movements are conjugate and the eyes move in the same direction, such movements are called *versions:*

- right gaze *(dextroversion)*: movement of both eyes to the patient's right
- left gaze *(levoversion)*: movement of both eyes to the patient's left
- *elevation,* or *upgaze (sursumversion):* upward rotation of both eyes
- *depression,* or *downgaze (deorsumversion):* downward rotation of both eyes
- *dextrocycloversion:* rotation of the superior pole of the vertical meridian of both eyes to the patient's right
- *levocycloversion*: movement of both eyes so that the superior pole of the vertical meridian rotates to the patient's left

The term *yoke muscles* refers to the 2 muscles (1 in each eye) that are the primary movers of their respective eyes into a given position of gaze. For example, when the eyes move into right gaze, the right lateral rectus muscle and the left medial rectus muscle are simultaneously innervated and contracted. These muscles are said to be "yoked" together. Each EOM in 1 eye has a yoke muscle in the other eye. Figure 3-1 shows the yoke muscles in the 6 cardinal positions of gaze.

Hering's law of motor correspondence states that when the eyes move into a gaze direction, there is a simultaneous and equal increase in innervation to the yoke muscles for that direction. Hering's law has important clinical implications when the practitioner is evaluating a paralytic or restrictive strabismus. Because the amount of innervation supplied to both eyes is always determined by the fixating eye, the angle of deviation varies according to which eye is fixating. When the sound eye is fixating (prism over the affected eye when the prism and alternate cover test is performed), the amount of misalignment is called the *primary deviation.* When the affected eye is fixating (prism over the sound eye when the prism and alternate cover test is performed), the amount of misalignment is called the *secondary deviation.* The secondary deviation is larger than the primary deviation because of the increased innervation necessary to move the affected eye to the position of fixation. This extra innervation is shared by the yoke muscle in the sound eye, which causes excessive action of that muscle and a larger angle of deviation. An example of primary and secondary deviations in monocular elevation deficiency is shown in Figure 3-6. Video 3-1 demonstrates this concept.

VIDEO 3-1 Primary and secondary deviations in monocular elevation deficiency.
Animation developed by Faruk H. Örge, MD, and David K. Epley, MD.

Vergences

When binocular eye movements are dysconjugate and the eyes move in opposite directions, such movements are known as *vergences:*

- *convergence:* movement of both eyes nasally relative to a given starting position; the medial rectus muscles are yoke muscles for convergence

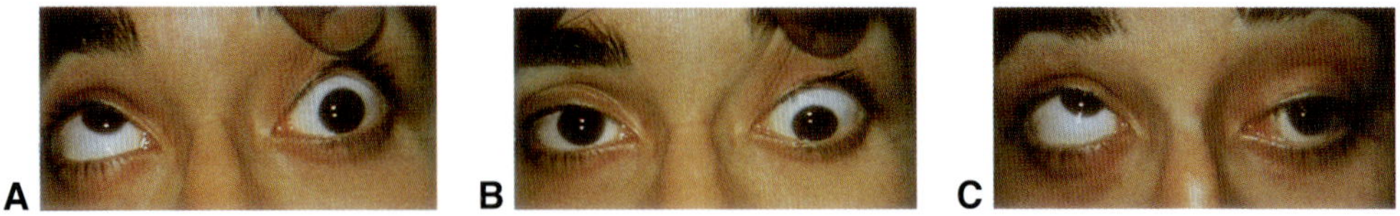

Figure 3-6 Demonstration of primary and secondary deviation in patient with a left monocular elevation deficiency. **A,** Patient looking to up gaze showing elevation deficit of the left eye. **B,** Patient in primary gaze fixating with nonparetic right eye showing the primary deviation of left hypotropia. **C,** Patient in primary gaze fixating with the paretic left eye showing the larger secondary deviation of right hypertropia.

- *divergence:* movement of both eyes temporally relative to a given starting position; the lateral rectus muscles are yoked for divergence
- *vertical vergence* movements: 1 eye moves upward, and the other moves downward
- *incyclovergence:* a rotation of both eyes so that the superior pole of the vertical meridian is rotated nasally
- *excyclovergence:* a rotation of both eyes so that the superior pole of the vertical meridian rotates temporally

Vergence movements are described further in the following sections.

Accommodative convergence of the visual axes Accommodative convergence (AC) is part of the near reflex (also called *near synkinesis, near triad*), which consists of accommodation, convergence, and miosis. A certain amount of AC occurs with each diopter of accommodation (A), giving the *accommodative convergence/accommodation (AC/A) ratio.*

Abnormalities of this ratio are common and are important causes of strabismus (see Chapter 7). If the AC/A ratio is abnormally high, the excess convergence tends to produce esotropia during near fixation that is greater than esotropia at distance. An abnormally low AC/A ratio tends to make the eyes less esotropic, or even exotropic, when the patient looks at near targets. Techniques for measuring this ratio are discussed in Chapter 6.

Fusional convergence A movement to converge and position the eyes so that similar retinal images project on corresponding retinal areas, fusional convergence is activated when a target in the midline is seen with bitemporal retinal image disparity. See also Chapter 4.

Proximal (instrument) convergence An induced convergence movement caused by a psychological awareness that the object of fixation is located at a near viewing distance, proximal convergence is particularly apparent when a person looks through an instrument such as a binocular microscope.

Tonic convergence The constant innervational tone to the EOMs when a person is awake and alert is called tonic convergence. Because of the anatomic shape of the bony orbits and the position of the rectus muscle origins, the position of the eyes during complete muscle paralysis is divergent.

CLINICAL PEARL

Convergence tone is normally necessary for the eyes to be aligned when an individual is awake. An esotropic patient under general anesthesia may become less esotropic or even exotropic with suspension of tonic convergence.

Voluntary convergence Voluntary convergence refers to conscious application of the near reflex.

Fusional divergence A movement to diverge and position the eyes so that similar retinal images project on corresponding retinal areas, fusional divergence is activated when a target in the midline is seen with binasal retinal image disparity. See also Chapter 4.

Fusional vertical vergence Fusional vertical vergence is the superior movement of 1 eye and inferior movement of the other to reduce vertical disparity so that similar images project on corresponding retinal areas.

Fusional cyclovergence This term refers to intorsion of both eyes (incyclovergence) or extorsion of both eyes (excyclovergence) to reduce torsional disparity so that similar retinal images project on corresponding retinal areas. Although it can be enhanced by special training, cyclovergence is normally very limited, and fusion of torsional disparity is mostly accomplished by sensory adaptation.

Supranuclear Control Systems for Eye Movement

Eye movements are directed and coordinated by several supranuclear systems. The *saccadic system* generates fast (up to 400°–500° per second) eye movements, such as eye movements of refixation. This system functions to place the image of an object of interest on the fovea or to shift gaze from 1 object to another. Saccadic movements require a sudden strong pulse of force from the EOMs to move the eye rapidly against the viscosity produced by the fatty tissue and the fascia in which the globe lies.

The *smooth-pursuit system* generates following, or pursuit, eye movements that maintain the image of a moving object on the fovea. Pursuit latency is shorter than saccade latency, but the maximum peak velocity of these slow pursuit movements is limited to 30°–60° per second. The involuntary *optokinetic system* utilizes smooth pursuit to track a moving object and then introduces a compensatory saccade to refixate. Tests of this system, performed with an optokinetic stimulus, are often used to detect visual responses in an infant or child with apparent vision loss, such as with ocular motor apraxia (see Chapter 11).

The *vergence system* controls dysconjugate eye movement, as in convergence or divergence. Supranuclear control of vergence eye movements is not yet fully understood.

There are also systems that integrate eye movements with body movements in order to stabilize the image on the retinas. The most clinically important of these systems is the *vestibular-ocular system.* Vestibular-ocular reflex responses are driven by the labyrinth, which involves the semicircular canals and otoliths (utricle and saccule) of the inner ears. The cervical, or neck, receptors also provide input for this reflex control. See BCSC Section 5, *Neuro-Ophthalmology,* for in-depth discussion of these systems.

CHAPTER 4

Sensory Physiology and Pathology

Highlights

- A healthy child with normal alignment who notices diplopia might actually be experiencing physiologic diplopia.
- Anomalous retinal correspondence and suppression are adaptations made by the immature visual system to avoid diplopia.
- Monofixation occurs when there is normal peripheral fusion and deficient bifoveal fusion; often mild amblyopia and a small strabismus are present.

The Physiology of Normal Binocular Vision

If an area of the retina is stimulated by any means—externally by light or internally by mechanical pressure or electrical processes—the resulting sensation is always one of light, and the light is subjectively localized as coming from a specific visual direction in space. The imaginary line connecting the fixation point and the fovea is termed the *visual axis,* and normally, with central fixation, it is subjectively localized straight ahead.

Retinal Correspondence

Retinal correspondence is the term used when a viewed target stimulates paired retinal areas in an individual's 2 eyes. These retinal locations are said to be *corresponding.* When the image of an object in space falls on corresponding points, it is perceived as a single object located in the same subjective or egocentric direction. On the other hand, stimulation of *noncorresponding* or *disparate* retinal points results in the sensation of 2 visual directions for the same target, or diplopia.

In *normal retinal correspondence,* the foveae of the 2 eyes are corresponding points. Retinal areas in each eye that are equidistant from the right or left and above or below the fovea are also corresponding points. The locus of points in space that stimulate corresponding points in each retina is known as the *horopter.*

The geometric relationship between corresponding points—for example, a point 1° nasal to the fovea in 1 eye would correspond to a point 1° temporal to the fovea in the other eye—creates a circle that passes through the nodal point of each eye and the point of fixation. This theoretical horopter is known as the *Vieth-Müller circle.* When the horopter is determined experimentally, the locus of points that are seen singly falls not on a circle but on a curve called the *empirical horopter* (Fig 4-1). A real-life application of the empirical horopter can be seen in the shape of the curved screen in 3-dimensional projection theaters.

The horopter exists in both the horizontal and vertical planes. Although it might seem that the horopter would be a surface in space, the horizontal separation of the eyes causes points in the oblique quadrants to be vertically disparate. For symmetric convergence, the 3-dimensional horopter of points that have both horizontal and vertical correspondence consists of a curved horizontal line and a sloped vertical line that intersect at the fixation point. Each fixation point has a unique horopter centered on that point.

If the horopter includes all points in space that stimulate corresponding retinal points, double vision would be expected when the target does not lie on the horopter. However, the visual system can combine slightly disparate points within a limited area surrounding the horopter, called *Panum's area of single binocular vision* (see Fig 4-1). Objects within Panum's area do not result in diplopia. Objects outside Panum's area stimulate widely disparate retinal points, resulting in physiologic diplopia (see eSidebar Steps to Experience Physiologic Diplopia online at www.aao.org/bcscsupplement_section06). If an object is distal to Panum's area, uncrossed physiologic diplopia will result; if an object is proximal to Panum's area, crossed physiologic diplopia will result (Fig 4-2). A healthy child without strabismus might notice this phenomenon and report diplopia.

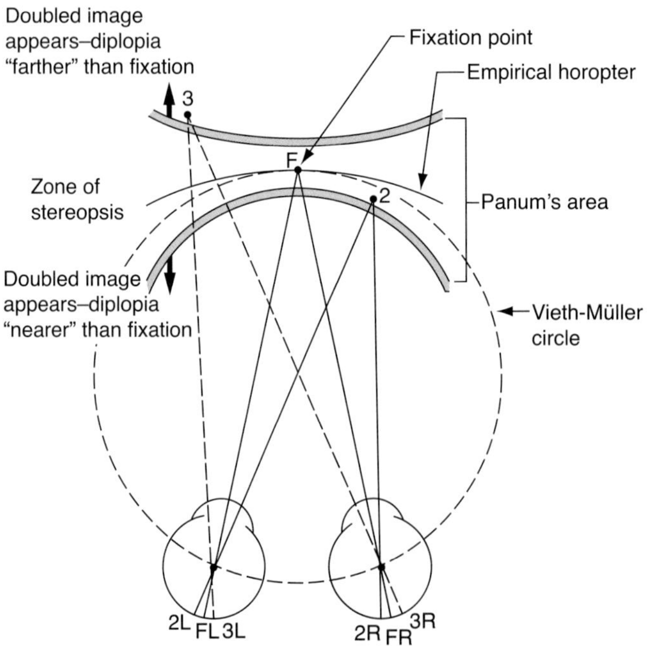

Figure 4-1 Empirical horopter. F = fixation point; FL and FR = left and right foveae, respectively. Point 2, falling within Panum's area, is seen singly and stereoscopically. Point 3 falls outside Panum's area and is therefore seen as double. *(©2021 The American Academy of Ophthalmology.)*

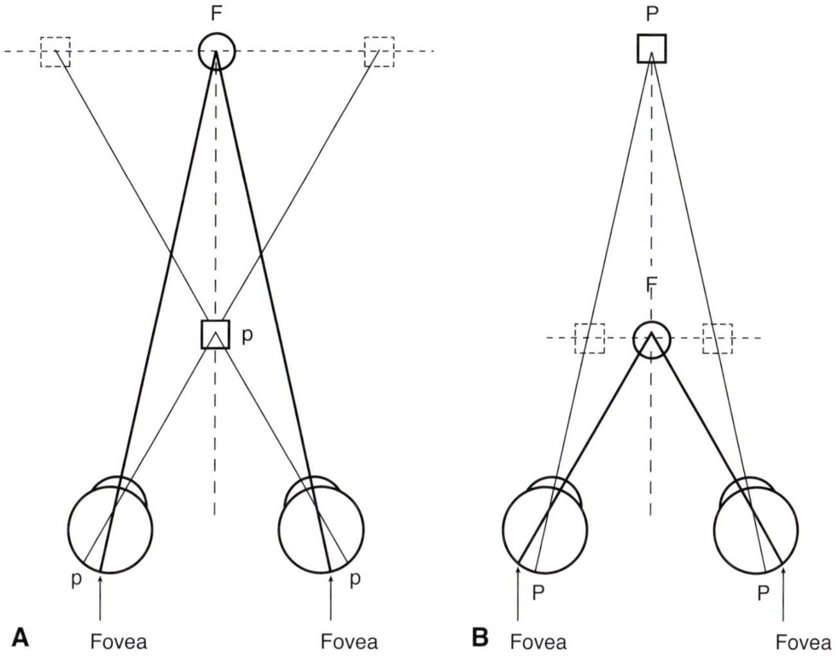

Figure 4-2 Diagram of physiologic diplopia. **A,** Crossed physiologic diplopia occurs when an object (p) is placed closer than the fixation point (F circle). The object p projects on the temporal retina in each eye, resulting in crossed diplopia (dotted-line squares). **B,** Uncrossed physiologic diplopia occurs when an object (P) is placed further than the fixation point (F circle). The object P projects on the nasal retina, resulting in uncrossed diplopia (dotted-line squares). *(Modified with permission from von Noorden GK, Campos EC.* Binocular Vision and Ocular Motility: Theory and Management of Strabismus. *6th ed. Mosby; 2002:19.)*

Fusion

Fusion is the cortical unification of 2 images of an object, 1 from each eye, into a single percept. For retinal images to be fused, they must be similar in size and shape. For fusion of macular images *(central fusion)* to occur, there can be very little dissimilarity between the images in each eye, because of the small receptive fields in the area near the fovea; otherwise, diplopia results.

CLINICAL PEARL

Adults with epiretinal membranes may experience double vision because of foveal distortion.

More image dissimilarity is tolerated in the periphery *(peripheral fusion)*, where the receptive fields are larger. Fusion has been artificially subdivided into sensory fusion, motor fusion, and stereopsis.

Sensory fusion

Sensory fusion is based on the innate, orderly topographic relationship between the retinas and the visual cortex, whereby images falling on corresponding (or nearly corresponding) retinal points in the 2 eyes are combined to form a single visual percept.

Motor fusion

Motor fusion is a vergence movement that allows similar retinal images to be maintained on corresponding retinal areas despite natural conditions (eg, heterophorias) or artificial causes that induce disparities. For example, when a progressive base-out prism is introduced in front of both eyes while a target is viewed, the retinal images move temporally over both retinas if the eyes remain in fixed position. However, because of a response called *fusional convergence* (see Chapter 3), the eyes instead converge, repositioning so that similar retinal images are projected on corresponding retinal areas. Measurement of fusional vergence amplitudes is discussed in Chapter 6.

Stereopsis

Stereopsis is a *binocular* sensation of relative depth caused by horizontal disparity of retinal images. It is the highest form of binocular cooperation. The region of points with binocular disparities that result in stereopsis is slightly wider than Panum's area, so stereopsis is not simply a by-product of combining the disparate images from a point into a single visual percept. The brain interprets nasal disparity between 2 similar retinal images of an object in the midline as indicating that the object is farther away from the fixation point, and temporal disparity as indicating that the object is nearer. Binasal or bitemporal images are not a requirement for stereopsis; objects not in the midline in front of or behind the horopter also elicit stereopsis, even though their images fall on the nasal retina in 1 eye and the temporal retina in the other. Stereoacuity reaches a high level (60 seconds of arc) by approximately age 5–6 months.

> **CLINICAL PEARL**
>
> Stereopsis and depth perception are not synonymous. Monocular cues—which include object overlap, relative object size, highlights and shadows, motion parallax, and perspective—also contribute to depth perception. Monocular patients can have excellent depth perception using these cues.

Selected Aspects of the Neurophysiology of Vision

The decussation of the optic nerves at the chiasm is essential for the development of binocular vision and stereopsis. With decussation, visual information from corresponding retinal areas in each eye runs through the lateral geniculate body (lateral geniculate nucleus) and optic tracts to the visual cortex, where the information from both eyes is commingled and modified by the integration of various inputs. See BCSC Section 5, *Neuro-Ophthalmology,* Chapter 1, for further discussion.

Visual Development

In the human retina, most of the ganglion cells are generated between 8 and 15 weeks' gestation, reaching a plateau of 2.2–2.5 million by week 18. After week 30, the retinal ganglion cell (RGC) population decreases dramatically during *apoptosis,* which lasts 6–8 weeks. Thereafter, RGC death continues at a low rate into the first few postnatal months. The RGC population is reduced to a final count of approximately 1.0–1.5 million. The loss of about 1 million RGC axons may serve to refine the topography and specificity of the retinogeniculate projection by eliminating inappropriate connections.

The continued development of visual function after birth is accompanied by major anatomical changes, which occur at all levels of the central visual pathways. The fovea is still covered by multiple cell layers and is sparsely packed with cones, which, in addition to neural immaturity, contributes to the estimated visual acuity of 20/400 in the newborn. During the first years of life, the photoreceptors redistribute within the retina, and foveal cone density increases fivefold to achieve the configuration found in the mature retina. In newborns, the white matter of the visual pathways and optic nerves is not fully myelinated. Myelin sheaths enlarge rapidly in the first 2 years after birth and then more slowly through the first decade of life. At birth, the neurons of the lateral geniculate body are only 60% of their average adult size. Their volume gradually increases until age 2 years. Refinement of synaptic connections in the striate cortex continues for many years after birth. The density of synapses declines by 40% over several years, attaining final adult levels at approximately age 10 years.

See BCSC Section 2, *Fundamentals and Principles of Ophthalmology,* for further discussion of ocular development.

Effects of Abnormal Visual Experience on the Retinogeniculocortical Pathway

Abnormal visual experience resulting from visual deprivation, anisometropia, or strabismus can powerfully affect retinogeniculocortical development. In studies of baby macaque monkeys, single-eyelid suturing usually produces axial myopia but no other significant anatomical changes in the eye. The lateral geniculate laminae that receive input from the deprived eye experience minor shrinkage, but these cells respond rapidly to visual stimulation, suggesting that a defect in the lateral geniculate body is not likely to account for amblyopia.

In the striate cortex, monocular visual deprivation causes the regions of the visual cortex driven predominantly by the closed eye (ocular dominance columns) to radically narrow (Fig 4-3). This occurs because the 2 eyes compete for synaptic contacts in the cortex. As a result, the deprived eye loses many of the connections already formed at birth with postsynaptic cortical targets. The open eye profits as the terminal arbors sprout beyond their usual boundaries to occupy territory relinquished by the deprived eye (Fig 4-4). However, the benefit derived from invading the cortical territory of the deprived eye is unclear, because visual acuity does not improve beyond normal. Positron emission tomography has shown that cortical blood flow and glucose metabolism are lower during stimulation of the amblyopic eye compared with the normal eye, suggesting the visual

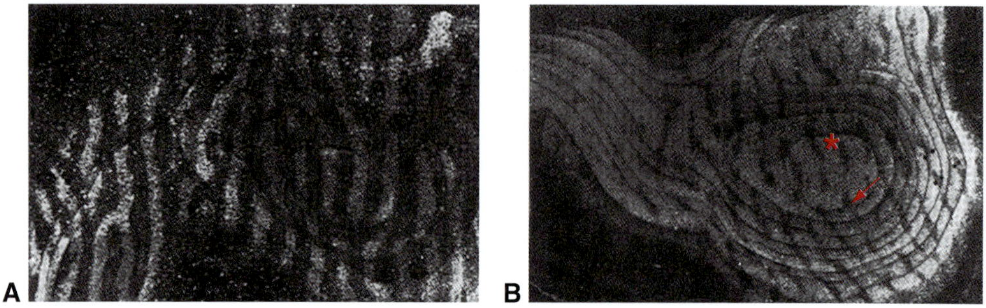

Figure 4-3 Change in ocular dominance columns in macaque visual cortex after monocular deprivation. Radioactive proline was injected into the normal eye and transported to the visual cortex to reveal the projections of that eye. In these sections, cut parallel to the cortical surface, white areas show labeled terminals. **A,** Normal monkey. There is roughly equal spacing of the stripes, which represent the injected eye (bright) and noninjected eye (dark). **B,** Monkey that had 1 eye sutured closed from birth for 18 months. The bright stripes (open, injected eye) are widened *(asterisk)* and the dark ones (closed eye) *(arrow)* are greatly narrowed, showing the devastating physical effect of deprivation amblyopia. *(Reproduced with permission from Kaufman PL, Alm A.* Adler's Physiology of the Eye. *10th ed. Mosby; 2002:699. Originally from Hubel DH, Wiesel TN, LeVay S. Plasticity of ocular dominance columns in monkey striate cortex.* Philos Trans R Soc Lond B Biol Sci. *1977;278(961):377–409.)*

cortex as the primary site of amblyopia. Monocular deprivation also devastates binocularity because few cells can be driven by both eyes.

There is a critical period in which visual development in the macaque is vulnerable to the effects of eyelid suturing. This period corresponds to the stage in which wiring of the striate cortex is still vulnerable to the effects of visual deprivation. During the critical period, the deleterious effects of suturing the right eyelid, for example, are correctable by reversal—that is, opening the sutured right eye and closing the left eye. After this reversal, the ocular dominance columns of the initially closed right eye appear practically normal, indicating that anatomical recovery of the initially shrunken columns was induced by opening the right eye and closing the left eye. However, when the right eye is sewn closed beyond the critical period, the columns of the right eye do not re-expand if the right eye is opened and the left eye closed.

Eyelid suturing in the baby macaque is a good model for visual deprivation amblyopia. In children, this condition can be caused by any dense opacity of the ocular media or significant occlusion by the eyelid. Visual deprivation can rapidly cause profound amblyopia.

Amblyopia in children can have other causes. Optical defocus resulting from anisometropia causes the cortical neurons driven by the defocused eye to be less sensitive (particularly to higher spatial frequencies, because they are most affected by blur) and to send out a weaker signal. This results in reduced binocular activity. The critical period for anisometropic amblyopia occurs later than that for strabismic amblyopia, and a prolonged period of unilateral blur is necessary before anisometropic amblyopia develops. Meridional (astigmatic) amblyopia does not develop during the first year of life and may not develop until age 3 years.

Strabismus can be artificially created in monkeys by the sectioning of an extraocular muscle. Alternating fixation develops in some monkeys after this procedure; they maintain normal acuity in each eye. Examination of the striate cortex reveals cells with normal

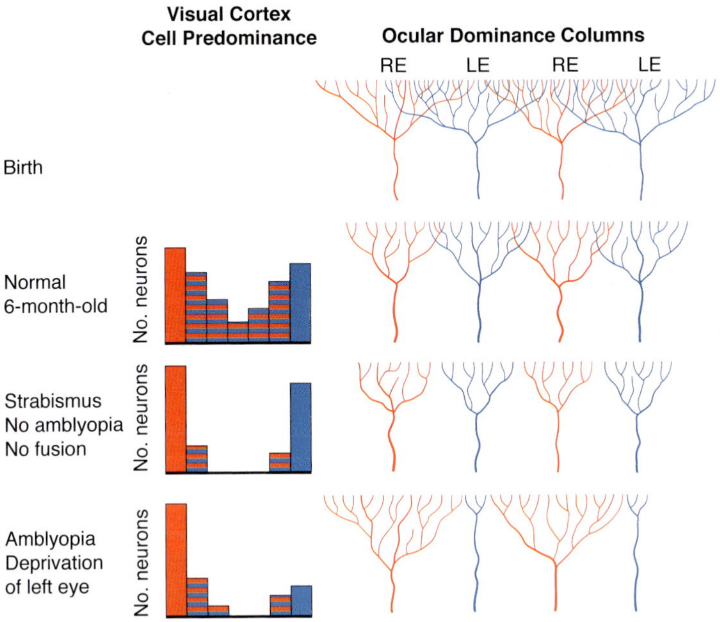

Figure 4-4 Anatomic and physiologic maturation of ocular dominance columns of the primary visual cortex in normal and deprived monkeys. **Birth:** Broad overlap of afferents from the lateral geniculate nucleus, hence little dominance by right eye (RE-red) versus left eye (LE-blue). **Normal 6-month-old:** Regression of overlapping afferents from both eyes with distinct areas of monocular dominance. The bar graph shows the distribution obtained by single-cell recordings from the visual cortex. About half the cells are driven predominantly by the right eye (red) and the other half by the left eye (blue). A small number are driven equally by the 2 eyes (red and blue stripes). **Strabismus:** Effect of artificial eye misalignment in the neonatal period on ocular dominance. The monkey alternated fixation (no amblyopia) and lacked fusion. Lack of binocularity is evident as exaggerated segregation into dominance columns. The bar graph shows the results of single-cell recordings obtained from this animal after age 1 year. Almost all neurons are driven exclusively by the right or left eye, with little binocular activity. **Amblyopia:** Effect of suturing the left eyelid shut shortly after birth. Dominance columns of the normal right eye are much wider than those of the amblyopic left eye. The bar graph shows markedly skewed ocular dominance and little binocular activity. *(Modified with permission from Tychsen L. Binocular vision. In: Hart WM, ed.* Adler's Physiology of the Eye: Clinical Application. *9th ed. Mosby; 1992:810.)*

receptive fields and an equal number of cells responsive to stimulation of either eye. However, the cortex is bereft of binocular cells (see Fig 4-4).

Following sectioning of an extraocular muscle, some of the monkeys studied were found to constantly fixate with the same eye, with amblyopia developing in the deviating eye. An important factor in the development of strabismic amblyopia is interocular suppression due to uncorrelated images in the 2 eyes. Strabismus prevents synchronous attainment of correlated images from the 2 foveae, resulting in abnormal input to the striate cortex. Another factor is the optical defocus of the deviated eye. The dominant eye is focused on the object of regard, while the deviated eye is oriented in a different direction; for the deviated eye, the object may be too near or too far to be in focus. Either mechanism can cause asynchrony or inhibition of 1 set of signals in the striate cortex. The critical period for development of strabismic amblyopia begins at approximately 4 months of age, during the time of ocular dominance segregation and sensitivity to binocular correlation.

Abnormal sensory input alone is sufficient to alter the normal anatomy of the visual cortex. Other areas of the cerebral cortex may also depend on sensory stimulation to form the proper anatomical circuits necessary for normal adult visual function, underscoring the importance of providing children with a stimulating sensory environment.

Abnormalities of Binocular Vision

When a manifest deviation of the eyes occurs, the corresponding retinal elements of the eyes are no longer directed at the same object. This places the patient at risk for 2 distinct visual phenomena: visual confusion and diplopia.

Visual Confusion and Retinal Rivalry

Visual confusion occurs when 2 objects separated in visual space both project images to corresponding retina areas. Clinically significant visual confusion is rare. Confusion may be a phenomenon of extrafoveal retinal areas only because the 2 foveal areas are physiologically incapable of simultaneous perception of dissimilar objects.

The closest foveal equivalent to confusion is *retinal rivalry,* wherein there is rapid alternation of the 2 perceived images (Fig 4-5).

Diplopia

Double vision, or *diplopia,* usually results from an acquired misalignment of the visual axes that causes an image to fall simultaneously on the fovea of 1 eye and on a nonfoveal point in the other eye. As stated earlier, the object that falls on these disparate retinal points must be outside Panum's area to appear double. The same object is perceived as having 2 locations in subjective space, and the foveal image is always clearer than the nonfoveal image of the nonfixating eye.

The perception of diplopia depends on the age at onset, its duration, and the patient's subjective awareness of it. The younger the child, the greater the ability to suppress, or inhibit, the nonfoveal image. Adults with acquired strabismus commonly present to the ophthalmologist because of diplopia.

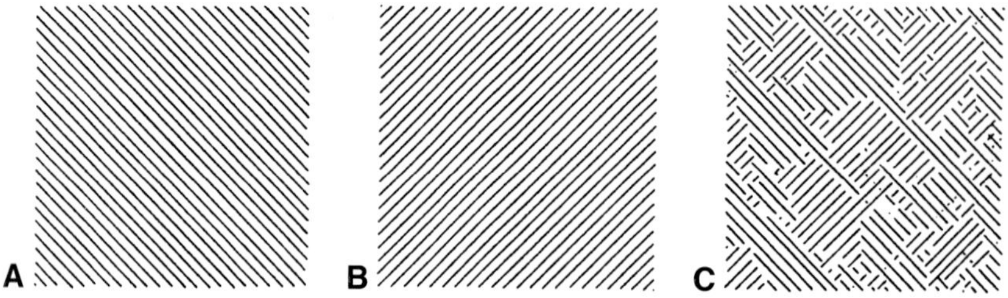

Figure 4-5 Rivalry pattern. **A,** Pattern seen by the left eye. **B,** Pattern seen by the right eye. **C,** Pattern seen binocularly from a rapid alteration of **A** and **B,** resulting in a dynamic pattern similar to that shown. *(Reproduced from Panum PL.* Physiologische Untersuchungen über das Sehen mit zwei Augen. *Kiel: Schwerssche Buchhandlung; 1858:52.)*

The loss of normal binocular fusion in an individual unable to suppress disparate retinal images results in intractable diplopia, referred to as *central fusion disruption (horror fusionis)*. It occurs in adults or visually mature children following traumatic brain injury or treatment of prolonged monocular visual deprivation (eg, uncorrected aphakia). Management is challenging.

Khan AO. Persistent diplopia following secondary intraocular lens placement in patients with sensory strabismus from uncorrected monocular aphakia. *Br J Ophthalmol.* 2008;92(1):51–53.

Sensory Adaptations in Strabismus

To avoid visual confusion and diplopia, the visual system uses the mechanisms of suppression and anomalous retinal correspondence (Fig 4-6). Pathologic suppression and anomalous retinal correspondence develop only in the immature visual system under binocular conditions.

Suppression

Suppression is the alteration of visual sensation that occurs when an eye's retinal image is prevented from reaching consciousness during binocular visual activity. Physiologic suppression is the mechanism that prevents physiologic diplopia (diplopia elicited by objects outside

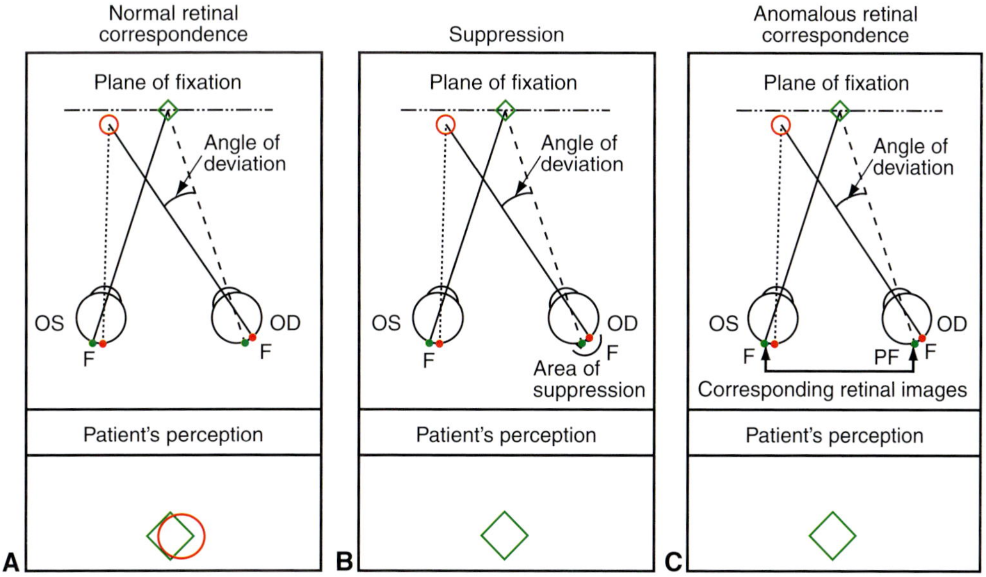

Figure 4-6 Retinal correspondence and suppression in strabismus. **A,** A patient with right esotropia with normal retinal correspondence (NRC) and without suppression would have diplopia because the fixated objects project to different points on the retinas, 1 foveal and 1 extrafoveal. **B,** The elimination of diplopia by suppression of the retinal images of the deviating/esotropic right eye. **C,** The elimination of diplopia by anomalous retinal correspondence (ARC), an adaptation of visual directions in the deviated right eye from the fovea to a pseudofovea so that the correspondence of the retinal images is anomalous. F = fovea; PF = pseudofovea. *(Adapted from Kaufman PL, Alm A.* Adler's Physiology of the Eye. *11th ed. Mosby; 2011:682. With permission from Elsevier.)*

Panum's area) from reaching consciousness. Pathologic suppression may develop because of strabismic misalignment of the visual axes or other conditions resulting in discordant images in each eye, such as cataract or anisometropia. Such suppression can be regarded as an active binocular adaptation within the immature visual system to avoid diplopia. If a patient with strabismus and normal retinal correspondence (NRC) does not have diplopia, suppression is present, provided the sensory pathways are intact. In less obvious situations, several simple tests are available for clinical diagnosis of suppression (see Chapter 6).

The following classification of suppression may be useful for the clinician:

- *Central versus peripheral.*
  - *Central suppression* is the mechanism that keeps the foveal image of the deviating eye from reaching consciousness, thereby preventing visual confusion.
  - *Peripheral suppression* eliminates diplopia by preventing awareness of the image that falls on the peripheral retina in the deviating eye, which corresponds to the image falling on the fovea of the fixating eye. When strabismus develops after visual maturation/in adults, peripheral suppression does not develop, and the patient is thus unable to eliminate the peripheral second image without closing or occluding the deviating eye.
- *Nonalternating versus alternating.*
  - *Nonalternating:* Suppression always causes the image from the dominant eye to be predominant over the image from the deviating eye; this may lead to amblyopia.
  - *Alternating:* Suppression switches between the 2 eyes; amblyopia is less likely.
- *Facultative versus constant.*
  - *Facultative:* Present only when the eyes are deviated; absent in all other states. Patients with intermittent exotropia, for instance, often experience suppression when the eyes are divergent but may experience high-grade stereopsis when the eyes are straight.
  - *Constant:* Always present, whether the eyes are deviated or aligned. The suppression scotoma in the deviating eye may be either *relative* (permitting some visual sensation) or *absolute* (permitting no perception of light).

Management

Therapy for suppression often includes the following:

- proper refractive correction
- amblyopia therapy using occlusion or pharmacologic treatment
- alignment of the visual axes, to permit simultaneous stimulation of corresponding retinal elements by the same object

Antisuppression orthoptic exercises may result in intractable diplopia and are not typically recommended.

Anomalous Retinal Correspondence

Anomalous retinal correspondence (ARC) is a cortical adaptation that restores some degree of binocular cooperation despite a (usually small) manifest strabismus. In ARC, an object projects to the fovea of the fixating eye and to a peripheral retinal element in the deviating eye without diplopia. Anomalous binocular vision is a functional state that is superior to total suppression. In the development of ARC, normal sensory development is replaced gradually and incompletely. The more long-standing the deviation, the greater the potential for ARC to become deeply rooted. The period during which ARC may develop probably extends through the first decade of life.

Paradoxical diplopia can occur when ARC persists after strabismus surgery. For example, when esotropic patients with straight or nearly straight ocular alignment after surgery report symptoms of a crossed diplopic localization of foveal or parafoveal stimuli, they are experiencing paradoxical diplopia (Fig 4-7). Paradoxical diplopia is typically a fleeting postoperative phenomenon, seldom lasting longer than a few days or weeks, but in rare cases it can persist much longer.

Testing

Testing for ARC is performed to determine how affected patients use their eyes in everyday life and to seek any vestiges of normal correspondence. As discussed earlier, ARC is a binocular sensory adaptation to abnormal ocular alignment. Because the depth of the sensory rearrangement can vary widely, an individual can demonstrate both NRC and ARC, depending on the testing method used. Tests that closely simulate everyday use of the eyes are more likely to elicit evidence of ARC. The more dissociative the test, the more likely it is to produce an NRC response, unless the ARC is deeply rooted.

Common tests for ARC (discussed at length in Chapter 6), in order of most dissociative to least dissociative, include:

- the Worth 4-dot test
- the red-glass test (dissociation increases with the density of the red filter)
- testing with an amblyoscope/synoptophore
- testing with Bagolini striated lenses

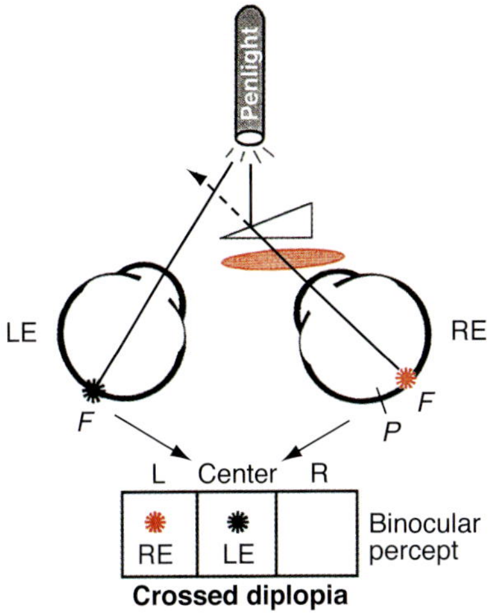

Figure 4-7 Paradoxical diplopia. Diagram of esotropia and ARC, with the esodeviation neutralized with a base-out prism over the right eye (RE). A red glass is placed over the right eye. The prism correction moves the retinal image of the penlight temporally, off the pseudofovea (P) to the true fovea (F). Because the pseudofovea is the center of orientation, the image is perceived to fall on the temporal retina and is projected to the opposite field, thus resulting in crossed diplopia. LE = left eye. *(Modified with permission from Wright KW, Spiegel PH.* Pediatric Ophthalmology and Strabismus: The Requisites in Ophthalmology. *Mosby; 1999:219.)*

If an anomalous localization response occurs in the more dissociative tests, the depth of ARC is greater.

Because ARC is a binocular phenomenon, it is tested for and documented in both eyes simultaneously. It is not necessarily related to eccentric fixation (see Chapter 5), which is a monocular phenomenon found by testing 1 eye alone. Because some tests for ARC depend on separate stimulation of each fovea, the presence of eccentric fixation can significantly affect the test results (see also Chapter 6).

Monofixation Syndrome

The term *monofixation syndrome* is used to describe a particular presentation of a sensory state in strabismus. The defining characteristic of this syndrome is the presence of peripheral fusion with the absence of bifoveal fusion due to a central scotoma. The term *microtropia* was introduced separately to describe small-angle strabismus with a constellation of findings that largely overlap those of monofixation syndrome.

A patient with monofixation syndrome may have no manifest deviation but usually has a small (≤8 prism diopters [Δ]) heterotropia; the heterotropia is most commonly an esotropia but is sometimes an exotropia or hypertropia. Stereoacuity is present but reduced. Amblyopia is a common finding.

Monofixation syndrome is a favorable outcome of infantile strabismus surgery and is present in a substantial minority of patients with intermittent exotropia. It can also be a primary condition that causes unilaterally decreased vision when no obvious strabismus is present. Monofixation syndrome can result from anisometropia or macular lesions as well.

Diagnosis

To diagnose monofixation syndrome, the clinician must demonstrate the absence of bimacular fusion by documenting a macular scotoma in the nonfixating eye under binocular conditions and the presence of peripheral binocular vision (peripheral fusion).

Testing stereoacuity is an important part of the monofixation syndrome evaluation. Any amount of gross stereopsis confirms the presence of peripheral fusion. Most patients with monofixation syndrome demonstrate stereopsis of 200–3000 seconds of arc. However, because some patients with this syndrome have no demonstrable stereopsis, other tests for peripheral fusion, such as the Worth 4-dot test and testing with Bagolini lenses, must be used in conjunction with stereoacuity measurement. Fine stereopsis (greater than 67 seconds of arc) is present only in patients with bifoveal fixation.

Management

If associated amblyopia is clinically significant, occlusion therapy is indicated. Monofixation may decompensate to a larger heterotropia in adulthood, resulting in diplopia. Strabismus surgery may be required to restore fusion.

Ing MR, Roberts KM, Lin A, Chen JJ. The stability of the monofixation syndrome. *Am J Ophthalmol.* 2014;157(1):248–253.

CHAPTER 5

Amblyopia

Highlights

- Amblyopia, a failure of normal neural development of the immature visual system, is the most common cause of unilateral vision loss in children.
- Amblyopia treatment is most effective during the critical childhood period; therefore, pediatric screening is essential.
- Neonatal visually significant anterior segment opacities result in irreversible amblyopia if not treated and managed in a timely manner.

Introduction

Amblyopia is a unilateral or, less commonly, bilateral reduction of best-corrected visual acuity (also referred to as *corrected distance visual acuity*) that cannot be attributed directly to the effect of any structural abnormality of the eye or visual pathways. Amblyopia signifies a failure of normal neural development in the immature visual system (see Chapter 4) and is caused by abnormal visual experience early in life resulting from 1 or a combination of the following:

- strabismus
- refractive error: anisometropia or bilateral high refractive error (isoametropia)
- visual deprivation in 1 or both eyes

Epidemiology

Amblyopia is responsible for more cases of childhood-onset unilateral decreased vision than all other causes combined, with a prevalence of 2%–4% in North America. It is also the most common cause of unilateral vision impairment in adults younger than 60 years. Amblyopia prevalence is increased in individuals born prematurely, in those with developmental delay, or in those who have a family history of amblyopia or strabismus.

Because amblyopia treatment is most effective during the critical childhood period, pediatric vision screening is essential. The timing of the critical period depends upon the visual function being assessed. For assessment of visual acuity, 3 periods of development can be considered:

1. when acuity develops (birth to 3–5 years of age)
2. when visual deprivation *can cause* amblyopia (a few months to 7–8 years of age)

3. when amblyopia treatment *may* still be effective (up to 9 years of age practically, but has been documented in patients at older ages)

Daw NW. Critical periods and amblyopia. *Arch Ophthalmol.* 1998;116(4):502–505.

Pathophysiology

In early postnatal development, there are critical periods of cortical development during which neural circuits display a heightened sensitivity to environmental stimuli and are dependent on natural sensory experience for proper formation (see also Chapter 4). During these periods, the developing visual system is vulnerable to abnormal input due to visual deprivation, strabismus, or significant blur resulting from anisometropia or isoametropia. Conversely, the visual system's plasticity early in development allows the greatest opportunity for amblyopia reversal. The window of opportunity for treatment depends on the type of amblyopia (see the section Classification). For example, the critical period for reversal of visual deprivation amblyopia (eg, due to infantile cataracts) is shorter than that for reversal of infantile strabismic or anisometropic amblyopia.

Amblyopic vision deficits result primarily from visual cortical changes. With abnormal visual experience early in life, cells of the primary visual cortex can lose their ability to respond to stimulation of 1 or both eyes, and the cells that remain responsive show significant functional deficiencies including abnormally large receptive fields. Visual cortex deficiencies may account for the crowding phenomenon, in which optotypes are easier to recognize when isolated than when surrounded by similar forms (see Chapter 1). Abnormalities are also found in neurons within the lateral geniculate body, but the retina and optic nerve(s) in individuals with amblyopia are essentially normal. Amblyopia is primarily a defect of central vision; the peripheral visual field is usually normal.

Functional Considerations

In addition to the difficulties and social stigma associated with having to wear a patch, amblyopic children may manifest abnormalities in visual processing, movement integration, perception and processing of shapes, Vernier acuity, and reading speeds (see Chapter 28).

Classification

Strabismic Amblyopia

Strabismic amblyopia results from competitive or inhibitory interaction between neurons carrying nonfusible input from the 2 eyes. Constant, nonalternating heterotropias are the deviations most likely to cause amblyopia. The visual cortex becomes dominated by input from the fixating eye, with reduced responsiveness to input from the nonfixating eye. In young children with strabismus, suppression develops rapidly. This visual adaptation serves to avoid diplopia and visual confusion (see Chapter 4), but in a child who does not alternate fixation, constant suppression of input from the same eye can lead to amblyopia.

Several features distinguish strabismic amblyopia from other types of amblyopia and other causes of decreased vision. *Grating acuity* (see Chapter 1), the ability to resolve uniformly spaced stripes, is often reduced less than recognition acuity. Measurements obtained with Teller Acuity Cards II (Precision Vision) and the LEA Grating Acuity Test (LEA Test Intl/Good-Lite Company) may overestimate recognition visual acuity. Visual acuity measured through a neutral density filter declines less sharply for patients with strabismic amblyopia than for those with ocular disease *(neutral density filter effect).*

Eccentric fixation is the consistent use of a nonfoveal region of the retina during monocular viewing. Minor degrees of eccentric fixation, detectable only with special tests such as visuoscopy, are present in many patients with strabismic amblyopia. Clinically evident eccentric fixation results in a decentered position of the corneal light reflex when the amblyopic eye is fixating monocularly and implies visual acuity of 20/200 or worse, as well as a poorer prognosis. It should not be confused with an abnormal angle kappa (see Chapter 6).

Refractive Amblyopia

Refractive amblyopia results from consistent retinal defocus in 1 or both eyes. Anisometropia causes unilateral amblyopia; isoametropia may cause bilateral amblyopia.

Anisometropic amblyopia

In anisometropic amblyopia, dissimilar refractive errors in the 2 eyes cause 1 retinal image to be chronically defocused. Considered more prevalent than strabismic amblyopia in some US studies, this condition is thought to result partly from the direct effect of image blur and partly from interocular competition or inhibition similar (but not identical) to that responsible for strabismic amblyopia. Levels of anisometropia that commonly lead to amblyopia are greater than 1.50 diopters (D) of anisohyperopia, 2.00 D of anisoastigmatism, and 3.00 D of anisomyopia. Higher levels are associated with greater risk. The eyes of a child with anisometropic amblyopia usually appear normal to the family and primary care physician, which may delay detection and treatment.

McKean-Cowdin R, Cotter SA, Tarczy-Hornoch K, et al; Multi-Ethnic Pediatric Eye Disease Study Group. Prevalence of amblyopia or strabismus in Asian and non-Hispanic White preschool children: Multi-Ethnic Pediatric Eye Disease Study. *Ophthalmology.* 2013;120(10):2117–2124.

Multi-Ethnic Pediatric Eye Disease Study Group. Prevalence of amblyopia and strabismus in African American and Hispanic children ages 6 to 72 months: the Multi-Ethnic Pediatric Eye Disease study. *Ophthalmology.* 2008;115(7):1229–1236.

Isoametropic amblyopia

Isoametropic amblyopia (bilateral ametropic amblyopia) is bilaterally decreased visual acuity resulting from chronically defocused retinal images, which are due to similarly large uncorrected refractive errors in both eyes. Hyperopia exceeding 4.00–5.00 D (at age >1 year) and myopia exceeding 5.00–6.00 D (any age) are risk factors. Bilateral high astigmatism may cause loss of resolving ability specific to the chronically blurred meridians *(meridional amblyopia).* Most ophthalmologists recommend correction for eyes with more than 2.00–3.00 D of astigmatism (Table 5-1).

Table 5-1 Guidelines for Refractive Corrections in Infants and Young Children

	Refractive Errors (Diopters)			
Condition	**Age <1 year**	**Age 1 to <2 years**	**Age 2 to <3 years**	**Age 3 to <4 years**
Isoametropia (similar refractive error in both eyes)				
Myopia	5.00 or more	4.00 or more	3.00 or more	2.50 or more
Hyperopia (no manifest deviation)	6.00 or more	5.00 or more	4.50 or more	3.50 or more
Hyperopia with esotropia	2.00 or more	2.00 or more	1.50 or more	1.50 or more
Astigmatism	3.00 or more	2.50 or more	2.00 or more	1.50 or more
Anisometropia (without strabismus)[a]				
Myopia	4.00 or more	3.00 or more	3.00 or more	2.50 or more
Hyperopia	2.50 or more	2.00 or more	1.50 or more	1.50 or more
Astigmatism	2.50 or more	2.00 or more	2.00 or more	1.50 or more

Note: These values were generated by consensus and are based solely on professional experience and clinical impressions, because there are no scientifically rigorous published data for guidance. These guidelines do not consider other aspects of the clinical examination, symptoms, and patient history. The exact values are unknown and may differ among age groups; they are presented as general guidelines that should be tailored to the individual child. Specific guidelines for older children are not provided because refractive correction is determined by the severity of the refractive error, visual acuity, and visual symptoms.

[a] The values represent the minimum difference in the magnitude of refractive error between eyes that would prompt refractive correction. Threshold for correction of anisometropia should be lower if the child has strabismus.

Courtesy of American Academy of Ophthalmology Pediatric Ophthalmology/Strabismus Panel, Hoskins Center for Quality Eye Care. Preferred Practice Pattern Guidelines. *Pediatric Eye Evaluations.* American Academy of Ophthalmology; 2017. www.aao.org/ppp

Visual Deprivation Amblyopia

The least common form of amblyopia, but the most severe and difficult to treat, is visual deprivation amblyopia (also known as *stimulus deprivation amblyopia, deprivation amblyopia, visual stimulus deprivation amblyopia*, and *form-vision deprivation amblyopia*), which is due to an eye abnormality that obstructs the visual axis or otherwise interferes with central vision. The most common cause is congenital or early-acquired cataract; other causes include severe blepharoptosis, periocular lesions obstructing the visual axis, corneal opacities, and vitreous hemorrhage. Visual deprivation amblyopia develops faster, and is deeper, than strabismic or anisometropic amblyopia. Unilateral visual deprivation tends to cause vision deficits in the affected eye that are more severe than the bilateral amblyopic deficits produced by bilateral deprivation of the same degree because interocular competition adds to the direct impact of image degradation (see Chapter 4). Even in bilateral cases, visual acuity can be 20/200 or worse if not treated early.

CLINICAL PEARL

In individuals with a dense neonatal anterior segment opacity (eg, congenital cataract), irreversible amblyopia can develop quickly if not treated early; however, surgery can be safely deferred until by approximately 6 weeks of age if unilateral and 10 weeks of age if bilateral.

In children younger than 6 years, dense cataracts occupying the central 3 mm or more of the lens can cause severe visual deprivation amblyopia. Similar lens opacities acquired after age 6 years are generally less harmful. Small anterior polar cataracts, around which retinoscopy can be readily performed, and lamellar cataracts, through which a reasonably good view of the fundus can be obtained, may cause mild to moderate amblyopia or have no effect on visual development. Unilateral anterior polar cataracts, however, are associated with anisometropia and subtle optical distortion of the surrounding clear portion of the lens, which may cause anisometropic and/or mild visual deprivation amblyopia.

Detection and Screening

With timely detection and intervention, amblyopia is preventable or reversible. Screening techniques include direct visual acuity measurement and testing for risk factors. Corneal light reflex tests and cover testing detect strabismus; the Brückner test (see Chapter 1) can reveal media opacities, strabismus, anisometropia, and isoametropia.

Instrument-based vision screening is becoming adopted more broadly in screening programs. The sensitivity and specificity of the screening instrument depend on the referral criteria, which are preset by the manufacturer and vary by age.

American Academy of Ophthalmology Pediatric Ophthalmology/Strabismus Panel, Hoskins Center for Quality Eye Care. Preferred Practice Pattern Guidelines. *Pediatric Eye Evaluations.* American Academy of Ophthalmology; 2017. www.aao.org/ppp

Donahue SP, Arthur B, Neely DE, Arnold RW, Silbert D, Ruben JB, POS Vision Screening Committee. Guidelines for automated preschool vision screening: a 10-year, evidence-based update. *J AAPOS.* 2013;17(1):4–8.

Donahue SP, Baker CN; Committee on Practice and Ambulatory Medicine, Section on Ophthalmology, American Academy of Pediatrics; American Association of Certified Orthoptists; American Association for Pediatric Ophthalmology and Strabismus; American Academy of Ophthalmology. Procedures for the evaluation of the visual system by pediatricians [epub ahead of print December 7, 2015]. *Pediatrics.* 2016;137(1): e20153597.

Evaluation

Amblyopia is diagnosed when a patient has a known risk factor and also decreased best-corrected visual acuity that cannot be explained by other diseases of the eye or visual pathways. Vision characteristics alone cannot differentiate amblyopia from other forms of vision loss. The crowding phenomenon, for example, is typical of amblyopia but not pathognomonic or uniformly demonstrable. Afferent pupillary defects should raise the suspicion for a possible optic nerve or retinal pathology, because they are not typical in amblyopia alone. Amblyopia sometimes coexists with vision loss that is directly caused by an uncorrectable structural abnormality of the eye such as optic nerve hypoplasia or coloboma. If amblyopia is suspected in such a case, it is appropriate to undertake a therapeutic trial of amblyopia treatment. Improvement in vision confirms that amblyopia was indeed present.

Multiple assessments of visual acuity are sometimes required to determine the presence and severity of amblyopia. (Assessment of visual acuity is discussed in Chapter 1.)

In some cases, the clinician may assume that amblyopia is present and initiate treatment before a quantitative evaluation of vision difference can be demonstrated. For example, if a clinician does not have access to a grating acuity test such as Teller Acuity Cards II, occlusion therapy may be started in a preverbal child in the presence of a high degree of anisometropia or shortly after surgery for a unilateral cataract.

When determining the severity of amblyopia in a young patient, the clinician should remember that both false-positive and false-negative errors may occur with fixation preference testing; a strabismic child may show a strong fixation preference despite having equal visual acuity, whereas an anisometropic child may alternate fixation despite having significant amblyopia. In addition, a young child's brief attention span frequently results in grating or recognition acuity measurements that fall short of the true limits of acuity; these measurements can mimic those of bilateral amblyopia or mask or falsely suggest a significant interocular difference. Finally, because test–retest variability can comprise up to a full line of letters in children, it is important for the clinician to evaluate trends when assessing response to treatment.

AlHarkan DH, Khan AO. False amblyopia prediction in strabismic patients by fixation preference testing correlates with contralateral ocular dominance. *J AAPOS.* 2014; 18(5):453–456.

Treatment

The Pediatric Eye Disease Investigator Group (PEDIG) has extensively studied amblyopia treatment; patching, atropine, and spectacle correction have been shown to be clinically effective and safe. Treatment involves the following steps:

1. Eliminate (if needed) any obstruction of the visual axis, such as a cataract.
2. Correct any significant refractive error.
3. Promote use of the amblyopic eye.

Cataract Removal

Cataracts capable of producing dense amblyopia require timely surgery. Removal of unilateral, visually significant congenital lens opacities within the first 6 weeks of life is necessary for optimal recovery of vision. In young children, significant cataracts with uncertain time of onset also deserve prompt and aggressive treatment if recent development is at least a possibility. For bilateral, dense congenital cataracts, surgery is recommended within the first 10 weeks of life. However, small partial cataracts may sometimes be managed nonsurgically; pharmacologic pupillary dilation may permit good vision despite a central opacity (see also the section Visual Deprivation Amblyopia, earlier in the chapter). Childhood cataract is discussed further in Chapter 22.

Refractive Correction

Refractive correction (see Table 5-1) plays a key role in the treatment of all types of amblyopia, not just refractive amblyopia. Anisometropic, isoametropic, and even strabismic amblyopia may improve or resolve with refractive correction alone. Many ophthalmologists thus initiate amblyopia treatment with refractive correction, adding occlusion or pharmacologic or optical treatment later if necessary (see the following sections). Refractive correction for aphakia following cataract surgery in childhood is initiated promptly to avoid prolonging visual deprivation. Unilateral aphakic spectacles can be used when contact lens correction is not possible. For patients with high refractive error that is amblyogenic who will not or cannot wear glasses or contact lenses, refractive surgery may be an alternative in select cases.

In general, refractive correction in amblyopia should be based on the cycloplegic refraction. It is important to consider the strabismic status of the patient (see Chapter 7). All significant anisometropia should be fully corrected. Also see BCSC Section 3, *Clinical Optics and Vision Rehabilitation.*

Writing Committee for the Pediatric Eye Disease Investigator Group; Cotter SA, Foster NC, Holmes JM, et al. Optical treatment of strabismic and combined strabismic-anisometropic amblyopia. *Ophthalmology.* 2012;119(1):150–158.

Occlusion Therapy

Occlusion therapy (patching) is commonly used to treat unilateral amblyopia. The sound eye is covered, obligating the child to use the amblyopic eye. Adhesive patches are usually employed, but spectacle-mounted occluders or opaque contact lenses are alternatives if skin irritation or inadequate adhesion is a problem. With spectacle-mounted occluders, close supervision is necessary to ensure that the patient does not peek around the occluder.

Full-time occlusion, defined as occlusion during all waking hours, can cause *reverse (occlusion) amblyopia* and strabismus (see the section Complications and Challenges of Therapy). If instituted, full-time occlusion should be monitored with a "rigid follow-up" of less than 1 week per year of age in children younger than 4 years.

> **CLINICAL PEARL**
>
> Most practitioners will not prescribe patching for more than half of a patient's waking hours to avoid the development of reverse amblyopia in young children.

For severe amblyopia, *part-time occlusion* of 6 hours per day achieves results similar to those obtained with prescribed full-time occlusion. The relative duration of patch-on and patch-off intervals should reflect the degree of amblyopia. For severe deficits (visual acuity of 20/125–20/400), 6 hours per day is preferred. For moderate deficits (visual acuity of 20/100 or better), 2 hours of daily patching may be effective. It is not necessary for the patient to engage in specific activities (eg, near work) while patched.

Follow-up timing depends on patient age and treatment intensity. Part-time treatment permits less frequent follow-up; reexamination 2–3 months after initiating treatment is typical. Subsequent visits can be at longer intervals, based on early response.

The desired endpoint of therapy for unilateral amblyopia is free alternation of fixation and/or linear recognition acuity that differs by no more than 1 line between the 2 eyes. The time required to complete treatment depends on amblyopia severity, treatment intensity, and patient adherence and age. More severe amblyopia and older children require more intensive or longer treatment. Occlusion during infancy may reverse substantial strabismic amblyopia in less than 1 month. In contrast, an older child who wears a patch only after school and on weekends may require several months to overcome a moderate deficit.

Adherence to occlusion therapy for amblyopia declines with increasing age. However, studies in older children and teenagers with strabismic or anisometropic amblyopia show that treatment can still be beneficial beyond the first decade of life. This is especially true in children who have not previously undergone treatment.

Pharmacologic or Optical Treatment

Alternatives to occlusion therapy involve pharmacologic and/or optical degradation of the better eye's vision such that it becomes temporarily inferior to the amblyopic eye's vision, promoting use of the amblyopic eye. For patients with orthotropia or small-angle strabismus, an advantage of these treatments over occlusion therapy is that they allow a degree of binocularity, which is particularly beneficial in children with latent nystagmus.

Pharmacologic treatment of moderate amblyopia (visual acuity of 20/100 or better) is as effective as patching and may also be successful in patients with more severe amblyopia (visual acuity of 20/125–20/400), particularly younger children. A cycloplegic agent (usually atropine sulfate solution, 1%) is administered to the better-seeing eye so that it is unable to accommodate. Vision in the better eye is thus blurred at near distance viewing and, if hyperopia is undercorrected, also for distance viewing. Atropine may be administered daily, but weekend administration is as effective for milder amblyopia. Regular follow-up is important to monitor for reverse amblyopia (see the section Complications and Challenges of Therapy).

Pharmacologic treatment is difficult for a child to thwart. It may not work well for patients with myopia, however, because clear near vision persists in the dominant eye despite cycloplegia if the distance correction is not worn. In some children, attempts to accommodate with the dominant eye in the face of cycloplegia can increase accommodative convergence, worsening any underlying esotropia during treatment. Parents and caregivers should be counseled regarding the adverse effects of atropine, including light sensitivity as well as potential systemic toxicity, the symptoms of which include fever, tachycardia, delirium, and dry mouth and skin (see Chapter 1).

Optical treatment involves the prescription of excessive plus lenses (fogging) or diffusing filters for the sound eye. This form of treatment avoids potential pharmacologic adverse effects and may be able to induce greater blur than cycloplegic agents. If the child wears glasses, a translucent filter, such as Scotch Magic Tape (3M) or a Bangerter occlusion foil (Ryser Optik AG), can be applied to the spectacle lens. Optical treatment may be more acceptable than occlusion therapy to many children and their parents, but patients must be closely monitored to ensure proper use (ie, no peeking) of spectacle-borne devices.

Binocular Treatment

Binocular amblyopia treatments showed early promise in amblyopic children with orthotropia or small-angle strabismus, but higher-level evidence has not yet been documented. In these treatments, the child engages in active or passive visual tasks that require simultaneous perception but require the amblyopic eye to perform the majority of the visual task. The treatments are performed on an electronic device under dichoptic viewing conditions, that is, high contrast to the amblyopic eye and low contrast to the fellow eye. The relative salience of amblyopic and fellow eye input can be adjusted over the course of treatment.

American Academy of Ophthalmology. *Binocular Treatment of Amblyopia.* Ophthalmic Technology Assessment. American Academy of Ophthalmology; 2019.

Complications and Challenges of Therapy

Reverse amblyopia and new strabismus

Both occlusion therapy and pharmacologic treatment carry a risk of overtreatment, which can result in reverse amblyopia in the sound eye. Strabismus can also develop or worsen with amblyopia treatment (although strabismus can also improve with amblyopia treatment).

As mentioned, full-time occlusion carries the greatest risk of reverse amblyopia and thus requires close monitoring. Consequently, most ophthalmologists do not use full-time occlusion in younger children. Children with binocular fusion, especially, may benefit from time spent viewing binocularly. The family of a strabismic child should be instructed to watch for a reversal of fixation preference with full-time occlusion and to report its occurrence promptly. Usually, iatrogenic reverse amblyopia can be treated successfully by judicious patching of the formerly worse-seeing, now better-seeing, eye. Sometimes, simply stopping treatment leads to equalization of vision.

During pharmacologic treatment, the risk of reverse amblyopia is greatest if daily treatment is coupled with undercorrection of hyperopic refractive error in the sound eye undergoing cycloplegia (see the section Refractive Correction, earlier in the chapter).

Poor adherence

Lack of adherence to the therapeutic regimen is a common problem that can prolong the treatment period or lead to outright failure. If difficulties derive from a particular treatment method, the clinician should seek a suitable alternative. Adhesive and cloth patches may not be covered by medical insurance in the United States; if treatment cost is a burden, pharmacologic treatment may facilitate adherence. If the skin becomes irritated from patch adhesives, switching to a different brand or applying skin lotion after patching may help. A barrier application of tincture of benzoin or milk of magnesia can protect the skin from contact with adhesive and help when patches do not adhere because of perspiration; however, this can make patch removal more traumatic.

Families who seem to lack sufficient motivation should be counseled concerning the importance of the therapy and the need for consistency in carrying it out. They can be reassured that once an appropriate routine is established, the daily effort required is likely to diminish, especially if the amblyopia improves. For an older child, it can also be helpful for the physician to explain and emphasize the importance of treatment adherence directly to the child in an age-appropriate manner. Further, it is important for the family to understand that amblyopia treatment is performed primarily to improve vision rather than ocular alignment and, conversely, that improving ocular alignment (with surgery or glasses) does not obviate the need for treatment of associated amblyopia.

Adherence to a patching regimen in older children can be improved by creating goals and offering rewards or by linking patching to play activities (eg, decorating the patch, patching while the child plays a video game, or applying patches to decorate a reward poster after use). For infants and toddlers, adherence to a patching regimen depends greatly on parental engagement and commitment. Arm splints and mittens are sometimes used as a last resort.

Unresponsiveness

Sometimes even conscientious application of an appropriate therapeutic program fails to improve vision at all or beyond a certain level. Complete or partial unresponsiveness to treatment occasionally affects younger children but more often occurs in patients older than 5 years. When there is a significant deviation from the expected treatment response despite good adherence, reexamination may reveal subtle optic nerve or retinal anomalies. Optical coherence tomography may be considered if an occult optic nerve or retinal pathology is suspected.

In a prognostically unfavorable situation, decisions about treatment should take into account the patient's and parents' wishes, as well as the effect of patching on the child's psychological development. Amblyopia is not always fully correctable, even in younger children. Primary therapy may reasonably be terminated if there is a lack of demonstrable progress over 3–6 months despite good treatment adherence. Progress or lack thereof may be harder to quantify in preverbal children, however, so longer treatment is appropriate in these patients. If a child does not respond to a treatment, a different modality could be added or used instead.

Recurrence

When amblyopia treatment is discontinued after complete or partial improvement of vision, up to one-third of patients show some degree of recurrence. Reducing the occlusion regimen (to 1–2 hours per day) or the frequency of pharmacologic treatment for a few months before cessation is associated with a decreased incidence of recurrence, although no randomized trial has compared tapered and nontapered cessation. If recurrence occurs, vision can usually be improved again with resumption of therapy. In a study of children who were between 7 and 12 years of age when treated for amblyopia, the vision improvements that occurred seemed to be mostly sustained after cessation of treatment other than spectacles. Younger patients may require periodic monitoring until vision is stable with spectacle treatment alone (eg, until age 8–10 years). With stable vision, 12-month examination intervals are acceptable.

Hertle RW, Scheiman MM, Beck RW, et al; Pediatric Eye Disease Investigator Group. Stability of visual acuity improvement following discontinuation of amblyopia treatment in children aged 7 to 12 years. *Arch Ophthalmol.* 2007;125(5):655–659.

CHAPTER 6

Diagnostic Evaluation of Strabismus and Torticollis

This chapter includes related videos. Go to www.aao.org/bcscvideo_section06 or scan the QR codes in the text to access this content.

This chapter includes a related activity. Go to www.aao.org/bcscactivity_section06 or scan the QR code in the text to access this content.

Highlights

- Surgeons often plan strabismus surgery based on prism and alternate cover test measurements, because this test captures both the tropic and phoric parts of the misalignment.
- Uncrossed and crossed diplopia can be associated with acquired esotropia and exotropia, respectively (the "x" in eXotropia helps to remind the clinician of crossed (X) diplopia).
- In the 3-step test, a right-left-right pattern (right hypertropia worse in left gaze and right tilt) is consistent with a right superior oblique palsy, and a left-right-left pattern (left hypertropia worse in right gaze and left tilt) is consistent with a left superior oblique palsy.

Obtaining a History in Cases of Strabismus or Torticollis

Both strabismus and torticollis are common presenting conditions in pediatric ophthalmology. Torticollis is an abnormal head position (AHP), such as a head turn or tilt. Torticollis is a common presenting sign of strabismus but can be caused by a wide variety of other ocular and nonocular conditions. There is broad overlap in the diagnostic assessment of strabismus and torticollis.

Key questions for the clinician to ask when obtaining a strabismus or torticollis history include the following:

- At what age did the deviation or AHP appear? (Reviewing old photographs may be helpful.)
- Did onset coincide with trauma or illness?
- Is the deviation or AHP constant or intermittent?

- Is it present for distance or near vision or both?
- Is it present only when the patient is inattentive or fatigued?
- Is it associated with double vision or eyestrain?
- If a deviation is noted, is it present in all positions of gaze?
- If a deviation is noted, is it unilateral or alternating?
- Does the patient close 1 eye?
- Is there a history of other ocular disease or ocular surgery?

It is important to review any previous treatment, such as amblyopia therapy, spectacle correction, and eye muscle surgery. The initial assessment also includes observation of the patient's habitual head position, head movement, and attentiveness. See Chapter 1 for a general discussion of examination of children.

In adults, reports of diplopia warrant taking additional history to determine whether the double vision has a monocular origin. Monocular diplopia can arise from corneal irregularities, cataract, uncorrected refractive error, and retinal distortion. Binocular and monocular diplopia can coexist.

Key additional questions for the clinician to ask when taking a history from a person who may have monocular diplopia include:

- Is double vision present when viewing with only 1 eye?
- Does 1 or both of the images appear to be distorted?
- Does the double vision resolve briefly with blinking?

Further information regarding differentiation of binocular and monocular diplopia can be found in BCSC Section 5, *Neuro-Ophthalmology.* Information regarding the contribution of retinal problems to strabismus can be found in Chapter 11.

Records RE. Monocular diplopia. *Surv Ophthalmol.* 1980;24(5):303–306.

Assessment of Ocular Alignment

Diagnostic Positions of Gaze

The *diagnostic positions of gaze* are a core set of 9 different gaze positions used in the comprehensive assessment of ocular alignment. They consist of

- *primary position:* The eyes fixate straight ahead on an object at infinity, which, for practical purposes, is considered to be 6 m, or 20 ft. For this position, the head should be straight.
- *6 cardinal positions:* Two muscles (1 in each eye) are the prime movers of their respective eyes into each of these positions of gaze (see Chapter 3).
- *straight up and straight down:* These positions do not isolate any single muscle, because the actions of both oblique and vertical rectus muscles affect elevation and depression from primary position (see Chapter 3).

For patients with vertical strabismus, the diagnostic positions of gaze also include forced head tilt toward the right shoulder and the left shoulder (see the section The 3-Step

Test, later in this chapter). Near fixation (usually 33 cm in the primary position ing position (depending on the patient's symptoms) complete the list of clinic tant test positions.

Finally, it can be useful to measure the alignment of a patient with torticollis while they are using their abnormal head posture even if this does not correspond to a diagnostic position of gaze. Comparison of alignment in the preferred gaze position to other gazes gives information regarding habitual control of any deviation and whether strabismus is the likely cause of the torticollis.

Tests for measuring ocular alignment can be grouped into 3 basic types: cover tests, corneal light reflex tests, and subjective tests.

Cover Tests

To undergo cover testing, the patient must

- have foveal fixation in each eye
- be able to pay attention and cooperate with the examiner
- be able to make eye movements

If the patient is unable to maintain constant fixation on an accommodative target, cover tests should not be used.

There are 3 main types of cover tests: cover-uncover, alternate cover, and simultaneous prism and cover. All can be performed at distance and near fixation.

The monocular *cover-uncover test* is the most important test for detecting manifest strabismus and for distinguishing a heterophoria (latent deviation) from a heterotropia (manifest deviation) (Video 6-1; Fig 6-1). As the patient views the target, 1 eye is covered for a few seconds and the opposite eye observed for any movement. The process is then repeated, covering the other eye. If either eye moves when the other is covered, a manifest misalignment or heterotropia (or tropia) exists.

VIDEO 6-1 The cover-uncover test.
Animation developed by Steven M. Archer, MD, and Kristina Tarczy-Hornoch, MD, DPhil.

A patient with a heterotropia starts with a deviated eye and, after testing, ends with the same eye or—in the case of an *alternating heterotropia*—the opposite eye deviated. In patients with intermittent heterotropia, the eyes may be straight before testing but become dissociated after occlusion.

Recovery from a heterophoria or phoria may be observed when an occluder is removed from a covered eye. If there is a shift of the newly uncovered eye to resume fixation following the period of occlusion, without a corresponding shift of the fellow eye, a phoria is present. If the patient has a heterophoria, the eyes will be straight before and after the cover-uncover test; the deviation appears during occlusion because of interruption of binocular vision.

The *alternate cover test* (Video 6-2; Fig 6-2A) detects both latent and manifest deviations (ie, both heterophorias and heterotropias). As the patient views the target, the

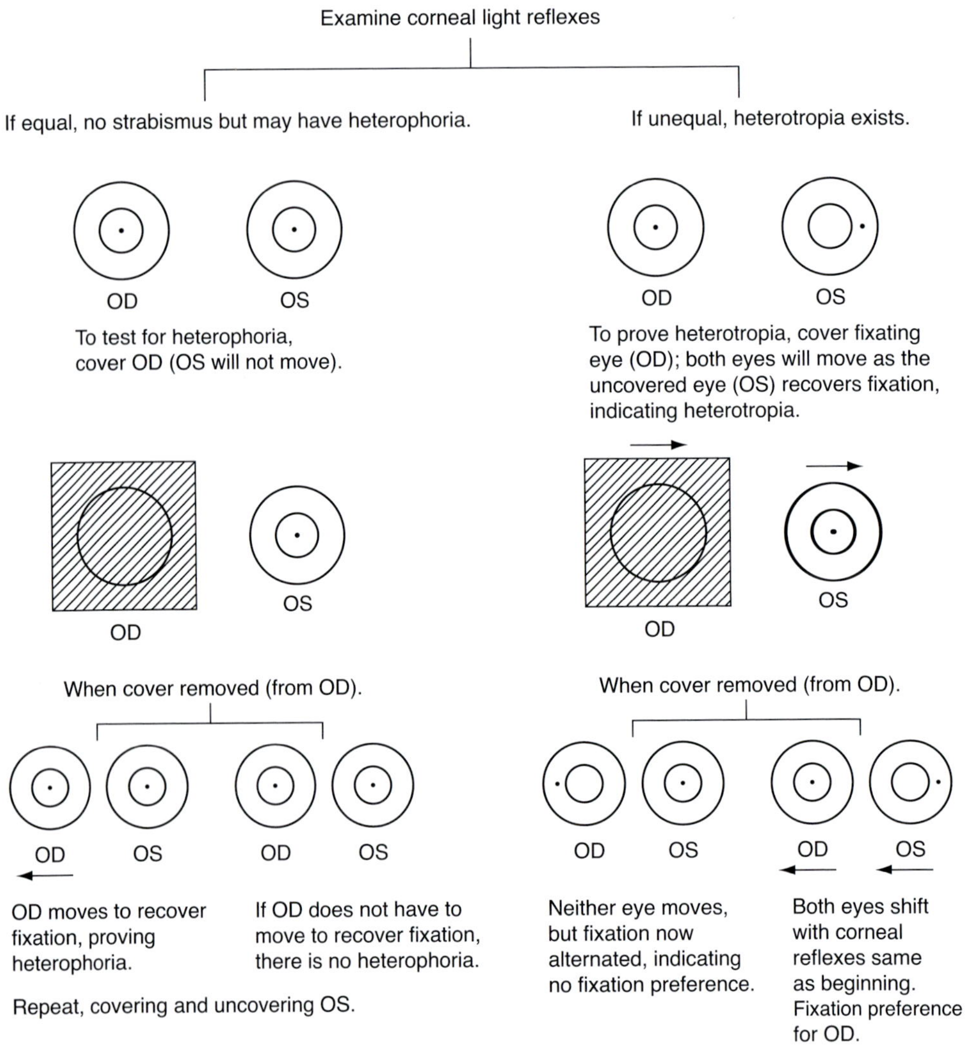

Figure 6-1 The monocular cover-uncover test. OD = oculus dexter; OS = oculus sinister.

examiner moves the occluder from 1 eye to the other, observing the direction of movement of each eye when it is uncovered. Because this test disrupts binocular fusion, dissociating the eyes, it does not distinguish between latent and manifest components.

VIDEO 6-2 The alternate cover test.
Animation developed by Steven M. Archer, MD, and Kristina Tarczy-Hornoch, MD, DPhil.

In the *prism and alternate cover test,* prisms of varying strengths are held over 1 eye or both eyes during alternate cover testing; the amount of prism that neutralizes the deviation, so that eye movement is no longer seen as the occluder is moved from 1 eye to the other, represents the magnitude of the deviation (Fig 6-2B; Video 6-3). It may be necessary

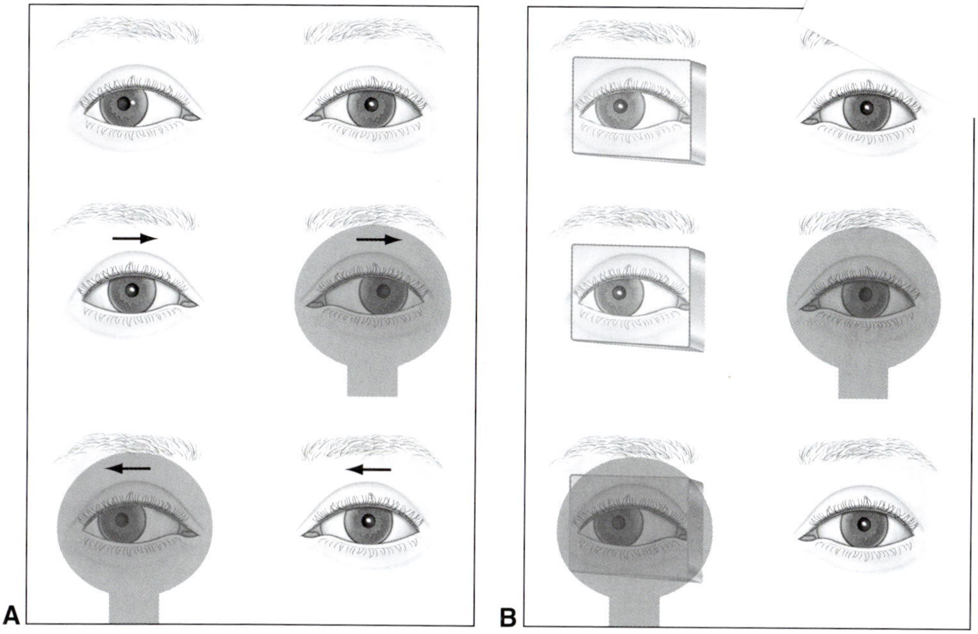

Figure 6-2 Alternate cover tests. **A,** The alternate cover test. *Top:* Exotropia, left eye fixating. *Middle and bottom:* Both eyes move each time the cover alternates from 1 eye to the other. **B,** The prism and alternate cover test. *Top:* The exotropia is neutralized with a prism of the correct power. *Middle and bottom:* The eyes do not move as the cover alternates from 1 eye to the other. *(Illustration developed by Steven M. Archer, MD; original illustration by Mark Miller.)*

to use both horizontal and vertical prisms. This test measures the total deviation (heterotropia plus heterophoria) and is often used as the strabismus surgery target angle.

VIDEO 6-3 The prism and alternate cover test.
Animation developed by Steven M. Archer, MD, and Kristina Tarczy-Hornoch, MD, DPhil.

Stacking 2 horizontal or 2 vertical prisms should be avoided as this can induce significant measurement error. Deviations larger than the largest-available single prism are best measured by placing 1 prism in front of each eye, although this is not perfectly additive either. A horizontal prism and a vertical prism may be stacked over the same eye, however.

Plastic prisms should always be held with the back surface (closest to the patient) in the patient's frontal plane. If the head is tilted, the prisms must be tilted accordingly. In patients with incomitant (paretic or restrictive) strabismus, the primary and secondary deviations are measured by holding the prism over the paretic or restricted eye and the sound eye, respectively.

The *simultaneous prism and cover test* (Video 6-4) measures the manifest deviation during binocular viewing (only the heterotropia). This test provides the best indication of the size of the deviation under real-life conditions. It is performed by placing a prism in front of the deviating eye and covering the fixating eye at the same time. The test is repeated using increasing prism powers until the deviated eye no longer shifts.

VIDEO 6-4 The simultaneous prism and cover test.
Animation developed by Steven M. Archer, MD, and Kristina Tarczy-Hornoch, MD, DPhil.

COVER TESTS IN MONOFIXATION SYNDROME

Under binocular conditions, patients with monofixation syndrome (see Chapter 4) often use peripheral fusion to exert some control over their deviation. Therefore, the heterotropia that is measured by the simultaneous prism and cover test is often smaller than the total deviation (heterotropia plus heterophoria) measured by the prism and alternate cover test.

CLINICAL PEARL

When the examiner needs both hands for prism and cover testing at near distances, a cooperative child can be asked to hold an accommodative near-fixation target, or a similar target in the form of a sticker can be placed on the examiner's nose.

See Activity 6-1 for an interactive simulator of the cover tests.

ACTIVITY 6-1 Strabismus simulator.
Courtesy of Faruk H. Örge, MD.

Thompson JT, Guyton DL. Ophthalmic prisms. Measurement errors and how to minimize them. *Ophthalmology.* 1983;90(3):204–210.

Corneal Light Reflex Tests

Corneal light reflex tests assess eye alignment using the location of the first Purkinje image, the image formed from reflection of a fixation light by the anterior corneal surface, which acts as a curved mirror. The Hirschberg and Krimsky tests are the main tests of this type. Though not as accurate as cover tests, they are useful for uncooperative patients and those with poor fixation, in whom cover testing is not possible.

The *Hirschberg test* is based on the correlation between the decentration of the corneal light reflection and the ocular deviation. The ratio is about 15 prism diopters (Δ) per millimeter of decentration but can vary between 12Δ and 27Δ. With an uncooperative child, it is not always possible to accurately measure the light reflex displacement, so gross estimates of the deviation are often used (although these are highly dependent on pupil size): 30Δ if the reflex is at the pupil margin, 60Δ if the reflex is in the middle of the iris, and 90Δ if the reflex is at the limbus (Fig 6-3).

The *Krimsky test* uses prisms to quantify the decentration of the corneal reflections from a handheld light. This is done by holding a prism over the deviating eye or the fixating eye *(modified Krimsky test)* and adjusting the prism power until the corneal reflection is positioned symmetrically in each eye to approximate the near deviation (Fig 6-4; Video 6-5).

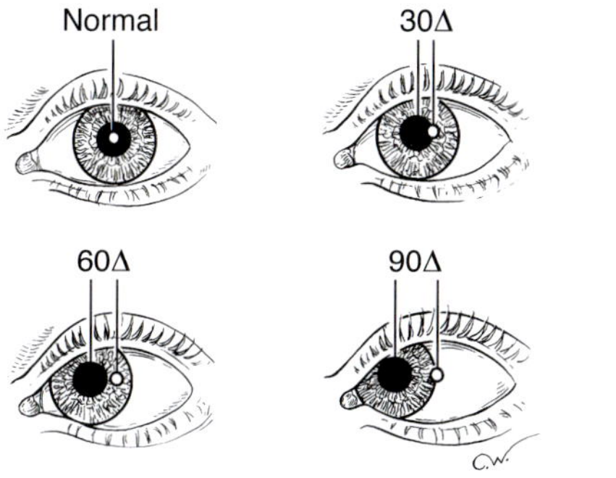

Figure 6-3 Hirschberg test, left eye. The extent to which the corneal light reflex is displaced from the center of an average-sized pupil provides an approximation of the angular size of the deviation (here, a left esotropia). Δ = prism diopter. *(Modified with permission from Simon JW, Calhoun JH.* A Child's Eyes: A Guide to Pediatric Primary Care. *Triad Publishing Company; 1997:72.)*

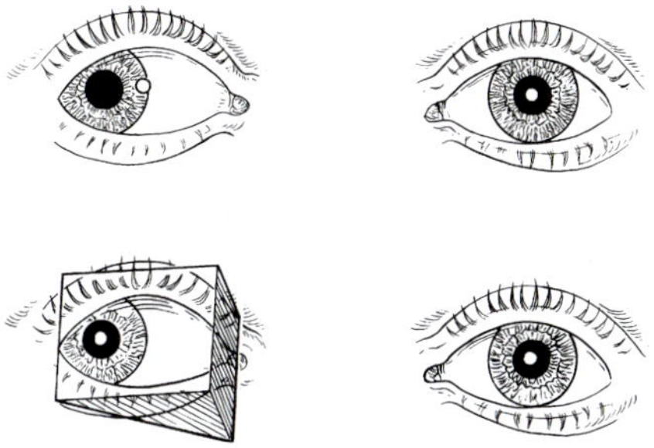

Figure 6-4 Krimsky test. The magnitude of the right exotropia is estimated by the power of the prism required to produce symmetric pupillary reflexes, as shown at bottom. *(Reprinted with permission from Simon JW, Calhoun JH.* A Child's Eyes: A Guide to Pediatric Primary Care. *Triad Publishing Company; 1997:72.)*

VIDEO 6-5 The Krimsky test.
Animation developed by Steven M. Archer, MD, and Kristina Tarczy-Hornoch, MD, DPhil.

CLINICAL PEARL

A translucent toy placed over a muscle light can function as an accommodative near target and simultaneously allow assessment of the corneal light reflexes.

The *angle kappa*, the angle between the visual axis and the anatomical pupillary axis of the eye (Fig 6-5), can affect corneal light reflex measurements. The fovea is usually slightly temporal to the pupillary axis, making the corneal light reflection slightly nasal to the center of the cornea. This is termed *positive angle kappa*. A large positive angle kappa (eg, from temporal dragging of the macula in cicatricial retinopathy of prematurity) can simulate exotropia. If the position of the fovea is nasal to the pupillary axis, the corneal light reflection will be temporal to the center of the cornea. This *negative angle kappa* simulates esotropia. The angle kappa does not affect any of the cover tests.

Subjective Tests of Ocular Alignment

The *Maddox rod test* assesses ocular alignment using the patient's perception of the relative position of the images seen by each eye. For the eye viewing through the Maddox rod, a series of parallel cylinders convert a point source of light into a line image perpendicular to the cylinders. Like alternate cover testing, the test is dissociating and precludes fusion; thus, this test cannot differentiate heterophorias and heterotropias. In addition, it cannot assess alignment in patients with anomalous retinal correspondence (ARC) or suppression.

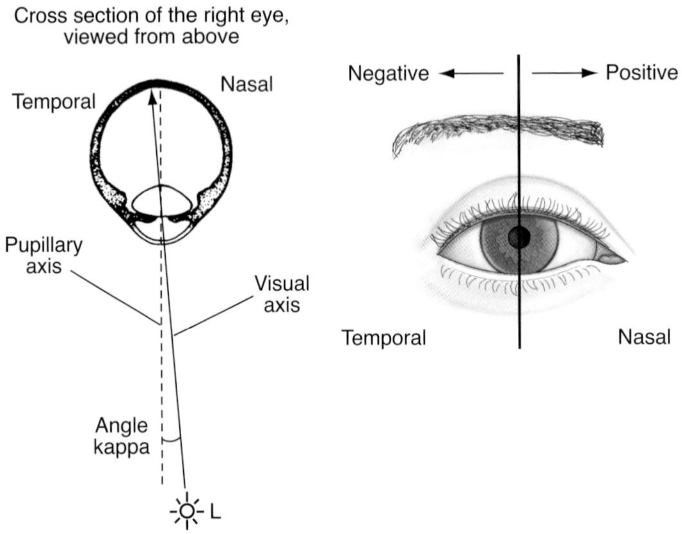

Figure 6-5 Angle kappa. A positive angle kappa (in which the corneal light reflex is nasally displaced; shown in cross section for the right eye), if large enough, simulates exotropia, whereas a negative angle (in which the light reflex is temporally displaced) simulates esotropia. L = examiner's light source, on which the patient fixates. *(Modified with permission from Parks MM.* Ocular Motility and Strabismus. *Harper & Row; 1975.)*

To test for horizontal deviations, the Maddox rod is held in front of 1 eye (eg, the right eye) so that the cylinders are horizontal. The patient, fixating on a point source of light, sees a vertical line with the right eye and the point source of light with the left eye. Assuming normal retinal correspondence (NRC), in orthophoria, the point superimposes on the line; in esodeviations, the light is seen to the left of the line; and in exodeviations, the light is to the right of the line. The deviation is measured by finding the prism power that superimposes the point source on the line. Note, however, that unlike in cover testing with an accommodative target, accommodative convergence is not controlled by this technique, so measurements of horizontal strabismus may be variable. Vertical deviations can be assessed by orienting the cylinders vertically (Fig 6-6).

The *double Maddox rod test* (Fig 6-7) is used to measure cyclodeviations. Two Maddox rods are placed in a trial frame or phoropter and aligned vertically so that the patient sees 2 horizontal lines. A small vertical prism may be introduced to help separate the lines. The rod axes are rotated until the patient sees parallel lines. The angle of rotation indicates the magnitude and direction (intorsion or extorsion) of cyclodeviation. Traditionally, a red Maddox rod was paired with a clear one, but this was thought to bias the patient's localization of the cyclodeviation toward the eye with the red rod. Using the same color bilaterally avoids this bias. In congenital conditions such as congenital superior oblique palsy, the patient may not subjectively appreciate torsion or indicate any torsion with the double Maddox rod test. In these cases, seeing fundus torsion on indirect ophthalmoscopy can aid diagnosis.

The *Lancaster red-green test* (and variations such as the Hess, Harms, and Lees screen tests) is useful for assessing ocular alignment in complicated incomitant strabismus in cooperative patients with NRC and no suppression (see Chapter 4), such as adults with

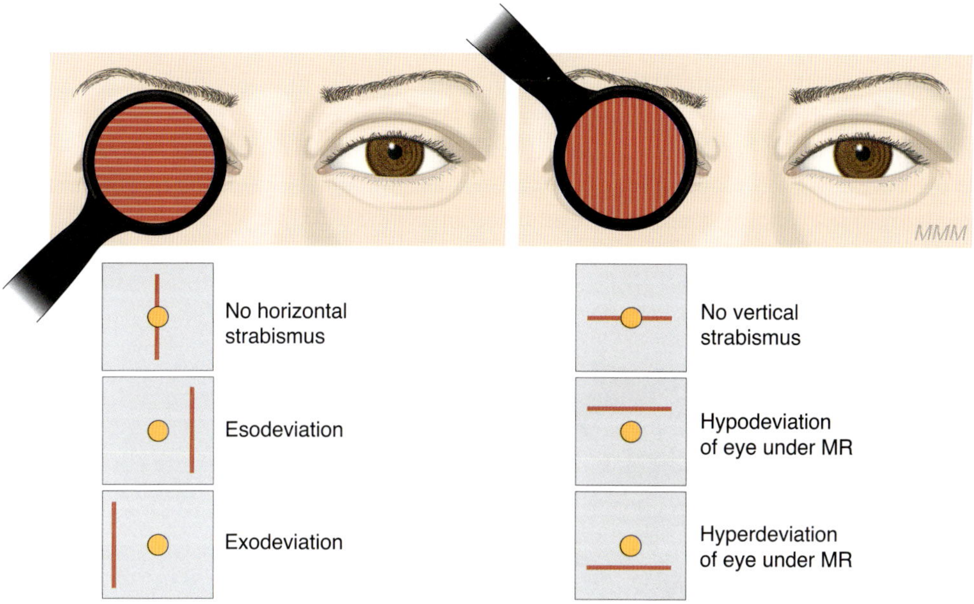

Figure 6-6 Maddox rod (MR) test for horizontal **(A)** and vertical **(B)** strabismus. If no horizontal or vertical strabismus is present, the patient sees the line and the light as superimposed. Patterns viewed by patients with horizontal and vertical heterotropias are also shown. *(Redrawn and modified with permission from Liu GT, Volpe NJ, Galetta SL. The neuro-ophthalmic examination. In:* Neuro-Ophthalmology. *3rd ed. Elsevier; 2019:29. With permission from Elsevier. Illustration by Mark Miller.)*

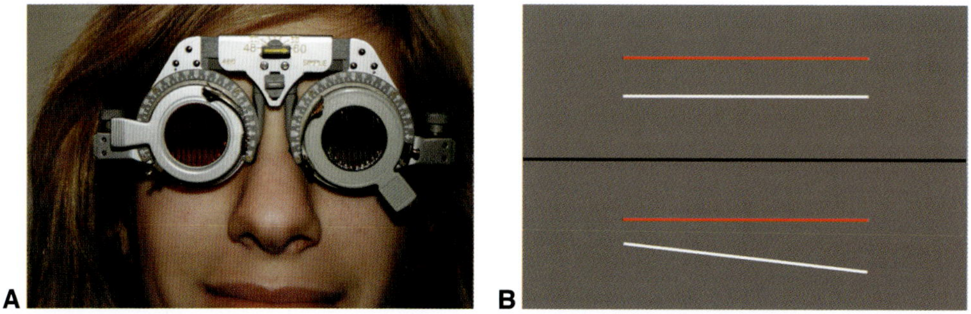

Figure 6-7 Double Maddox rod test. **A,** The cylinders are aligned vertically, so that a patient with normal binocular vision sees 2 superimposed horizontal lines. **B,** *Top:* View seen by a patient with a small left hypertropia and no torsion. *Bottom:* View seen by a patient with a small left hypertropia and extorsion. *(Part A courtesy of Scott Olitsky, MD; part B courtesy of Steven M. Archer, MD.)*

acquired strabismus. Reversible red-green goggles, red-slit and green-slit projectors, and a grid projected or marked on a screen or wall are used in the test. With the red filter in front of the patient's right eye, the examiner projects a red slit onto the grid; the patient places the green slit so that it appears superimposed on the red slit. The relative positions of the streaks are recorded. The test is repeated for the 9 diagnostic positions of gaze, and the goggles are reversed to record deviations with the fellow eye fixating.

The *major amblyoscope* or synoptophore (Fig 6-8A) can be used to measure ocular alignment both objectively and subjectively. It may be particularly useful in adults with strabismus, as it allows neutralization of torsional diplopia to assess fusional responses and can help detect ARC. Separate, dissimilar targets are presented to each eye simultaneously, and the amblyoscope is adjusted until the patient sees the images superimposed. If the patient has NRC, the horizontal, vertical, and torsional deviations can be read directly from the calibrated scale of the amblyoscope (Fig 6-8B).

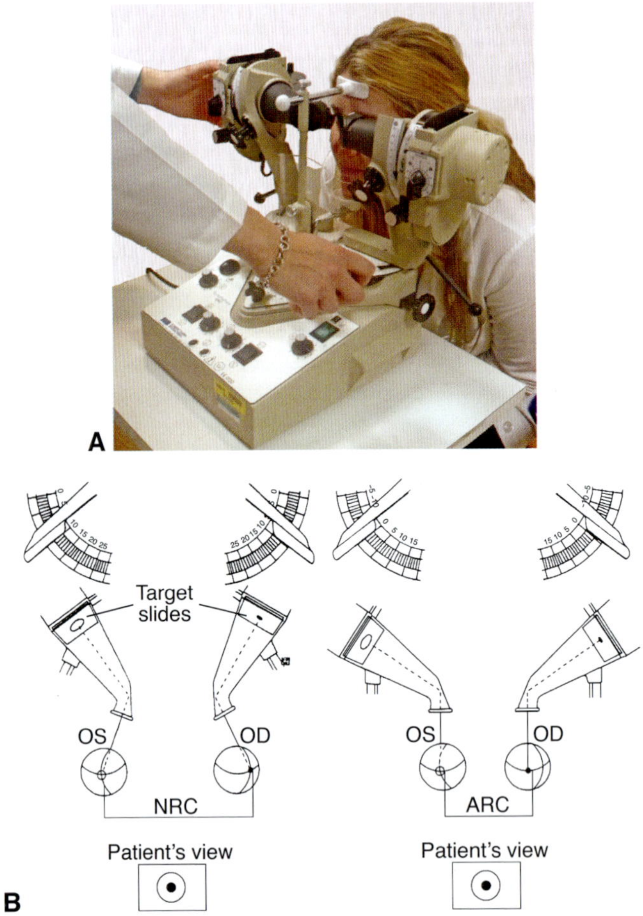

Figure 6-8 The major amblyoscope (synoptophore). **A,** Targets can be placed in each arm of the device to be presented separately to each eye. The arms can then be moved to compensate for ocular misalignment. **B,** Testing for retinal correspondence in a patient with 20Δ of esotropia. The examiner has moved the arms of the instrument so that the circle and dot are subjectively superimposed. The scales on each arm of the instrument correspond to the prism-diopter offset. NRC = normal retinal correspondence, with a fused percept when the angle of strabismus is fully compensated (ie, scale = 20), presenting targets to the fovea of each eye; ARC = anomalous retinal correspondence, with a fused percept in the absence of any compensation for the angle of strabismus (ie, scale = 0), with 1 eye viewing the target foveally and the other extrafoveally. *(Part A courtesy of Steven M. Archer, MD; part B modified with permission from von Noorden GK.* Atlas of Strabismus. *4th ed. Mosby; 1983.)*

Assessment of Eye Movements

Ocular Rotations

Generally, versions are tested first; both eyes' movements into the 9 diagnostic positions of gaze are assessed. Limitations of movement and asymmetric excursion of the 2 eyes (such as "overaction") are noted. To elicit vestibular-stimulated eye movements, the clinician may spin the child or rotate the child's head side to side (doll's head maneuver). If versions are not full, the examiner should test duction movements for each eye separately (Video 6-6). BCSC Section 5, *Neuro-Ophthalmology,* also discusses testing of the ocular motility system.

VIDEO 6-6 Versions and ductions.

Convergence

To determine the *near point of convergence,* the patient fixates on an object in the midsagittal plane, and the object, positioned initially at 40 cm, is moved toward the patient until 1 eye loses fixation and turns out. The distance from the object to the patient is then measured, giving the near point of convergence, which is normally 8–10 cm or less. The eye that maintains fixation is considered the dominant eye. This test does not distinguish between fusional convergence and accommodative convergence.

Accommodative convergence/accommodation ratio

The *accommodative convergence/accommodation (AC/A) ratio* is defined as the amount of convergence (in prism diopters) per unit change in accommodation (in diopters). The normal AC/A ratio is 3:1–5:1. There are 2 methods of clinical measurement (see also BCSC Section 3, *Clinical Optics and Vision Rehabilitation*):

1. The *gradient method* derives the AC/A ratio by stimulating a change in accommodation using lenses and dividing the resulting change in deviation (in prism diopters) by the change in lens power. An accommodative target must be used, and the working distance (typically 33 cm or 6 m) is held constant. Plus or minus lenses (eg, +1.00, +2.00, +3.00, −1.00, −2.00, −3.00) are used to vary the accommodative requirement (plus lenses at distance can be used only in patients with uncorrected hyperopia).
2. In the *heterophoria method,* the deviation in prism diopters with the fixation target viewed at 6 m is subtracted from the deviation at 33 cm, assigning positive values to esodeviations and negative values to exodeviations. The difference, divided by the change in accommodative demand (~3.00 D) and added to the interpupillary distance in cm, gives the AC/A ratio. As a rough clinical estimate, in accommodative esotropia, a near deviation exceeding distance deviation by 10Δ or more is considered a high AC/A ratio. Note, however, that in intermittent exotropia, the near deviation may be smaller than the distance deviation despite a normal AC/A ratio, because of *tenacious proximal fusion* (see Chapter 8).

Both methods measure the *stimulus AC/A ratio,* which may differ from the *response AC/A ratio.* The latter can be determined only by simultaneously measuring the refractive state of the eyes to quantify the change in accommodation actually occurring.

Fusional Vergence

Vergences are movements of the 2 eyes in opposite directions (see Chapter 3). Fusional vergences are motor responses that eliminate horizontal, vertical, and, to a limited degree, torsional image disparity.

- *Fusional convergence* eliminates bitemporal retinal image disparity and controls an exophoria.
- *Fusional divergence* eliminates binasal retinal image disparity and controls an esophoria.
- *Vertical fusional vergence* controls a hyperphoria or hypophoria.
- *Torsional fusional vergence* is cyclovergence that controls an incyclophoria or excyclophoria.

Fusional vergence can be measured using an amblyoscope/synoptophore, rotary prism, or prism bar; the prism power is gradually increased until diplopia occurs. Accommodation must be controlled during fusional vergence testing. Normal fusional vergence amplitudes are listed in Table 6-1. Fusional vergence can be altered by the following:

- *Compensatory mechanisms:* As a deviation evolves, a larger-than-normal fusional vergence develops. Large fusional vergences are common in compensated, long-standing vertical deviations and exodeviations.
- *Change in vision:* An improvement in vision may facilitate the fusional vergence mechanism and change a symptomatic intermittent deviation to an asymptomatic heterophoria.
- *State of awareness:* Fatigue, illness, or drug or alcohol ingestion may decrease the fusional vergence mechanism, converting a heterophoria to a heterotropia.
- *Orthoptics:* Orthoptic exercises may increase the magnitude of the fusional vergence mechanism (mainly fusional convergence). This treatment works best for near fusional convergence, particularly in convergence insufficiency.
- *Optical stimulation of fusional vergence:* In controlled accommodative esotropia, reducing the strength of the hyperopic or bifocal correction induces an esophoria that stimulates compensatory fusional divergence. In convergence insufficiency, base-out prism stimulates fusional convergence. Similarly, the power of prisms used to control diplopia may be decreased gradually to stimulate compensatory fusional vergence.

Table 6-1 Average Normal Fusional Vergence Amplitudes in Prism Diopters (Δ)

Testing Distance	Convergence	Divergence	Vertical
6 m	14	6	2.5
25 cm	38	16	2.6

Forced Duction, Active Force Generation, and Saccadic Velocity

Other methods to assess eye movements include the following:

- In the *forced duction test,* the eye is moved into various positions with the use of forceps to detect resistance to passive movement. This is usually done intraoperatively but can be done in the clinic with topical anesthesia in cooperative patients.
- In the *active force generation test,* the awake patient is asked to move a topically anesthetized eye while the examiner grasps it with forceps. If the muscle tested is paretic, the examiner feels less-than-normal tension.
- *Saccadic velocity* can be measured with instruments that track and record eye movement (eg, using magnetic search coils or video-based eye tracking). This measurement is useful for distinguishing paresis from restriction. For paretic muscles, saccadic velocity is low throughout the movement, whereas for restricted muscles, the velocity is initially normal but drops rapidly when the eye reaches the limit of its excursion. Clinical observation of saccadic velocity is qualitative: slow, "floating" saccades indicate muscle paresis.

See also BCSC Section 5, *Neuro-Ophthalmology.*

The 3-Step Test

There are 8 cyclovertical extraocular muscles (4 in each eye). The 2 *depressors* of each eye are the *inferior rectus (IR)* and *superior oblique (SO) muscles;* the 2 *elevators* of each eye are the *superior rectus (SR)* and *inferior oblique (IO) muscles.* Cyclovertical (especially superior oblique) muscle weakness often causes vertical deviations.

The *3-step test* (also called the *Parks-Bielschowsky 3-step test*) is an algorithm that helps identify a weak cyclovertical muscle. However, it is not always diagnostic, and results can be misleading, especially in patients with 1 or more of the following: more than 1 paretic muscle, previous strabismus surgery, skew deviation, restrictions, or dissociated vertical deviation (see Chapter 10). The 3-step test is performed as follows (Fig 6-9; see also Chapter 10, Fig 10-4):

- *Step 1:* Determine which eye is higher using the cover-uncover test (see Fig 6-1). Step 1 narrows the number of possible underacting muscles from 8 to 4. In the example shown in Figure 6-9, the right eye is higher than the left eye. This indicates weakness in 1 of the 2 depressors of the right eye (RIR, RSO) or 1 of the 2 elevators of the left eye (LIO, LSR). Draw an oval around these 2 muscle groups (see Fig 6-9A).
- *Step 2:* Determine whether the vertical deviation is greater in right gaze or in left gaze. In the example shown in the figure, the deviation is larger in left gaze, which implicates 1 of the 4 vertically acting muscles used in left gaze. Draw an oval around these (see Fig 6-9B). At the end of step 2, the 2 remaining possible muscles (1 in each eye) are either both intortors or both extortors and are either both superior or both inferior muscles (1 rectus and 1 oblique). In the example shown in Figure 6-9B, the increased left-gaze deviation eliminates 2 inferior muscles and implicates 2 superior muscles.

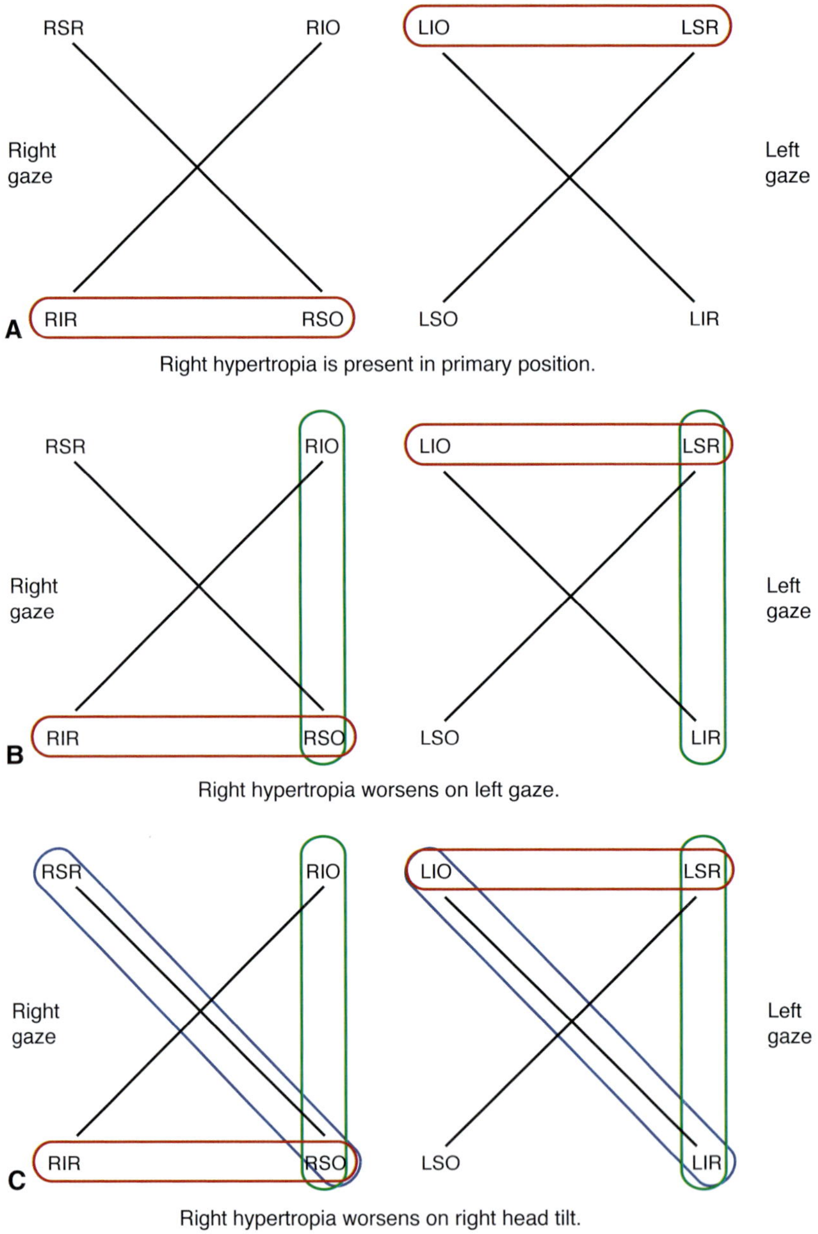

Figure 6-9 The 3-step test. The cyclovertical muscles are represented in their fields of action (see text for explanation). LIO = left inferior oblique; LIR = left inferior rectus; LSR = left superior rectus; RIR = right inferior rectus; RSO = right superior oblique; RSR = right superior rectus.

- *Step 3:* Known as the *Bielschowsky head tilt test,* the final step involves tilting the head toward the right shoulder and the left one during distance fixation. Head tilt to the right stimulates intorsion of the right eye (RSR, RSO) and extorsion of the left eye (LIR, LIO). Head tilt to the left stimulates extorsion of the right eye (RIR,

RIO) and intorsion of the left eye (LSR, LSO). Normally, the 2 intortors and the 2 extortors of each eye have *opposite* vertical actions that cancel each other. If 1 intortor or 1 extortor is weak, the vertical action of the other ipsilateral torting muscle becomes manifest during the torsional response to head tilt. In the example shown in Figure 6-9C, the right hypertropia increases when the head is tilted to the right. This suggests that the vertical action of the right superior rectus muscle is unopposed, causing the right eye to move upward as it attempts to intort to maintain fixation. Thus, the right superior oblique muscle is likely the weak muscle. (See also Chapter 10, Fig 10-3.)

Tests of Sensory Adaptation and Binocular Function

Sensory binocularity involves the use of both eyes together to form a unified perception. Ideally, testing of this function is performed before occlusion disrupts binocularity or ocular alignment. The sensory response to strabismus is diplopia, suppression, or ARC (see Chapter 4). While a variety of tests can assess these sensory responses, the Worth 4-dot and stereopsis tests are the ones typically used in clinical practice. Sensory tests must be performed in conjunction with cover tests to determine whether a fusion response is due to normal alignment or ARC. Also, the clinician should remember that no sensory test can perfectly replicate habitual viewing conditions; the more dissociative the test, the greater the risk that it does not reflect habitual binocular function.

The Red-Glass (Diplopia) Test

In a strabismic patient, a red glass or filter is placed before the fixating eye while the patient views a white light to stimulate the fovea of the fixating eye and an extrafoveal area of the fellow eye (Fig 6-10). The following results are possible:

- An esotropic patient with NRC and no suppression will experience *homonymous* or *uncrossed* diplopia (see Chapter 4) (with the red glass over the *left* eye, the red light is perceived to the *left* of the white light—the *same* side as the red lens; see Fig 6-10A).
- A patient with exotropia with NRC and no suppression will have *heteronymous* or *crossed* diplopia (with the red glass over the *left* eye, the red light is perceived to the *right* of the white light—the side *opposite* that of the red lens; see Fig 6-10B). The "x" in eXotropia helps to remind the clinician of crossed diplopia.
- A patient with harmonious ARC will see the 2 lights superimposed so that they appear pinkish despite a measurable deviation (not shown in Fig 6-10).
- A patient with esotropia and suppression will see only 1 light (either red or white) (see Fig 6-10C).
- A 5.00 D or 10.00 D base-up prism placed in front of the deviated eye can move the image out of the suppression scotoma, causing the patient to experience diplopia. In a patient with esotropia and NRC, the white light will be localized below and to one side of the red light. In a patient with esotropia and ARC, the white light will be localized directly below the red light, indicative of a pseudofovea (see Fig 6-10D).

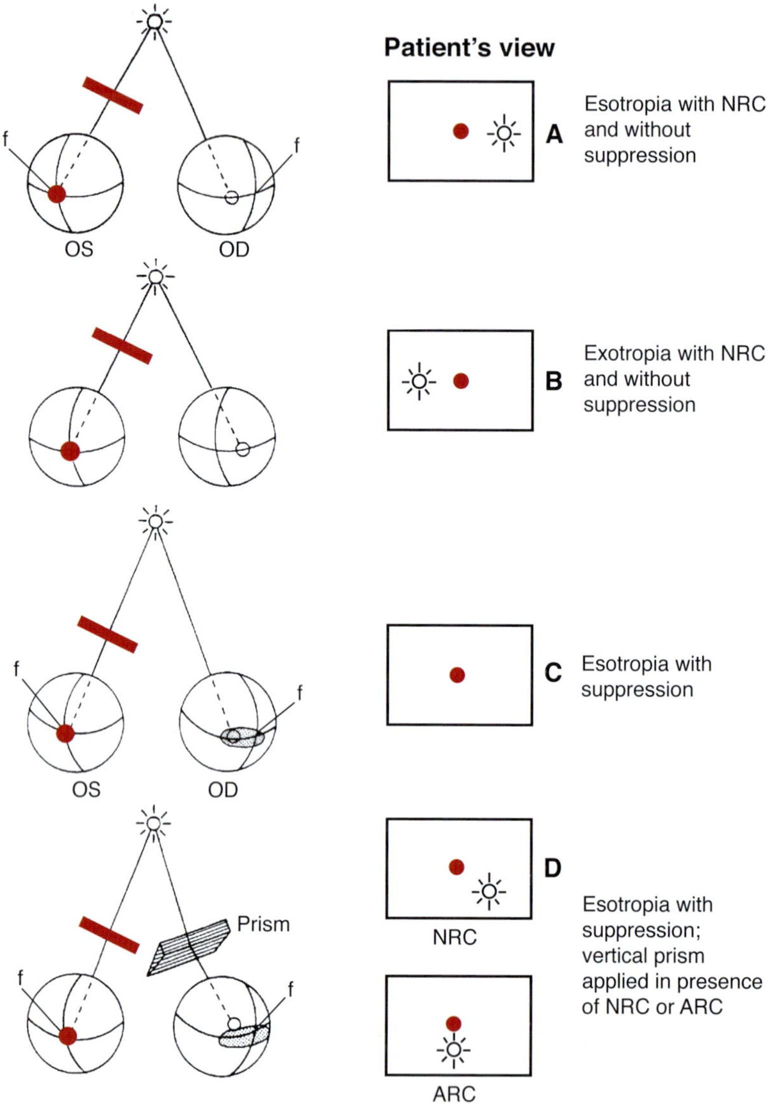

Figure 6-10 Red-glass test findings in esotropia and exotropia, with and without suppression, in the presence of NRC or ARC (see text for explanation; see also Chapter 4, Fig 4-6). The suppression scotoma is represented by the shaded area in **(C)** and **(D)**. f = fovea. *(Modified with permission from von Noorden GK.* Atlas of Strabismus. *4th ed. Mosby; 1983.)*

Bagolini Lenses

Bagolini lenses have many narrow, parallel striations that, like Maddox rods, cause a point source of light to appear as a streak perpendicular to the striations. The lenses are usually placed with the striations at an angle of 135° (patient's view) for the right eye and at an angle of 45° for the left eye, and the patient is asked to fixate on a distant light. Orthotropic patients will see 2 line segments crossing at their centers, forming an "X." Figure 6-11 illustrates a range of possible subjective results. For a patient with monofixation syndrome

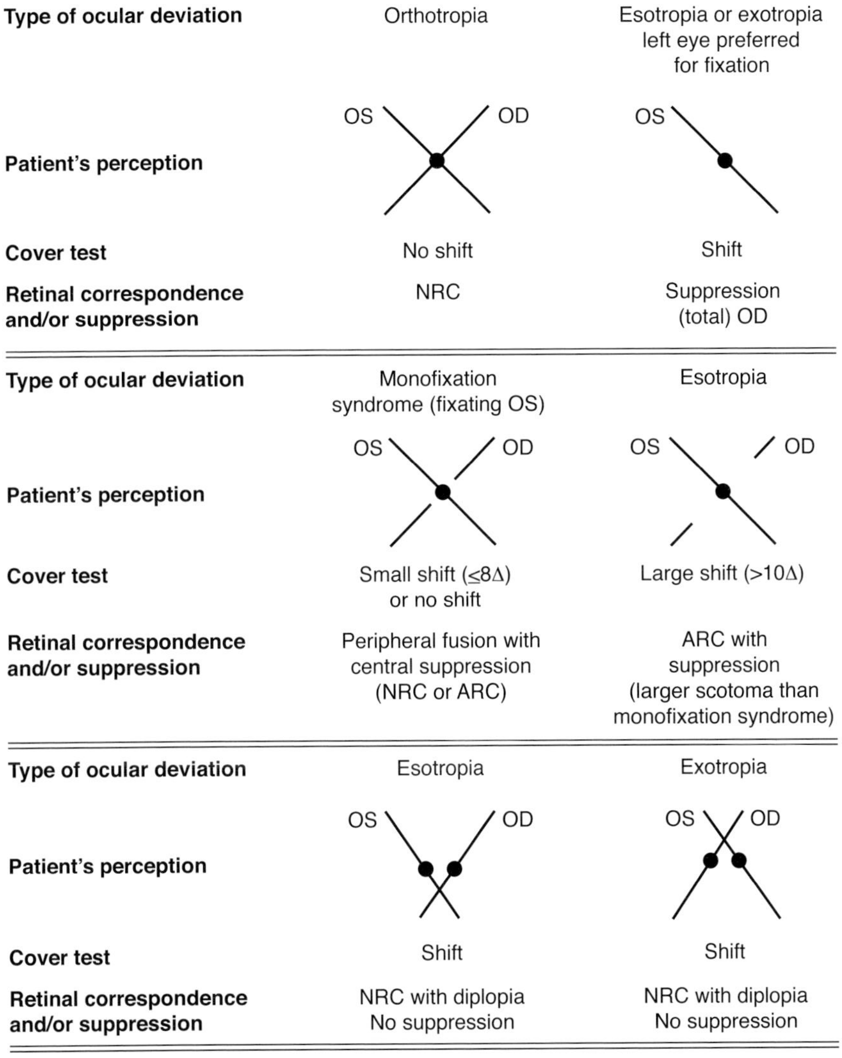

Figure 6-11 Bagolini striated lens test for retinal correspondence and suppression. For these figures, the Bagolini lens striations are oriented at 135° in front of the right eye (patient's view) and at 45° in front of the left eye, so that the patient sees a line segment at an angle of 45° with the right eye and a line segment at an angle of 135° with the left eye. The perception of the oblique lines seen by each eye under binocular conditions is shown. Examples of the types of strabismus in which these responses are commonly found are given.

and a central scotoma, 1 of the lines will be perceived as having a gap, corresponding to the scotoma.

Like Maddox rods, parallel Bagolini lenses can also assess torsion, but unlike Maddox rods, which are more dissociating, Bagolini lenses permit close-to-normal viewing and fusion and therefore reveal only manifest torsion; in addition, cover testing can be performed simultaneously.

The 4Δ Base-Out Prism Test

The 4Δ base-out prism test can identify a small facultative scotoma in a patient with monofixation syndrome and no manifest deviation (see Chapter 4). In this test, a 4Δ base-out prism is placed before 1 eye during binocular viewing, while motor responses are observed (Fig 6-12); the test is then repeated with the prism over the other eye. Patients with bifixation usually show a refixation version movement toward the apex of the prism (see Fig 6-12A), followed by a fusional convergence movement in which the eye with the prism maintains fixation while the fellow eye moves nasally to restore fusion (see Fig 6-12B). A similar response occurs regardless of which eye has the prism. In patients with monofixation, typically no movement is seen when the prism is placed before the nonfixating eye. When the prism is placed before the fixating eye, a refixation version movement occurs, but without any subsequent fusional convergence (see Fig 6-12C).

The 4Δ base-out prism test is the least reliable method of documenting a central suppression scotoma. Patients with bifixation may recognize diplopia when the prism is placed before an eye but make no convergence movement to correct for it. Patients with monofixation may switch fixation each time the prism is placed and show no version movement, regardless of which eye is tested.

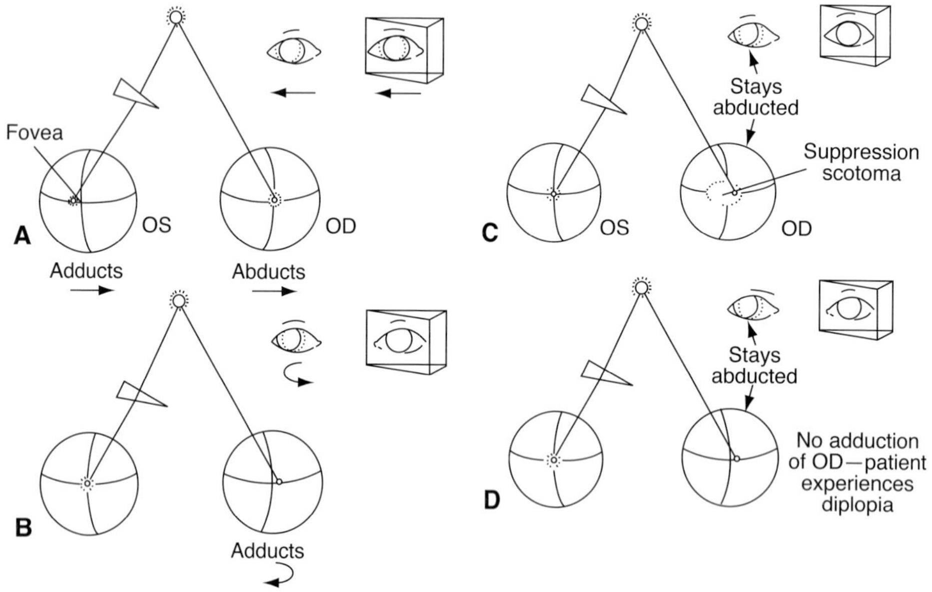

Figure 6-12 The 4Δ base-out prism test. **A,** When a prism is placed over the left eye, dextroversion of both eyes is driven by refixation of the left eye, indicating absence of foveal suppression in the left eye. If a suppression scotoma is present in the left eye, neither eye will move when the prism is placed before the left eye. **B,** Slow fusional adduction movement of the right eye is then observed, indicating absence of foveal suppression in the right eye. **C,** Foveal suppression in the right eye. In this case, following dextroversion of both eyes, there is no adduction movement of the right eye because the image has fallen in the suppression scotoma of the right eye. The patient does not experience diplopia. **D,** Weak fusion can also cause absence or delay of adduction movement, but in this case, diplopia is present (ie, no suppression scotoma). *(Modified with permission from von Noorden, GK. Present status of sensory testing. In: Burian HM, ed.* Symposium on Strabismus. *Transactions of the New Orleans Academy of Ophthalmology. Mosby, 1978:57. With permission from Elsevier.)*

The Afterimage Test

In the afterimage test, the macula of each eye is stimulated by h a linear light filament separately, which produces a different h eye: 1 horizontal and 1 vertical. Because suppression scotomata typical horizontal retinal meridian and may obscure most of a horizontal afterimage afterimage is induced in the deviating eye and the horizontal afterimage in the eye. The patient is then asked to draw the relative positions of the perceived afterimage A patient with NRC with or without manifest strabismus will view the images in a crossed configuration, as shown in Fig 6-13A. The configuration of the images in patients with ARC and horizontal strabismus are shown in Figs 6-13B and C. In patients with eccentric fixation (see Chapter 5), the afterimage is extrafoveal, and the test cannot be interpreted. The afterimage test is very dissociative; demonstration of ARC indicates that it is dense.

Amblyoscope Testing

An amblyoscope/synoptophore can neutralize torsion and is therefore useful for distinguishing between central fusion disruption (see Chapter 4) and an inability to fuse because of a large cyclodeviation. The amblyoscope can also assess fusion ability, suppression, retinal correspondence, fusional amplitudes, and stereopsis. In addition, it may be used in exercises designed to overcome suppression and increase fusional amplitudes.

The Worth 4-Dot Test

The Worth 4-dot test (Fig 6-14) is often considered a test of sensory fusion; however, it does not evaluate sensory fusion directly as there is no fusible feature in the test. Its best use is to identify a suppression scotoma. The test uses red-green glasses and a target consisting of 4 illuminated dots: 1 red, 2 green, and 1 white. By convention, the red lens is placed in front of the right eye and the green lens in front of the left. The red lens blocks

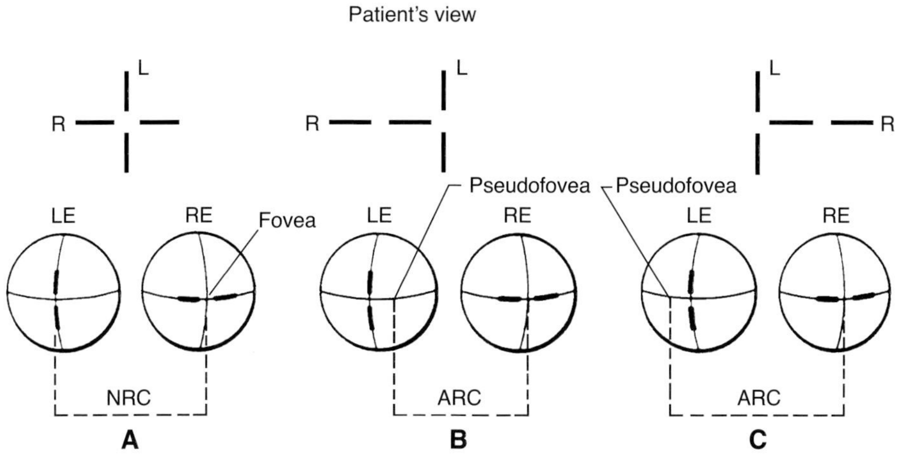

Figure 6-13 Afterimage test. **A,** NRC. **B,** ARC in a case of esotropia. **C,** ARC in a case of exotropia. *(Modified with permission from von Noorden GK.* Atlas of Strabismus. *4th ed. Mosby; 1983.)*

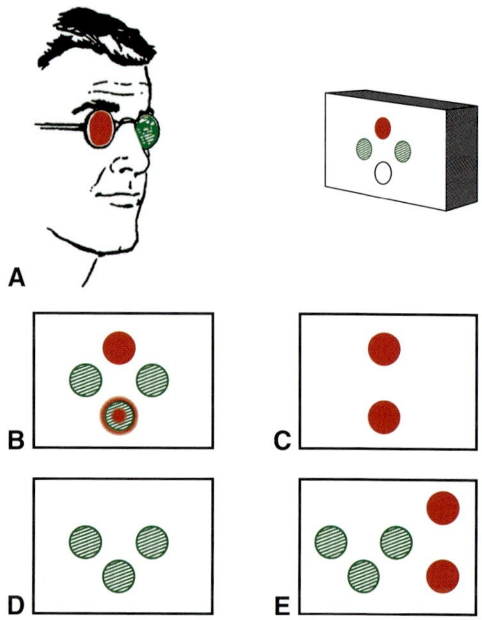

igure 6-14 Worth 4-dot test. **A,** Looking through a pair of red-green glasses, the patient views 4 illuminated dots (1 red, 2 green, 1 white) at 6 m (projected, or mounted in a box) and at 33 cm (on a Worth 4-dot flashlight). The possible responses are given in parts **B** through **E. B,** Patient sees all 4 dots: peripheral fusion with orthophoria or strabismus with ARC. The dot in the 6 o'clock position is seen in color rivalry or, depending on ocular dominance, as predominantly red or predominantly green. **C,** Patient sees 2 red dots: suppression in left eye. **D,** Patient sees 3 green dots: suppression in right eye. **E,** Patient sees 5 dots: uncrossed diplopia with esotropia if the red dots appear to the right of the green dots, as in this figure; crossed diplopia with exotropia if the red dots appear to the left. *(Modified with permission from von Noorden GK.* Atlas of Strabismus. *4th ed. Mosby; 1983.)*

the green light, and the green lens blocks the red light, so the red and green dots are each seen by only 1 eye. The white dot is the only feature seen by both eyes, but in a patient with fusion it is seen in color rivalry (see Fig 6-14B). The *polarized Worth 4-dot test* uses polarized glasses rather than red and green ones. The stimulus lights can be presented in a wall-mounted display or with a Worth 4-dot flashlight. The test should be administered in good ambient light so that peripheral features in the room can stimulate motor fusion. The number of dots that the patient reports seeing indicates the diagnosis as follows:

- Seeing 2 dots indicates a suppression scotoma in the left eye (see Fig 6-14C).
- Seeing 3 dots indicates a suppression scotoma in the right eye (see Fig 6-14D).
- Seeing 4 dots indicates that if there is a suppression scotoma, it must subtend a smaller visual angle than the test target. The perception of 4 dots indicates some degree of sensory fusion, either NRC (if there is no manifest strabismus, or small-angle strabismus consistent with monofixation and peripheral fusion; see below) or ARC (if there is larger-angle manifest strabismus) (see Fig 6-14B).
- Seeing 5 dots indicates diplopia, usually from larger-angle manifest strabismus without suppression or ARC (see Fig 6-14E).

In a patient with monofixation syndrome (see Chapter 4), the Worth 4-dot test can demonstrate both the presence of peripheral fusion and the absence of bifixation. The standard Worth 4-dot flashlight projects onto a central retinal area of 1° or less when viewed at 3 m (10 ft), well within the 1°–4° scotoma characteristic of monofixation syndrome, so patients with monofixation syndrome report seeing 2 or 3 lights, depending on fixation preference. As the Worth 4-dot flashlight is brought closer to the patient, the dots project onto more peripheral retina outside the central monofixation scotoma and a fusion response (4 lights) is obtained. This usually occurs between 0.67 and 1 m (2–3 ft).

Stereoacuity Tests

Stereopsis occurs when the 2 retinal images of an object in front of or behind the plane of fixation—which have small disparities due to the horizontal separation of the eyes—are cortically integrated, resulting in a perception of relative depth. Both *contour stereopsis* and *random-dot stereopsis tests* present horizontally displaced copies of the same stimulus to each eye separately (usually by having the patient wear polarized or red-green glasses). Contour stereopsis tests present horizontally displaced figures (1 to each eye) that are recognizable to each eye individually. For contour stereoscopic figures with larger disparities, monocular cues in the form of decentration of the image are present, which can enable some patients to pass the test despite limited stereopsis. *Random-dot stereopsis tests* avoid such artifacts by embedding the stereoscopic figure in a background of similarly random dots; the dots in the area of the figure but not those in the background are shifted between the eyes, so that there is a stereoscopic percept, but neither eye alone can perceive the figure.

In the *Titmus test,* contour stereopsis is tested at near using polarized glasses. The ability to detect elevation of the fly's wings above the plane of the card indicates gross stereopsis (3000 seconds of arc). Finer levels of stereoacuity can also be demonstrated using stereoscopic images employing less horizontal disparity; at each level, the patient must identify the 1 stereoscopically presented figure out of a group of otherwise similar figures.

Clinically useful random-dot near stereopsis tests include the *Randot test,* which requires polarized glasses and measures stereoacuity down to 20 seconds of arc; the *TNO test,* which requires red-green glasses and measures stereoacuity down to 15 seconds of arc; the *Random-Dot E test,* a forced-choice test also requiring polarized glasses and employed mainly in pediatric vision-screening programs; and the *Lang stereopsis tests,* which do not require glasses to produce a random-dot stereoscopic effect and therefore may be useful in children who are not willing to put on glasses for testing.

Stereopsis can also be measured at distance using a chart projector with a vectographic slide, the Smart System PC-Plus (M&S Technologies, Inc.), or the Frisby Davis Distance Stereotest (Stereotest Ltd). Distance stereoacuity tests may be helpful in monitoring control of intermittent exotropia.

Assessment of the Field of Single Binocular Vision

The field of single binocular vision may be tested using a Goldmann perimeter or tangent screen. This assessment is useful for following recovery of a paretic muscle or measuring the outcome of surgery to alleviate diplopia. A small, white test object is followed by both eyes in the cardinal positions throughout the visual field. When the patient indicates that the test object is seen double, the point is plotted. The field of binocular vision normally measures about 45°–50° from the fixation point except where it is blocked by the nose (Fig 6-15). Weighted templates reflecting the greater importance of single binocular vision in primary and reading positions can be used to quantify the findings.

Sullivan TJ, Kraft SP, Burack C, O'Reilly C. A functional scoring method for the field of binocular single vision. *Ophthalmology.* 1992;99(4):575–581.

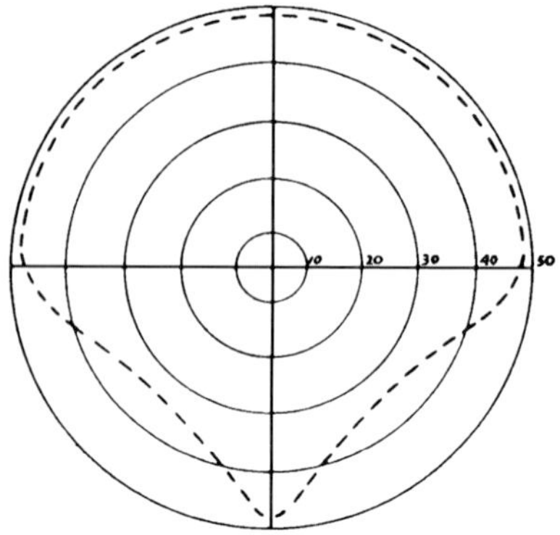

Figure 6-15 The normal field of single binocular vision.

The Prism Adaptation Test

In the prism adaptation test, binocular function is tested with prisms to align the visual axes to help predict whether fusion may be restored with surgical or prismatic alignment, especially in adults. This test is distinct from the use of prolonged prism adaptation to unmask a larger angle of deviation in acquired esotropia, as described in Chapter 7.

Torticollis: Differential Diagnosis and Evaluation

Torticollis is an abnormal head position (AHP): head turn, chin-up or chin-down, head tilt, or any combination of these. Ocular torticollis results from strabismus or other eye conditions; see Table 6-2 for the differential diagnosis of both ocular and nonocular torticollis.

Early diagnosis and correction of ocular conditions resulting in torticollis are important because prolonged AHP (primarily head tilt) in children can cause facial asymmetry or secondary musculoskeletal changes. Note, however, that facial asymmetry coexisting with head tilt is not always caused by the head tilt. For example, unicoronal craniosynostosis can result in strabismus with ocular torticollis and also directly cause facial asymmetry independent of the torticollis.

Ocular Torticollis

Sometimes an AHP and associated ocular abnormality simply have a shared underlying cause (eg, ocular tilt reaction), but more often, the AHP compensates for the ocular condition.

Incomitant strabismus (eg, superior oblique palsy, Duane syndrome, Brown syndrome, blowout fractures, thyroid eye disease) can cause an AHP that improves binocularity. Chin-up positioning in unilateral ptosis likewise enables binocularity. In rare cases, patients with superior oblique palsy present with paradoxical head tilt to the wrong side, possibly to increase the separation between diplopic images when fusion is not possible.

Table 6-2 Differential Diagnosis of Torticollis

Ocular Torticollis	Nonocular Torticollis
Nystagmus	Congenital muscular torticollis
Infantile nystagmus syndrome (congenital motor or sensory nystagmus; null point)	Skeletal abnormalities
Periodic alternating nystagmus (alternating null point)	Congenital abnormalities (eg, Klippel-Feil anomaly)
Fusion maldevelopment nystagmus syndrome (less in adduction)	Traumatic abnormalities
Spasmus nutans	Neurologic conditions
Acquired adult jerk nystagmus	Syringomyelia
A- or V-pattern esotropia or exotropia	Dystonia
Paretic strabismus	Posterior fossa lesions
Superior oblique palsy	Deafness in 1 ear
CN VI palsy	Sandifer syndrome
CN III palsy	Psychogenic disease
Inferior oblique palsy	
Restrictive strabismus	
Brown syndrome	
Thyroid eye disease	
Orbital fracture	
Congenital cranial dysinnervation disorders	
Duane syndrome	
Congenital fibrosis of extraocular muscles	
Supranuclear disorders	
Monocular elevation deficiency	
Dorsal midbrain syndrome	
Gaze palsy	
Dissociated vertical deviation	
Ocular tilt reaction	
Monocular blindness (with fusion maldevelopment nystagmus syndrome, or for centration of remaining field)	
Homonymous hemianopia	
Ptosis	
Refractive error	

CN = cranial nerve.

In infantile nystagmus syndrome (congenital motor or sensory nystagmus) with a null point away from primary position, an AHP improves vision (see Chapter 12). In patients with fusion maldevelopment nystagmus syndrome, vision improves with an AHP that brings the fixating eye into adduction. In those with bilateral duction deficits (eg, congenital fibrosis of extraocular muscles) or bilateral ptosis, an AHP may be needed for foveation. Refractive errors may also cause an AHP.

Finally, monocular individuals and patients with homonymous hemianopia may have a variable head turn toward their blind side, perhaps to better center (relative to the body) the total field of view that is accessible through eye movements.

Diagnostic evaluation of ocular torticollis

To identify ocular causes of an AHP, motility testing with particular attention to gaze positions opposite those favored is essential. Nystagmus is usually obvious, but subtle nystagmus may be visible only during slit-lamp or fundus examination. Fundus examination may reveal extorsion suggestive of superior oblique palsy, or conjugate torsion (extorsion in 1 eye and intorsion in the other), as seen in the ocular tilt reaction. If placing the patient in the supine position eliminates the head tilt, a musculoskeletal etiology is unlikely. If both right eye monocular occlusion and left eye monocular occlusion eliminate the AHP, then the torticollis probably serves binocular fusion.

CHAPTER 7

Esodeviations

Highlights

- Acquired esotropia in a toddler is often accommodative and responsive to full hyperopic refractive correction; however, more ominous causes must be ruled out.
- A child's preference for cross-fixation can be mistaken as an abduction defect.
- In an infant, incomitant esotropia from Duane syndrome is more common than and can be confused with incomitant esotropia from cranial nerve VI palsy.

Introduction

An *esodeviation* is a latent or manifest convergent misalignment of the visual axes. Esodeviations are the most common type of childhood strabismus in North America, accounting for more than 50% of ocular deviations in the pediatric population. In adults, esodeviations and exodeviations are equally prevalent.

Repka MX, Yu F, Coleman A. Strabismus among aged fee-for-service Medicare beneficiaries. *J AAPOS.* 2012;16(6):495–500.

Epidemiology

Globally, esodeviations occur with equal frequency in males and females; in the United States, they are more common in African Americans and White ethnic groups than in Asian ethnic groups. Risk factors include anisometropia, hyperopia, neurodevelopmental impairment, prematurity, low birth weight, craniofacial or chromosomal abnormalities, maternal smoking during pregnancy, and a family history of strabismus. The prevalence of esotropia increases with age (higher prevalence at 48–72 months compared with 6–11 months), moderate anisometropia, and moderate hyperopia. Some families show mendelian inheritance. Amblyopia develops in approximately 50% of children who have esotropia.

Esodeviations can result from innervational, anatomical, mechanical, refractive, or accommodative factors. They may be classified by subtype and by whether the deviation is comitant or incomitant (Table 7-1, Fig 7-1).

American Academy of Ophthalmology Pediatric Ophthalmology/Strabismus Panel, Hoskins Center for Quality Eye Care. Preferred Practice Pattern Guidelines. *Esotropia and Exotropia.* American Academy of Ophthalmology; 2017. www.aao.org/ppp

Table 7-1 Major Types of Esodeviation

Comitant Esotropia
Accommodative
Normal AC/A ratio
High AC/A ratio
Partially accommodative
Infantile (congenital)
Acquired nonaccommodative
Basic
Cyclic
Sensory
Divergence insufficiency
Primary (adult-onset distance)
Secondary
Spasm of the near reflex
Convergence excess
Consecutive
Spontaneous
Postsurgical
Incomitant Esotropia
CN VI palsy
Slipped or lost lateral rectus muscle following surgery
Globe prolapse associated with high myopia
Congenital cranial dysinnervation disorders (CCDDs; see Chapter 11)
Postsurgical and periocular implants
Medial rectus muscle restriction
Thyroid eye disease
Medial orbital wall fracture with entrapment
Following excessive resection
Nystagmus and Esotropia
Fusion maldevelopment nystagmus syndrome
Nystagmus blockage syndrome

AC/A = accommodative convergence/accommodation; CN = cranial nerve.

Cotter SA, Varma R, Tarczy-Hornoch K, et al; Joint Writing Committee for the Multi-Ethnic Pediatric Eye Disease Study and the Baltimore Pediatric Eye Disease Study Groups. Risk factors associated with childhood strabismus: the Multi-Ethnic Pediatric Eye Disease and Baltimore Pediatric Eye Disease studies. *Ophthalmology.* 2011;118(11): 2251–2261.

Pseudoesotropia

Pseudoesotropia refers to the appearance of esotropia when the visual axes are actually aligned. The appearance may be caused by a flat and broad nasal bridge, prominent epicanthal folds, a narrow interpupillary distance, or a negative angle kappa (see Chapter 6). Less than the expected amount of sclera is seen nasally, creating the impression that the eye is deviated inward (Fig 7-2). This is especially noticeable when the child gazes to either side. Results of both corneal light reflex testing and cover testing are normal. In 1 study of

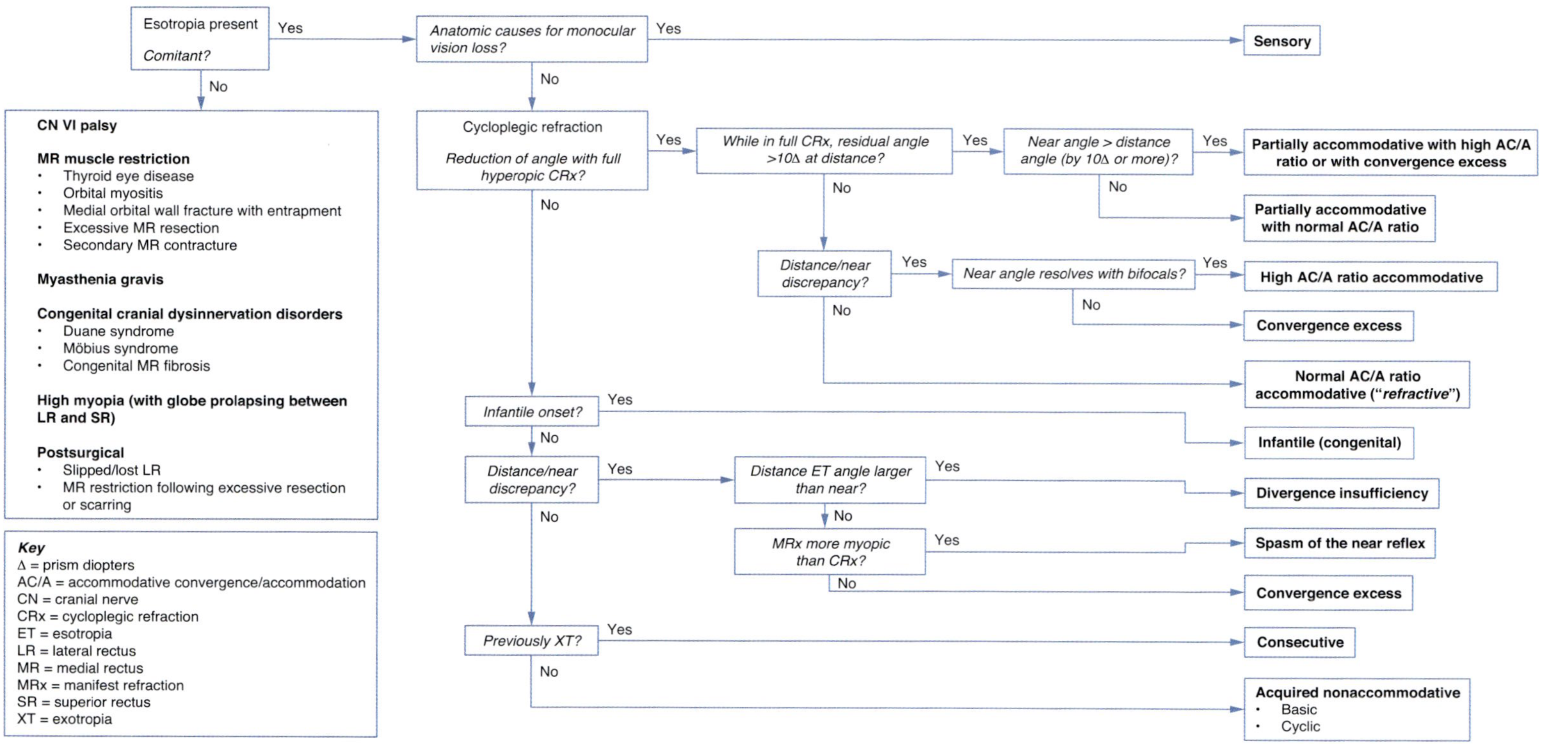

Figure 7-1 Diagnostic algorithm and classification of esodeviations. *(Courtesy of Ta Chen Peter Chang, MD, on behalf of Childhood Glaucoma Research Network (CGRN) and the Samuel & Ethel Balkan International Pediatric Glaucoma Center, Bascom Palmer Eye Institute, University of Miami.)*

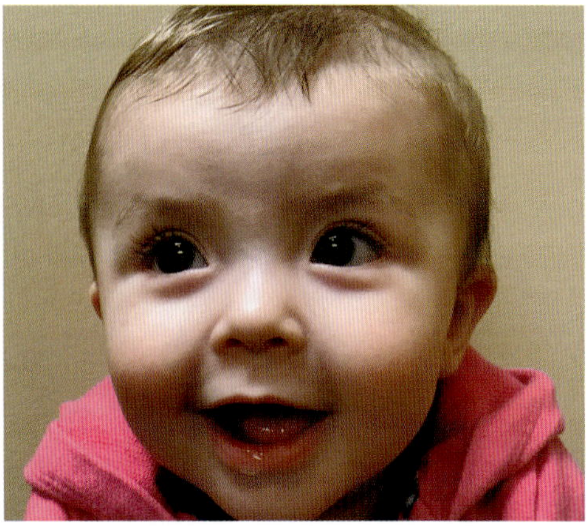

Figure 7-2 Infant girl with pseudoesotropia. The child is looking to right gaze, and the broad epicanthal folds create the appearance of a left esotropia. *(Courtesy of Katherine A. Lee, MD, PhD.)*

children initially diagnosed with pseudoesotropia under the age of 3 years, 12% were later found to have developed strabismus or mild refractive amblyopia. Thus, it is important to monitor children with pseudoesotropia.

Silbert AL, Matta NS, Silbert DI. Incidence of strabismus and amblyopia in preverbal children previously diagnosed with pseudoesotropia. *J AAPOS.* 2012;16(2):118–119.

Accommodative Esotropia

Accommodative esotropia is a convergent deviation of the eyes associated with activation of the accommodative reflex. The accommodative convergence/accommodation (AC/A) ratio (see Sidebar and Chapter 6) can be normal or high. All accommodative esodeviations are acquired and can be characterized as follows:

- onset from 4 months to 7 years of age; typically 2–3 years of age
- usually intermittent at onset, later becoming constant
- comitant
- often familial
- sometimes precipitated by trauma or illness
- frequently associated with amblyopia
- diplopia may be present (especially with onset at an older age); it usually disappears with the development of a facultative suppression scotoma in the deviating eye
- deviation angle decreases to less than 10 prism diopters (Δ) with proper refractive correction (if the residual angle is larger, the patient has partially accommodative esotropia; see Table 7-2 and the section Partially Accommodative Esotropia later in this chapter)

It is important to discover and treat all hyperopia in patients with accommodative esotropia. If residual esotropia persists with hyperopic refractive correction, atropine refraction should be considered.

ACCOMMODATIVE CONVERGENCE/ACCOMMODATION RATIO

When a near-fixation stimulus is presented, it activates the near reflex, which consists of 2 parallel sets of *simultaneous* actions (accommodative convergence and accommodation). In accommodative convergence, the medial rectus muscles in both eyes contract, converging the visual axes to allow the near stimulus image to fall on both foveae. In accommodation, the ciliary muscles contract, relax the zonular fibers, increase the axial thickness of the lenses, and allow the near stimulus image to focus on the fovea. The AC/A ratio is the ratio of accommodative convergence (measured in prism diopters, Δ) per unit of accommodation (measured in lens diopters; the amount depends on the eye's refractive state and the distance of the near stimulus). The AC/A ratio is an innate quality of an individual's near reflex. As a person's ability to accommodate and converge changes over time, so does the AC/A ratio. See also Chapter 6 and BCSC Section 3, *Clinical Optics and Vision Rehabilitation*.

Pathogenesis and Types of Accommodative Esotropia

Normal AC/A ratio accommodative esotropia

The mechanism of accommodative esotropia with *normal AC/A ratio* (also referred to as refractive accommodative esotropia) involves 3 factors:

1. uncorrected hyperopia
2. accommodative convergence
3. insufficient fusional divergence

Because of uncorrected hyperopia, the patient must accommodate to focus the retinal image. Accommodation is accompanied by the other components of the near reflex, namely convergence and miosis. If the patient's fusional divergence mechanism is insufficient to compensate for the increased convergence tonus, esotropia results. The angle of esotropia is approximately the same at distance and near fixation and is generally between 20Δ and 30Δ. Patients with refractive accommodative esotropia have an average of +4.00 diopters (D) of hyperopia.

High AC/A ratio accommodative esotropia

Patients with *high AC/A ratio* accommodative esotropia (also referred to as nonrefractive accommodative esotropia) have an excessive convergence response for the amount of accommodation required to focus while wearing their full cycloplegic correction. In this form of esotropia, the deviation is present only at near fixation or is much larger at near (by 10Δ or more). The refractive error in high AC/A ratio accommodative esotropia averages +2.25 D. However, this esotropia can occur in patients with a normal level of hyperopia or high hyperopia, with emmetropia, or even with myopia.

Evaluation

The 2 eyes can have equal vision, or amblyopia can be present. Versions and ductions may be normal, or overelevation in adduction or dissociated strabismus complex (discussed in

Chapter 10) may be present. The examiner measures the deviation using an accommodative target at distance and at near fixation. Alternate cover testing at the initial examination typically reveals an intermittent comitant esotropia.

Management

Normal AC/A ratio accommodative esotropia

Treatment of refractive accommodative esotropia consists of correction of the full amount of hyperopia, as determined under cycloplegia. If binocular fusion is maintained, the refractive correction can later be decreased to 1.00–2.00 D less than the full cycloplegic refraction. Amblyopia, if present, may respond to spectacle correction alone, but treatment with occlusion or atropine may be necessary if the amblyopia persists after a period of spectacle wear (see Chapter 5).

Parents must understand not only that full-time wear of the glasses is important but also that the refractive correction can only help control the strabismus, not "cure" it. Once full-time wear has begun, the esotropia may increase when the child is not wearing glasses, because the child makes a strong accommodative effort to produce an image that is as clear as the one experienced with refractive correction. Discussing these issues with the parents at the time the prescription is given is helpful.

High AC/A ratio accommodative esotropia

A high AC/A ratio can be managed optically or surgically; it can also be observed.

Bifocals Plus lenses for uncorrected hyperopia reduce accommodation and therefore accommodative convergence. Bifocal glasses further reduce or eliminate the need to accommodate for near fixation. Not all ophthalmologists advocate bifocal glasses if the distance angle is controlled. Considerations for bifocals include the following:

- Flat-top style bifocals are prescribed initially (see the chapter on clinical refraction in BCSC Section 3, *Clinical Optics and Vision Rehabilitation*).
- The clinician should use lowest plus power needed (up to +3.00 D) to achieve ocular alignment at near fixation.
- The bifocal segment should be set high enough that the top of the bifocal segment bisects the pupil.
- Progressive bifocal lenses have been used successfully in older children after they have learned how to use bifocal glasses.
- Some children with convergence excess do not have a high AC/A ratio and thus do not respond to bifocals.

An ideal response to bifocal glasses is restoration of normal binocular function (fusion and stereopsis) at both distance and near fixation. An acceptable response is fusion at distance and less than 10Δ of residual esotropia at near with bifocals (signifying the potential for fusion). Although some children improve spontaneously with time, others need to be slowly weaned from bifocal glasses. The process of reducing the bifocal power in 0.50–1.00 D steps can be started at about age 7 or 8 years and can allow weaning by age 10–12 years. If a child cannot be weaned from bifocals, surgery may be considered.

Surgery Surgical management of high AC/A ratio accommodative esotropia is controversial. Some ophthalmologists advocate surgery (medial rectus muscle recessions with or without posterior or pulley fixation) to normalize the AC/A ratio, which may allow the discontinuation of bifocal use. The risk of overcorrection at distance is low (<10%). Some ophthalmologists use prism adaptation, which entails using prisms preoperatively to neutralize a deviation for a certain length of time. The prism neutralization can then be used to predict the outcome of surgery and determine the maximum deviation.

Observation Some ophthalmologists observe the near deviation as long as the distance alignment allows for the development of peripheral fusion. Many patients show a decrease in the near deviation with time, and binocular vision at both distance and near fixation ultimately develops.

General considerations For the long-term management of both normal and high AC/A ratio accommodative esotropia, it is important to remember that hyperopia usually increases until age 5–7 years before it starts to decrease. Therefore, if the esotropia with correction increases, the cycloplegic refraction should be repeated and the full correction prescribed. If glasses fully correct the esotropia, the hyperopia is low, and some degree of sensory binocular cooperation or fusion is present, the clinician may begin to reduce the hyperopic correction to create a small esophoria, which is thought to stimulate fusional divergence. An increase in the fusional divergence, combined with the natural decrease of both the hyperopia and the high AC/A ratio, may enable the patient to eventually maintain straight eyes without bifocals or glasses altogether. This does not apply to children with high hyperopia.

Partially Accommodative Esotropia

Partially accommodative esotropia is similar to accommodative esotropia in that a significant component of the esotropia results from accommodative convergence. However, unlike pure accommodative esotropia, patients with partially accommodative esotropia show a reduction in the angle of esotropia when wearing glasses but have a residual esotropia despite provision of the full hyperopic correction. Undercorrection of hyperopia due to insufficient cycloplegia should be ruled out as the cause of residual esotropia, especially in eyes with dark irides. In some cases, partially accommodative esotropia results from decompensation of a pure normal or high AC/A ratio accommodative esotropia. This is more likely to occur if there is a long delay in refractive correction. In other instances, an initial nonaccommodative esotropia subsequently develops an accommodative component.

Treatment of partially accommodative esotropia consists of strabismus surgery for the deviation that persists while the patient wears the full hyperopic correction. It is important that the patient and parents understand *before* surgery that its purpose is to produce straight eyes with spectacle wear—not to enable the child to discontinue wearing glasses altogether. In older patients, refractive surgery may be considered to both reduce the hyperopic refractive error and improve the ocular alignment. Before proceeding with surgery, it is important

Table 7-2 Different Types of Esotropia with Accommodative Component

	Normal AC/A ratio	High AC/A ratio
(Pure) accommodative	• High hyperopia, usually +4.00 D or more • Distance angle = near angle • In full CRx = little or no residual ET (<10Δ) • Treat alignment with single-vision hyperopic correction; treat amblyopia (if any)	• Moderate hyperopia, emmetropia, or myopia • Distance angle < near angle • In full CRx with BF = little or no residual ET (<10Δ) • Treat alignment with bifocal correction; treat amblyopia (if any)
Partially accommodative	• High hyperopia, usually +4.00 D or more • Distance angle = near angle • In full CRx = improved ET but with residual ET ≥10Δ • Prescribe full CRx; rule out missed hyperopia; surgery to correct residual angle	• Moderate hyperopia, emmetropia, or myopia • Distance angle < near angle • In full CRx = improved ET but with residual ET ≥10Δ • Prescribe full CRx, rule out missed hyperopia; surgery to correct residual angle (ET surgery augmented with posterior fixation to normalize AC/A ratio)

AC/A = accommodative convergence/accommodation; BF = bifocals; CRx = cycloplegic refraction; D = diopters; ET = esotropia; Δ = prism diopters.

to recheck the cycloplegic refraction to rule out latent uncorrected hyperopia. Table 7-2 summarizes the different types of esotropia with accommodative component.

Infantile (Congenital) Esotropia

Infantile esotropia is defined as an esotropia that is present by 6 months of age. Some ophthalmologists refer to this disorder as *congenital esotropia,* although the deviation is usually not manifest at birth.

Variable, transient, intermittent strabismus is commonly noted in the first 2–3 months of life. Also, it is common to see both intermittent esotropia and exotropia in the same infant (termed *ocular instability of infancy*). This condition usually resolves by 3 months of age but sometimes persists, especially in premature infants. If an esotropia is present after age 2 months, is constant, and measures 30Δ or more, it is unlikely to resolve and will probably require surgical intervention.

Patients with infantile esotropia often have a family history of esotropia or other strabismus, but well-defined genetic patterns are unusual. Infantile esotropia occurs more frequently in children born prematurely and in up to 30% of children with neurologic and developmental problems, including cerebral palsy and hydrocephalus.

Pathogenesis

The cause of infantile esotropia remains unknown. It has been hypothesized that the primary problem in infantile esotropia is associated with motor development and is potentially curable if ocular alignment is achieved in infancy. Several authors have reported favorable sensory results in infants operated on between 6 months and 2 years of age, and these encouraging results have become the basis for the practice of early surgery for infantile esotropia.

Clinical Features and Evaluation

Versions and ductions

Versions and ductions are often normal. Overelevation in adduction and dissociated strabismus complex develop in more than 50% of patients, usually after 1–2 years of age. There may be an apparent (pseudo-) abduction deficit because of cross-fixation; children with equal vision in both eyes have no need to abduct either eye on side gaze. The infant's ability to abduct each eye can be demonstrated with the doll's head maneuver or by observation after patching either of the patient's eyes. The clinician can also hold the infant and spin in a circle, which stimulates the vestibular-ocular reflex and helps demonstrate full abduction. Eyes with long-standing infantile esotropia may develop a small abduction deficit from a relative tightening of the medial rectus muscles, in which case, cranial nerve (CN) VI palsy should be ruled out. The deviation is comitant and characteristically larger than 30Δ.

Visual acuity

The eyes may have equal vision, in which case alternate fixation or cross-fixation will be present. Cross-fixation, the use of the adducted eye for fixation of objects in the contralateral visual field, is associated with large-angle esotropias (Fig 7-3). If amblyopia is present, a fixation preference can be observed; the better-seeing eye will fixate in all fields of gaze, making the amblyopic eye appear to have an abduction deficit unless duction is assessed with the doll's head maneuver or when the better-seeing eye is patched. A severe form of infantile esotropia, referred to as *Ciancia syndrome,* consists of large-angle esotropia (>50Δ), abducting nystagmus, and mild abduction deficits. Children with this syndrome uniformly use cross-fixation.

Associated anomalies

Asymmetry of monocular horizontal smooth pursuit is normal in infants up to 6 months of age, with the nasal-to-temporal direction less well developed than the temporal-to-nasal.

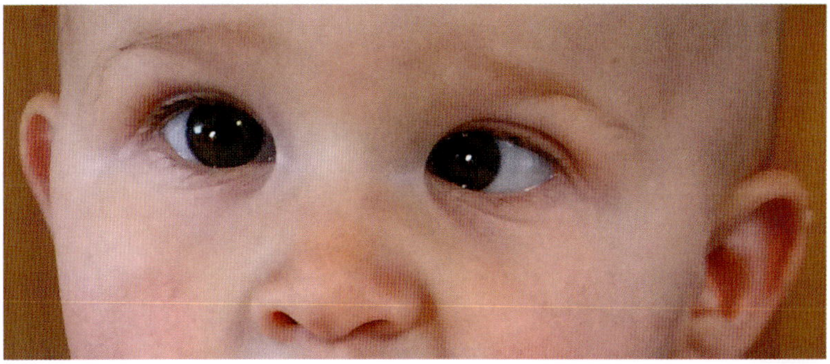

Figure 7-3 Infant boy with left esotropia. Cross-fixation of the right eye from the adducted position. *(Courtesy of Katherine A. Lee, MD, PhD.)*

Patients with infantile esotropia, however, have persistent smooth-pursuit asymmetry throughout their lives. Fusion maldevelopment nystagmus syndrome is also a commonly associated motility anomaly. Cycloplegic refraction characteristically reveals low hyperopia (+1.00 to +2.00 D). Hyperopia greater than 2.00 D warrants consideration of spectacle correction; reduction of the strabismic angle with glasses indicates the presence of an accommodative component.

Management

Management goals

Ocular alignment is rarely achieved without surgery in infantile esotropia. The goal of surgical treatment is to reduce the deviation to orthotropia or as close to it as possible. In the presence of normal vision, this ideally results in the development of some degree of sensory fusion. Alignment within 10Δ of orthotropia frequently results in the development of the monofixation syndrome, characterized by peripheral fusion, central suppression, and favorable alignment (see Chapter 4). Even though bifoveal fusion is not achieved, this small-angle strabismus generally represents a stable, functional surgical outcome and thus a successful surgical result. In addition, after the eyes are straightened the child's psychological and motor development may improve and accelerate.

Timing of surgery

The Congenital Esotropia Observational Study found that when patients present with constant esotropia of at least 40Δ after 10 weeks of age, the deviations are unlikely to resolve spontaneously. Most ophthalmologists in North America agree that surgery should be undertaken early, before age 2 years, to optimize binocular cooperation. Surgery can be performed in healthy children as early as age 4 months. Previously, it was thought that concurrent amblyopia should be fully treated before surgery. However, it has been shown that successful postoperative alignment is as likely to occur in patients with mild to moderate amblyopia at the time of surgery as it is in those whose amblyopia has been fully treated preoperatively. When ocular alignment is achieved earlier, there may be the added benefits of better fusion, stereopsis, and long-term stability. A prospective, multicenter European study comparing early (age 6–24 months) versus delayed (age 32–60 months) strabismus surgery showed a small improvement in gross binocularity in the early-surgery group; however, a higher number of procedures were performed in the early-surgery group.

Surgical approach

The most commonly performed initial procedure is recession of both medial rectus muscles. Recession of a medial rectus muscle combined with resection of the ipsilateral lateral rectus muscle is also effective. Two-muscle surgery spares the other horizontal rectus muscles for subsequent surgery should it be necessary, which is common. For infants with large deviations (typically >60Δ), some surgeons operate on 3 or even 4 horizontal rectus muscles at the time of the initial surgery, or they add botulinum toxin injection to the medial rectus muscle recession. Significant inferior oblique muscle overaction can be treated at the time of the initial surgery. Chapter 13 discusses surgical procedures in detail.

Alternatives to surgery

Injection of botulinum toxin to the medial rectus muscles has also been used as primary treatment of infantile esotropia. In one study, botulinum toxin injection was associated with a substantially higher reoperation rate than was strabismus surgery, and children treated with botulinum toxin were found to have a higher rate of postoperative abnormal binocularity. Botulinum toxin may be most useful for smaller deviations.

Leffler CT, Vaziri K, Schwartz SG, et al. Rates of reoperation and abnormal binocularity following strabismus surgery in children. *Am J Ophthalmol.* 2016;162:159–166.e9.

Pediatric Eye Disease Investigator Group. The clinical spectrum of early-onset esotropia: experience of the Congenital Esotropia Observational Study. *Am J Ophthalmol.* 2002;133(1): 102–108.

Simonsz HJ, Kolling GH, Unnebrink K. Final report of the early vs late infantile strabismus surgery study (ELISSS), a controlled, prospective, multicenter study. *Strabismus.* 2005;13(4): 169–199.

Acquired Nonaccommodative Esotropia

Several types of comitant esotropia not associated with activation of the accommodative reflex may develop in later infancy (>6 months), childhood, or even adulthood. The causes of these acquired nonaccommodative esotropias are varied.

Basic Acquired Nonaccommodative Esotropia

Basic acquired nonaccommodative esotropia is a comitant esotropia that develops after age 6 months and is not associated with an accommodative component. As in infantile esotropia, the amount of hyperopia is not significant, and the angle of deviation is similar when measured at distance and near. Acquired esotropia may be acute in onset. In such cases, the patient immediately becomes aware of the deviation and may have diplopia. A careful evaluation is important to rule out an accommodative or paretic component. Temporary but prolonged disruption of binocular vision—such as that resulting from a hyphema, preseptal cellulitis, mechanical ptosis, or prolonged patching for amblyopia—is a known precipitating cause of acquired nonaccommodative esotropia. Prolonged use of devices at near fixation is also a risk factor. In patients with acquired nonaccommodative esotropia, fusion is thought to be tenuous, so this temporary disruption of binocular vision upsets the balance, resulting in esotropia. Because the onset of nonaccommodative esotropia in an older child may be a sign of an underlying neurologic disorder, neuroimaging and neurologic evaluation may be indicated, especially when other symptoms or signs of neurologic abnormality are present, such as lateral incomitance, deviation greater at distance than near, small V-pattern incomitance, abnormal head position, or concomitant headache.

Many patients with acquired nonaccommodative esotropia have a history of normal binocular vision; thus, the prognosis for restoration of single binocular vision with prisms and/or surgery is good. Therapy consists of amblyopia treatment, if necessary, and surgical correction or botulinum toxin injection as soon as possible after the onset of the deviation. The Prism Adaptation Study showed a smaller undercorrection rate (approximately 10% less) when the amount of surgery was based on the prism-adapted angle.

Jacobs SM, Green-Simms A, Diehl NN, Mohney BG. Long-term follow-up of acquired nonaccommodative esotropia in a population-based cohort. *Ophthalmology.* 2011; 118(6):1170–1174.

Repka MX, Connett JE, Scott WE. The one-year surgical outcome after prism adaptation for the management of acquired esotropia. *Ophthalmology.* 1996;103(6):922–928.

Cyclic Esotropia

Cyclic esotropia is a rare form of strabismus; other forms of cyclic strabismus occur but are even rarer. Onset of cyclic esotropia is typically during the preschool years. The esotropia is comitant and intermittent, usually occurring every other day (48-hour cycle). Variable intervals and 24-hour cycles have also been documented.

Fusion and binocular vision are usually absent or defective on the strabismic day, with marked improvement or normalization on the orthotropic day. Occlusion therapy may convert the cyclic deviation into a constant one.

Surgical treatment of cyclic esotropia is usually effective. The amount of surgery is based on the maximum angle of deviation present when the eyes are esotropic.

Sensory Esotropia

Monocular vision loss (due to cataract, corneal clouding, optic nerve or retinal disorders, or various other entities) may cause sensory (deprivation) esotropia. Conditions preventing clear and focused retinal images and symmetric visual stimulation must be identified and remedied promptly, if possible, to prevent irreversible amblyopia. If surgery or botulinum toxin injection is indicated for strabismus, it is generally performed only on the eye with a significant vision deficit.

Divergence Insufficiency

In divergence insufficiency, the characteristic finding is an esodeviation that is greater at distance than at near. The deviation is horizontally comitant, and fusional divergence is reduced.

Primary divergence insufficiency is an increasingly diagnosed type of adult strabismus. In one form, *adult-onset distance esotropia,* the entity is a slowly progressing, benign condition that occurs predominantly in patients older than 50 years. Affected individuals report a gradual onset of horizontal diplopia that is present at distance but not at near. Imaging may demonstrate thinning, elongation, and rupture of the connective tissue between the lateral and superior rectus muscles and sagging and elongation of the lateral rectus muscles. Management consists of base-out prisms, botulinum toxin injection of the medial rectus muscles, and strabismus surgery. In patients with adult-onset distance esotropia, reestablishment of binocular fusion generally occurs following treatment. Another, more recently recognized form of primary divergence insufficiency is acquired distance esotropia associated with myopia in the young adult, usually resulting from prolonged near work.

The secondary form of divergence insufficiency is rare and is associated with neurologic abnormalities, including pontine tumors, increased intracranial pressure, or severe head trauma. In these secondary cases, the divergence insufficiency is probably due to a mild CN VI paresis. In patients with secondary divergence insufficiency, neuroimaging is required to rule out treatable intracranial lesions.

Chaudhuri Z, Demer JL. Sagging eye syndrome: connective tissue involution as a cause of horizontal and vertical strabismus in older patients. *JAMA Ophthalmol.* 2013;131(5): 619–625.

Spasm of the Near Reflex

Spasm of the near reflex (also known as *ciliary spasm* or *convergence spasm*) is a spectrum of abnormalities of the near response. The etiology is generally thought to be functional, related to psychological factors such as stress and anxiety. In rare cases, it can be associated with organic disease. Patients present with varying combinations of excessive convergence, increased accommodation, and miosis. Patients may present with acute esotropia alternating with orthotropia. Substitution of a convergence movement for a gaze movement with horizontal versions is characteristic. Monocular abduction is normal despite marked limitation of abduction on version testing. Pseudomyopia may occur.

Treatment consists of cycloplegic agents such as atropine or homatropine, hyperopic correction, and bifocal glasses. Counseling to address underlying psychological issues may be helpful. If the spasm cannot be broken, botulinum toxin injection of the medial rectus muscles and strabismus surgery may be considered with caution.

Kaczmarek BB, Dawson E, Lee JP. Convergence spasm treated with botulinum toxin. *Strabismus.* 2009;17(1):49–51.

Consecutive Esotropia

Consecutive esotropia refers to an esotropia that follows a history of exotropia. It can arise spontaneously, or it can develop after surgery for exotropia. Spontaneous consecutive esotropia is rare and almost always occurs in patients with neurologic disorders or with very poor vision in 1 eye. Postsurgical consecutive esotropia, on the other hand, is common. Fortunately, it often resolves over time without treatment. In fact, an initial small overcorrection is desirable after surgery for exotropia, as it is associated with an improved long-term success rate. Treatment options for consecutive esotropia include base-out prisms, hyperopic correction, alternating occlusion, botulinum toxin injection, and strabismus surgery. In postsurgical consecutive esotropia, unless the deviation is very large or a slipped or "lost" muscle is suspected, surgery or botulinum toxin injection may be postponed for several months after onset because of the possibility of spontaneous improvement.

A slipped or lost lateral rectus muscle (discussed in Chapter 13) produces various amounts of esotropia and incomitance, depending on the amount of slippage, and should be suspected in consecutive esotropia following lateral rectus recession surgery if a significant abduction deficit is present. However, if the ipsilateral medial rectus muscle was resected at the time of the lateral rectus recession, the consecutive esotropia could be due to a tight medial rectus muscle. Forced duction testing can help differentiate between these 2 causes. In cases of a slipped or lost lateral rectus muscle, surgical exploration is required (see Chapter 13).

Incomitant Esotropia

Several positional, restrictive, and innervational abnormalities of the extraocular muscles may result in incomitant esotropia (see Table 7-1).

Cranial Nerve VI Palsy

General considerations and differential diagnoses

Weakness of the lateral rectus muscle due to palsy of the abducens nerve results in incomitant esotropia. CN VI palsy occurring in the neonatal period is rare and usually transient. Most cases of suspected congenital CN VI palsy are actually infantile esotropia with cross-fixation. Congenital CN VI palsy may be difficult to differentiate from the congenital cranial dysinnervation disorder (CCDD) esotropic Duane syndrome, which is more common in young infants (see Chapter 11), as the unique retraction feature of this syndrome may not yet be evident. A distinguishing characteristic is that for an equal amount of abduction deficit, the deviation in primary position is usually much larger in CN VI palsy than it is in esotropic Duane syndrome.

Pathogenesis

Congenital CN VI palsy is usually benign and transient and may be caused by the increased intracranial pressure associated with the birth process. CN VI palsy in older children is associated with intracranial lesions in approximately one-third of cases; these cases have additional neurologic findings. Other cases may be related to infectious or immunologic processes involving CN VI. The most common cause of isolated, transient CN VI palsy in a child is thought to be a virus; in an adult, it is a microvascular occlusive event.

Clinical features

Older children and adults may report diplopia. Often there is a compensatory head turn toward the side of the paralyzed lateral rectus muscle, adopted to place the eyes in a position where they are best aligned. If a child presents soon after the onset of the deviation, vision in the eyes is usually equal. The esotropia increases in gaze toward the side of the paralyzed lateral rectus muscle, and versions show limited or no abduction of the affected eye (Fig 7-4). Results of the saccadic velocity test show slowing of the affected lateral rectus muscle, and active force generation tests document weakness of that muscle.

Evaluation

It is important to take a careful history that includes antecedent infections, head trauma, and hydrocephalus, as well as hypertension and diabetes in adults. Considering the high prevalence of associated intracranial lesions in children with CN VI palsy, neurologic evaluation and magnetic resonance imaging of the head and orbit are usually indicated, even in the absence of other focal neurologic findings.

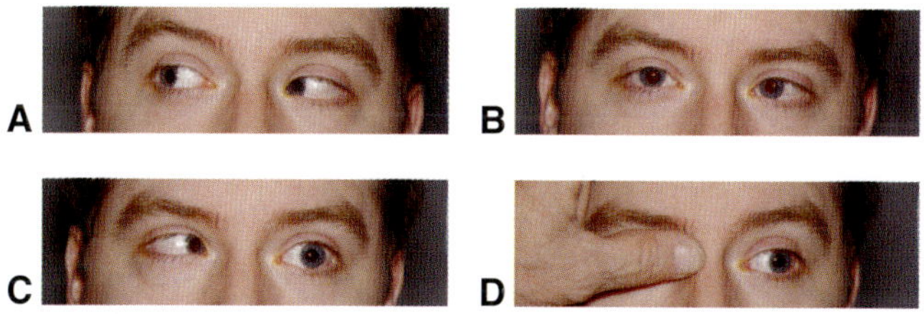

Figure 7-4 Cranial nerve (CN) VI palsy, left eye. **A,** Right gaze. **B,** Esotropia in primary position. **C,** Limited abduction, left eye. **D,** Abduction is still incomplete, but there is further abduction when the left eye is fixating, an important finding for the surgical correction plan. *(Courtesy of Edward L. Raab, MD.)*

Management

Patching may be necessary to prevent or treat amblyopia if the child is not using a compensatory head posture or if the child is very young. Press-on prisms are sometimes used to correct diplopia in primary position. Correction of a significant hyperopic refractive error may help prevent the development of an associated accommodative esotropia. Botulinum toxin injection of the ipsilateral medial rectus muscle is sometimes employed to temporarily decrease the esotropia. If the deviation does not resolve after 6 months of treatment, surgery may be indicated. Options include horizontal rectus muscle surgery if abduction is at least partially preserved or vertical rectus muscle transposition surgery if abduction is absent (see Chapter 13).

See BCSC Section 5, *Neuro-Ophthalmology,* for further discussion of CN VI palsy.

Other Forms of Incomitant Esotropia

Medial rectus muscle restriction may result from thyroid eye disease, orbital myositis, medial orbital wall fracture with medial rectus entrapment, excessive medial rectus muscle resection, or CCDDs. For CCDDs such as Duane syndrome and Möbius syndrome, secondary restriction of the medial rectus may develop later. In patients with high myopia, esotropia may develop because of prolapse of the posterior globe between displaced lateral and superior rectus muscles. Periocular implants, such as scleral buckles or glaucoma drainage devices, can also produce incomitant esotropia.

For further discussion of these special forms of strabismus, see Chapter 11 in this volume and BCSC Section 5, *Neuro-Ophthalmology.*

Nystagmus and Esotropia

Several types of nystagmus are associated with esotropia. *Fusion maldevelopment nystagmus syndrome* is a common feature of infantile esotropia. Ciancia syndrome (discussed earlier in this chapter) is a severe form of infantile esotropia associated with an abducting nystagmus. *Nystagmus blockage syndrome* occurs in children with congenital motor nystagmus, who use convergence to “dampen” or decrease the amplitude or frequency of their nystagmus (null position in convergence), resulting in esotropia. See also Chapter 12.

CHAPTER 8

Exodeviations

Highlights

- The classification of intermittent exotropia is based on the difference between distance and near deviations.
- The form of exotropia that responds to orthoptic exercises is convergence insufficiency exotropia with diplopia.
- Infants with constant exotropia have increased risk of associated neurologic impairment or craniofacial disorders.

Introduction

An exodeviation is a manifest (exotropia) or latent (exophoria) divergent strabismus. Risk factors for exotropia include maternal substance abuse and smoking during pregnancy, premature birth, perinatal morbidity, genetic anomalies, family history of strabismus, and uncorrected refractive errors.

Pseudoexotropia

The term *pseudoexotropia* refers to an appearance of exodeviation when the eyes are actually aligned. Pseudoexotropia is much less common than pseudoesotropia (see Chapter 7 for discussion of pseudoesotropia) and may occur when there is a wide interpupillary distance or a positive angle kappa with or without other ocular abnormalities (see the discussions of angle kappa in Chapter 6 of this volume and in BCSC Section 3, *Clinical Optics and Vision Rehabilitation*).

Exophoria

Exophoria is a relatively common exodeviation that is controlled by fusion under normal binocular viewing conditions. An exophoria is detected when binocular vision is interrupted, such as during an alternate cover test or monocular visual acuity testing. Patients with exophoria are usually asymptomatic, although they may experience asthenopia with prolonged near work. Decompensation of an exophoria to an exotropia may occur when the patient is ill or under the influence of sedatives or alcohol. Treatment is recommended when the exophoria becomes symptomatic.

Intermittent Exotropia

Intermittent exotropia is the most common type of manifest exodeviation; major types include (Fig 8-1)

- basic intermittent exotropia
- exotropia with high accommodative convergence/accommodation (AC/A) ratio
- divergence excess exotropia
- convergence insufficiency exotropia

Clinical Characteristics

The onset of intermittent exotropia is usually before age 5 years, and the exotropia typically continues into adulthood. The exodeviation becomes manifest during times of visual inattention, fatigue, stress, or illness. Parents of affected children often report that the exotropia occurs late in the day or when the child is daydreaming or tired. Exposure to bright light often triggers exodeviation and a reflex closure of 1 eye (which is why strabismus is sometimes referred to as a "squint").

Exodeviations are usually larger when the patient views distant targets, and they may be difficult to elicit at near fixation. Because most parental interactions with young children occur at near, parents of a child with intermittent exotropia may not notice it initially. Intermittent exotropia can be associated with small hypertropias, A and V patterns, and overelevation and underelevation in adduction (see Chapter 9).

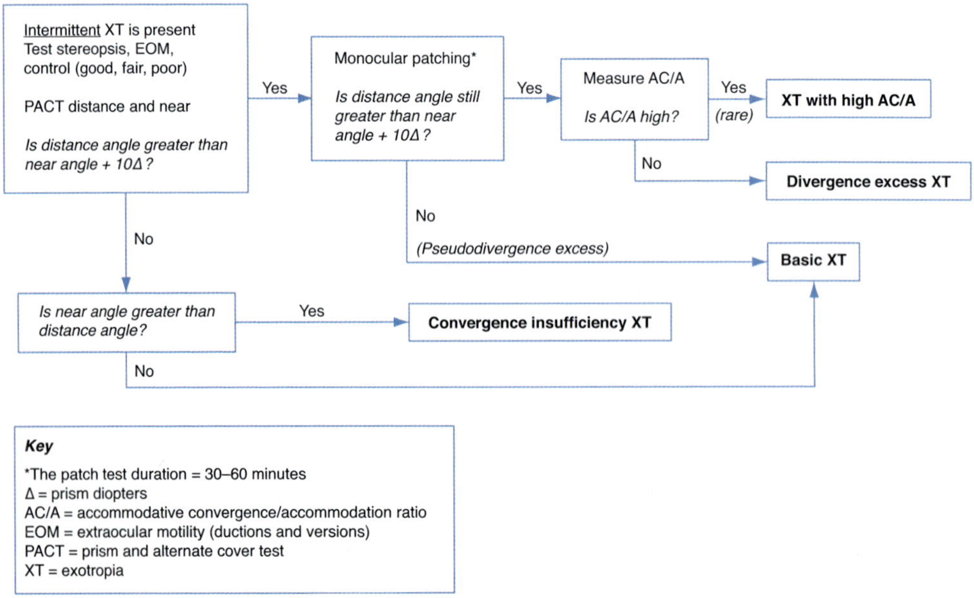

Figure 8-1 Diagnostic algorithm and classification of intermittent exotropia. *(Courtesy of Ta Chen Peter Chang, MD.)*

Left untreated, intermittent exotropia may remain stable, resolve, or progress, sometimes to constant exotropia. Because of suppression, children younger than 10 years with intermittent exotropia rarely report diplopia. They retain normal retinal correspondence and good binocular function when orthotropic. Loss of stereoacuity may occur if the strabismus is poorly controlled or becomes constant. Amblyopia is uncommon. Adults with poorly controlled intermittent or constant exotropia often experience significant psychological stress, anxiety, and depression because of their strabismus. Adults with strabismus often report reduced quality of life, obtain lower levels of education, and may have limited career choices and advancement opportunities.

Evaluation

History

Important aspects of history include the age at onset of the strabismus, frequency and duration of misalignment, circumstances under which the deviation is manifest, and whether the exotropia is becoming more frequent with time. The clinician should determine whether symptoms such as diplopia, asthenopia, or difficulty with interpersonal interactions secondary to ocular misalignment are present.

Examination

Because visual acuity and alignment tests are dissociating and may adversely affect assessment of strabismus control, sensory tests for stereopsis and fusion are typically performed first (see Chapter 6). A typical examination order is:

1. stereopsis (distance and near)
2. duction and version
3. exodeviation control
4. alignment angle
5. visual acuity

Exotropia control can be categorized as

- *Good:* Exotropia manifests only after cover testing; the patient resumes fusion rapidly without blinking or refixating.
- *Fair:* Exotropia manifests after fusion is disrupted by cover testing; the patient resumes fusion only after blinking or refixating.
- *Poor:* Exotropia manifests spontaneously; it may remain manifest for an extended time.

Prism and alternate cover testing is used to evaluate the exodeviation at fixation distances of 6 m and 33 cm. A far-distance measurement at 30 m or greater (eg, at the end of a long hallway or out a window) may uncover a latent deviation or elicit an even larger one. At this point, several findings are possible:

- The distance exotropia angle is similar (within 10 prism diopters [Δ]) to the near exotropia angle.
- The distance exotropia angle is greater than the near exotropia angle by at least 10Δ.
- The near exotropia angle is greater than the distance exotropia angle.

Classification

Distance exotropia angle is similar to near exotropia angle

If the distance exotropia angle is similar to the near exotropia angle, the diagnosis is *basic intermittent exotropia.*

Distance exotropia angle is greater than near exotropia angle

When the distance angle is greater than the near angle by at least 10Δ, this difference is usually due to *tenacious proximal fusion* (a slow-to-dissipate fusion mechanism at near) causing *pseudodivergence excess* in a patient with basic intermittent exotropia. The difference may sometimes be due to a high accommodative convergence/accommodation (AC/A) ratio; however, a high AC/A ratio occurs much less commonly in exotropia than in esotropia (see Chapter 6, which discusses measurement of AC/A ratios). Thus, when the exodeviation at distance is larger than the deviation at near fixation by 10Δ or more, the near exodeviation should be remeasured after 1 eye is occluded for 30–60 minutes (the patch test). This test eliminates the effects of tenacious proximal fusion and distinguishes pseudodivergence excess from true divergence excess. A patient with pseudodivergence excess has similar distance and near measurements after the patch test. A patient with true divergence excess continues to have a significantly larger exodeviation at distance. Many patients with true divergence excess also have a high AC/A ratio. For these patients, the AC/A ratio can be determined by measuring the near deviation with and without +3.00 diopter (D) lenses (while the patient wears corrective lenses, if necessary), after the patch test is completed. The measurements are then compared. Alternatively, the distance deviation can be measured with and without −2.00 D lenses to determine the AC/A ratio.

Near exotropia angle is greater than distance exotropia angle

Convergence insufficiency (CI) is an exodeviation that is greater at near fixation than at distance fixation. It is characterized by poor fusional convergence amplitudes and a remote near point of convergence (normal fusional vergence amplitudes are given in Chapter 6, Table 6-1). This sometimes results in symptoms of asthenopia, blurred near vision, and diplopia during near work, usually in older children or adults. Convergence insufficiency is a common complication of Parkinson disease. Rarely, accommodative spasms occur when accommodation and convergence are stimulated in an effort to overcome the CI.

American Academy of Ophthalmology Pediatric Ophthalmology/Strabismus Panel, Hoskins Center for Quality Eye Care. Preferred Practice Pattern Guidelines. *Esotropia and Exotropia.* American Academy of Ophthalmology; 2017. www.aao.org/ppp

Treatment

It is important to monitor all patients with exodeviations as some will require treatment. Opinions vary widely regarding the timing of surgery and the use of nonsurgical treatments. Patients who have well-controlled, asymptomatic intermittent exotropia and good binocular fusion can be observed. Untreated strabismus often results in poor self-esteem in both adults and children. Adults with strabismus report a wide range of difficulties with social interactions, which improve significantly after surgery.

Nonsurgical management

Correction of refractive errors Corrective lenses should be prescribed for significant refractive errors. Correction of even mild myopia may improve control of the exodeviation. Mild-to-moderate degrees of hyperopia are not routinely corrected in children with intermittent exotropia because refractive correction may worsen the deviation. Children with marked hyperopia (> +4.00 D) may be unable to sustain accommodation, which results in a blurred retinal image and manifest exotropia. In these patients, correction of refractive errors with glasses or contacts may improve retinal image clarity and help control the exodeviation.

In some cases, overcorrection of myopia by 2.00–4.00 D can stimulate accommodative convergence to help control the exodeviation. It can be effective as a temporizing measure to promote fusion and delay surgery in children with an immature visual system. However, in school-aged children this therapy may cause asthenopia, which may limit its usefulness. For patients whose initial overcorrection results in control, the prescription can be gradually tapered and surgery may be avoided.

Occlusion therapy Occlusion therapy (patching) for amblyopia may improve exotropic deviations. For patients without amblyopia, part-time patching of the dominant (nondeviating) eye or alternate patching (alternating which eye is patched each day) in the absence of a strong ocular preference can improve control of small- to moderate-sized deviations, particularly in young children. The improvement is often temporary, however, and many patients eventually require surgery.

Prisms Although they can be used to promote fusion in intermittent exotropia, base-in prisms are seldom chosen for long-term management because they can cause a reduction in fusional vergence amplitudes. In older adults with CI, base-in prism reading glasses may alleviate symptoms of asthenopia.

Orthoptic exercises Treatment of symptomatic CI typically involves orthoptic exercises such as stereograms, "pencil push-ups," and computer-based or office-based convergence training programs. In children and young adults, randomized controlled trials found that office-based vergence and accommodative therapies were effective in improving motor outcomes but had conflicting results in alleviating CI symptoms.

CITT-ART Investigator Group. Treatment of symptomatic convergence insufficiency in children enrolled in the Convergence Insufficiency Treatment Trial—Attention and Reading Trial: a randomized clinical trial. *Optom Vis Sci.* 2019;96(11):825–835.

Surgical treatment

Factors influencing the decision to proceed with surgery include strabismus that is frequently manifest, poorly controlled, worsening (especially at near), symptomatic; decreased stereoacuity in the distance before near; poor self-image; and difficulty with personal or professional relationships. Strabismus surgery is reconstructive, not cosmetic, and may alleviate anxiety and depression in some patients.

Surgical treatment of exotropia typically consists of bilateral lateral rectus muscle recession or unilateral lateral rectus muscle recession combined with medial rectus muscle resection. Large (>50Δ) deviations may require surgery on 3 or 4 muscles; for small deviations, single-muscle recession is sometimes performed. The optimal age for surgery and the choice of procedure are debatable. Caution is advised when surgery is considered for a patient with true divergence excess exotropia, especially with a high AC/A ratio, because of the associated risk of postoperative diplopia and esotropia at near.

Adams GG, McBain H, MacKenzie K, Hancox J, Ezra DG, Newman SP. Is strabismus the only problem? Psychological issues surrounding strabismus surgery. *J AAPOS.* 2016;20(5):383–386.

Joyce KE, Beyer F, Thomson RG, Clarke MP. A systematic review of the effectiveness of treatments in altering the natural history of intermittent exotropia. *Br J Ophthalmol.* 2015;99(4):440–450.

Postoperative alignment A small-angle esotropia in the immediate postoperative period tends to resolve and is desirable because of its association with a reduced risk of recurrent exotropia and with higher success rates. Preoperatively, it is important to advise patients that they may experience diplopia while esotropic. An esodeviation that persists beyond 3–4 weeks or that develops 1–2 months after surgery *(postsurgical esotropia)* may require further treatment, such as hyperopic correction, base-out prisms, patching to prevent amblyopia, or additional surgery. Bifocal glasses can be used in patients with a high AC/A ratio and should be discussed preoperatively with these patients. Unless deficient ductions suggest a slipped or "lost" muscle, a delay of a few months is recommended before reoperation for postsurgical esotropia, because spontaneous improvement may occur.

Because of the possibility of persistent consecutive esodeviations, some ophthalmologists prefer to delay surgery in young children who have good preoperative visual acuity and stereopsis. Others, however, consider surgical delay a risk factor for recurrence of strabismus. Long-term follow-up studies of the effectiveness of surgical treatment of intermittent exotropia show high recurrence rates. Patients may require multiple surgeries to maintain ocular alignment long term.

Astudillo PP, Cotesta M, Schofield J, Kraft S, Mireskandari K. The effect of achieving immediate target angle on success of strabismus surgery in children. *Am J Ophthalmol.* 2015;160(5):913–918.

Constant Exotropia

Constant exotropia is encountered most often in older patients with sensory exotropia or in patients with a history of long-standing intermittent exotropia that has decompensated. Constant exotropia also occurs in persons with infantile or consecutive exotropia. A patient with an exotropia that is constant can have basic, pseudodivergence excess, or true divergence excess exotropia—the same forms seen in intermittent exotropia.

Some patients with constant exotropia have an enlarged field of peripheral vision because they have large areas of nonoverlapping visual fields. These patients may notice a field constriction when the eyes are straightened.

Surgical treatment is the same as that for intermittent exotropia, discussed earlier in the chapter.

Infantile Exotropia

Infantile exotropia is much less common than infantile esotropia. Constant infantile exotropia is apparent before age 6 months as a large-angle deviation (Fig 8-2). The risk of amblyopia is higher in constant exotropia than in intermittent exotropia. Although infants with constant exotropia may be otherwise healthy, the risk of associated neurologic impairment or craniofacial disorders is increased in these patients. A careful developmental history is thus important, and referral for neurologic assessment should be considered if there are indications of developmental delay. Patients with constant infantile exotropia undergo surgery early in life, and surgical outcomes are similar to those for infantile esotropia (see Chapter 7). Early surgery can lead to monofixation with gross binocular vision, but restoration of normal binocular function is rare. Dissociated vertical deviations and overelevation in adduction may develop (see Chapter 10).

Sensory Exotropia

Esotropia or exotropia may develop as a result of any condition that severely reduces vision or the visual field in 1 eye. It is not known why some individuals become esotropic and others exotropic after unilateral vision loss. In addition, although both sensory esotropia and sensory exotropia occur in infants and young children, the latter predominates in older children and adults. If the vision in the exotropic eye can be improved, peripheral fusion may be reestablished after surgical realignment, provided the sensory exotropia has not been present for an extended period. Loss of fusional abilities, known as *central fusion disruption,* can lead to constant and permanent diplopia despite anatomical realignment when adult-onset sensory exotropia has been present for several years before vision rehabilitation.

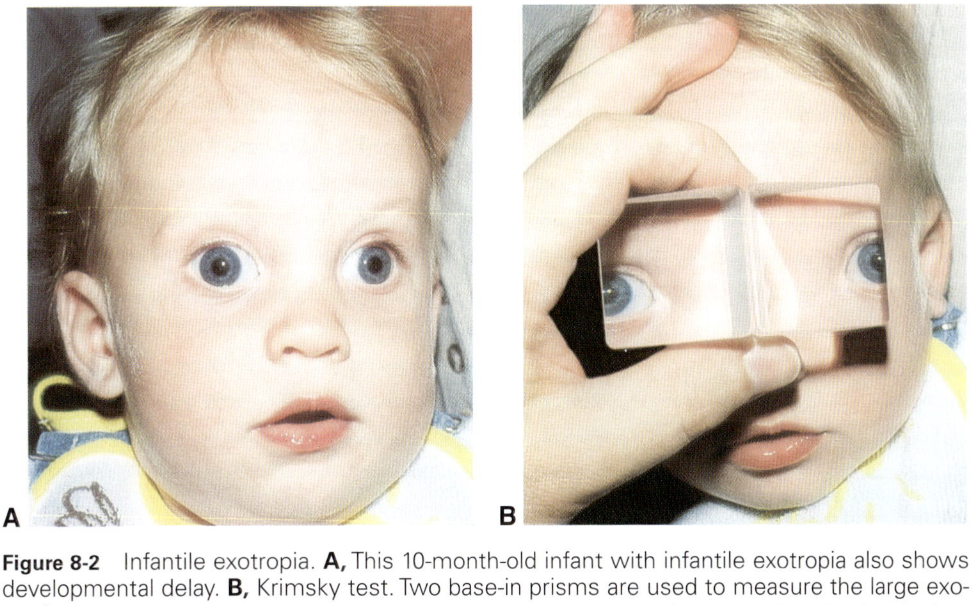

Figure 8-2 Infantile exotropia. **A,** This 10-month-old infant with infantile exotropia also shows developmental delay. **B,** Krimsky test. Two base-in prisms are used to measure the large exotropia. *(Reproduced from Wilson ME. Exotropia.* Focal Points: Clinical Modules for Ophthalmologists. *American Academy of Ophthalmology; 1995, module 11.)*

Consecutive Exotropia

Exotropia that occurs after a period of esotropia is called *consecutive exotropia.* In rare cases, exotropia may develop spontaneously in a patient who was previously esotropic and never underwent strabismus surgery. Much more commonly, consecutive exotropia develops after previous surgery for esotropia *(postsurgical exotropia),* usually within a few months or years after the initial surgery. However, in some patients who had surgery for infantile esotropia, consecutive exotropia may not develop until adulthood. Consecutive exotropia may be intermittent or constant.

Other Forms of Exotropia

Exotropic Duane Syndrome

The most widely used classification of Duane syndrome defines 3 types. Patients with type 2 can present with exotropia, usually accompanied by deficient adduction and a head turn away from the affected side. See Chapter 11 for further discussion.

Neuromuscular Abnormalities

A constant exotropia may result from cranial nerve (CN) III nerve palsy, internuclear ophthalmoplegia, or myasthenia gravis. These conditions are discussed in Chapter 11 of this volume and in BCSC Section 5, *Neuro-Ophthalmology.*

Dissociated Horizontal Deviation

Dissociated strabismus complex may include vertical, horizontal, and/or torsional components (see Chapter 10 and the Appendix). It may be associated with infantile esotropia. When a dissociated abduction movement is predominant, the condition is called *dissociated horizontal deviation (DHD).* Though not a true exotropia, DHD can be confused with a constant or intermittent exotropia and may be incomitant when fixation is switched from 1 eye to the other. Dissociated vertical deviation and latent nystagmus often coexist with DHD (Fig 8-3). In rare cases, patients may manifest both DHD and intermittent esotropia. DHD must be differentiated from anisohyperopia associated with intermittent

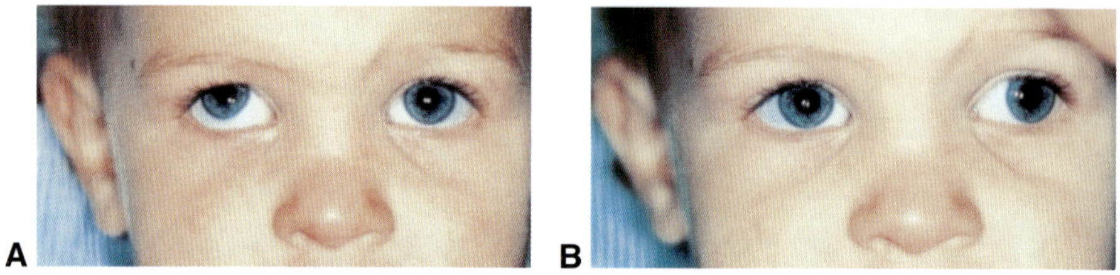

Figure 8-3 Dissociated strabismus complex. **A,** When the patient fixates with the left eye, a prominent vertical deviation is observed in the right eye. **B,** However, when the patient fixates with the right eye, a prominent horizontal deviation is noted in the left eye. *(Reproduced from Wilson ME. Exotropia.* Focal Points: Clinical Modules for Ophthalmologists. *American Academy of Ophthalmology; 1995, module 11.)*

exotropia, in which the exotropic deviation is present during fixation with the normal eye but is masked during fixation with the hyperopic eye because of accommodative convergence. Treatment of DHD usually consists of unilateral or bilateral lateral rectus recession in addition to any necessary oblique or vertical muscle surgery.

Convergence Paralysis

Convergence paralysis is distinct from convergence insufficiency and is usually secondary to an intracranial lesion, most commonly in association with dorsal midbrain syndrome (see BCSC Section 5, *Neuro-Ophthalmology*). It is characterized by normal adduction and accommodation, with exotropia and diplopia present at attempted near fixation only. Apparent convergence paralysis due to malingering or lack of effort can be distinguished from true convergence paralysis by the presence of pupillary constriction with attempted near fixation in true convergence paralysis and its absence in malingering or lack of effort.

Treatment of convergence paralysis is difficult and often limited to use of base-in prisms at near to alleviate the diplopia. Plus lenses may be required if accommodation is limited. Monocular occlusion is indicated if diplopia cannot be otherwise treated.

CHAPTER 9

Pattern Strabismus

Highlights

- Oblique muscle weakening can correct pattern strabismus associated with oblique muscle overaction.
- In the absence of oblique muscle dysfunction, vertical transposition of the medial recti toward the apex or the lateral recti toward the base of the pattern can correct the pattern.
- Pseudo-inferior oblique overaction with a Y pattern is often a disorder of anomalous innervation; in this situation inferior oblique recession is of no benefit.

Introduction

Pattern strabismus is a horizontal deviation in which there is a difference in the magnitude of deviation between upgaze and downgaze. *V pattern* describes a horizontal deviation that is more divergent (less convergent) in upgaze than in downgaze, while *A pattern* describes a horizontal deviation that is more divergent (less convergent) in downgaze than in upgaze. An A or V pattern is found in 15%–25% of horizontal strabismus cases. Less common variations of pattern strabismus include Y, X, and λ (lambda) patterns.

Etiology

The following conditions are associated with various types of pattern strabismus or considered causes of these patterns:

- *Oblique muscle dysfunction.* Inferior oblique muscle overaction is associated with *overelevation in adduction (OEAd;* see Chapter 10) and V patterns (Fig 9-1), and superior oblique muscle overaction is associated with *overdepression in adduction (ODAd)* and A patterns (Fig 9-2). These associations may be due to the tertiary abducting action of these muscles in upgaze and downgaze, respectively; however, oblique dysfunction is frequently associated with ocular torsion that can also contribute to A or V patterns (see below).
- *Orbital pulley system abnormalities.* Extraocular muscle pulley heterotopy (see Chapter 2), in which horizontal rectus muscle pulleys are shifted superiorly or inferiorly or vertical rectus muscle pulleys are shifted nasally or temporally from their typical locations, can result in altered muscle paths and thus altered direction of pull. This altered direction of pull can simulate oblique muscle overaction, resulting

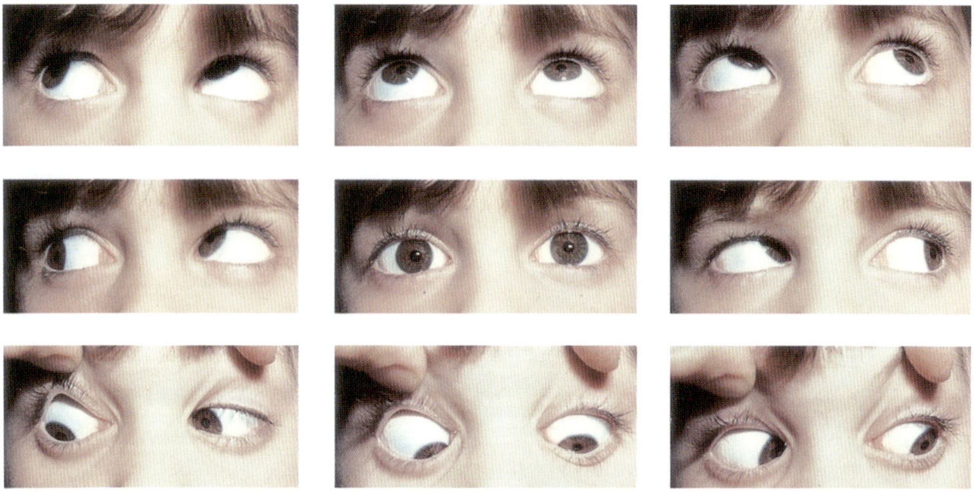

Figure 9-1 V pattern with exotropia in upgaze and esotropia in downgaze. Note bilateral over-elevation in adduction and limitation of depression in adduction.

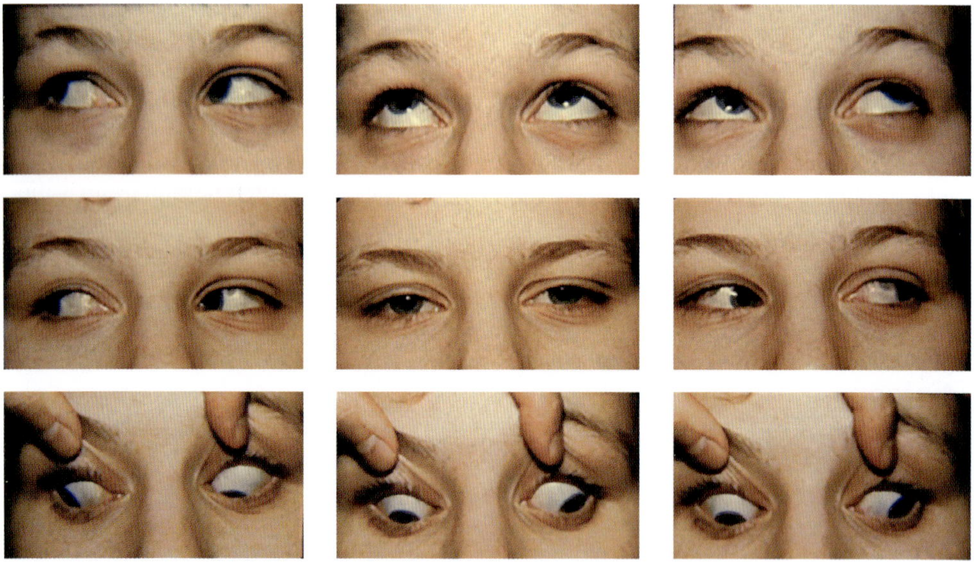

Figure 9-2 A-pattern exotropia worse in downgaze. Note marked bilateral overdepression in adduction and milder bilateral underelevation in adduction. *(Modified with permission from Levin A, Wilson T, eds.* The Hospital for Sick Children's Atlas of Pediatric Ophthalmology and Strabismus. *Lippincott Williams & Wilkins; 2007:11.)*

in A or V patterns. These pulley effects may help explain why patients with upward- or downward-slanting palpebral fissures (Fig 9-3) may show A or V patterns, respectively; an underlying variation in orbital configuration is reflected in the orientation of the fissures. Similarly, patients with craniofacial anomalies (see Chapter 17) may have a V-pattern strabismus with marked elevation of the adducting eye as a manifestation of excyclorotation of the orbits, pulley system, and muscle pathways.

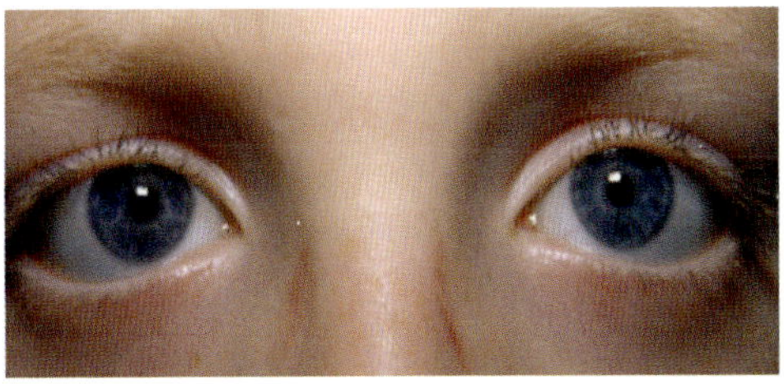

Figure 9-3 Palpebral fissures that slant downward temporally, sometimes associated with a V-pattern horizontal deviation. *(Courtesy of Edward L. Raab, MD.)*

- *Ocular torsion.* Ocular torsion displaces the insertions of the vertical rectus muscles relative to the orbit; studies of the normal compensatory torsional response to head tilt show that it is also associated, to a lesser extent, with displacement of the pulley system. Torsion thus shifts the anterior paths of the muscles: extorsion displaces the superior rectus muscle temporally and the inferior rectus muscle nasally, which tends to produce a V pattern; conversely, intorsion tends to produce an A pattern.
- *Restricted horizontal rectus muscles.* Contracture of the lateral rectus muscles in patients with large-angle exotropia may result in an X pattern, with globe slippage above or below the tight muscle.
- *Anomalous innervation.* Sometimes seen in isolation and sometimes associated with other congenital cranial dysinnervation disorders (see Chapter 11), this most commonly produces a Y pattern.
- *Compartmentalized innervation of superior and inferior compartments of the horizontal rectus muscles* (see Chapter 2). It is conceivable that compartmentalized innervation could contribute to A and V patterns if there were also differential relative activation of the 2 compartments in upgaze and downgaze, but this is currently speculative.

Clinical Features and Identification of Pattern Strabismus

To identify pattern strabismus, the examiner measures alignment with appropriate refractive correction using prism and alternate cover testing while the patient fixates at distance in primary position and in straight upgaze and downgaze, approximately 25° from the primary position. It is also important to note any associated apparent oblique muscle overaction (OEAd or ODAd).

An A, Y, or λ pattern is considered clinically significant when the difference in measurement between upgaze and downgaze is at least 10 prism diopters (Δ). For a V pattern, this difference must be at least 15Δ, because slightly more physiologic convergence in downgaze is normal.

V Pattern

The most common type of pattern strabismus is the V pattern, which is frequent in patients with infantile esotropia. It is usually not present when the esotropia first develops but becomes apparent during the first year of life or later. V patterns may also occur in patients with superior oblique palsies, particularly if they are bilateral, and in patients with craniofacial malformations.

A Pattern

The second most common type of pattern strabismus, the A pattern occurs most frequently in patients with exotropia and in persons with spina bifida.

Y Pattern

In patients with Y patterns (pseudo-overaction of the inferior oblique muscle), the ocular alignment may be normal in primary position and downgaze, but the eyes diverge in upgaze. Although these patients appear to have overaction of inferior oblique muscles, the deviation is thought to be due to anomalous innervation, with activation of the lateral rectus muscles during upgaze. Clinical features of this form of strabismus include the following:

- The overelevation is not seen when the eyes are moved directly horizontally, but it becomes manifest when the eyes are moved horizontally and slightly into upgaze.
- There is no fundus torsion.
- There is no difference in vertical deviation with head tilts.
- There is no superior oblique muscle underaction.

Kushner BJ. Pseudo inferior oblique overaction associated with Y and V patterns. *Ophthalmology.* 1991;98(10):1500–1505.

X Pattern

In X-pattern strabismus, an exodeviation is present in primary position and increases in both upgaze and downgaze. This pattern is usually associated with OEAd and ODAd when the eye moves slightly above or below direct side gaze. X patterns are most commonly seen in patients with large-angle exotropia.

λ Pattern

This rare pattern is a variant of A-pattern exotropia. In λ-pattern strabismus, the horizontal deviation is the same in primary position and upgaze but becomes more divergent in downgaze. The λ pattern is usually associated with ODAd.

Management

Clinically significant patterns (see the section Clinical Features and Identification of Pattern Strabismus) are typically treated surgically, in combination with correction of the underlying horizontal deviation.

Surgical Correction of Pattern Deviations: General Principles

The following are strategies for surgical correction of pattern deviations. See Chapter 13 for further discussion of some of the procedures and concepts mentioned here.

Weakening of the oblique muscles

For pattern strabismus (other than Y pattern) associated with corresponding apparent overaction of the oblique muscles (OEAd, ODAd), weakening of the oblique muscles is performed. There is uncertainty over whether oblique muscle weakening significantly affects the horizontal deviation in the primary position.

Vertical transposition of horizontal rectus muscles

For patients with no apparent overaction of the oblique muscles or a pattern inconsistent with oblique dysfunction, vertical transposition of the horizontal muscles is performed. The muscles are transposed from one-half to a full tendon width. Medial rectus muscles are always moved toward the "apex" of the pattern (ie, downward in V patterns and upward in A patterns). Lateral rectus muscles are moved toward the open end (ie, upward in V patterns and downward in A patterns) (Fig 9-4). These rules apply whether the horizontal rectus muscles are weakened or tightened.

CLINICAL EXAMPLE 9-1

How does vertical transposition of the rectus muscles help correct a pattern deviation?

Consider the example of combining vertical transposition of the medial rectus muscles with bilateral medial rectus muscle recession for a V-pattern esotropia. The surgeon would transpose the medial rectus muscles inferiorly, toward the apex of the pattern. Transposing a medial rectus muscle insertion inferiorly makes the muscle's path length different depending on whether the eye is looking up or down. When the front of the globe is rotated downward, moving the inferiorly transposed attachment point more posteriorly, the muscle's path length is shorter, making the muscle more slack. Conversely, when the front of the globe is rotated upward, moving the inferiorly transposed attachment point more anteriorly, the muscle's path length becomes longer, putting the muscle on stretch. The adducting effect of the muscle thus becomes relatively weaker in downgaze and stronger in upgaze, tending to correct any underlying V pattern.

Vertical transposition can also be used to correct a pattern in monocular horizontal rectus muscle recession-resection surgery, transposing the medial and lateral muscles in

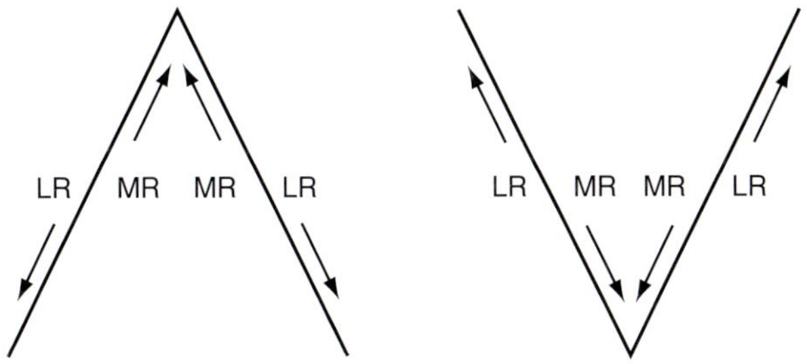

Figure 9-4 Direction of displacement of medial rectus (MR) and lateral rectus (LR) muscles in procedures to treat A-pattern *(left)* and V-pattern *(right)* deviations. *(Modified with permission from von Noorden, GK.* Atlas of Strabismus. *4th ed. Mosby;1983.)*

opposite directions; this has little if any net vertical effect in primary position. This procedure should be used with caution in patients with binocular fusion because it can produce symptomatic torsion.

CLINICAL PEARL

A useful mnemonic for horizontal rectus muscle transposition to treat pattern strabismus is MALE: *m*edial rectus muscle to the *a*pex, *l*ateral rectus muscle to the *e*mpty space.

If transposition of horizontal rectus muscles is used to treat pattern strabismus when there is associated ocular torsion, it may exacerbate the torsion (adding to preexisting extorsion when used to correct a V pattern and adding further intorsion when used to correct an A pattern); this may even undermine the effect of transposition, because torsion itself can contribute to the pattern. Conversely, when rectus muscle transposition is used to treat torsion, it will make any associated pattern strabismus worse.

Horizontal transposition of vertical rectus muscles

Surgery on the vertical rectus muscles (eg, temporal displacement of the superior rectus muscles for A-pattern esotropia or temporal displacement of the inferior rectus muscles for V-pattern esotropia) is used only in rare cases; transposition of the horizontal rectus muscles that are being operated on for the underlying esotropia or exotropia is usually sufficient.

Surgical Treatment of Specific Patterns

Table 9-1 summarizes the surgical treatment of pattern strabismus (see also Chapter 13).

V pattern

For V-pattern esotropia or exotropia associated with OEAd, weakening of the inferior oblique muscles is performed. For patients with V-pattern esotropia or exotropia not associated with OEAd, appropriate vertical transposition of the horizontal rectus muscles is performed (see Fig 9-4).

A pattern

For A-pattern exotropia or esotropia associated with ODAd, weakening of the superior oblique muscles is performed. Tenotomy of the posterior 7/8 of the insertions is an effective method for treating up to 20Δ of A pattern, without a significant effect on torsion. Lengthening of the oblique tendon by recession, insertion of a spacer, or a split-tendon lengthening procedure may also be used to weaken the superior oblique muscles. Bilateral superior oblique complete tenotomy is a very powerful procedure that may correct up to 40Δ–50Δ of A pattern. There is a risk of induced torsion with this procedure, which may be symptomatic for patients with binocular fusion.

For patients with A-pattern exotropia or esotropia not associated with ODAd, appropriate vertical transposition of the horizontal rectus muscles is performed (see Fig 9-4).

Table 9-1 Surgical Treatment of Pattern Strabismus

Type of Pattern	Most Common Clinical Association	Treatment: With OEAd or ODAd	Treatment: Without OEAd or ODAd	Other
V pattern	Infantile esotropia	Weakening of inferior oblique muscles	Vertical transposition of horizontal rectus muscles	
A pattern	Exotropia	Weakening of superior oblique muscles	Vertical transposition of horizontal rectus muscles	
Y pattern	Pseudo-inferior oblique overaction			Superior transposition of lateral rectus muscles
X pattern	Large-angle exotropia (pseudo-overaction due to contracture of lateral rectus muscles)			Recession of lateral rectus muscles
λ pattern	Variant of A-pattern exotropia	Weakening of superior oblique muscles	Vertical transposition of horizontal rectus muscles	

ODAd = overdepression in adduction; OEAd = overelevation in adduction.

Y pattern

If there is no deviation in primary position and downgaze, surgery may not be needed; however, a Y pattern can also coexist with a horizontal deviation in primary position. Because Y patterns are not caused by overaction of the inferior oblique muscles, weakening these muscles is not an effective treatment. Superior transposition of the lateral rectus muscles can improve this pattern but does not eliminate it.

X pattern

X patterns are usually due to pseudo-overaction of the oblique muscles, which is caused by contracture of the lateral rectus muscles in large-angle exotropia. Recession of the lateral rectus muscles alone usually improves the pattern.

λ pattern

This pattern is typically associated with ODAd, for which appropriate superior oblique weakening procedures may be used. Vertical transposition of horizontal rectus muscles may be considered if ODAd is not present.

CHAPTER 10

Vertical Deviations

This chapter includes related videos. Go to www.aao.org/bcscvideo_section06 or scan the QR codes in the text to access this content.

Highlights

- Overelevation and overdepression in adduction can be caused by overaction of the oblique muscles or by mechanical factors, such as extraocular muscle pulley heterotopia or restricted eye muscles.
- Surgeons often aim for a small undercorrection of a unilateral superior oblique palsy because patients can typically easily fuse small undercorrections, whereas overcorrections can cause disabling diplopia.
- Orbital floor trauma can be associated with an ipsilateral hyper- or hypotropia, depending on whether the inferior rectus muscle is paretic or restricted.
- Dissociated vertical deviation can sometimes be managed by optically encouraging fixation of the affected (or more affected) eye.

Introduction

A vertical deviation refers to a hyperdeviation of the higher eye or a hypodeviation of the lower, fellow eye. Vertical deviations are typically named according to the hypertropic eye. However, the term *hypotropia of the nonfixating eye* is used to describe the patient who has a strong fixation preference for the hypertropic eye.

Surgical treatment of these conditions is discussed in Chapter 13.

A Clinical Approach to Vertical Deviations

Vertical deviations can be challenging to evaluate because their magnitude often varies with gaze position (incomitance). In addition, if *dissociated vertical deviation (DVD)* is present, the direction and magnitude of deviation can differ depending on which eye is fixating.

In a patient with a completely *comitant deviation,* there is no movement of either eye on prism alternate cover testing with the same amount of prism used for either eye (prism placed base down over 1 eye or base up over the other).

When an individual has an *incomitant hyperdeviation* due to restriction or cyclovertical muscle paresis, the amount of prism needed to neutralize the deviation may be different depending on which eye is fixating in primary position. This is the difference between a primary and a secondary deviation according to Hering's law (see Chapter 3). Once the neutralizing prism for a given eye is found, however, neither eye moves when alternate cover testing is performed, as long as DVD is *not* present.

By contrast, in patients with DVD, each eye drifts upward whenever it is not fixating; this appears to violate Hering's law.

EXAMINING A PATIENT WITH RIGHT HYPERTROPIA AND LEFT DVD

- *Step 1:* The examiner neutralizes the patient's right hypertropia with prism. As the occluder shifts to the left eye, there is no movement of the right eye under the prism as it picks up fixation.
- *Step 2:* When the occluder moves from the left eye back to the right eye, there is a slow downward drift of the left eye as it resumes fixation, indicating DVD on the left. The DVD becomes manifest when the left eye is covered/not fixating.

Some patients have both a *"true" hypertropia* and a *superimposed* DVD. For instance, if a deviation is always a left hyperdeviation but has a different magnitude depending on which eye is fixating, then left hypertropia and DVD are both present (Video 10-1).

VIDEO 10-1 Hypertropia and DVD.
Courtesy of Inas Makar, MD.

In these patients, there is no way to quantify how much of the deviation is DVD and how much is true hypertropia. In practice, however, often 1 is usually predominant and the other, smaller component can be ignored. For the sake of simplicity, this chapter does not discuss true hypertropia and DVD in combination but only as separate entities.

Vertical Deviations With Marked Horizontal Incomitance

Many vertical deviations are characterized by a hypertropia that is much greater on gaze to 1 side. They are often, but not exclusively, associated with oblique muscle abnormalities.

Overelevation and Overdepression in Adduction

There are several causes of overelevation in adduction (OEAd) (Table 10-1) and overdepression in adduction (ODAd) (Table 10-2) or both (Table 10-3). These causes include true overaction and underaction of the oblique muscles, as well as several conditions that can simulate oblique muscle overactions.

In some patients, such as those with large-angle exotropia or thyroid eye disease, clinical examination of versions appears to show overaction of both the superior and the inferior oblique muscles. In such cases, elevation or depression of the vertical rectus muscle

Table 10-1 Causes of Overelevation in Adduction

Inferior oblique muscle overaction (primary or secondary)
Dissociated vertical deviation
Anti-elevation syndrome after contralateral inferior oblique muscle anterior transposition
Contralateral inferior rectus muscle restriction (eg, after orbital floor fracture, in thyroid eye disease)

Table 10-2 Causes of Overdepression in Adduction

Superior oblique muscle overaction (primary or secondary)
Brown syndrome (in rare cases)
Contralateral superior rectus muscle contracture (eg, after muscle resection)

Table 10-3 Causes of Overelevation and/or Overdepression in Adduction

Large-angle exotropia
Rectus muscle pulley heterotopia
Orbital dysmorphism (eg, craniofacial syndromes)
Duane syndrome
Skew deviation

of the opposite, abducting eye is restricted in the lateral portion of the bony orbit. The clinical findings can be explained as an attempt by the vertical rectus muscle to overcome this restriction through extra innervational activation, which, according to Hering's law, is distributed to the yoke oblique muscle as well (see Chapter 3). Alternatively, overelevation may be due to slippage of the globe relative to a tight lateral rectus muscle as the eye adducts (see Chapter 9).

Malposition of the rectus muscle pulleys can lead to anomalous movements that can simulate oblique muscle overactions. This can be seen in craniofacial syndromes. An inferiorly displaced lateral rectus muscle pulley can cause depression in abduction or, if this is the fixating eye, OEAd of the contralateral eye and a V-pattern deviation that simulate inferior oblique muscle overaction. A superiorly displaced lateral rectus muscle can produce ODAd—simulating a superior oblique overaction—along with an A-pattern deviation. Lateral and medial malpositioning of vertical rectus muscles can also create pseudo-overactions of oblique muscles. Apparent oblique dysfunction or A and V patterns associated with anomalous pulley positions respond poorly to oblique muscle surgery.

Other causes of OEAd and ODAd include

- the upshoots and downshoots of Duane syndrome
- superior or inferior rectus muscle restriction (causing extra innervation of contralateral oblique muscles)
- limitation of elevation in abduction of the contralateral eye after inferior oblique anterior transposition (anti-elevation syndrome)
- rare cases of Brown syndrome

Inferior oblique muscle overaction

Overaction of the inferior oblique muscle can cause OEAd. The eye is elevated in adduction, both on horizontal movement and in upgaze (Fig 10-1). The overaction can be primary or secondary according to the following criteria:

- *primary:* not associated with superior oblique muscle palsy
- *secondary:* accompanies palsy of the superior oblique muscle or the contralateral superior rectus muscle

One explanation for primary overaction relates to vestibular factors governing postural tonus of the extraocular muscles. Some authors have questioned whether primary inferior oblique overaction truly exists, preferring to describe the movement merely as OEAd.

Clinical features Primary inferior oblique muscle overaction develops between ages 1 and 6 years in up to two-thirds of patients with infantile strabismus (esotropia or exotropia). It sometimes occurs with acquired esotropia or exotropia and, occasionally, in patients with no other strabismus. In side gaze, there is a hypertropia of the adducting eye. In bilateral cases there is a right hypertropia in left gaze and a left hypertropia in right gaze. Bilateral overaction can be asymmetric, often in patients with poor vision in 1 eye, which leads to greater overaction in that eye. V-pattern horizontal deviation (see Chapter 9) and extorsion are common with overaction of the inferior oblique muscles.

Management When inferior oblique overaction produces V-pattern strabismus, hypertropia in primary position, or symptomatic hypertropia in side gaze, a procedure to weaken the inferior oblique muscle (recession, disinsertion, myectomy, myotomy, or anterior transposition) is indicated. Some surgeons grade the weakening procedure according to the severity of the overaction. There is uncertainty about how weakening the oblique muscle changes the patient's horizontal alignment in the primary position; many surgeons believe the effect is insignificant.

Superior oblique muscle overaction

Superior oblique muscle overaction is 1 of several causes of ODAd.

Clinical features Overaction of the superior oblique muscle causes a hypotropia of the adducting eye, which is accentuated in the lower field of gaze (Fig 10-2). A vertical deviation in primary position often occurs with unilateral or asymmetric bilateral overaction of the superior oblique muscles. In unilateral cases, the lower eye has the overacting superior

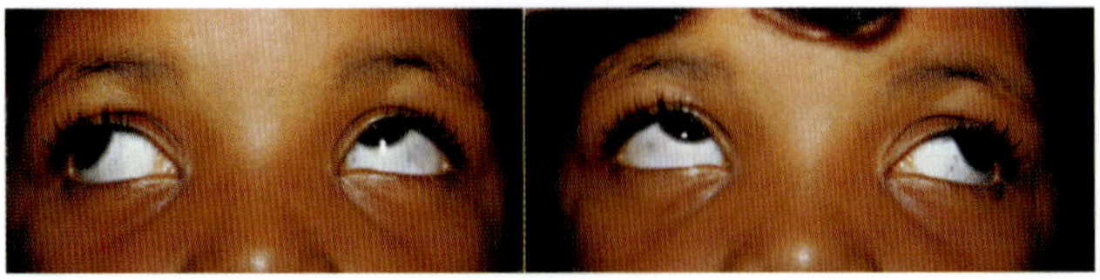

Figure 10-1 Bilateral inferior oblique muscle overaction. Overelevation in adduction, seen best in the upper fields of gaze. *(Courtesy of Edward L. Raab, MD.)*

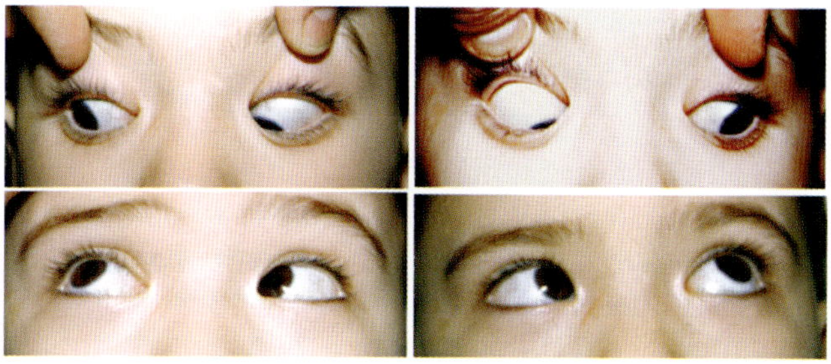

Figure 10-2 *Top row,* Bilateral superior oblique muscle overaction. Overdepression in adduction, seen best in the lower fields of gaze. *Bottom row,* Associated bilateral inferior oblique underaction. *(Courtesy of Edward L. Raab, MD.)*

oblique muscle; in bilateral cases, the lower eye has the more prominently overacting superior oblique muscle. A horizontal deviation, most often A-pattern exotropia, may be present (see Chapter 9). Intorsion is common with superior oblique muscle overaction. Most cases of bilateral superior oblique overaction are primary overactions.

Management In a patient with clinically significant hypertropia or hypotropia or an A pattern, a procedure to weaken the superior oblique tendon (recession, tenotomy, tenectomy, or lengthening by split-tendon lengthening or by insertion of a silicone spacer or nonabsorbable suture) is appropriate. Significant intorsion will also be reduced with any of these procedures. Many surgeons are reluctant to perform superior oblique tendon weakening in patients with fusion because torsional or asymmetric vertical effects can cause diplopia. As in cases of inferior oblique muscle overaction, a horizontal deviation can be corrected during the same operative session. Some surgeons, anticipating a small convergent effect in primary position, alter the amount of horizontal rectus muscle surgery when simultaneously weakening the superior oblique muscles.

Superior Oblique Muscle Palsy

The most common paralysis of a single cyclovertical muscle is cranial nerve (CN) IV (trochlear) palsy, which involves the superior oblique muscle. The palsy can be congenital or acquired; if the latter, it is usually a result of closed head trauma or, less commonly, vascular problems of the central nervous system, diabetes, or a brain tumor. Direct trauma to the tendon or the trochlear area is an occasional cause of unilateral superior oblique muscle palsy. Results of 1 study showed that most patients with congenital superior oblique palsy had an absent ipsilateral trochlear nerve and varying degrees of superior oblique muscle hypoplasia.

The same clinical features (discussed in the next section) can be observed when there is a congenitally lax, attenuated, or even absent superior oblique tendon or an unusual course of the muscle, or when there are malpositioned orbital pulleys—although, strictly speaking, these are not paralytic entities. Superior oblique muscle underaction can also occur in several craniofacial abnormalities (see Chapter 17).

DIFFERENTIATION OF A CONGENITAL FROM AN ACQUIRED SUPERIOR OBLIQUE MUSCLE PALSY

1. Examine childhood photographs of the patient for a preexisting compensatory head tilt; however, note that manifestations of congenital palsy sometimes become apparent only later in life.
2. Evaluate for the presence of a large vertical fusional amplitude, which supports a diagnosis of congenital superior oblique palsy.
3. Evaluate for any associated neurologic disorders (eg, closed head trauma) that suggest an acquired condition.
4. Look for facial asymmetry that results from a long-standing head tilt.

Diagnostic evaluation, including neuroimaging, often fails to identify an etiology but may still be warranted for acquired superior oblique palsy without a history of trauma. Neurologic aspects of superior oblique muscle palsy are discussed in BCSC Section 5, *Neuro-Ophthalmology.*

Yang HK, Kim JH, Hwang JM. Congenital superior oblique palsy and trochlear nerve absence: a clinical and radiological study. *Ophthalmology.* 2012;119(1):170–177.

Clinical features, evaluation, and diagnosis

Either the unaffected or the affected eye can be preferred for fixation. Examination of versions usually reveals underaction of the involved superior oblique muscle and overaction of its antagonist inferior oblique muscle; however, the action of the superior oblique muscle can appear normal (Fig 10-3).

CLINICAL PEARL

If depression in adduction cannot be evaluated because the eye is unable to adduct (eg, in CN III palsy), superior oblique muscle function can still be evaluated by observing whether the eye intorts, as judged by the movement of surface landmarks, or by examination of the fundus, when the patient attempts to look downward and inward from primary position.

Unilateral superior oblique palsy In a unilateral palsy, the hyperdeviation is typically incomitant, especially in the acute stages. Over time, contracture of the ipsilateral superior rectus or contralateral inferior rectus muscle can lead to "spread of comitance," resulting in minimal difference in the magnitude of the hypertropia when the patient looks from 1 side to the other.

Weakness of the superior oblique muscle also results in extorsion of the eye. If the degree of extorsion is large enough, then subjective incyclodiplopia, in which the patient describes the image as appearing to tilt inward, can occur.

The diagnosis of unilateral superior oblique muscle palsy can be further established by means of results of testing such as the 3-step test (also called the *Parks-Bielschowsky*

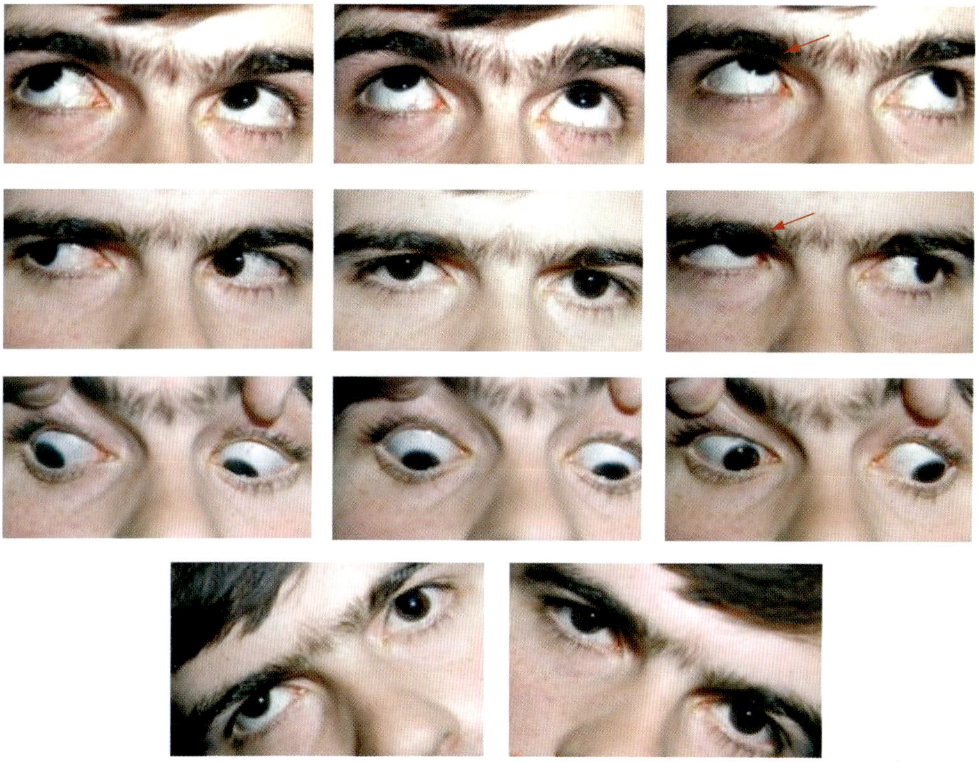

Figure 10-3 Right superior oblique palsy. There is a right hypertropia in primary position that increases in left gaze and with head tilt to the right. Note accompanying overaction of the right inferior oblique muscle *(arrows)*. *(Courtesy of Edward L. Raab, MD.)*

3-step test) (see Fig 10-3; see also Chapter 6, Fig 6-9) and the double Maddox rod test to measure torsion (see Chapter 6, Fig 6-7). Some ophthalmologists document serial changes in the deviation by means of the Hess screen test or the Lancaster red-green test or by plotting the field of single binocular vision. See Chapter 6 for further discussion of some of the tests mentioned in this section.

> **CLINICAL PEARL**
>
> Note that the results of the 3-step test can be confounded by DVD, muscle restriction, additional paretic muscles, previous strabismus surgery, or skew deviation.

INHIBITIONAL PALSY OF THE CONTRALATERAL ANTAGONIST Patients who fixate with the paretic eye can exhibit so-called *inhibitional palsy of the contralateral antagonist* (Fig 10-4). If a patient with right superior oblique palsy uses the right eye to fixate on an object that is located up and to the left, the innervation of the right inferior oblique muscle required to move the eye into this gaze position is reduced because the right inferior oblique muscle

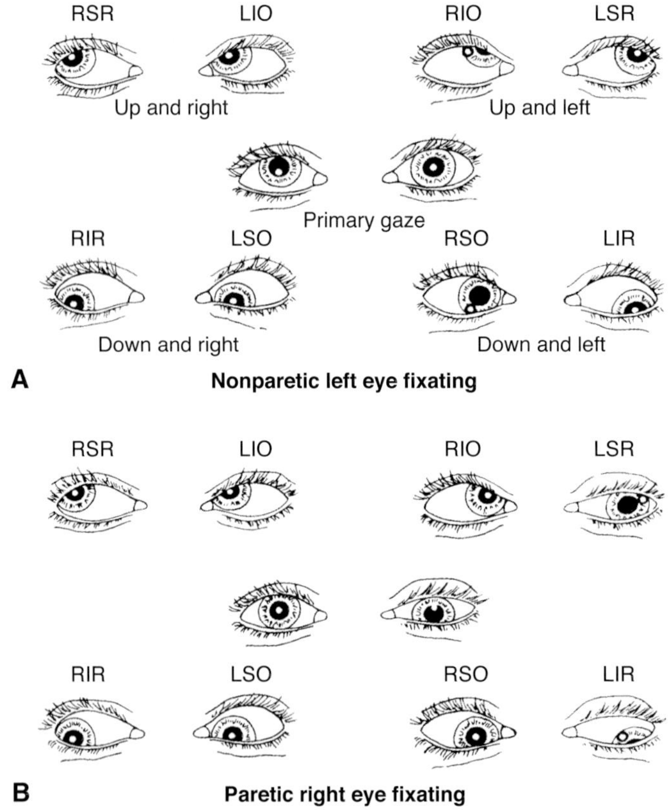

Figure 10-4 Palsy of right superior oblique muscle. **A,** In primary position, the right eye is elevated because of unopposed elevators. With the unaffected left eye fixating, no vertical difference appears in the right field of gaze. When gaze is up and left, the RIO shows marked overaction because its antagonist RSO is palsied. The action of the LSR is normal. When gaze is down and left, normal innervation required by the fixating normal eye does not suffice to fully move the palsied eye into that field of gaze (see also Chapter 6, Fig 6-9.) **B,** With the palsied right eye fixating, a left hypotropia may be present in primary position because the right elevators require less innervation to stabilize the eye, and thus the left elevators will receive less-than-normal innervation. Little or no vertical difference appears between the 2 eyes in the right field of gaze. When gaze is up and left, the RIO needs less-than-normal innervation to elevate the right eye because its antagonist, the RSO, is palsied. Consequently, its yoke, the LSR, will be receive reduced innervation and will be underacting: inhibitional palsy of the contralateral antagonist. When gaze is toward the field of action of the palsied RSO muscle, down and left, maximum innervation is required to move the right eye down during adduction, and thus the yoke LIR will be overacting. LIO = left inferior oblique; LIR = left inferior rectus; LSO = left superior oblique; LSR = left superior rectus; RIO = right inferior oblique; RIR = right inferior rectus; RSO = right superior oblique; RSR = right superior rectus. *(Modified with permission from von Noorden GK.* Atlas of Strabismus. *Mosby; 1983:24–25.)*

does not have to overcome the normal antagonistic effect of the right superior oblique muscle (Sherrington's law). According to Hering's law, less innervation is also received by the yoke muscle of the right inferior oblique muscle, which is the left superior rectus muscle. This decreased innervation can lead to underelevation of the left eye in this gaze position, simulating paresis of the left superior rectus muscle.

Bilateral superior oblique palsy Bilateral superior oblique palsy occurs commonly after head trauma but is sometimes congenital. It can be differentiated from unilateral superior oblique muscle palsy by the criteria shown in Table 10-4.

MASKED BILATERAL SUPERIOR OBLIQUE PALSY Markedly asymmetric bilateral superior oblique palsy that initially appears to be unilateral is called *masked bilateral palsy.* Signs of masked bilateral palsy include bilateral objective fundus extorsion, esotropia in downgaze, and even the mildest degree of oblique muscle dysfunction on the presumably uninvolved side. Masked bilateral palsy is more common in patients with head trauma. Surgical overcorrection of unilateral superior oblique palsy can produce a pattern of hypertropia and 3-step-test findings similar to those of superior oblique palsy in the contralateral eye; these should not be mistaken for masked bilateral palsy.

Management

For small, symptomatic deviations that lack a prominent torsional component—especially those that have become comitant—prisms that compensate for the hyperdeviation in primary position may be used to overcome diplopia.

Abnormal head position, significant vertical deviation, diplopia, and asthenopia are indications for surgery. Common operative strategies are discussed in the following sections (see Chapter 13 for details of the procedures as well as related videos).

Unilateral superior oblique muscle palsy There are many options for surgical treatment of a unilateral palsy. Any of the 4 cyclovertical muscles in each eye could potentially be operated on to correct the hypertropia. The following sections discuss some of the surgical strategies.

ONE-SIZE-FITS-ALL APPROACH Some surgeons use a *uniform approach,* choosing to weaken the ipsilateral antagonist inferior oblique muscle in all cases.

APPROACH BASED ON TENDON LAXITY For other surgeons, the surgical plan is informed by *superior oblique tendon laxity.* Tendon laxity is assessed at the time of surgery by forced duction testing, in which the globe is pushed (translated) posteriorly into the orbit while it is simultaneously extorted, thus placing the superior oblique tendon on stretch (Video 10-2). If the tendon is lax, a superior oblique tightening procedure is performed; if it is not, an inferior oblique weakening procedure is typically performed. Other ophthalmologists use tendon laxity only as diagnostic confirmation of superior oblique palsy.

Table 10-4 Comparison of Unilateral and Bilateral Superior Oblique (SO) Palsies

	Unilateral SO Palsy	Bilateral SO Palsy
V pattern	Minimal if any	Usually present
Downgaze excyclotorsion	<10° in downgaze	≥10° in downgaze, >15° in primary gaze
Bielschowsky head tilt	Positive to affected side	Positive to both sides
Abnormal head posture	Tilt away from affected side	Chin down
Oblique muscle dysfunction	Affected side only	Bilateral
Hypertropia in primary gaze	Variable in size	Small or none if palsies symmetric
Subjective incyclodiplopia	Uncommon	Common if acquired

VIDEO 10-2 Oblique muscle forced duction testing.

CLINICAL PEARL

Some surgeons believe that superior oblique tightening is the most effective procedure for addressing a marked head tilt in children with congenital superior oblique palsy.

APPROACH BASED ON PATTERN OF DEVIATION Many surgeons take *a tailored approach* that considers the variety of hypertropia patterns that may occur in association with superior oblique palsy. Because each of the 8 cyclovertical muscles has a somewhat different field of action, the surgeon may choose the muscles to operate based on the field of gaze in which the deviation is largest. Table 10-5 lists the procedures commonly used in different situations.

APPROACH IN THE PRESENCE OF SYMPTOMATIC TORSION *Extorsion* in unilateral superior oblique palsy rarely produces symptoms. When it does, it can be corrected with a *Harada-Ito procedure.*

APPROACH WHEN THE HYPERDEVIATION IS LARGE If the hyperdeviation is greater than 15 prism diopters (Δ) in primary position, surgery on more than 1 muscle may be required. Ipsilateral inferior oblique weakening and superior oblique tightening can be a particularly effective combination but carry an increased risk of problematic iatrogenic Brown syndrome or overcorrection. In the unusually severe case in which a vertical deviation is greater than 35Δ in primary position, 3-muscle surgery is usually required.

CLINICAL PEARL

Undercorrection of a long-standing unilateral superior oblique palsy is often well tolerated because there are typically generous vertical fusional amplitudes. However, it is important to avoid overcorrection of a long-standing unilateral superior oblique muscle palsy. Because there are often no sensory or motor adaptations to hypertropia in the opposite direction, disabling diplopia can result.

Table 10-5 Surgical Treatment of Unilateral Superior Oblique Palsy

	Magnitude of Incomitance (Difference in Hypertropia Between Right and Left Gaze)	
Pattern of Incomitance	**Large (Incomitance >15Δ)**	**Moderate (Incomitance <15Δ)**
Greater deviation in (contralateral) upgaze	Inferior oblique weakening	Inferior oblique weakening Ipsilateral superior rectus recession Contralateral superior rectus tightening (in rare cases)
Greater deviation in (contralateral) downgaze	Superior oblique tightening	Contralateral inferior rectus recession Ipsilateral superior rectus recession (if restricted)

Δ = prism diopters.

Bilateral superior oblique muscle palsy Surgical planning for treatment of bilateral superior oblique muscle palsy can be complex. If the paresis is asymmetric, hypertropia in primary position may be present, requiring many of the same considerations as hypertropia in unilateral palsy. In addition, there is often symptomatic extorsion or a V pattern that needs to be addressed.

If the palsies are symmetric (minimal hypertropia in primary position), both inferior oblique muscles can be weakened if they are overacting and hypertropia is present in side gaze. Bilateral superior oblique muscle tightening should be performed when hypertropia in side gaze is accompanied by V-pattern esotropia or symptomatic extorsion, especially in downgaze.

If there is symptomatic extorsion but minimal hypertropia in side gaze, bilateral Harada-Ito procedures can be performed. Other, less commonly used approaches, such as bilateral inferior rectus muscle recessions, may add extra innervational drive on downgaze to help overcome the superior oblique deficits.

Brown Syndrome

Brown syndrome causes limited elevation in adduction; it is discussed in detail in Chapter 11.

Inferior Oblique Muscle Palsy

The existence of inferior oblique muscle palsy (Fig 10-5) is controversial. Most cases are considered to be congenital or posttraumatic.

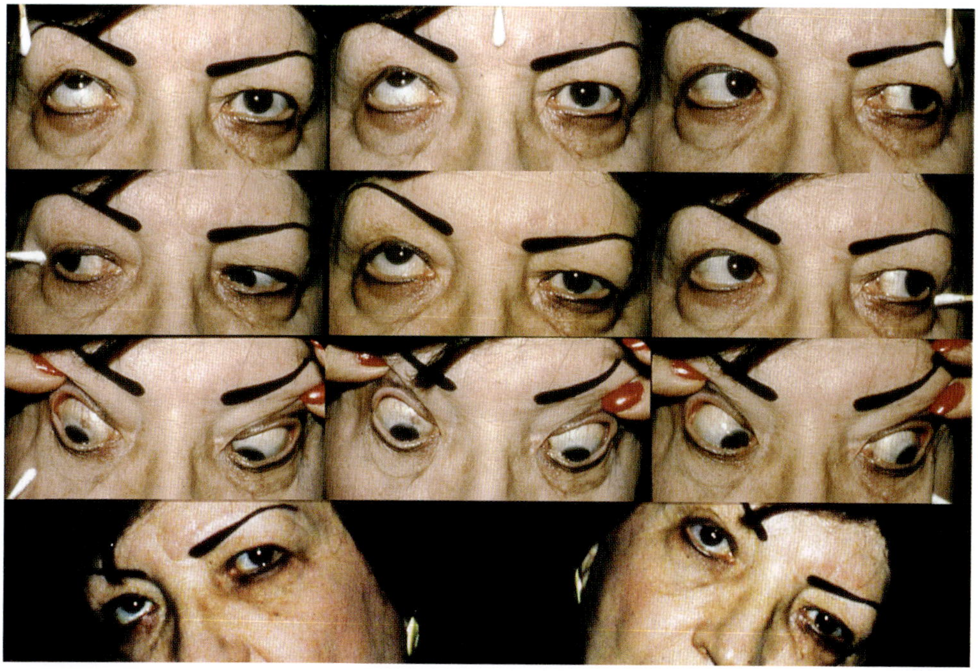

Figure 10-5 Left inferior oblique palsy. When the patient fixates with the paretic eye, there is a right hypertropia in primary position that is also most prominent in right gaze and with head tilt to the right—the 3-step test is consistent with this diagnosis. This patient had no abnormal neurologic findings. *(Courtesy of Steven M. Archer, MD.)*

Table 10-6 Comparison of Inferior Oblique Muscle Palsy and Brown Syndrome

Feature	Inferior Oblique Muscle Palsy	Brown Syndrome
Forced duction test	Negative	Positive
Strabismus pattern	A pattern	None or V pattern
Superior oblique muscle overaction	Usually significant	None or minimal
Torsion	Intorsion	None
Head-tilt test	Positive	Negative

Clinical features

Inferior oblique palsy is suspected when the patient has hypotropia and the 3-step-test results are consistent with this diagnosis. As with Brown syndrome, a prominent feature is deficient elevation when the eye is in adduction. The features that distinguish inferior oblique palsy from Brown syndrome are listed in Table 10-6.

Management

Indications for treatment of inferior oblique muscle palsy are abnormal head position, vertical deviation in primary position, and diplopia. Management consists of weakening either the ipsilateral superior oblique muscle or the contralateral superior rectus muscle.

Skew Deviation

Skew deviation is an acquired vertical strabismus that can mimic superior or inferior oblique palsy. The deviation is due to peripheral or central asymmetric disruption of supranuclear input from the otolith organs. Intorsion of the hypertropic eye on fundus examination—rather than the extorsion expected in cases of superior oblique palsy—suggests skew deviation, particularly when there are associated neurologic findings.

In addition, if the patient is placed in a supine position, the vertical tropia is more likely to decrease with skew deviation than with superior oblique palsy. Similarly, if there is extorsion of the hypotropic eye on fundus examination—instead of the intorsion expected in inferior oblique palsy—then skew deviation is the likely diagnosis. See BCSC Section 5, *Neuro-Ophthalmology,* for additional discussion.

Other Conditions With Incomitant Vertical Deviations

Incomitant hypertropia may occur in several other conditions. These include innervational problems, such as CN III palsy with aberrant regeneration and the upshoots and downshoots in Duane syndrome, as well as mechanical disorders, such as Brown syndrome and thyroid eye disease or those due to orbital tumors and orbital implants (eg, tube shunts, scleral buckles). These topics are discussed elsewhere in this book and in other BCSC Sections.

Vertical Deviations With Horizontal Comitance

Most patients with vertical deviations demonstrate some lateral incomitance. However, in vertical deviations not associated with apparent oblique muscle dysfunction, the difference between the deviations in right gaze and left gaze is usually less than 10Δ.

Monocular Elevation Deficiency

In monocular elevation deficiency (previously termed *double-elevator palsy*), there is a limitation of upward gaze with a hypotropia that is similar in adduction and abduction. The 3 forms of this motility pattern each have a different cause:

1. restriction of the inferior rectus muscle
2. deficient innervation of elevator muscles (paresis of 1 or both elevator muscles or a monocular supranuclear gaze disorder)
3. a combination of restriction and elevator muscle deficit

Clinical features

All 3 forms of monocular elevation deficiency are characterized by hypotropia of the involved eye with limited elevation, a chin-up head position with binocular fusion in downgaze, and ptosis or pseudoptosis (Fig 10-6). True ptosis is present in 50% of affected patients. Because these are also features of CN III palsy, if any other feature of CN III palsy is present, that condition should be suspected rather than monocular elevation deficiency.

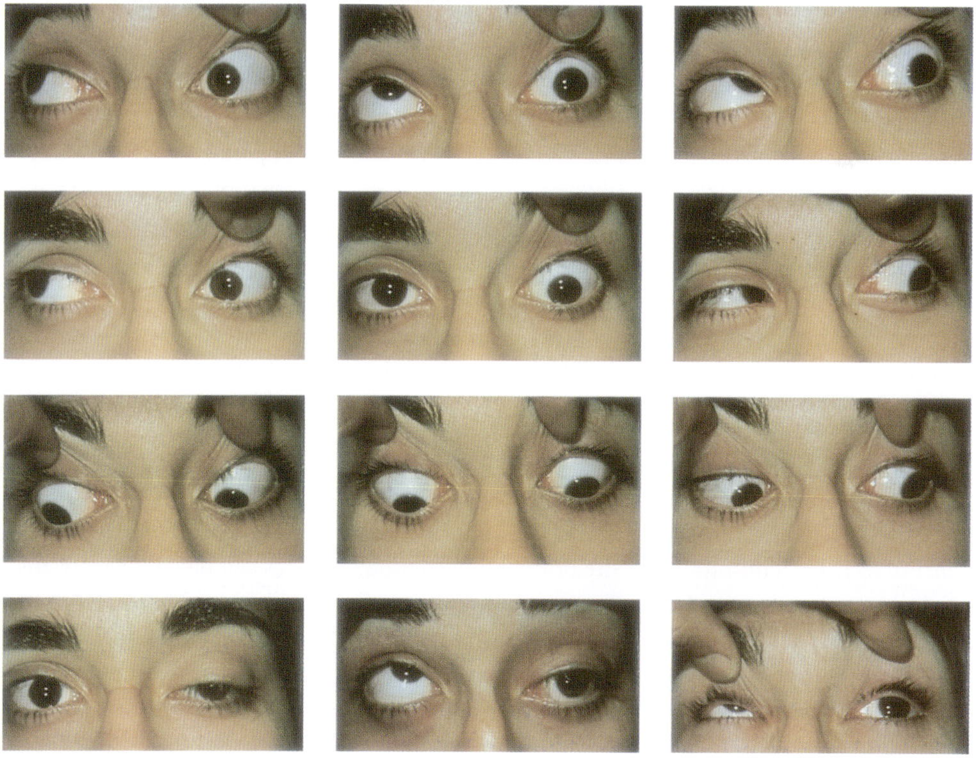

Figure 10-6 Monocular elevation deficiency of the left eye. *Top row,* No voluntary elevation of the left eye above horizontal. *Second row,* Hypotropia of the left eye across the horizontal fields of gaze. *Third row,* Depression of the left eye is unaffected. *Bottom row, left,* Ptosis (true and pseudo-) of the left upper eyelid during fixation with the right eye (in the top 3 rows, the left upper eyelid is elevated manually). *Bottom row, center,* Persistence of ptosis and marked secondary overelevation of the right eye during fixation with the left eye. *Bottom row, right,* Bell phenomenon, with the left eye elevating above the horizontal on forced eyelid closure.

The clinical features of each form of monocular elevation deficiency are as follows:

- *Restriction*
  - positive forced duction on elevation
  - normal force generation and saccadic velocity (no muscle paralysis)
  - often an extra or deeper lower eyelid fold on attempted upgaze
  - poor or absent Bell phenomenon
- *Elevator muscle innervational deficit*
  - negative forced duction on elevation
  - reduced force generation and saccadic velocity
  - preservation of Bell phenomenon (indicating a supranuclear cause) in many cases
- *Combination of restriction and elevator muscle deficit*
  - positive forced duction on elevation
  - reduced force generation and saccadic velocity

Management

Indications for treatment include a large vertical deviation in primary position, with or without ptosis, and an abnormal chin-up head position. *If restriction originating inferiorly is present,* the inferior rectus muscle should be recessed. *If there is no restriction*, the medial and lateral rectus muscles can be transposed toward the superior rectus muscle *(Knapp procedure).* Alternatively, the surgeon can recess the ipsilateral inferior rectus and either recess the contralateral superior rectus muscle or resect the ipsilateral superior rectus muscle.

Ptosis surgery should be deferred until the vertical deviation has been corrected and the pseudoptosis component eliminated.

Orbital Floor Fractures

Clinical features and management of orbital floor fractures are discussed in Chapter 26 of this volume and in BCSC Section 7, *Oculofacial Plastic and Orbital Surgery.* The discussion in this chapter focuses on motility abnormalities in patients with these fractures.

Clinical features

Diplopia in the immediate postinjury stage is common and is not necessarily an indication for urgent intervention. Indications and timing for surgical repair of fractures are discussed in Chapter 26 of this volume and in BCSC Section 7, *Oculofacial Plastic and Orbital Surgery.* Depending on the site of the bony trauma, muscles can be either restricted due to entrapment or paretic due to muscle contusion or nerve damage. "Flap tears" of the inferior rectus muscle have also been described by some authors as a cause of limitation of elevation, depression, or both. Paresis of a muscle may resolve over several months. If the fracture requires surgery, the range of eye movements may improve. By contrast, fibrosis after trauma may cause restriction to persist even after successful repair of the fracture.

Management

Treatment of strabismus is usually necessary when diplopia persists in primary position or downgaze or there is an associated compensatory head position. Some mild limitations of eye movements can be managed with prisms.

Planning of eye muscle surgery depends on the fields where diplopia is present and on the relative contributions of muscle restriction and paresis. It is important to repair any flap tear discovered on exploration of the inferior rectus muscle. For hypotropia in primary position (Fig 10-7), recession of the ipsilateral inferior rectus muscle can be effective, especially if the muscle is restricted on forced duction testing. Similarly, an incomitant esotropia (with diplopia on side gaze) due to restriction on the medial side may be improved by recession of the ipsilateral medial rectus muscle.

Initially, hypertropia due to weakness of the inferior rectus muscle without entrapment is managed with observation as the weakness may improve with time. If recovery is not complete within 6–12 months of the injury and there is at least a moderate degree of active force, resection of the affected muscle can be performed. If the hypertropia is large, the procedure can be combined with recession of the ipsilateral superior rectus muscle or recession of the contralateral inferior rectus muscle, with or without the addition of a posterior fixation suture *(fadenoperation)* or resection *(combined recession-resection procedure)*. Transposition of the ipsilateral medial and lateral rectus muscles to the inferior rectus muscle *(inverse Knapp procedure)* may be necessary for treatment of complete, chronic inferior rectus muscle palsy or when a crippling amount of recession has been necessary to relieve restriction.

Other Conditions With Comitant Vertical Deviations

Other conditions and disorders featuring a hypertropia that does not change markedly from right to left gaze include innervational problems, such as superior division (partial) CN III palsy, and mechanical disorders, such as thyroid eye disease, congenital fibrosis of the extraocular muscles, and orbital tumors. These topics are discussed elsewhere in this volume and in other BCSC Sections.

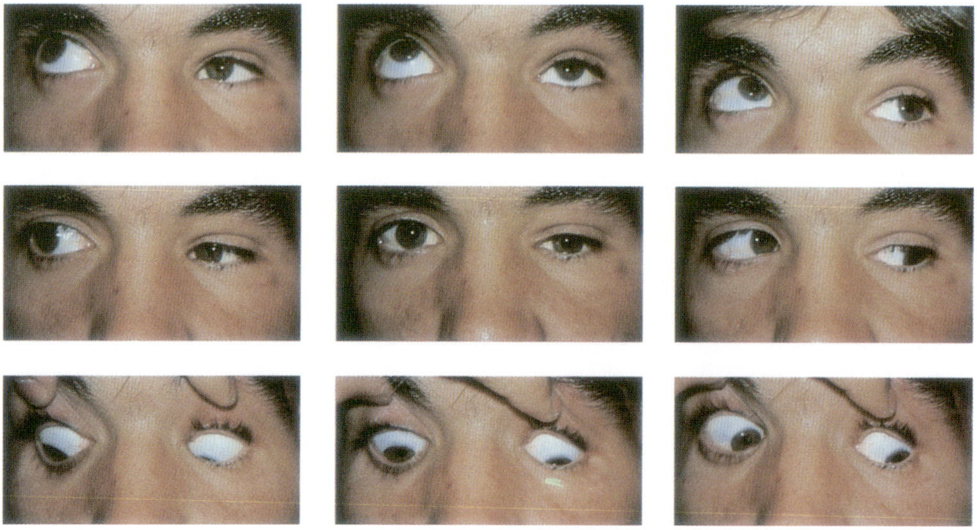

Figure 10-7 Old orbital floor fracture, left eye, with inferior rectus muscle entrapment. Note limitation of elevation of the left eye and pseudoptosis from enophthalmos. The eyelids are elevated manually in the bottom row.

Dissociated Vertical Deviation

Dissociated vertical deviation (DVD) is an innervational disorder found in more than 50% of patients with infantile strabismus (esotropia or exotropia). It is typically associated with other sequelae of deficient binocular vision, including fusion maldevelopment nystagmus syndrome and inferior oblique overaction. There are 2 theories to explain the origin of DVD:

1. The vertical vergence movement of DVD is harnessed to dampen fusion maldevelopment nystagmus syndrome and thereby improve vision, with the oblique muscles playing the principal role (Video 10-3).
2. Deficient fusion allows the primitive dorsal light reflex, which is prominent in other species, to emerge.

VIDEO 10-3 DVD and fusion maldevelopment nystagmus syndrome.
Courtesy of Guyton DL. Ocular torsion reveals the mechanisms of cyclovertical strabismus: The Weisenfeld Lecture. Invest Ophthalmol Vis Sci. *2008;49:847–857.*

Brodsky MC. Dissociated vertical divergence: a righting reflex gone wrong. *Arch Ophthalmol.* 1999;117(9):1216–1222.

Guyton DL. Ocular torsion reveals the mechanisms of cyclovertical strabismus: the Weisenfeld lecture. *Invest Ophthalmol Vis Sci.* 2008;49(3):847–857.

Clinical Features

Dissociated vertical deviation usually presents by age 2 years, whether or not any underlying horizontal strabismus has been surgically corrected. Either eye slowly drifts upward and outward, with simultaneous extorsion, when occluded or during periods of visual inattention (Video 10-4, Fig 10-8). Some patients have an associated head tilt, for reasons that are unclear.

VIDEO 10-4 Bilateral DVD in a person with esotropia.
Courtesy of Susana Gamio, MD.

DVD is usually the most prominent component of the *dissociated strabismus complex (DSC),* but sometimes the principal dissociated movement is one of abduction *(dissociated horizontal deviation, DHD)* (Video 10-5), and occasionally it is almost entirely a torsional movement *(dissociated torsional deviation, DTD)* (Video 10-6). DVD is usually bilateral

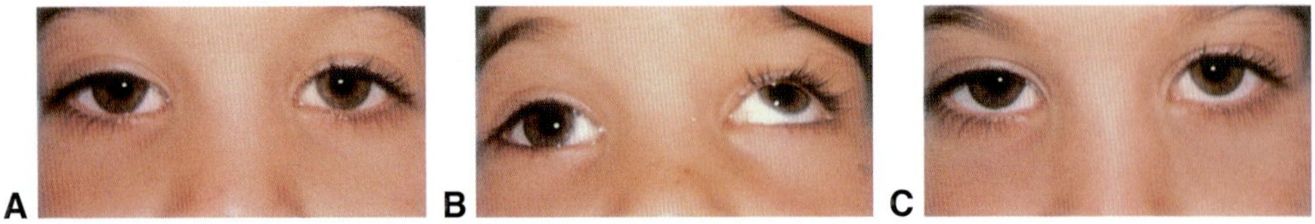

Figure 10-8 Dissociated vertical deviation, left eye. **A,** Straight eyes during binocular viewing conditions. **B,** Large left hyperdeviation immediately after the eye is covered and then uncovered. **C,** The left eye comes back down to primary position without a corresponding right hypotropia.

but is frequently asymmetric. It may occur spontaneously (manifest DVD) or only when 1 eye is occluded (latent DVD).

VIDEO 10-5 DHD in right eye and DVD in left eye.
Courtesy of Inas Makar, MD.

VIDEO 10-6 Bilateral torsional DVD.
Courtesy of Inas Makar, MD.

CLINICAL PEARL

Even in the absence of true inferior oblique overaction, an eye with latent DVD may overelevate in adduction, because it is occluded by the nose. Because DVD can mimic OEAd, distinguishing it from simple overaction of the inferior oblique muscles is important, as the surgical approaches to these 2 conditions may differ. In addition, the 2 conditions may coexist.

Measurement of vertical deviations in the presence of DVD cannot be performed with standard prism and alternate cover testing, because no single prism neutralizes the vertical refixation movement in both directions of the cover test. One approach is to measure the deviations when the left eye is fixating and when the right eye is fixating separately: a prism is placed in front of the nonfixating eye while it is behind an occluder. The occluder is then switched to the initially fixating eye. The prism power is adjusted until the deviating eye shows no vertical movement to refixate. These steps are then repeated for the other eye. The measurement taken when a given eye is fixating reflects the combined effect of the DVD in the fellow eye and any coexisting true hypertropia.

Management

Treatment of DVD is indicated if the deviation is noticeable (generally more than 6Δ–8Δ) and occurs frequently during the day. When DVD is unilateral or highly asymmetric, encouraging fixation by the eye with greater DVD by optically blurring the fellow eye is sometimes sufficient.

Surgery on vertical muscles can make DVD less noticeable but rarely eliminates it. For constant DVD of 1 eye in a child who never alternates fixation, vertical muscle surgery on the affected eye can mask the deviation. However, in a child with bilateral DVD and alternating fixation, any vertical eye muscle surgery that would mask the DVD in 1 eye would worsen the appearance of the DVD in the fellow eye. Treatment in this situation therefore involves bilateral procedures that limit the vertical excursions of each eye. These usually consist of large (6–10 mm) recessions of the superior rectus muscles, or anterior transposition of the inferior oblique muscles (especially if inferior oblique overaction is present). If there is residual DVD, inferior rectus muscle resection or plication can be performed.

CHAPTER 11

Special Motility Disorders

This chapter includes related videos. Go to www.aao.org/bcscvideo_section06 or scan the QR codes in the text to access this content.

Highlights

- Duane syndrome, congenital fibrosis of the extraocular muscles, and Möbius syndrome are different forms of congenital cranial dysinnervation.
- Thyroid eye disease is an autoimmune disorder; it is not caused by thyroid dysfunction.
- Myasthenia gravis does not affect the pupils.

See BCSC Section 5, *Neuro-Ophthalmology,* for additional discussion of several entities covered in this chapter; see Chapter 13 in this volume for discussion of some of the surgical procedures mentioned in this chapter.

Congenital Cranial Dysinnervation Disorders

Congenital cranial dysinnervation disorders (CCDDs) are developmental defects of 1 or more cranial nerves (CNs), with associated nuclear hypoplasia, nerve misdirection, and/or absent nerves. Abnormal innervation often results in secondary structural changes of the extraocular muscles (eg, stiffening or contracture). CCDDs include Duane syndrome, congenital fibrosis of the extraocular muscles, Möbius syndrome, some cases of congenital CN IV palsy (see Chapter 10), and possibly congenital Brown syndrome.

Gutowski NJ, Chilton JK. The congenital cranial dysinnervation disorders. *Arch Dis Child.* 2015;100(7):678–681.

Duane Syndrome

Duane syndrome (DS) is characterized by reduced lateral rectus function on attempted abduction, and anomalous co-contraction of both lateral and medial rectus muscles on attempted adduction, which causes the globe to retract. Both abduction and adduction may be limited. An upshoot or downshoot on attempted adduction may occur, caused by 1–2 mm of vertical slippage of the contracted lateral rectus muscle or, less commonly, anomalous vertical rectus muscle activation.

Although many affected patients have isolated DS, possible associated congenital anomalies include Goldenhar syndrome (hemifacial microsomia, ocular dermoids, ear anomalies, preauricular skin tags, and eyelid colobomas) and Wildervanck syndrome (sensorineural hearing loss and Klippel-Feil anomaly with fused cervical vertebrae).

Most cases of DS are sporadic; however, 5%–10% show autosomal dominant inheritance. Discordance in monozygotic twins suggests the intrauterine environment may play a role. The occurrence of DS in infants whose mothers were exposed to thalidomide while pregnant indicates that the developmental defect develops between 4 and 6 weeks of gestational age. DS is more common in females and shows a predilection for the left eye.

Anatomic, imaging, and electromyographic studies indicate an absent or hypoplastic CN VI nucleus (Fig 11-1), with aberrant innervation of the lateral rectus muscle by a branch of CN III. Tight and broadly inserted medial rectus muscles and fibrotic lateral rectus muscles are often encountered during surgery.

Clinical features

> **KEY POINTS 11-1**
>
> DS is a continuous spectrum characterized by independently varying degrees of lateral rectus (1) hypoinnervation by CN VI and (2) misinnervation by CN III.

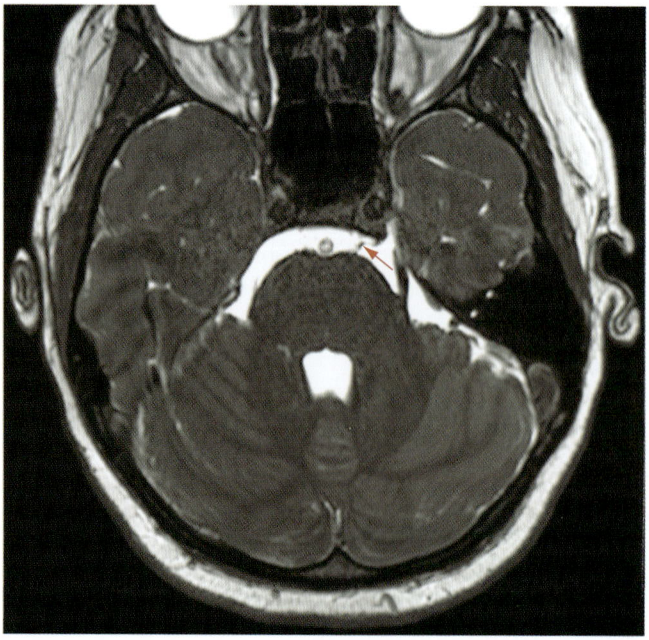

Figure 11-1 Magnetic resonance imaging (MRI) of a patient with Duane syndrome (DS) on the right side, showing an absent right cranial nerve (CN) VI and normal left CN VI *(arrow)*, with corresponding hypoplasia of the right lateral rectus muscle compared to the left lateral rectus muscle. *(Reprinted by permission from Brodsky MC. Congenital optic disc anomalies. In:* Pediatric Neuro-Ophthalmology. *2nd ed. Springer-Verlag; 2010.)*

Although DS is a continuous spectrum, it is often classified into 3 types:

1. *Type 1:* poor abduction, frequently with esotropia in primary position (Fig 11-2)
2. *Type 2:* poor adduction, with exotropia; less lateral rectus hypoinnervation than in type 1; and more misinnervation and co-contraction (Fig 11-3)
3. *Type 3:* poor abduction and adduction (Fig 11-4)

Approximately 15% of cases are bilateral, often asymmetric (Video 11-1).

VIDEO 11-1 Bilateral Duane syndrome.
Courtesy of Michael S Vaphiades, DO.

CLINICAL PEARL

Type 1 DS has limited abduction (1 "d" in "abduction"); type 2 has limited adduction (2 "d"s in "adduction"); type 3 has limitations in both.

In addition, *synergistic divergence* is a rare CCDD often classified as a type of Duane syndrome. There is usually exotropia, and with attempted contralateral gaze, the affected eye, instead of adducting, abducts even further ("the ocular splits"; Video 11-2). Synergistic divergence can be a result of biallelic *COL25A1* mutations.

VIDEO 11-2 Synergistic divergence.
Courtesy of Michael C. Brodsky, MD.

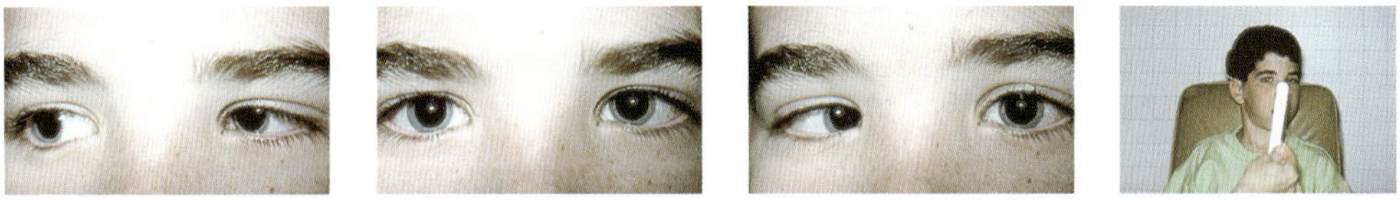

Figure 11-2 Type 1 DS with esotropia, left eye, showing limitation of abduction, almost full adduction, and retraction of the globe with resulting palpebral fissure narrowing on adduction. *Far right,* Compensatory left head turn. *(Courtesy of Edward L. Raab, MD.)*

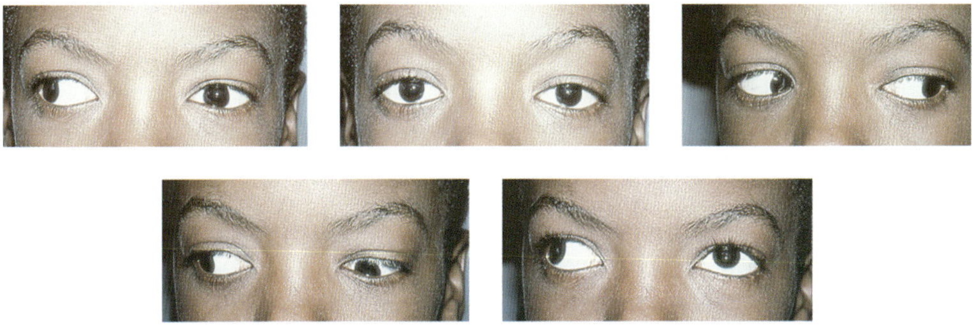

Figure 11-3 Type 2 DS, left eye. *Top row,* Marked limitation of adduction and full abduction of the left eye. *Bottom row,* Variable upshoot and downshoot of the left eye with extreme right-gaze effort. The typical primary position exotropia is not present. *(Courtesy of Edward L. Raab, MD.)*

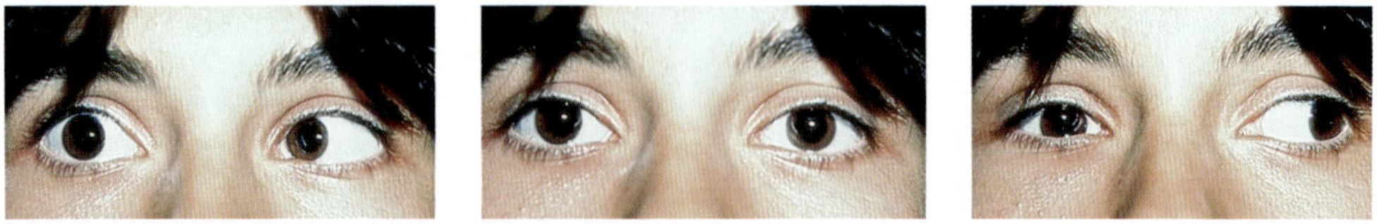

Figure 11-4 Type 3 DS, right eye. Severe limitation of abduction and adduction, with palpebral fissure narrowing even though adduction cannot be accomplished. There is no deviation in primary position. *(Courtesy of Edward L. Raab, MD.)*

Type 1 DS is most common, constituting 50%–80% of cases. Patients and families may believe the unaffected eye is inappropriately turning in, not realizing that the involved eye is failing to abduct. To differentiate type 1 DS from CN VI palsy without neuroimaging, the clinician can look for the following:

- globe retraction on adduction
- small esotropia in primary position (usually <30 prism diopters) and orthotropia with just a small face turn, despite a severe abduction deficit
- a small exotropia on gaze contralateral to the affected eye. Many patients have good stereopsis with their preferred head posture, and diplopia on gaze ipsilateral to the affected eye is rare.

CLINICAL PEARL

Spinning an infant can help the clinician evaluate horizontal ductions and globe retraction. Globe retraction can also be appreciated by viewing the patient from above. For patients able to undergo slit-lamp examination, globe retraction may be seen as disruption of the vertical slit-lamp beam cast from the cornea onto the lower eyelid during adduction.

Management

For patients achieving orthotropia and sensory fusion with only a small anomalous head posture, conservative management is appropriate, even in patients with large duction deficits. Coexisting accommodative esotropia is treated with refractive correction. Use of a prism may be helpful in some instances.

Surgery cannot normalize ductions. Surgery may alleviate primary position deviations, head turns required for fusion, marked globe retraction, or large upshoots or downshoots.

For unilateral type 1 DS, recession of the ipsilateral medial rectus muscle can reduce the primary position deviation and head turn; it does not usually improve abduction. Because of misinnervation, the effect of contralateral medial rectus muscle recession is harder to predict. When the contralateral eye is brought to primary position, increased ipsilateral CN VI activity might drive the ipsilateral lateral rectus muscle (depending on the degree of hypoinnervation), and reduced ipsilateral CN III activity will relax the ipsilateral medial rectus muscle; however, due to misinnervation, reduced CN III activity also reduces innervational drive to the ipsilateral lateral rectus muscle, offsetting the benefit.

Although most surgeons avoid lateral rectus muscle resection, which can exacerbate globe retraction, occasionally, patients with minimal co-contraction may benefit from small resections (<3–4 mm). Partial or full lateral transposition of both vertical rectus muscles or of the superior rectus alone, usually with medial rectus recession, sometimes improves abduction.

Type 2 DS is usually treated with ipsilateral lateral rectus muscle recession. Some surgeons recess both lateral rectus muscles in patients with large-angle exotropia, but as described above, the net effect of contralateral muscle surgery is difficult to predict in patients with anomalous innervation.

Severe globe retraction may warrant surgery even when patients are aligned near the primary position, as in patients with type 3 DS. Large lateral rectus muscle recession with simultaneous medial rectus muscle recession can lessen globe retraction and can improve upshoot and downshoot. Upshoot or downshoot can also be treated with a Y-splitting procedure or retroequatorial fixation of the lateral rectus muscle, or disinsertion and periosteal fixation of the muscle combined with a vertical rectus muscle transposition procedure.

Doyle JJ, Hunter DG. Transposition procedures in Duane retraction syndrome. *J AAPOS.* 2019;23(1):5–14.

Congenital Fibrosis of the Extraocular Muscles

Congenital fibrosis of the extraocular muscles (CFEOM) is a group of rare developmental defects of cranial nerves and their nuclei, resulting in dysinnervation and secondary abnormal EOM structure, with restriction caused by fibrous tissue replacing hypoplastic muscles.

Clinical features

The dominantly inherited CFEOM1 phenotype (which predominantly involves CN III) is typically characterized by bilateral ptosis, severe restriction to upgaze, exotropia, and a chin-up head posture (Fig 11-5). It can be caused by mutations in *KIF21A*. CFEOM2, with bilateral CN III and IV dysgenesis, is rare and recessively inherited. It is associated with *PHOX2A* mutations and sometimes with retinal dystrophy. CFEOM3 is dominantly inherited with variable penetration, can be unilateral or asymmetric, and is often associated with other neurological abnormalities. *TUBB3* mutations can cause CFEOM3, including monocular elevation deficiency (see Chapter 10). Tukel syndrome is a form of CFEOM associated with limb abnormalities.

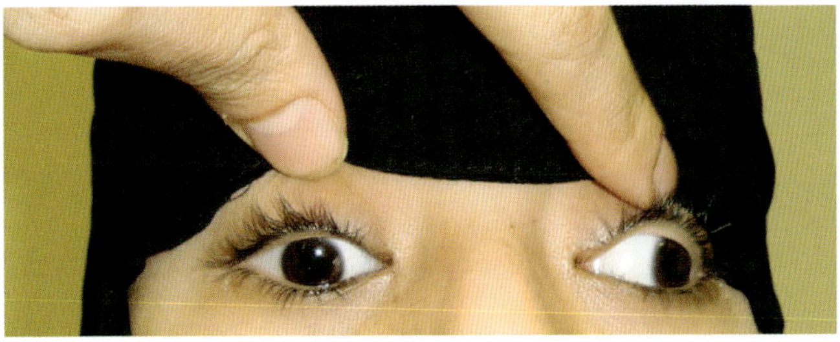

Figure 11-5 Congenital fibrosis of the extraocular muscles type 1 (CFEOM1), in forced primary position, with bilateral ptosis, hypotropia, exotropia, and partial ophthalmoplegia (upper eyelids are elevated manually). *(Courtesy of Arif O. Khan, MD.)*

Management

Surgery for CFEOM is challenging and requires release of the restricted muscles (ie, weakening procedures). Fibrosis of the adjacent tissues may also be present. A good surgical result aligns the eyes in primary position, but full ocular rotations cannot be restored. Multiple surgeries are often required.

Sener EC, Taylan Sekeroglu H, Ural O, Oztürk BT, Sanaç AS. Strabismus surgery in congenital fibrosis of the extraocular muscles: a paradigm. *Ophthalmic Genet.* 2014;35(4):208–225.

Möbius Syndrome

Clinical features

Möbius syndrome is a rare condition characterized by both CN VI and CN VII dysgenesis, the latter causing masklike facies. Horizontal gaze palsy resulting from involvement of both the paramedian pontine reticular formation (PPRF) and the CN VI nucleus can occur. Limb, chest, and tongue defects are common.

Patterns of ocular motility in Möbius syndrome include

- orthotropia in primary position with marked deficits in abduction and adduction (Fig 11-6)
- esotropia with cross-fixation and sparing of convergence
- large exotropia with absence of convergence (least common)

Some patients appear to have palpebral fissure changes on adduction or vertical EOM involvement. A syndrome that resembles Möbius syndrome but also includes exotropia and vertical limitation is due to *TUBB3* mutations.

MacKinnon S, Oystreck DT, Andrews C, Chan WM, Hunter DG, Engle EC. Diagnostic distinctions and genetic analysis of patients diagnosed with Moebius syndrome. *Ophthalmology.* 2014;121(7):1461–1468.

Management

Medial rectus muscle recession may improve large-angle esotropia, but caution is warranted in patients with severe adduction deficits. Vertical rectus muscle transposition procedures have also been combined with medial rectus muscle recession.

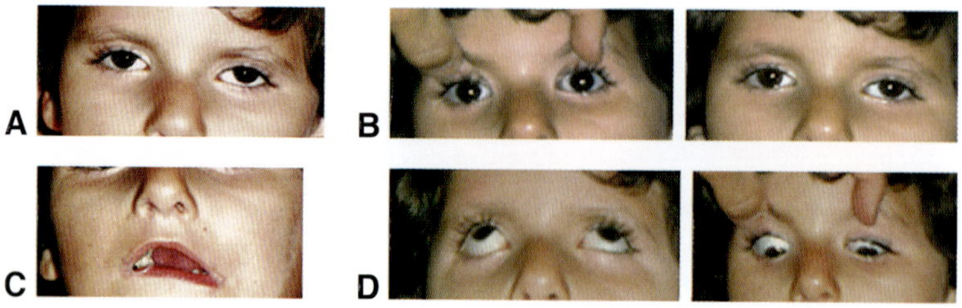

Figure 11-6 Möbius syndrome. **A,** Straight eyes in primary position. **B,** Attempted right and left gaze, showing bilaterally absent adduction and severely limited abduction. **C,** The patient cannot smile because of bilateral CN VII palsy. **D,** Vertical movements are not affected. *(Courtesy of Edward L. Raab, MD.)*

Special Types of Strabismus With Congenital and Acquired Forms

This section discusses Brown syndrome and CN III palsy. CN palsies that involve a single EOM are discussed elsewhere in this volume. Diagnosis and treatment of CN IV palsy are discussed in Chapter 10, with vertical deviations. Diagnosis and treatment of CN VI palsy are discussed in Chapter 7, with esotropia. See also BCSC Section 5, *Neuro-Ophthalmology*.

Brown Syndrome

Brown syndrome causes vertical deviations (see Chapter 10) with characteristic restriction of elevation in adduction due to abnormalities of the tendon–trochlea complex (see Chapter 2). It is bilateral in approximately 10% of cases. Most cases are congenital, and some may be a form of CCDD.

Acquired Brown syndrome can result from peritrochlear trauma, scleral buckles, tube shunt surgery, orbital tumors, or sinusitis. Systemic inflammatory conditions such as rheumatoid arthritis often cause intermittent Brown syndrome, which may resolve spontaneously. Orbit and sinus imaging is advisable in acute-onset cases of unknown etiology. Instability of the lateral rectus pulley can present an identical clinical picture (pseudo–Brown syndrome).

Clinical features

Deficient elevation in adduction improves in abduction, but often not completely (Fig 11-7). In mild cases, no hypotropia is present in primary position. Severe cases with primary position hypotropia often cause a chin-up head position or a head turn away from the side of the affected eye.

Several findings differentiate Brown syndrome from underelevation in adduction due to inferior oblique muscle paresis (see Chapter 10, Table 10-6). Ipsilateral superior oblique overaction is typical of inferior oblique muscle paresis but is rare in Brown syndrome. In Brown syndrome, attempts at elevation straight upward may cause divergence (V pattern) due to

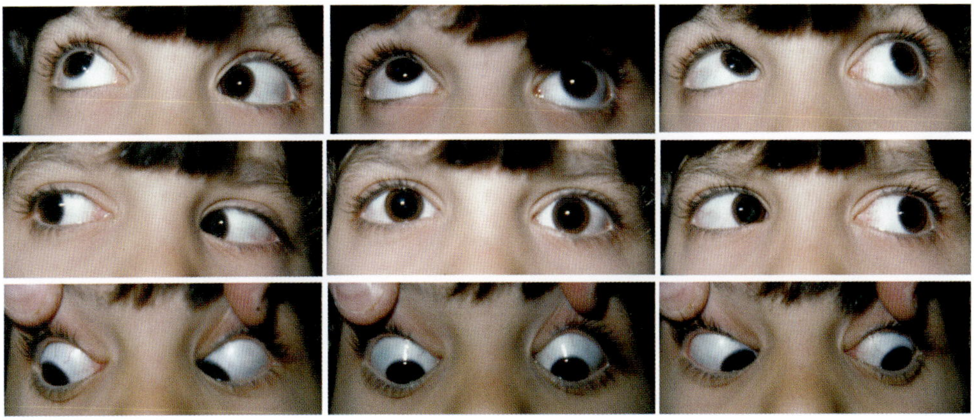

Figure 11-7 Brown syndrome, left eye. There is no elevation of the left eye when adducted; left eye is depressed instead. Elevation is also severely limited in straight-up gaze and moderately so even in up-and-left gaze. Note the characteristic divergence in straight-up gaze and lack of ipsilateral superior oblique overaction. *(Courtesy of Edward L. Raab, MD.)*

slippage of the globe laterally as it meets resistance from the tight superior oblique tendon (see Fig 11-7), whereas inferior oblique muscle paresis is more likely to exhibit an A pattern.

Forced duction testing demonstrates restricted passive elevation in adduction, accentuated by retropulsion of the globe, which stretches the superior oblique tendon. By contrast, inferior rectus muscle restriction is accentuated by proptosis of the eye rather than by retropulsion.

Management

Mild congenital Brown syndrome does not require treatment, particularly because the condition may improve spontaneously over time, often after many years. Surgery is indicated for more severe congenital cases, for example, if a child with binocular visual potential is not achieving fusion or requires a large anomalous head posture for fusion. Superior oblique tenotomy nasal to the superior rectus muscle is effective; however, because it is likely to cause consecutive superior oblique muscle paresis, it is often combined with inferior oblique recession. Superior oblique tendon lengthening (using a suture or silicone spacer, or via split-tendon lengthening) is preferred by some; this procedure can be reversed if necessary (see Chapter 13).

When Brown syndrome is secondary to rheumatoid arthritis or other systemic inflammatory diseases, resolution may occur as systemic treatment brings the underlying disease into remission or when corticosteroids are injected near the trochlea.

Dawson E, Barry J, Lee J. Spontaneous resolution in patients with congenital Brown syndrome. *J AAPOS.* 2009;13(2):116–118.

Cranial Nerve III Palsy

In children, CN III palsy can be congenital, in which case it is more appropriately considered a CCDD. Acquired cases can be caused by trauma, inflammation, viral infection, or a mass lesion. It can result from a steroid-responsive condition known as *ophthalmoplegic migraine,* also termed *recurrent ophthalmoplegic cranial neuropathy.* CN III palsy in children can also occur after vaccination or as a result of a benign or malignant tumor. Aneurysm causing isolated CN III palsy in a child is rare. Acquired CN III palsy of unknown etiology in a child is an indication for neuroimaging.

In adults, the usual causes are intracranial aneurysm, microvascular infarction, inflammation, trauma, infection, or tumor. See BCSC Section 5, *Neuro-Ophthalmology,* for further discussion of the causes and manifestations of CN III palsy.

Gelfand AA, Gelfand JM, Prabakhar P, Goadsby PJ. Ophthalmoplegic "migraine" or recurrent ophthalmoplegic cranial neuropathy: new cases and a systematic review. *J Child Neurol.* 2012;27(6):759–766.

Clinical features

CN III involvement may be partial or complete. Complete paralysis causes limited adduction, elevation, and depression of the eye, with exotropia and hypotropia, because the remaining unopposed muscles are the lateral rectus (abductor) and the superior oblique (abductor and depressor), unless there is also paralysis of the nerves supplying these muscles. Upper eyelid ptosis is present, often with additional pseudoptosis due to the depressed position of the involved eye (Fig 11-8).

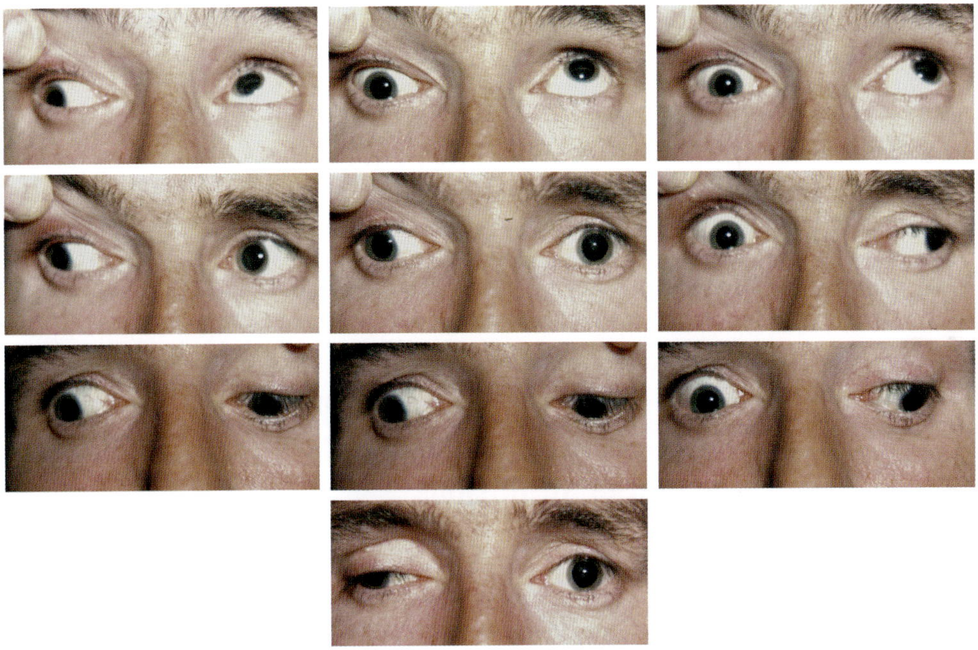

Figure 11-8 CN III palsy, right eye, with ptosis *(bottom photo)* and limited adduction, elevation, and depression (upper eyelid is elevated manually in top 9 photos). *(Courtesy of Edward L. Raab, MD.)*

The clinical findings and treatment may be complicated by misdirection (aberrant regeneration) of the damaged nerve, presenting as anomalous eyelid elevation, pupil constriction, or vertical excursion of the globe—any or all of which can occur upon attempted rotation into the field of action of the EOMs supplied by the injured nerve. A miotic pupil is sometimes noted in congenital cases, regardless of whether there is aberrant regeneration. Adults with acquired CN III palsy report experiencing incapacitating diplopia unless the involved eye is occluded by ptosis or other means.

Management

Because the visual system is still developing in pediatric patients, amblyopia is a common finding that must be treated aggressively. Impaired accommodation may result in functional anisometropia that further contributes to amblyopia and may require refractive correction.

CN III palsy presents difficult surgical challenges because multiple EOMs, including the levator muscle, are involved. Replacing all the lost rotational forces on the globe is impossible. The incidence of diplopia in patients younger than 8 years is low because of suppression (see Chapter 4), but in adults with acquired CN III palsy and previously normal binocularity, the goal of surgery is adequate alignment for binocular function in primary position and in slight downgaze for reading. In acquired cases, it is advisable to allow 6 or even 12 months for spontaneous recovery before surgical correction. Because ptosis may be preventing incapacitating diplopia, ptosis repair should not be done without ensuring the patient will be able to achieve binocular vision.

The surgical approach depends on the degree of paralysis of different muscles and on the presence or absence of misinnervation. In partial paresis, a large recession-resection of the horizontal rectus muscles can correct the exodeviation, with supraplacement of both for coexisting hypotropia. For vertical deviations, the vertical rectus muscles may be operated on if they have partially preserved function. Superior oblique tenotomy can reduce hypotropia. In some cases, superior oblique tendon transposition, with tenotomy medial to the superior rectus muscle border and reinsertion 2–3 mm anterior to the medial pole of the superior rectus muscle insertion, may be helpful. For complete paralysis, it may be necessary to completely inactive the lateral rectus muscle, either with extirpation or with disinsertion and reattachment to the lateral orbital periosteum. Splitting and transposition of the lateral rectus muscle to the nasal side of the globe has also been described. Most surgeons correct ptosis only after strabismus surgery is complete.

Special Types of Acquired Strabismus

Thyroid Eye Disease

This chapter focuses on motility disturbances in thyroid eye disease (TED). Other aspects of TED are discussed in BCSC Section 5, *Neuro-Ophthalmology,* and Section 7, *Oculofacial Plastic and Orbital Surgery.*

TED causes edema, inflammation, and fibrosis of the EOMs due to lymphocytic infiltration, restricting motility. Massively enlarged muscles can also contribute to compressive optic neuropathy. Muscle enlargement can be seen on orbital imaging (Fig 11-9).

TED myopathy is not caused by thyroid dysfunction; rather, both conditions result from a common autoimmune disease. Thyroid-stimulating immunoglobulins likely mediate TED and may be a biomarker for TED. Some patients have coexisting myasthenia

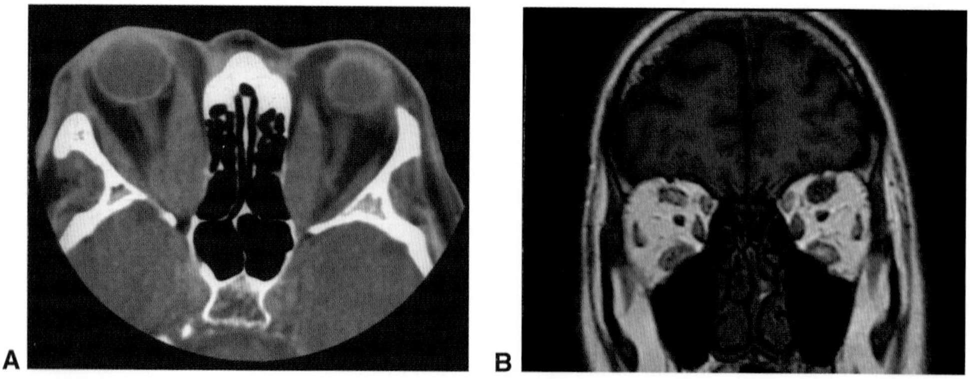

Figure 11-9 Thyroid eye disease (TED). **A,** Axial computed tomography (CT) scan of a patient with marked bilateral medial rectus muscle enlargement. **B,** Coronal MRI of a different patient with enlargement of multiple extraocular muscles. The greatest abnormalities are seen in the left superior and right inferior rectus muscles. *(Part A © 2021 American Academy of Ophthalmology; part B courtesy of Knights of Templar Pediatric Ophthalmology Education Center; Howard MA.* Considerations in Surgical Correction of Adult Strabismus. *American Academy of Ophthalmology; 2020. Accessed February 9, 2022. www.aao.org/disease-review/considerations-in-surgical-correction-of-adult-str)*

gravis (discussed in the following section), complicating the clinical findings. Smoking increases TED severity, doubling the hazard ratio for strabismus surgery in patients with thyroid disease.

Clinical features

The muscles affected in TED, in decreasing order of severity and frequency, are the inferior rectus, medial rectus, superior rectus, and lateral rectus. The condition is usually bilateral but is often asymmetric. Forced duction testing shows restriction of involved muscles.

A typical patient may present with upper eyelid retraction, proptosis, hypotropia, and esotropia (Fig 11-10). TED is a common cause of acquired vertical strabismus in adults, especially women, but rarely causes motility problems in children.

Management of strabismus

Treatment of TED with systemic steroids, radiation, or teprotumumab; treatment of co-existing thyroid disease; and management of the nonstrabismic complications associated with TED are discussed in BCSC Section 5, *Neuro-Ophthalmology,* and Section 7, *Oculofacial Plastic and Orbital Surgery.*

Diplopia and abnormal head posture are the principal indications for strabismus surgery in TED. It is best to perform surgery after strabismus measurements and thyroid function tests have been stable for 6 months. In studies of surgery performed to alleviate severely abnormal head posture before stability was achieved, surgery was effective, but half the patients required further surgery. If orbital decompression is necessary, strabismus surgery should be delayed until afterward. Prisms may help alleviate diplopia. Botulinum toxin may reduce the severity of fibrosis when injected into tight muscles in the acute phase.

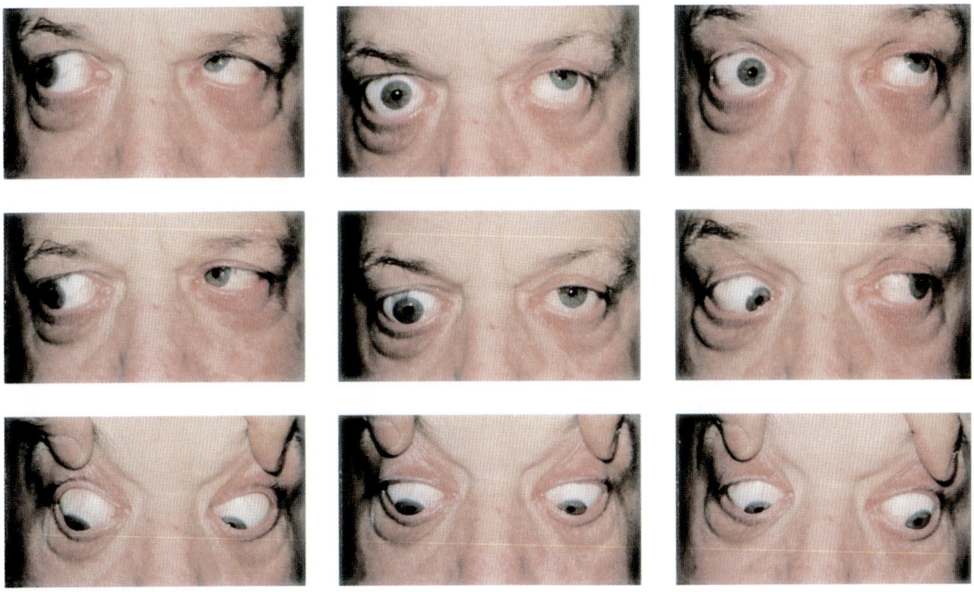

Figure 11-10 TED. Note right upper eyelid retraction and restrictive right hypotropia with very limited elevation. Other rotations are not affected in this patient.

Strabismus surgery in TED may eliminate diplopia in primary gaze but rarely restores normal motility because of the restrictive myopathy, the large recessions sometimes required to bring the eye to primary position, and the ongoing underlying disease. Recession of affected muscles is the preferred treatment; although resection procedures usually worsen restriction, they may be helpful in carefully selected cases. Standard guidelines for the amount of surgery required for a given angle of strabismus may not apply to TED. Surgeons sometimes use adjustable or semi-adjustable sutures. With *intraoperative relaxed muscle positioning,* the restricted muscle is reattached wherever it comes into contact with the globe in primary position when the muscle is not under tension.

Late progressive overcorrection is common with unilateral inferior rectus muscle recessions, due to factors such as asymmetric bilateral inferior rectus restriction, ipsilateral superior rectus restriction, or suboptimal apposition of the recessed muscle to the globe; thus, slight initial undercorrection of hypotropia is desirable. Bilateral surgery may be required, although large bilateral inferior rectus muscle recessions can cause limited depression of the eyes, interfering with bifocal use. They may also cause an A-pattern exotropia in downgaze with intorsion. Bilateral inferior rectus restriction can cause esotropia that improves with recession of the restricted inferior rectus muscles, but esotropia can also be due to medial rectus restriction, requiring horizontal muscle surgery. Imaging may help with surgical planning. Because proptosis and eyelid retraction can increase after EOM surgery, eyelid surgery is best delayed until after strabismus surgery is completed.

Myasthenia Gravis

Myasthenia gravis is an autoimmune disorder in which antibodies directed against acetylcholine receptors cause dysfunction in striated muscle. Onset is usually in adulthood but can occur in childhood. A transient neonatal form, caused by placental transfer of antibodies, can occur in infants of mothers with myasthenia gravis.

The disease may be purely ocular or part of a systemic disorder involving other striated muscles. Generalization to systemic myasthenia is less common with childhood-onset ocular myasthenia than with the adult-onset form.

See BCSC Section 5, *Neuro-Ophthalmology,* and the website of the Myasthenia Gravis Foundation of America (www.myasthenia.org) for further discussion.

Clinical features

Myasthenia gravis can cause weakening of any combination of the EOMs, including the levator muscle. Most cases (90%) exhibit both ptosis and limited ocular rotations (Fig 11-11).

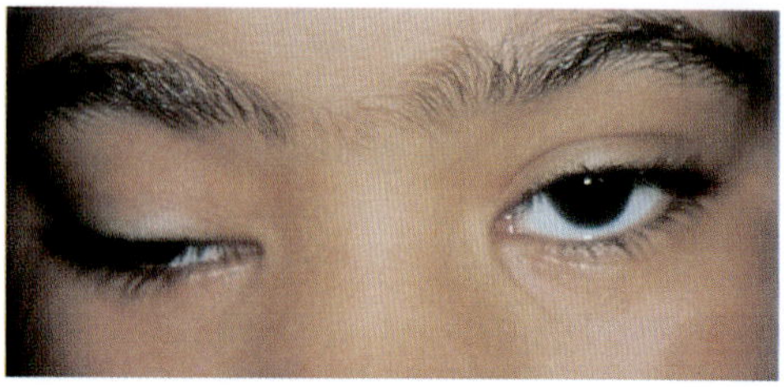

Figure 11-11 Myasthenia gravis. Bilateral ptosis (right more than left) with right hypotropia.

The ocular signs can mimic those of any unilateral or bilateral ophthalmoplegia, including internuclear ophthalmoplegia. Myasthenia gravis does not affect the pupil. Myasthenia gravis should be suspected when multiple EOMs are affected in a pattern that is inconsistent with other etiologies (eg, cranial nerve palsies) and when EOMs show fatigability or variability of deficits.

Management

Systemic treatment options include pyridostigmine, immunosuppression, and thymectomy if there is an associated thymoma (see BCSC Section 5, *Neuro-Ophthalmology*). In adults, the ocular manifestations are frequently resistant to systemic treatments. However, pediatric ocular myasthenia is often successfully managed with pyridostigmine alone. In adults and children in whom the ocular deviation has stabilized, strabismus surgery can restore binocular function in at least some gaze positions. Ptosis occasionally requires surgical repair.

Chronic Progressive External Ophthalmoplegia

Chronic progressive external ophthalmoplegia (CPEO) is a rare mitochondrial cytopathy that can affect various body systems. CPEO may be sporadic or familial. A number of nuclear-encoded mitochondrial genes have been associated with CPEO, but the genetic panel remains of moderate sensitivity.

For additional information on mitochondrial disorders, see BCSC Section 2, *Fundamentals and Principles of Ophthalmology;* Section 5, *Neuro-Ophthalmology;* and Section 12, *Retina and Vitreous.*

Clinical features

CPEO usually begins in childhood with ptosis and slowly progresses to bilateral total paralysis of all EOMs. Although profound retinal dysfunction is rare in CPEO, retinal pigmentary changes, constricted visual fields, and electrophysiologic abnormalities can occur. The diagnosis of CPEO is confirmed by a muscle biopsy that shows ragged red fibers or by detection of specific mitochondrial DNA alterations. *Kearns-Sayre syndrome* is characterized by retinal pigmentary changes, CPEO, and cardiomyopathy (especially heart block).

Management

Patients with CPEO require cardiac evaluation, because life-threatening arrhythmias can occur in Kearns-Sayre syndrome. Treatment options for ocular dysmotility are limited; long-term undercorrection is common. Cautious surgical suspension of the upper eyelids can lessen a severe chin-up head position.

Internuclear Ophthalmoplegia

Conjugate horizontal eye movements depend on connections between the CN VI nucleus and contralateral CN III nucleus via the *medial longitudinal fasciculus (MLF)* (discussed in BCSC Section 5, *Neuro-Ophthalmology*). MLF lesions may result in *internuclear ophthalmoplegia (INO).* INO is common in patients with demyelinating disease but may also occur in those who have had cerebrovascular accidents or brain tumors.

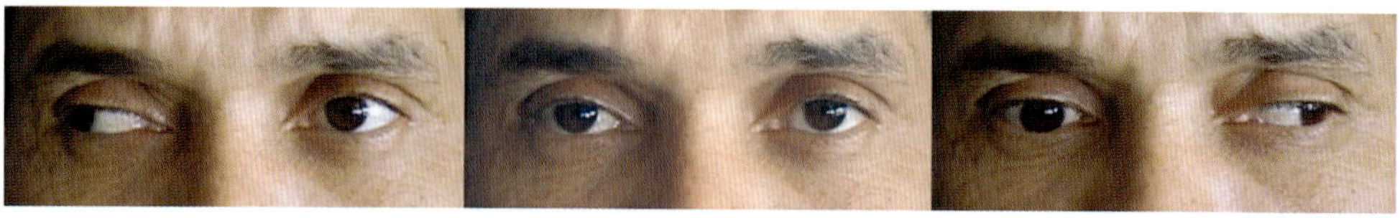

Figure 11-12 Bilateral internuclear ophthalmoplegia. *(Courtesy of Prem S. Subramanian, MD, PhD.)*

Clinical features

On horizontal versions, the eye ipsilateral to the MLF lesion adducts slowly and incompletely or not at all (Fig 11-12, Video 11-3), whereas the abducting eye exhibits a characteristic horizontal jerk nystagmus (see Chapter 12). Both eyes adduct normally on convergence. Skew deviation may be present, in addition to exotropia.

VIDEO 11-3 Internuclear ophthalmoplegia.
Courtesy of M. Tariq Bhatti, MD.

Management

If exotropia persists, medial rectus muscle resection and unilateral or contralateral lateral rectus muscle recession (to limit exotropia in lateral gaze) can help eliminate diplopia, particularly in bilateral cases.

Heavy Eye Syndrome

In highly myopic patients, extremely increased axial length can cause the elongated globe to herniate between the superior and lateral rectus muscles. High-resolution magnetic resolution imaging (MRI) studies show stretching and dehiscence of the intermuscular septum between these 2 muscles, with inferior slippage of the lateral rectus pulley, and medial displacement of the superior rectus. These anomalies cause a progressively worsening hypotropia and esotropia known as *heavy eye syndrome,* also referred to as *myopic strabismus fixus* in severe cases with limited motility (Fig 11-13). The medial rectus is often tight, exacerbating the esotropia.

Various surgical procedures can stabilize the position of the lateral rectus muscle. An effective option is a joining of the superior and lateral rectus muscles, usually with a nonabsorbable suture, to reposition the globe. Recession of the medial rectus muscle may also be necessary if the muscle is tight.

Hennein L, Robbins SL. Heavy eye syndrome: myopia-induced strabismus. *Surv Ophthalmol.* 2021;66(1):138–144.

Sagging Eye Syndrome

Dehiscence of the intermuscular septum between the superior and lateral rectus muscles can also result from age-related increases in connective tissue laxity in the absence of high myopia (Fig 11-14). The resulting small-angle vertical strabismus with esotropia usually worse at distance fixation is known as *sagging eye syndrome.*

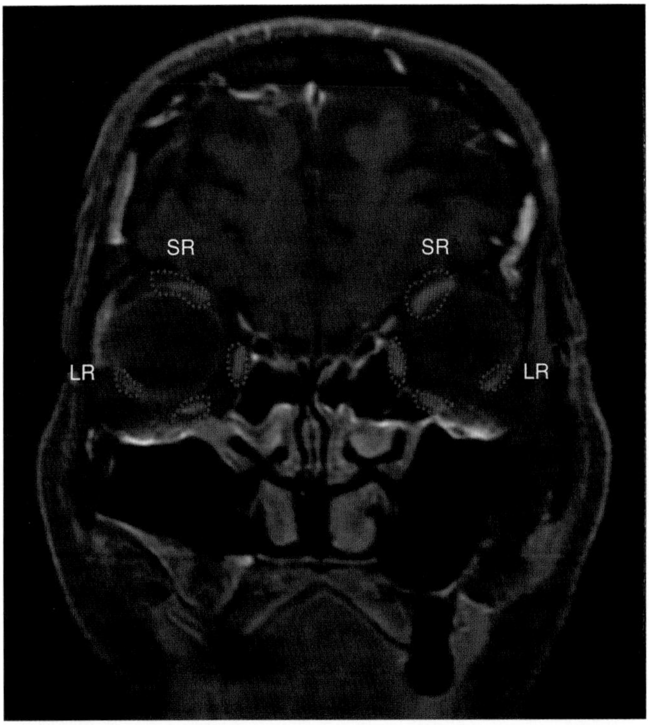

Figure 11-13 MRI scan of a patient with heavy eye syndrome. Rectus muscles are outlined in red, showing how herniation of the elongated globe between the lateral rectus (LR) and superior rectus (SR) muscles bilaterally results in displacement of the rectus muscles. *(Reprinted from Hennein L, Robbins SL. Heavy eye syndrome: myopia-induced strabismus.* Surv Ophthalmol. *2021;66(1):138–144. Copyright 2021, with permission from Elsevier.)*

Strabismus Associated With Other Ocular Surgery

Refractive surgery that produces monovision, facilitating visual clarity at distance and near without optical aids (mainly in presbyopic adults; see BCSC Section 13, *Refractive Surgery*), can result in dissimilar sensory input to the 2 eyes. This can impair motor fusion, particularly in patients with marginally controlled heterophorias, causing diplopia.

In a patient with preexisting childhood-onset strabismus, a refractive change that induces the patient to switch fixation to the nondominant eye during binocular viewing can cause *fixation-switch* diplopia, even if the preexisting strabismus is unchanged.

Retinal distortion from an epiretinal membrane or following retinal detachment repair can distort the retinal image (metamorphopsia, micropsia, or macropsia), impairing fusion and causing diplopia. The *dragged-fovea diplopia syndrome* occurs when an epiretinal membrane decenters the fovea within the retina, so that when the retinal periphery is aligned between the 2 eyes, the foveae are misaligned, and vice versa. Prism and alternate cover testing demonstrates a small heterotropia corresponding to the foveal displacement. But under binocular conditions, that prism eliminates the diplopia only briefly, until a fusion movement brings the peripheral retinae back into alignment. The diplopia may

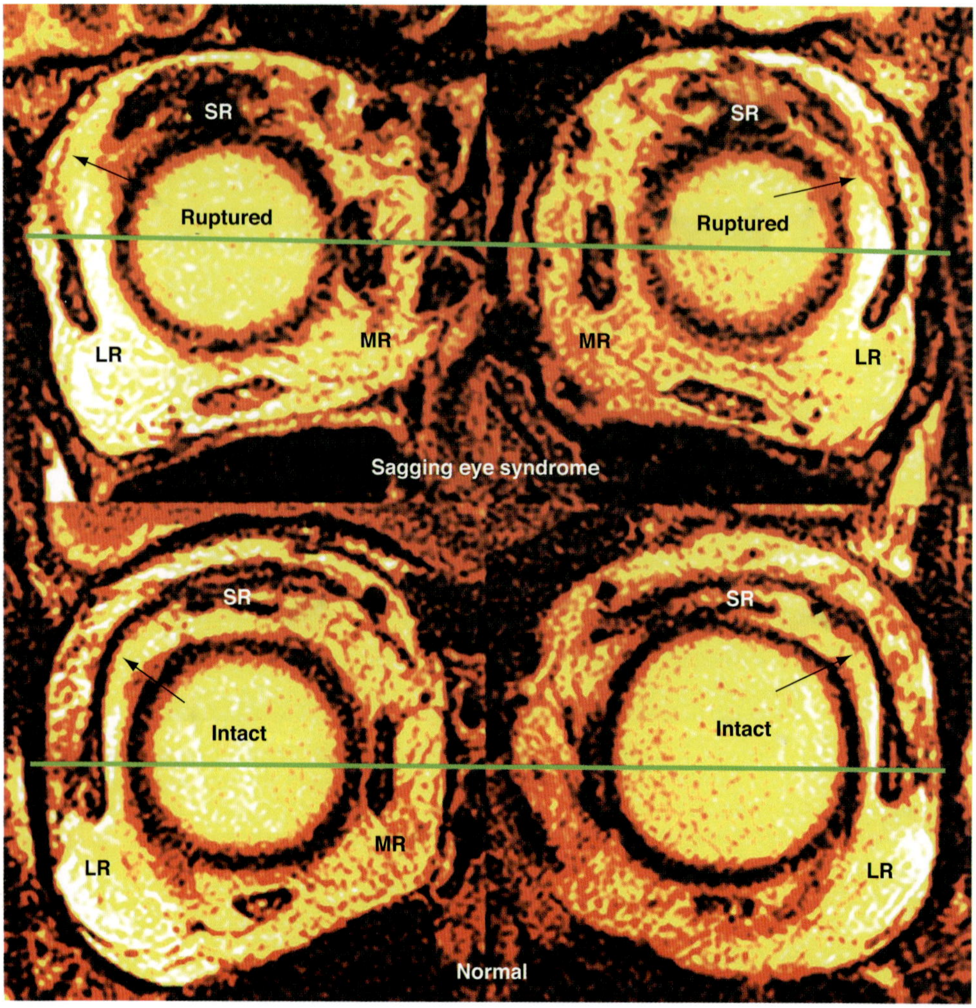

Figure 11-14 High-resolution MRI shows dehisced and ruptured intermuscular septum between the superior rectus (SR) and lateral rectus (LR) muscles in a patient with sagging eye syndrome *(top),* in contrast to the intact intermuscular septum in an unaffected individual *(bottom). (Courtesy of Joe L. Demer, MD, PhD.)*

sometimes improve with surgery for the epiretinal membrane, but often requires fogging the eye with a translucent filter or tape, sometimes in combination with a small amount of prism.

Surgery for retinal detachment can lead to restricted rotations and scarring from dissection of the EOMs and scleral buckles (see BCSC Section 12, *Retina and Vitreous*). Surgical correction of the resultant strabismus is often difficult. Consultation with a retina surgeon is recommended prior to considering removal of a scleral buckle.

Tube shunt surgery can cause scarring and interference with ocular rotations (see BCSC Section 10, *Glaucoma*). Treatment may require removal, relocation, or substitution of the device, which creates a dilemma if it has been functioning well.

The EOMs can be damaged by retrobulbar injections, by either direct injury to EOMs or toxicity of the injected material. Because injections are usually placed inferiorly, the inferior rectus muscle is the most vulnerable. The characteristic pattern is an initial hypertropia of the affected eye due to an induced inferior rectus muscle weakness, followed by a hypotropia of the affected eye from subsequent inferior rectus muscle scarring and restriction. Injection of botulinum toxin into the eyelids can result in diffusion of this substance and a transient paralysis of any EOM.

Laceration or inadvertent excision of a section of the medial rectus muscle can occur as a complication of pterygium removal or endoscopic sinus surgery. Surgical restoration of function can be extremely challenging.

Conjunctival scarring and symblepharon can result in restrictive strabismus after pterygium surgery or other surgery or trauma involving the conjunctiva, particularly in the lateral canthal area. Treatment involves lysis or excision of the fibrotic band, coupled with conjunctival recession, conjunctival transposition, or an amniotic membrane graft.

De Pool ME, Campbell JP, Broome SO, Guyton DL. The dragged-fovea diplopia syndrome. *Ophthalmology.* 2005;112(8):1455–1462.

Hatt SR, Leske DA, Klaehn LD, Kramer AM, Iezzi R Jr, Holmes JM. Treatment for central-peripheral rivalry-type diplopia ("dragged-fovea diplopia syndrome"). *Am J Ophthalmol.* 2019;208:41–46.

Other Special Motility Disorders

Ocular Motor Apraxia

Ocular motor apraxia (OMA), or *saccadic initiation failure,* is a rare supranuclear disorder of ocular motility. The congenital form may be familial, usually autosomal dominant.

OMA has been associated with premature birth and developmental delay. Bilateral lesions of the frontoparietal cortex, agenesis of the corpus callosum, hydrocephalus, and Joubert syndrome (developmental delay, microcephaly, cerebellar vermis hypoplasia, and retinal dysplasia, among other anomalies) are also associated with OMA. OMA may occur in childhood neurodegenerative conditions such as type 3 Gaucher disease and ataxia-telangiectasia. Several case reports describe OMA with mass lesions of the cerebellum that compress the rostral brainstem. Neurodevelopmental evaluation and neuroimaging are advisable in children with OMA, especially if there is also vertical apraxia.

Acquired OMA in adults can result from conditions that affect voluntary saccades, including degenerative diseases such as Huntington chorea.

Clinical features

In OMA, normal voluntary horizontal saccades cannot be generated. Horizontal vestibular and optokinetic nystagmus are also impaired. Vertical saccades and random eye movements are usually intact. Voluntary changes in horizontal fixation are accomplished by a head thrust that overshoots the target, followed by a rotation of the head back in the opposite direction once fixation is established. The initial thrust serves to break fixation; an associated blink serves the same purpose. Video 11-4 shows head-thrusting behavior to change gaze direction in a child with OMA associated with cerebellar vermis hypoplasia and abnormal brainstem motor fiber decussation; the child also has periodic alternating side gaze. The head thrust may improve in later childhood. See BCSC Section 5, *Neuro-Ophthalmology.*

VIDEO 11-4 Ocular motor apraxia.
Courtesy of Michael C. Brodsky, MD; Suresh Kotagal, MD; Pavel N. Pichurin, MD; and Mai-Lan Ho, MD.

Superior Oblique Myokymia

Superior oblique myokymia is a rare entity whose cause is poorly understood. Some evidence indicates that it is caused by ephaptic transmission between CN IV fibers, perhaps due, in some cases, to damage by vascular compression.

Clinical features

In superior oblique myokymia, there are abnormal torsional movements of the eye that cause diplopia and monocular oscillopsia (Video 11-5). Usually, patients are otherwise neurologically normal. Recurrences may persist indefinitely.

VIDEO 11-5 Superior oblique myokymia.
Courtesy of Paul H. Phillips, MD.

Management

Treatment is not necessary if the patient is not disturbed by the visual symptoms. Various systemic medications (eg, carbamazepine, phenytoin, propranolol, baclofen, gabapentin) and topical timolol have produced inconsistent results but have been advocated as first-line treatment because some patients will benefit, at least in the short term. Surgical treatment requires disconnecting the superior oblique muscle from the globe by generous tenectomy, sometimes coupled with simultaneous inferior oblique muscle weakening to mitigate the resulting superior oblique palsy.

CHAPTER 12

Childhood Nystagmus

This chapter includes related videos. Go to www.aao.org/bcscvideo_section06 or scan the QR codes in the text to access this content.

Highlights

- Nystagmus is a sign, not a diagnosis, and requires an evaluation for the underlying cause.
- Childhood nystagmus is often associated with visual sensory defects but can also result from neurologic abnormalities.
- Treatment options for some forms of nystagmus include the use of prisms or eye muscle surgery.

Introduction

Nystagmus is an involuntary, rhythmic oscillation of the eyes. It is a sign, not a diagnosis, and requires an evaluation. Nystagmus can be related to

- instability in the damping portion of the smooth pursuit system, which can be due to a motor defect that is compatible with relatively good vision
- an ocular abnormality that is associated with poor vision or fusion
- a neurologic abnormality

Distinguishing among these underlying diagnoses can be challenging. See BCSC Section 5, *Neuro-Ophthalmology,* for additional discussion of nystagmus.

General Features

The plane of nystagmus can be horizontal, vertical, torsional, or a combination of these. The condition is often characterized as either *jerk nystagmus,* which has a slow and a fast component, or *pendular nystagmus,* in which the eyes oscillate with equal velocity in each direction. By convention, jerk nystagmus is described by the direction of its fast-phase component; for example, a right jerk nystagmus consists of a slow movement to the left, followed by a fast movement (jerk) to the right. Nystagmus is conjugate (as opposed to dysconjugate) when its direction, frequency (number of oscillations per unit of time), and amplitude (magnitude of the eye movement) are the same in both eyes.

Nystagmus characteristics may change with gaze direction. Pendular nystagmus can become jerk nystagmus on side gaze. Jerk nystagmus can have a *null point* or *null zone* (gaze position in which the intensity [frequency × amplitude] is diminished and the vision improves), or it can decrease in intensity with gaze in the direction opposite that of the fast-phase component (analogous to Alexander's law for vestibular nystagmus). The abnormal head position that patients assume in order to reduce nystagmus can be the most prominent manifestation of their condition.

Nomenclature

The National Eye Institute (NEI) has classified eye movement abnormalities, including nystagmus. This chapter uses the terms recommended by the NEI-sponsored Committee for the Classification of Eye Movement Abnormalities and Strabismus.

CEMAS Working Group. A National Eye Institute sponsored workshop and publication on the classification of eye movement abnormalities and strabismus (CEMAS). In: Hertle RW, ed. *The National Eye Institute Publications.* National Eye Institute, National Institutes of Health; 2001.

Types of Childhood Nystagmus

Infantile Nystagmus Syndrome

Infantile nystagmus syndrome (INS) is a binocular, conjugate nystagmus with several distinctive features (Table 12-1, Video 12-1). It can be related to visual sensory defects or idiopathic. It is often recognized in the first few months of life. The nystagmus is uniplanar (ie, the plane of the nystagmus remains the same in all positions of gaze) and is most often horizontal. When INS has a jerk waveform, it shows an exponential increase in velocity during the slow phase (Fig 12-1). A null point may be present, with a change in the direction of the nystagmus to the right or the left of the null point (ie, right jerk nystagmus to the right of the null point and left jerk to the left of the null point). If the null point is not in primary position, the patient may adopt an abnormal head position to improve vision by placing the eyes near the null point. This head position becomes more pronounced as the child approaches school age. Head bobbing or movement may be present initially but commonly decreases with age if there is no progressive visual deficit.

Table 12-1 Features of Infantile Nystagmus Syndrome

Conjugate
Horizontal
Uniplanar
Worsens with attempted fixation
Improves with convergence
Null point often present with abnormal head position
"Inverted" optokinetic nystagmus response in two-thirds of patients
Oscillopsia usually not present

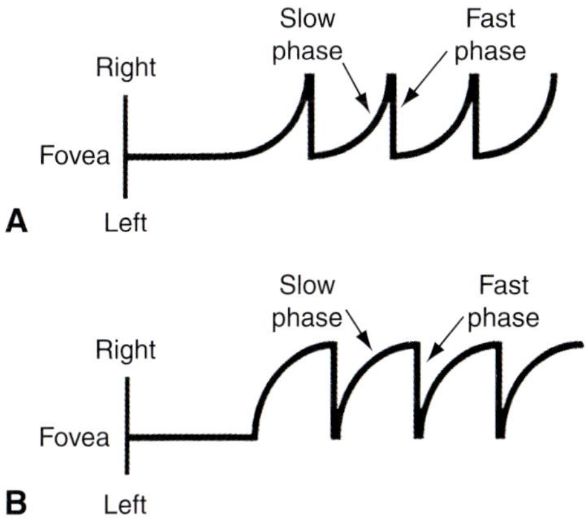

Figure 12-1 Left jerk nystagmus. **A,** Electronystagmographic evaluation of infantile nystagmus syndrome (INS) shows an exponential increase in velocity during the slow phase. **B,** An exponential decrease in velocity during the slow phase is the waveform characteristic of fusion maldevelopment nystagmus syndrome.

VIDEO 12-1 Infantile nystagmus syndrome.
Courtesy of Paul H. Phillips, MD.

INS worsens with fixation and may worsen with illness or fatigue. Convergence damps (reduces the intensity of) the nystagmus. Thus, near visual acuity is often better than distance acuity in these patients. Occasionally, children with INS overconverge to damp the nystagmus *(nystagmus blockage syndrome),* resulting in esotropia. INS can be confused with nystagmus blockage syndrome in which esotropia and nystagmus happen to coexist or with cases of infantile strabismus with fusion maldevelopment nystagmus syndrome (discussed later in this chapter). Patients with this condition characteristically present with an esotropia that "eats up prism" as the strabismic deviation increases upon attempted measurement, and with nystagmus that is least apparent when the deviation is largest.

Approximately two-thirds of INS patients exhibit a paradoxical inversion of the optokinetic nystagmus (OKN) response. Typically, when a patient with right jerk nystagmus views an optokinetic drum rotating to the patient's left (eliciting a "pursuit left, jerk right" response), the intensity of the right jerk nystagmus increases. However, patients with INS exhibit a damped right jerk nystagmus or possibly even a left jerk nystagmus when viewing an optokinetic drum rotating to the left.

The waveform is identical in INS whether it is related to visual sensory defects or is idiopathic. Given that the visual behavior of an infant with a central scotoma is not that different from that of an infant with normal visual acuity, all cases of INS should be presumed to be related to sensory issues and deserve a workup (see the following section).

INS with visual sensory defects

INS with visual sensory defects is associated with an early-onset, bilateral abnormality of the pregeniculate afferent visual pathway. Inadequate retinal image formation interferes with the normal development of the fixation reflex. If the visual deficit is present at birth, the resulting nystagmus becomes apparent in the first 3 months of life. Its severity is somewhat correlated with the degree of vision loss. The waveform of sensory nystagmus can be pendular or jerk.

Searching, slow, or wandering conjugate eye movements may also be observed. Searching nystagmus—defined as a roving or drifting, typically horizontal movement of the eyes without fixation (Video 12-2)—is usually seen in children whose visual acuity is worse than 20/200. Pendular nystagmus typically occurs in patients with visual acuity better than 20/200 in at least 1 eye. Jerk nystagmus is often associated with visual acuity between 20/60 and 20/100.

VIDEO 12-2 Roving eye movements.
Courtesy of Mays El-Dairi, MD. Narration by Robert Clay, COT.

The reason for the sensory abnormality may be obvious, as with cataracts; subtle, as with mild optic nerve hypoplasia or foveal hypoplasia; or not visible on examination, as with some forms of foveal hypoplasia, retinal dystrophies, or a retrobulbar pathology such as an optic pathway glioma (these topics are further discussed elsewhere in this volume).

Idiopathic infantile nystagmus

Idiopathic infantile nystagmus (IIS) is a form of INS that is not associated with visual dysfunction. Because the nystagmus waveform and clinical examination are almost identical to those of INS with visual sensory deficit, IIS should be considered a diagnosis of exclusion. Genetic testing for the gene *FRMD7* can be performed to evaluate for X-linked INS, which can be mistaken for IIS.

Central Vestibular Instability Nystagmus

Central vestibular instability nystagmus (also called *periodic alternating nystagmus; PAN*) is an unusual form of jerk nystagmus that can be congenital or acquired (the latter especially in those with cerebellar abnormalities or Arnold-Chiari malformation). The nystagmus periodically changes direction due to a shifting null point (Video 12-3). The cycle begins with a typical jerk nystagmus, which slowly damps; this leads to a 10- to 20-second period of no nystagmus, followed by jerk nystagmus in the opposite direction. The cycle repeats every few minutes. Some children adopt an alternating head turn to take advantage of the changing null point.

VIDEO 12-3 Central vestibular instability nystagmus (periodic alternating nystagmus).
Courtesy of Edward G. Buckley, MD.

Fusion Maldevelopment Nystagmus Syndrome

Fusion maldevelopment nystagmus syndrome (FMNS) is a conjugate, horizontal jerk nystagmus and a marker of fusion maldevelopment, which occurs as a result of infantile-onset strabismus or (less commonly) decreased vision in 1 eye. When either eye is occluded, a conjugate jerk nystagmus develops. The fast-phase component is directed toward the uncovered eye: left jerk nystagmus occurs upon covering the right eye, and right jerk nystagmus upon covering the left (Video 12-4). This is the only nystagmus that reverses direction depending on which eye is fixating. The nystagmus damps when the fixating eye is in adduction, so the

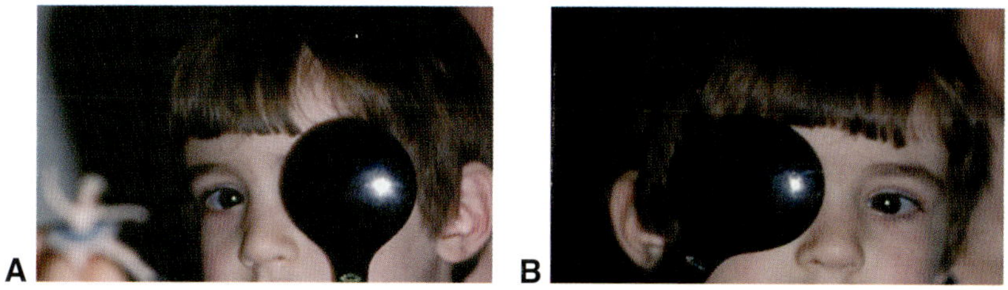

Figure 12-2 Fusion maldevelopment nystagmus syndrome. **A,** A right head turn occurs during fixation with the right eye. **B,** The head turn reverses direction during fixation with the left eye. The nystagmus damps with the fixating eye in adduction. *(Courtesy of Edward L. Raab, MD.)*

preferred head turn also reverses direction with change of fixation (Fig 12-2). Amplitude, frequency, and velocity of the nystagmus can also vary depending on which eye is fixating.

VIDEO 12-4 Fusion maldevelopment nystagmus syndrome.
Courtesy of Robert W. Hered, MD.

Fusion or binocular viewing damps FMNS, and disruption of fusion (eg, by occlusion) increases it. FMNS may manifest even when both eyes are open if only 1 eye is being used for viewing (eg, the other eye is suppressed or amblyopic). Electronystagmographic evaluation of both fully latent and manifest forms of FMNS shows similar waveforms, with a slow phase of constant or exponentially decreasing velocity (see Fig 12-1B). Like other hallmarks of infantile strabismus with which it is associated (dissociated vertical deviation and oblique muscle overaction), FMNS becomes more prominent with age.

Richards M, Wong A, Foeller P, Bradley D, Tychsen L. Duration of binocular decorrelation predicts the severity of latent (fusion maldevelopment) nystagmus in strabismic macaque monkeys. *Invest Ophthalmol Vis Sci.* 2008;49(5):1872–1878.

Acquired Nystagmus

Spasmus nutans syndrome

Spasmus nutans syndrome (spasmus nutans) is an idiopathic acquired nystagmus that manifests during the first 2 years of life, presenting as a triad of generally small-amplitude, high-frequency ("shimmering"), dysconjugate nystagmus; head nodding; and torticollis. The nystagmus is binocular but often asymmetric, sometimes appearing to be monocular. The plane of the nystagmus can be horizontal, vertical, or torsional; the nystagmus can vary with gaze position, and it is occasionally intermittent. The head nodding and torticollis appear to be compensatory movements that maximize vision. Typically, the abnormal head and eye movements diminish by 3–4 years of age. Spasmus nutans syndrome is a benign disorder in most cases, but there is a high incidence of associated strabismus, amblyopia, and developmental delay.

Spasmus nutans–like nystagmus has been seen with chiasmal or suprachiasmal tumors, hypomyelinating leukodystrophies (eg, Pelizaeus-Merzbacher disease) and retinal dystrophies such as cone dystrophy with supranormal rod response. Because the retina can appear normal despite abnormal function, electroretinography is part of the diagnostic evaluation. Neuroradiologic investigation is warranted when there is any evidence of optic nerve dysfunction or any sign of neurologic abnormality.

Khan AO. Recognizing the *KCNV2*-related retinal phenotype. *Ophthalmology*. 2013;120(11): e79–80.

See-saw nystagmus

See-saw nystagmus is an unusual but dramatic type of dysconjugate nystagmus that has both vertical and torsional components. If the 2 eyes are envisioned as being placed on an imaginary see-saw, 1 at either end, they "roll down the plank" as 1 end of the see-saw rises, with the high eye intorting and the low eye extorting. As the direction of the see-saw changes, so does that of the eye movement. Thus, the eyes make alternating movements of elevation and intorsion, followed by depression and extorsion (Video 12-5).

VIDEO 12-5 See-saw nystagmus.
Courtesy of Agnes M.F. Wong, MD, PhD.

This type of nystagmus is often associated with rostral midbrain or suprasellar lesions, most often craniopharyngioma in children. Confrontation visual field testing may elicit a bitemporal defect. Neuroradiologic evaluation is necessary. A congenital form of see-saw nystagmus can be seen in disorders of decussation (usually associated with optic nerve hypoplasia and temporal visual field defects), such as those sometimes seen in Joubert syndrome.

Vertical nystagmus

Vertical nystagmus is uncommon. Congenital vertical nystagmus, often upbeat, can occur in infants with inherited retinal dystrophies (Video 12-6). Downbeat nystagmus (Video 12-7) can be part of a neurologic ataxia syndrome. When vertical nystagmus is acquired and associated ocular sensory defect has been ruled out, neurological workup is indicated, including investigation of structural abnormalities such as Arnold-Chiari malformations. Acquired vertical nystagmus can also be related to medications such as codeine, lithium, anxiolytics, and anticonvulsants. (See BCSC Section 5, *Neuro-Ophthalmology*.)

VIDEO 12-6 Upbeat nystagmus.
Courtesy of Arif O. Khan, MD.

VIDEO 12-7 Downbeat nystagmus.
Courtesy of Janet C. Rucker, MD.

Monocular nystagmus

Monocular nystagmus has been reported to occur in severely amblyopic or blind eyes *(Heimann-Bielschowsky phenomenon)*. The oscillations are pendular, chiefly vertical, slow, variable in amplitude, and irregular in frequency.

Nystagmus-Like Disorders

See Chapter 10 in BCSC Section 5, *Neuro-Ophthalmology,* for more discussion of the topics in this section.

Induced Convergence-Retraction (Convergence-Retraction Nystagmus)

Induced convergence-retraction (convergence-retraction nystagmus) is not a true nystagmus; rather, the abnormal eye movements are saccades. In children and adults, induced convergence-retraction is part of the dorsal midbrain syndrome, which is associated with paralysis of upward gaze, eyelid retraction, and pupillary light–near dissociation. In children, it commonly occurs secondary to congenital aqueductal stenosis or a pinealoma. The phenomenon is best elicited by having the patient attempt an upgaze saccade (eg, track a downward-rotating optokinetic drum) (Video 12-8). Co-contraction of all horizontal extraocular muscles occurs upon attempted upgaze, causing globe *retraction. Convergence* also occurs, because the medial rectus muscles overpower the lateral rectus muscles (voluntary convergence, however, may be impaired).

VIDEO 12-8 Induced convergence-retraction (convergence-retraction nystagmus).
Courtesy of Edward G. Buckley, MD.

Saccadic Oscillations

Saccadic pulses, ocular flutter, and *opsoclonus* are not a true nystagmus (there is no slow phase). Saccadic pulses are horizontal saccadic intrusions that occur in a series or doublets with an intersaccadic interval. Ocular flutter consists of involuntary rapid horizontal saccades. *Opsoclonus* consists of involuntary rapid and multidirectional saccades and is often accompanied by somatic dyskinesias (Video 12-9). Causes of saccadic oscillations in children include acute postinfectious myoclonic encephalopathy of infants, cerebellar ataxia, viral encephalitis, and paraneoplastic manifestations of neuroblastoma.

VIDEO 12-9 Opsoclonus.
Courtesy of Arif O. Khan, MD.

Evaluation

History

The patient history should include questions about the pregnancy and birth because factors such as intrauterine exposure to infection, maternal use of drugs or alcohol, prematurity, and other prenatal or perinatal events can affect development of the visual system and contribute to nystagmus. Family history may aid diagnosis and provide prognostic information; many potential causes of INS are inherited.

For children older than 3 months, parental observations regarding head tilts, head movements, gaze preference, and viewing distances can aid in functional assessment.

Ocular Examination

Visual acuity

The level of visual function does not help determine the cause of the nystagmus, especially in an infant. INS with visual sensory defects such as an isolated central scotoma can behave exactly like IIS.

Because monocular occlusion can increase nystagmus intensity, particularly in cases of FMNS, monocular acuity should be tested with at least 1 of the following:

- fogging, either with a fogging occluder, using >+5.00 diopters greater than the refractive error, or with translucent tape placed over the patient's prescription glasses over the nontested eye)
- polarizing lenses with a polarized chart
- an occluder positioned several inches in front of the nontested eye

Binocular visual acuity is often better than monocular acuity and should be measured at distance and near fixation, with any desired head position permitted, to assess the child's true functional vision. Near visual acuity is usually better than distance. Children with a distance acuity below 20/400 can sometimes read as well as at the 20/40 to 20/60 level at near fixation.

In preverbal children, the optokinetic drum can be used to estimate visual acuity. If vertical rotation of an optokinetic drum elicits a vertical nystagmus superimposed on the child's underlying nystagmus, the visual acuity is usually 20/400 or better. Preferential looking tests such as Teller Acuity Cards II (Stereo Optical, Inc.) can also be used (see Chapter 1); in patients with horizontal nystagmus, the responses can be more easily assessed with the cards held vertically.

Pupils

Sluggish or absent responses to light, or a relative afferent pupillary defect in asymmetric cases, indicate a bilateral anterior visual pathway abnormality such as optic nerve or retinal dysfunction. However, normal responses can be seen with some sensory abnormalities such as foveal hypoplasia and achromatopsia.

The normal response to darkness is the immediate dilation of the pupil. If, instead of dilating, the pupils paradoxically constrict, optic nerve or retinal disease may be present (Video 12-10). To test for a paradoxical pupil, the clinician can use a retinoscope from a distance to see the red reflex while turning the room light on and off.

VIDEO 12-10 Paradoxical pupil.
Courtesy of Arif O. Khan, MD.

Anterior segment

Examination of the anterior segment may reveal a direct cause of decreased vision (eg, congenital cataracts, corneal opacities) or clues to the cause of decreased vision (eg, aniridia or iris transillumination in albinism, both of which are associated with foveal hypoplasia).

Ocular motility

Nystagmus may be associated with strabismus for a variety of reasons. Early-onset strabismus may cause FMNS; convergence may be used to damp nystagmus; or poor vision may be the underlying cause of both the nystagmus and the strabismus.

Fundus

Optic nerve hypoplasia and foveal hypoplasia are common causes of congenital sensory nystagmus that may be diagnosed on fundus examination. However, mild optic nerve hypoplasia and optic atrophy may be difficult to appreciate on an examination, especially when the nerve is moving at high speed. Some types of retinal dystrophy may present with vascular attenuation or optic nerve head pallor; however, the fundus typically appears normal in an infant with Leber congenital amaurosis.

If handheld optical coherence tomography is available, it can help the clinician rule out optic atrophy (eg, optic pathway glioma), foveal hypoplasia, or outer retinal changes (Fig 12-3); if electroretinography is available, it can help rule out Leber congenital amaurosis. If neither technology is available and vision is normal, genetic testing can reveal *FRMD7*-associated INS.

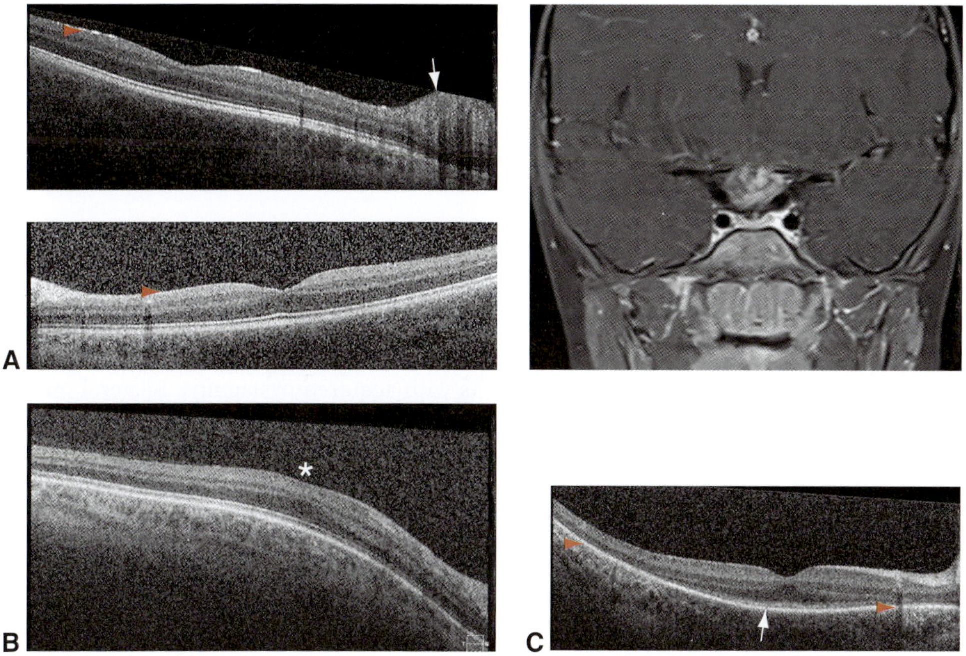

Figure 12-3 Optical coherence tomography (OCT) of 3 INS cases. **A,** A 4-year-old boy with nystagmus since infancy that was initially misdiagnosed as idiopathic. Visual acuity was not correctable to better than 20/300. OCT shows attenuation of the ganglion cell layer *(arrowheads)* and elevated optic nerves *(arrow)* in both eyes. Magnetic resonance imaging (MRI) shows an optic pathway glioma. **B,** Foveal hypoplasia *(asterisk)* due to Hermansky-Pudlack syndrome (visual acuity is 20/25). **C,** A 6-year-old girl with nystagmus due to Leber congenital amaurosis *(CEP290)*. OCT shows marked thickening of the ellipsoid zone centrally *(arrow)* and attenuation of the outer nuclear layer in the periphery *(arrowheads)*. *(Courtesy of Mays El-Dairi, MD.)*

Treatment

The first step in treating nystagmus is to address the primary cause, especially if vision is threatened (eg, with causes such as cataract or optic pathway glioma).

Prisms

The use of prisms can improve anomalous head positions by shifting the perceived object location toward the null point. For a patient with a left head turn and a null point in right gaze, the prism held before the right eye should be oriented base-in, and the prism held before the left eye oriented base-out. This shifts the retinal images to the patient's left and the perceived object location to the right; objects in front of the patient are now imaged on the fovea when the patient is in right gaze, reducing the amount of head turn required to use the null point gaze position.

In patients with binocular fusion, bilateral base-out prisms can improve vision by inducing convergence, which damps nystagmus (amounts are determined by trial and error).

Prisms can be used as the sole treatment of nystagmus or as a trial to predict surgical success. With powers ranging up to 40 prism diopters, Press-On (Fresnel) prisms, inexpensive plastic pieces that can be cut and then applied to glasses, can be used for both purposes. Ground-in prisms cause less distortion and are preferred for patients who require only small amounts of prism.

Other nonsurgical treatment options for nystagmus are discussed in BCSC Section 5, *Neuro-Ophthalmology.*

Surgery

Extraocular muscle surgery for nystagmus may correct a stable anomalous head position by shifting the null point closer to the primary position; this is achieved with medial rectus recession in 1 eye and lateral rectus recession in the other *(Anderson procedure)* or a recession-resection procedure in both eyes *(Kestenbaum procedure).* Surgery can similarly alleviate compensatory head positions in adults with acquired nystagmus. Bilateral medial rectus recession can treat esotropia resulting from nystagmus blockage syndrome (using larger-than-normal recessions for the amount of esotropia, sometimes in combination with posterior fixation sutures). Extraocular muscle surgery may also improve vision in nystagmus by increasing foveation time, as has been reported with recession or tenotomy and reattachment of all 4 horizontal rectus muscles. See Chapter 13 for further discussion of the surgical techniques mentioned in this chapter.

In a Kestenbaum or Anderson procedure, the eyes are rotated toward the direction of the head turn and away from the preferred gaze position, moving both eyes in the same direction. For patients with INS, a left head turn, and null point in right gaze, the eyes are surgically rotated to the left by recessing the right lateral and left medial rectus muscles and resecting the right medial and left lateral rectus muscles (exotropia surgery for the right eye and esotropia surgery for the left eye). The right-gaze effort, which damps nystagmus, now brings the eyes from this leftward-rotated position to primary position, instead of from primary position into right gaze; in other words, the null point has been shifted toward the primary position (Fig 12-4).

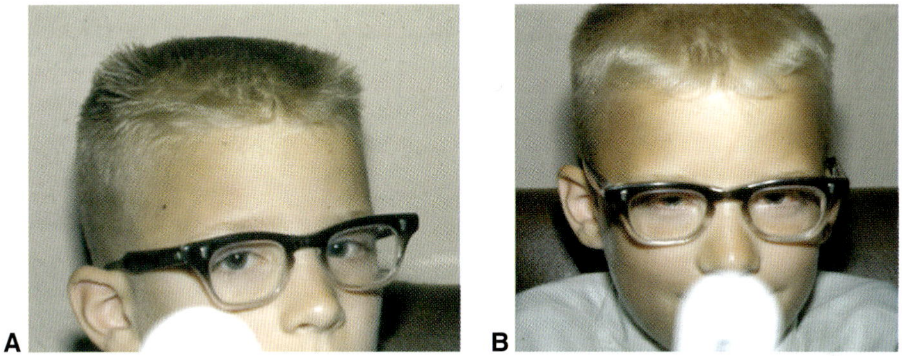

Figure 12-4 Shifting the null point in INS. **A,** Infantile nystagmus syndrome with the null point in right gaze. **B,** Null point shifted by the Kestenbaum procedure, reducing the head turn. *(Courtesy of Edward L. Raab, MD.)*

Suggested amounts of recession and resection are listed in Table 12-2. The total amount of surgery for each eye (in millimeters) is equal in order to rotate each globe an equal amount. Nonaugmented numbers are sufficient for head turn that is less than 20°. For head turns of 30°, 40% augmentation is recommended; for turns of 45°, 60% augmentation is used. Augmentation may restrict motility, but this is usually necessary to achieve a satisfactory result.

Similarly, chin-up or chin-down positions may be ameliorated by use of a vertical prism (apex toward the null point) or surgery on vertical rectus or oblique muscles, rotating the eyes away from the preferred gaze position. For a chin-up, eyes-down position, the inferior rectus muscles are recessed and the superior rectus muscles resected, usually by 8–10 mm in each eye. Alternatively, the surgeon can combine weakening of a vertical rectus muscle and an oblique muscle in each eye. For a chin-up position, the inferior rectus and superior oblique muscles are weakened; for a chin-down position, the superior rectus and inferior oblique muscles are weakened. Improvement of head tilt in nystagmus has been reported with torsional surgery involving the oblique muscles or transposition of the vertical or horizontal rectus muscles. Although surgery for downbeat nystagmus can significantly improve head posture and central vision, it has a lower success rate than does surgery for horizontal nystagmus.

Table 12-2 Amount of Recession and Resection for Kestenbaum Procedure, With Modifications[a]

Procedure	Kestenbaum, mm (Head Turn 20°–30°)	40% Augmented, mm (Head Turn 30°–40°)	60% Augmented, mm (Head Turn ≥45°)
Eye adducted in null point			
Recess medial rectus	5.0	7.0	8.0
Resect lateral rectus	8.0	11.0	12.5
Eye abducted in null point			
Recess lateral rectus	7.0	10.0	11.0
Resect medial rectus	6.0	8.5	9.5

[a]Amounts listed are for the original Kestenbaum procedure plus 2 modifications in which the amount of surgery is increased.

For nystagmus patients with strabismus, surgery to shift the null point is performed on the dominant eye; surgery on the nondominant eye is then adjusted to account for the strabismus. For example, a patient who is right-eye dominant with a right head turn and null point in left gaze would undergo right medial rectus recession and right lateral rectus resection, as shown in Table 12-2. This would contribute to reducing the angle of an esodeviation or increasing the angle of an exodeviation. Surgery would then be performed on the nonpreferred eye to correct the residual or resultant deviation. Prisms can be used to estimate the target angle.

Other types of nystagmus surgery are less widely practiced. The goal of recession of all 4 horizontal rectus muscles to a position posterior to the equator (8- to 10-mm recessions of medial rectus muscles and 10- to 12-mm recessions of lateral rectus muscles) is to improve vision. Simple 4-muscle tenotomy, in which the horizontal rectus muscles are disinserted and reattached without recession or resection, has produced similar results, improving recognition time and foveation time on electronystagmography, with modest improvements in visual acuity (approximately 1 line on average).

Hertle RW, Dell'Osso LF, FitzGibbon EJ, Thompson D, Yang D, Mellow SD. Horizontal rectus tenotomy in patients with congenital nystagmus: results in 10 adults. *Ophthalmology.* 2003; 110(11):2097–2105.

CHAPTER 13

Surgery of the Extraocular Muscles

This chapter includes related videos. Go to www.aao.org/bcscvideo_section06 or scan the QR codes in the text to access this content.

Highlights

- Strabismus surgery can improve the functional and psychosocial well-being of pediatric and adult patients.
- It is important for patients and families to understand the goals, expectations, and risks of the strabismus surgery.
- Botulinum toxin A can be a primary or adjunctive treatment for some forms of strabismus.

Evaluation

The patient history, general ophthalmologic examination, and sensorimotor evaluation guide the surgeon's plan for strabismus surgery. Evaluation may include sensory binocularity testing, forced duction testing, active force generation, and saccadic velocity measurement. Simulation of the target postoperative alignment with prisms or an amblyoscope may be used to assess the risk of diplopia and the potential for single binocular vision (see Chapter 6 for discussion of these tests). In preoperative discussions it is important to address the expectations of the patient and family, as well as the risks and potential complications of strabismus surgery, especially if surgery on the only eye with good vision is under consideration.

Indications for Surgery

Although refractive correction, orthoptic exercises, or prism glasses treat some forms of strabismus, many require incisional surgery. Surgery of the extraocular muscles (EOMs) is performed to improve visual function, improve head posture, restore the eyes to their normal anatomical position, improve patient well-being, improve patient nonverbal communication and social interactions, or any combination of these. It may relieve asthenopia (a sense of ocular fatigue) in patients with heterophorias or intermittent heterotropias, or it may relieve the diplopia that often accompanies adult-onset strabismus. Alignment of the visual axes can establish or restore binocular fusion and stereopsis, especially if the preoperative deviation is intermittent or of recent onset. Correction of esotropia expands the binocular visual field. For those patients who have adopted an abnormal head position to relieve diplopia or to improve vision, surgical treatment may not only increase the field of binocular vision but also shift it to a more useful, centered location. Correction of strabismus is reconstructive rather than cosmetic, as it has many functional and psychosocial benefits.

Gunton KB. Impact of strabismus surgery on health-related quality of life in adults. *Curr Opin Ophthalmol.* 2014;25(5):406–410.

Planning Considerations

Vision

When a child has amblyopia, some surgeons prefer to treat the amblyopia before strabismus surgery; others believe that the prognosis for binocular vision is better if surgery is not delayed. If a patient has dense amblyopia or permanent vision loss due to other causes, when possible, surgery is usually performed only on the eye with poor vision.

General Considerations

Symmetric surgery

The amount of surgery performed is based on the size of the preoperative deviation. Table 13-1 gives a commonly used dosage guide for medial rectus muscle recession or lateral rectus muscle resection for esodeviations (also see the section Rectus Muscle Tightening Procedures, later in this chapter). Surgical options for infants with large-angle esotropia (>60 prism diopters [Δ]) include combined recession-resection of 3 or 4 horizontal rectus muscles or large bilateral medial rectus muscle recessions. The latter can be augmented with botulinum toxin.

Table 13-2 provides a commonly used dosage guide for exodeviation. Some surgeons use bilateral lateral rectus muscle recessions of 9.0 mm or greater for deviations larger

Table 13-1 Surgical Guide for Esodeviation

Angle of Esotropia, Δ	Recession MR OU, mm	or	Resection LR OU, mm
15	3.0		4.0
20	3.5		5.0
25	4.0		6.0
30	4.5		7.0
35	5.0		8.0
40	5.5		9.0
50	6.0		9.0

LR = lateral rectus; MR = medial rectus; OU = both eyes *(oculi uterque).*

Table 13-2 Surgical Guide for Exodeviation

Angle of Exotropia, Δ	Recession LR OU, mm	or	Resection MR OU, mm
15	4.0		3.0
20	5.0		4.0
25	6.0		5.0
30	7.0		6.0
40	8.0		7.0

LR = lateral rectus; MR = medial rectus; OU = both eyes *(oculi uterque).*

than 40Δ. Others prefer to limit lateral rectus recession to no more than 8.0 mm and add resection of 1 or both medial rectus muscles for larger-angle exotropias.

Monocular horizontal rectus recession-resection procedures

The values given in Tables 13-1 and 13-2 may also be used in unilateral recession-resection procedures; the surgeon selects the appropriate number of millimeters for each muscle. For example, for an esotropia measuring 30Δ, the surgeon would recess the medial rectus muscle by 4.5 mm and resect the lateral rectus muscle by 7.0 mm. For an exodeviation measuring 15Δ, the surgeon would recess the lateral rectus muscle by 4.0 mm and resect the antagonist medial rectus muscle by 3.0 mm. Unilateral surgery for exotropia beyond the given values (ie, >40Δ) is likely to result in a limited rotation; this can be avoided with a 3- or 4-muscle procedure.

Incomitance

When the size of the deviation varies in different gaze positions, the surgical plan should be designed with a goal of making the postoperative alignment more comitant.

Vertical incomitance of horizontal deviations

The treatment of horizontal deviations that differ in magnitude in upgaze and downgaze—such as *A* or *V patterns*—is discussed in Chapter 9.

Horizontal incomitance

When the size of the esodeviation or exodeviation changes significantly between right and left gaze, paresis, paralysis, or restriction is likely. In general, restrictions must be relieved for surgery to be effective, and the surgical amounts usually used to correct a misalignment of a given size may not be applicable.

When there is no restriction to account for an incomitant deviation, the deviation is treated as if it were caused by a weak muscle, whether from neurologic, traumatic, or other causes. If the weak muscle exhibits little or no force generation, transposition procedures are usually indicated. Otherwise, treatment consists of some combination of resection of the weak muscle (or advancement if it has been previously recessed) and weakening of its direct antagonist and/or yoke muscle.

In some cases, both restriction and weakness are present, particularly in long-standing paretic or paralytic strabismus, and a combination of treatment strategies is necessary. Forced duction and active force generation testing are helpful in these cases.

Distance–near incomitance

Treatment of horizontal distance–near incomitance has classically consisted of medial rectus muscle surgery for deviations greater at near fixation and lateral rectus muscle surgery for deviations greater at distance fixation. Evidence suggests that, regardless of which muscles are operated on, the improvement in distance–near incomitance is similar.

Archer SM. The effect of medial versus lateral rectus muscle surgery on distance-near incomitance. *J AAPOS.* 2009;13(1):20–26.

Cyclovertical Strabismus

In many patients with cyclovertical strabismus, the deviation differs between right and left gaze and, on the side of the greater deviation, often between upgaze and downgaze as well. In general, surgery is performed on those muscles whose field of action corresponds to the greatest vertical deviation unless forced duction testing reveals contracture that requires weakening a restricted muscle. For example, for a patient with a right hypertropia that is greatest in downgaze and to the patient's left, the surgeon can consider either tightening the right superior oblique muscle or weakening the left inferior rectus muscle. (Tightening and weakening of the oblique muscles are discussed later in this chapter.) If the right hypertropia is the same in left upgaze, straight left gaze, and left downgaze, then any of the 4 muscles whose greatest vertical action is in left gaze may be chosen for surgery. In this example, the left superior rectus muscle or right superior oblique muscle could be tightened, or the left inferior rectus muscle or right inferior oblique muscle could be weakened. Larger deviations may require surgery on more than 1 muscle.

Prior Surgery

In the surgical treatment of residual or recurrent strabismus after previous surgery, procedures on EOMs that have not undergone prior surgery are technically easier and somewhat more predictable than on those that have. Unfortunately, when previous surgery has resulted in muscle restriction or weakness with limited duction (due to excessive recession, a slipped or "lost" muscle, or formation of a pseudotendon or stretched scar), reoperation on the involved muscle is usually necessary. If restriction results from retinal detachment surgery, correction can usually be accomplished without removal of scleral explants. For an eye that has previously undergone glaucoma surgery (eg, trabeculectomy or tube shunt surgery), strabismus surgery should be planned to minimize the risk of disrupting the filtering bleb.

Consent for Strabismus Surgery

It is important to review the surgical goals and patient expectations during the consent process. Some parents may incorrectly assume that surgery will obviate the need for glasses and/or patching. Postoperative "normal" alignment is not necessarily the goal of surgery. For example, in a patient with incomitant paralytic or restrictive strabismus and diplopia, the surgical aim is to center and improve the binocular field of single vision; diplopia would still be expected in certain gazes. It is also important to review anesthetic and surgical risks (outlined later in this chapter) with the patient and family.

Surgical Techniques for the Extraocular Muscles and Tendons

Step-by-step descriptions of each surgical procedure are beyond the scope of this volume. See the Basic Texts section of this volume for a list of texts describing surgical technique.

Approaches to the Extraocular Muscles

Fornix incision

The fornix incision (Video 13-1) is made in either the superior or, more frequently, the inferior quadrant. The incision is located on bulbar conjunctiva, not actually in the fornix, 1–2 mm to the limbal side of the cul-de-sac, so that bleeding is minimized. The incision is made parallel to the fornix and is approximately 8–10 mm in length.

VIDEO 13-1 Fornix incision.

Bare sclera is exposed by incising the Tenon capsule deep to the conjunctival incision. Through this opening, the surgeon engages the muscle with a succession of muscle hooks. The conjunctival incision is pulled over the hook that has passed under the muscle. All 4 rectus muscles and both oblique muscles can be explored, if necessary, through inferotemporal and superonasal conjunctival incisions.

When properly placed, the 2-plane incision can be self-closing at the end of the operation by gentle massage of the tissues into the fornix, with the edges of the incision splinted by the overlying eyelid. Some surgeons prefer to close the incision with conjunctival sutures.

Limbal incision

In this approach, the fused layer of conjunctiva and Tenon capsule is cleanly severed from the limbus. Some surgeons make the limbal incision *(peritomy)* 1–2 mm posterior to the limbus to spare limbal stem cells (Video 13-2). A short radial incision is made at each end of the peritomy so that the flap of conjunctiva and Tenon capsule can be retracted to expose the muscle. At the completion of the operation, the flap is reattached, without tension, close to its original position with a single suture at each corner. If the conjunctiva is restricted from prior surgery or shortened by a long-standing deviation, closure involves recession of the anterior edge.

VIDEO 13-2 Limbal incision.

Rectus Muscle Weakening Procedures

Table 13-3 defines various procedures to reduce the force exerted by an EOM on the globe and describes when each procedure is used. The most common is simple recession (Video 13-3); typical amounts of recession for esotropia and exotropia are given in Tables 13-1 and 13-2, respectively. Because of the risk of perforation associated with the

Table 13-3 Weakening Procedures Used in Strabismus Surgery

Procedure	Indications
Myotomy: cutting across a muscle *Myectomy:* removal of a portion of muscle	Used by some surgeons to weaken the inferior oblique muscle
Marginal myotomy: cutting partway across a muscle, usually following a maximal recession	Usually used to further weaken a rectus muscle during recession
Tenotomy: cutting across a tendon *Tenectomy:* removal of a portion of tendon	Both used routinely to weaken the superior oblique muscle; some surgeons interpose a spacer to control the weakening effect
Recession: removal and reattachment of a muscle (rectus or oblique) so that its insertion is closer to its origin	The standard weakening procedure for rectus muscles
Denervation and extirpation: ablation of the entire portion of the muscle, along with its nerve supply, within the Tenon capsule	Used only on severely or recurrently overacting inferior oblique muscles
Recession and anteriorization: transposition of the inferior oblique muscle's insertion to a position next to the insertion of the inferior rectus muscle	Used on the inferior oblique muscle to reduce its elevating action; particularly useful with coexisting inferior oblique overaction and DVD
Posterior fixation suture (fadenoperation): attachment of a rectus muscle to the sclera 11–18 mm posterior to the insertion using a nonabsorbable suture; fixation to the muscle's pulley may be an alternative for medial rectus muscles	Used to weaken a muscle by selectively decreasing its mechanical advantage in its field of action; often used in conjunction with recession; sometimes used in high AC/A ratio accommodative esotropia and in incomitant strabismus
Disinsertion and periosteal fixation: attachment of a rectus muscle to the lateral orbital tubercle or medial wall using a nonabsorbable suture	Used to totally incapacitate a muscle by attaching it to orbital bone, preventing its reattachment to the globe; often used when the antagonist muscle has no function

AC/A = accommodative convergence/accommodation; DVD = dissociated vertical deviation.

conventional rectus muscle recession technique, which involves passing sutures within thin sclera, some surgeons prefer a *hang-back recession,* in which the recessed tendon is suspended by sutures that pass through the thicker stump of the original insertion.

VIDEO 13-3 Recession of extraocular rectus muscle.
Courtesy of Scott A. Larson, MD; Ronald Price, MD; and George Beauchamp, MD.

Rectus Muscle Tightening Procedures

Although they are also referred to as strengthening procedures, muscle tightening procedures (defined in Table 13-4) do not actually give the muscles more strength. Rather, they increase tension to offset the action of the antagonist muscle. For this purpose, surgeons usually use the *resection* technique (Video 13-4); typical amounts of surgery for esotropia and exotropia are given in Tables 13-1 and 13-2, respectively. *Plication* of the muscle is an alternative that produces a similar effect. A previously recessed rectus muscle can also be tightened by *advancing* its insertion toward the limbus.

Table 13-4 Tightening Procedures Used in Strabismus Surgery

Procedure	Indication
Resection: removal of a segment of muscle followed by reattachment to the original insertion	The standard tightening procedure for rectus muscles
Advancement: movement of a previously recessed muscle toward its insertion	Used to correct a consecutive deviation
Tuck: folding and securing, reducing tendon length	Used on the superior oblique tendon
Plication: folding and securing to the sclera	Used on rectus muscles to impart an effect similar to resection

VIDEO 13-4 Resection of extraocular rectus muscle.
Courtesy of Scott A. Larson, MD, and Johanna Beebe, MD.

Rectus Muscle Surgery for Hypotropia and Hypertropia

For comitant vertical deviations, recession and resection of vertical rectus muscles are appropriate. Recessions are generally preferred as a first procedure. Approximately 3Δ of correction in primary position can be expected for every millimeter of vertical rectus muscle recession. For comitant vertical deviations less than 10Δ that accompany horizontal deviations, displacement of the reinsertions of the horizontal rectus muscles in the same direction, by approximately one-half the tendon width (up for hypotropia, down for hypertropia), performed during a recession-resection procedure, is often sufficient.

Adjustable Sutures

Some surgeons feel that adjustable sutures increase surgical success. In this procedure, surgeons use externalized sutures and slip knots that enable the position of the surgical muscle to be altered during the early postoperative period (Video 13-5). As long as anesthetic agents that affect ocular motility are avoided, adjustment can also be done intraoperatively if surgery is performed on an awake adult. Surgery with adjustable sutures can be challenging in patients with scarred or restricted muscles. This surgery can be used in children; however, general anesthesia is usually required for adjustment.

VIDEO 13-5 Adjustable sutures for extraocular rectus muscles.
Courtesy of Scott A. Larson, MD.

The success of a surgery with adjustable sutures requires knowing what angle should be targeted in the immediate postoperative period to ensure the desired long-term result, taking into account typical postoperative drift in the first few weeks after surgery.

Oblique Muscle Weakening Procedures

Weakening the inferior oblique muscle

Muscle weakening procedures (see Table 13-3) are most commonly used for treatment of overelevation in adduction that is believed to be due to inferior oblique muscle overaction.

In all these procedures, the surgeon must be sure that the entire inferior oblique muscle is identified, because the distal portion and the insertion can be anomalously duplicated (Videos 13-6, 13-7).

VIDEO 13-6 Strabismus surgery: inferior oblique—partial and complete hooking.
Courtesy of John D. Ferris, MBChB, and Peter E.J. Davies, MBBS, MPH.

VIDEO 13-7 Inferior oblique weakening procedures.

In cases in which there is asymmetry of the overactions of the inferior oblique muscles and no superior oblique muscle paralysis, unilateral surgery only on the muscle with the more prominent overaction can unmask a significant degree of overaction in the fellow eye. Therefore, some surgeons recommend bilateral inferior oblique muscle weakening even for asymmetric cases. A symmetric result is the rule and overcorrections are rare; however, inferior oblique muscles that are not overacting at all—even when there is overaction in the fellow eye—should not be weakened.

Secondary overaction of the inferior oblique muscle occurs in many patients who have superior oblique muscle paralysis. A weakening of that inferior oblique muscle typically corrects up to 15Δ of vertical deviation in primary position. The amount of vertical correction is roughly proportional to the degree of preoperative overaction (see Chapter 10). Frequently, a weakening procedure is performed on each inferior oblique muscle for V-pattern strabismus (see Chapter 9).

In standard recession of the inferior oblique muscle, the muscle is reattached close to its normal anatomical path; however, if both poles of the inferior oblique muscle are anteriorly transposed to the level of the inferior rectus insertion, contraction of the muscle actually results in depression rather than elevation of the globe, with the neurofibrovascular bundle along the lateral border of the inferior rectus muscle functioning as the origin of the muscle (Fig 13-1; also see Chapter 2). Full *anterior transposition* or *anteriorization* of the inferior oblique muscle can create a restrictive anti-elevation effect. This procedure is effective for treatment of dissociated vertical deviation (DVD) and is especially useful when DVD and inferior oblique overaction coexist (see Chapter 10).

Weakening the superior oblique muscle

Procedures to weaken the superior oblique muscle include tenotomy (Video 13-8); tenectomy; split-tendon lengthening; placement of a spacer of silicone, fascia lata, or nonabsorbable suture between the cut edges of the tendon to functionally lengthen it; and recession. Like split-tendon lengthening, spacers limit overcorrection and facilitate reversal compared to tenotomy or tenectomy, but they may cause adhesions, which can alter motility. Unilateral weakening of a superior oblique muscle is not commonly performed, except as treatment for Brown syndrome (see Chapter 11) or for isolated inferior oblique muscle weakness, which is rare. Unilateral superior oblique muscle weakening can affect not only vertical alignment but also torsion, potentially creating

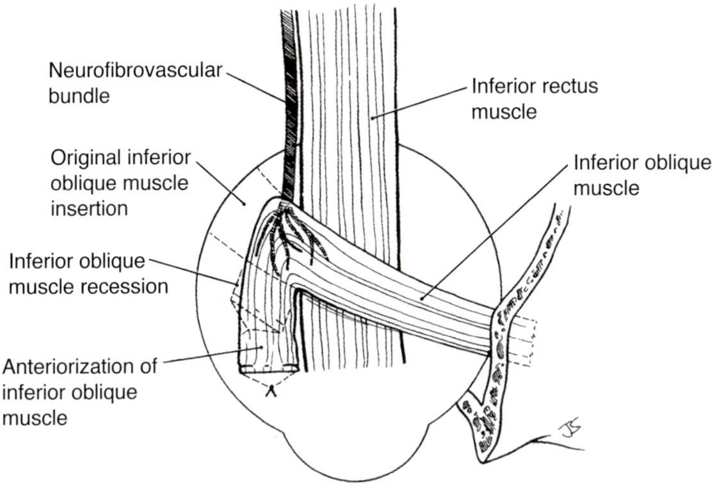

Figure 13-1 Inferior view, left eye, of anteriorization of the inferior oblique muscle, compared to standard recession and the original anatomical path of the muscle. *(Courtesy of Del Monte AM, Archer SM.* Atlas of Pediatric Ophthalmology and Strabismus Surgery. *Churchill Livingstone; 1993:88.)*

undesired extorsion. Many ophthalmologists favor a tenotomy of only the posterior 75%–80% of the tendon to preserve the torsional action, which is controlled by the most anterior tendon fibers.

VIDEO 13-8 Superior oblique muscle tenotomy.

Bilateral weakening of the superior oblique muscle can be performed in patients with A-pattern deviations and can cause an eso-shift in downgaze and almost no change in upgaze. If this procedure is performed on patients with normal binocularity, it may cause vertical or torsional strabismus with subsequent diplopia; this must be considered and discussed with the patient preoperatively.

Oblique Muscle Tightening Procedures

Tightening the inferior oblique muscle

Inferior oblique muscle tightening is seldom performed. To be effective, advancement of the inferior oblique muscle requires reinsertion more posteriorly and superiorly, which is technically difficult and exposes the macula to possible injury.

Tightening the superior oblique muscle

Tightening the superior oblique tendon is discussed in Chapter 10. Tucking the superior oblique tendon enhances both its vertical and torsional effects (Video 13-9). In the *Fells modification of the Harada-Ito procedure,* the anterior half of the superior oblique tendon alone is advanced temporally and somewhat anteriorly to reduce extorsion in patients with superior oblique muscle paralysis (Video 13-10).

VIDEO 13-9 Superior oblique tucking.

VIDEO 13-10 Strabismus surgery: Fells modification of the Harada-Ito procedure.
Courtesy of John D. Ferris, MBChB, and Peter E.J. Davies, MBBS, MPH.

Rectus Muscle Transposition Procedures

Transposition procedures involve redirection of the paths of the EOMs. In the treatment of conditions such as cranial nerve (CN) VI palsy, Duane syndrome, or monocular elevation deficiency, 1 or both neighboring muscles are transposed adjacent to the underacting muscle to provide a tonic force vector (Video 13-11). The effect of the transposition can be augmented by resecting the transposed muscles or by using offset posterior fixation sutures *(Foster modification).* Vertical deviations are a possible complication of vertical rectus muscle transposition surgery.

VIDEO 13-11 Strabismus surgery: lateral rectus and medial rectus inferior full-tendon transfers.
Courtesy of John D. Ferris, MBChB, and Peter E.J. Davies, MBBS, MPH.

Posterior Fixation

In posterior fixation, a rectus muscle is sutured to the sclera far posterior to its insertion. The result is weakening of the muscle in its field of action with little or no effect on the alignment in primary position. This procedure is particularly useful for treatment of incomitant strabismus. A similar effect may be achieved by combined recession-resection, or, at least for a medial rectus muscle, by fixation to the muscle pulley.

Anesthesia for Extraocular Muscle Surgery

Methods

General anesthesia is necessary for children and is often used for adults as well, particularly for those undergoing bilateral surgery. Neuromuscular blocking agents such as succinylcholine, which are administered to facilitate intubation for general anesthesia, can temporarily affect the results of a traction test. Nondepolarizing agents, which do not have this effect, can be used instead.

In cooperative patients, topical anesthetic eyedrops alone (eg, tetracaine 0.5%, proparacaine 0.5%, lidocaine 2%) are effective for most steps in an EOM surgical procedure. Topical anesthesia is not effective for control of the pain produced by pulling on or against a restricted muscle or for cases in which exposure is difficult.

Both peribulbar and retrobulbar anesthesia make most EOM procedures pain-free and can be considered in adults for whom general anesthesia may pose an undue hazard. The administration of a short-acting hypnotic by an anesthesiologist just before retrobulbar injection greatly improves patient comfort. Even when surgery is done under general anesthesia, sub-Tenon anesthetic injection can improve postoperative pain control.

Because injected anesthetics may influence alignment during the first few hours after surgery, suture adjustment is best delayed for at least half a day.

Oculocardiac Reflex

The oculocardiac reflex is a slowing of the heart rate caused by traction on the EOMs, particularly the medial rectus muscle. In its most severe form, the reflex can produce asystole. The surgeon should be aware of the possibility of inducing the oculocardiac reflex when manipulating a muscle and should be prepared to release tension if the patient's heart rate drops excessively. Intravenous atropine and other agents can protect against this reflex.

Malignant Hyperthermia

Pediatric ophthalmologists need to be aware of *malignant hyperthermia (MH)* because at-risk patients can have strabismus. MH is a defect of calcium binding by the sarcoplasmic reticulum of skeletal muscle that can occur sporadically or be dominantly inherited with incomplete penetrance. When MH is triggered by inhalational anesthetics or the muscle relaxant succinylcholine, unbound intracellular calcium concentration increases, which stimulates muscle contracture, causing massive acidosis. In its fully developed form, MH is characterized by extreme heat production, resulting from the hypermetabolic state.

MH can be fatal if diagnosis and treatment are delayed. The earliest sign is unexplained elevation of end-tidal carbon dioxide concentration. As soon as the diagnosis is made, surgery should be terminated, even if incomplete. Treatment is in the province of the anesthesiologist. See also BCSC Section 1, *Update on General Medicine.*

Postoperative Nausea and Vomiting

Eye muscle surgery is a risk factor for postoperative nausea and vomiting. This risk can be reduced by prophylaxis with dexamethasone and serotonin type 3 (5-HT_3) antagonists (eg, ondansetron), propofol use, adequate hydration, and reduced use of inhalation anesthetics and opioid analgesia.

Complications of Strabismus Surgery

Lost and Slipped Muscles

A rectus muscle that is traumatically transected or that retracts out of the sutures or instruments while unattached to the globe during an operation can retract through the Tenon capsule and become inaccessible ("lost") posteriorly in the orbit. This consequence is most severe when it involves the medial rectus muscle, because, lacking attachments to other EOMs, that muscle is the most difficult to recover.

The surgeon should immediately attempt to find the lost muscle, if possible, with the assistance of a surgeon experienced in this potentially complex surgery. Malleable retractors and a headlight are helpful. Minimal manipulation should be used to bring into view the anatomical site through which the muscle and its sheath normally penetrate the Tenon capsule. It is there that the proximal end of the muscle can be recognized and captured. If inspection does not reliably indicate that the muscle has been identified, sudden bradycardia when traction is exerted can be confirmatory. Recovery of the medial rectus muscle has been achieved by using a transnasal endoscopic approach through the ethmoid sinus or by performing a medial orbitotomy. Transposition surgery may be required if the lost muscle is not found, but anterior segment ischemia may be a risk. Where to reattach the recovered muscle depends on whether it was lost due to trauma or during surgery.

A slipped muscle is the result of inadequate imbrication of the muscle during strabismus surgery, which allows it to recede posteriorly within its capsule postoperatively. Clinically, the patient manifests a weakness of that muscle immediately postoperatively, with limited rotations and possibly decreased saccades in its field of action (Fig 13-2). Surgery should be performed as soon as possible in order to secure the muscle before further retraction and contracture take place.

Pulled-in-Two Syndrome

Dehiscence of a muscle during surgery has been termed *pulled-in-two syndrome (PITS).* The dehiscence usually occurs at the tendon–muscle junction; the inferior rectus may be the most frequently affected muscle. Advanced age, various myopathies, previous surgery, trauma, or infiltrative disease may predispose a muscle to PITS by weakening its structural integrity. Treatment is recovery, when possible, using techniques similar to those used for lost muscles, and re-anastomosis of the muscle.

Perforation of the Sclera

During reattachment of an EOM, a needle may penetrate the sclera and pass into the suprachoroidal space or perforate the choroid and retina. Perforation can lead to retinal detachment or endophthalmitis; in most cases, it results in only a small chorioretinal scar, with no effect on vision. Most perforations are unrecognized unless specifically looked for by ophthalmoscopy. If a retinal hole is identified on intraoperative binocular indirect ophthalmoscopy, the surgeon may consider applying immediate laser or cryotherapy. Topical antibiotics are generally given during the immediate postoperative period. Ophthalmoscopy during the postoperative period is an appropriate precaution, with referral to a retina consultant if needed.

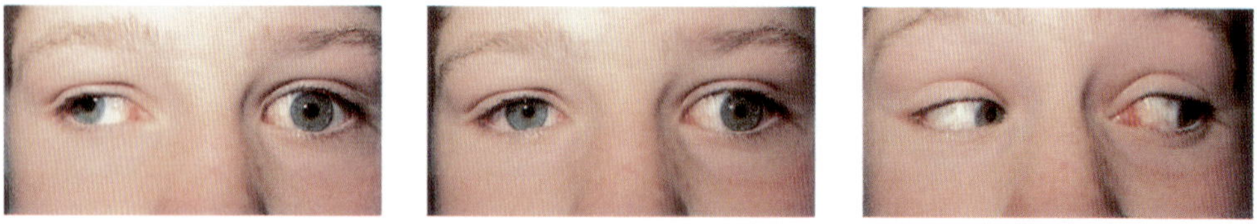

Figure 13-2 Slipped left medial rectus muscle. *Left,* Gaze right shows inability to adduct the left eye. *Center,* Exotropia in primary position. *Right,* Gaze left shows full abduction. Note that the left palpebral fissure is wider than the right, especially with attempted adduction.

Postoperative Infections

Postoperatively, mild conjunctivitis may develop in some patients; it may be caused by allergy to suture material or postoperative medications, as well as by infectious agents. Preseptal and orbital cellulitis with proptosis, eyelid swelling, chemosis, and fever are rare following strabismus surgery (Fig 13-3). Intraocular infection is even rarer. It is important to warn patients and caregivers of the signs and symptoms of orbital cellulitis and endophthalmitis and instruct them to seek emergency consultation if necessary. These conditions usually develop 2–3 days after surgery. Cellulitis generally responds well to systemic antibiotics; endophthalmitis, however, carries a poor prognosis.

Anterior Segment Ischemia

The blood supply to the anterior segment of the eye is mostly provided by the anterior ciliary arteries that travel with the 4 rectus muscles. Simultaneous surgery on 3 rectus muscles, or even 2 rectus muscles in patients with poor blood circulation, may therefore lead to anterior segment ischemia (ASI). The earliest signs of this complication are cells and flare in the anterior chamber. More severe cases are characterized by corneal edema and an irregular pupil (Fig 13-4). This complication may lead to anterior segment necrosis and phthisis bulbi. No universally agreed-upon treatment exists for ASI. Because the signs of ASI are similar to those of uveitis, most ophthalmologists treat with topical, subconjunctival, or systemic corticosteroids, although there is no firm evidence supporting this approach.

It is possible to recess, resect, or transpose a rectus muscle while sparing its anterior ciliary vessels. Though difficult and time consuming, this technique may be indicated in high-risk cases. Staging surgery, with an interval of several months between procedures, may also be helpful. Because the anterior segment is partially supplied by the conjunctival

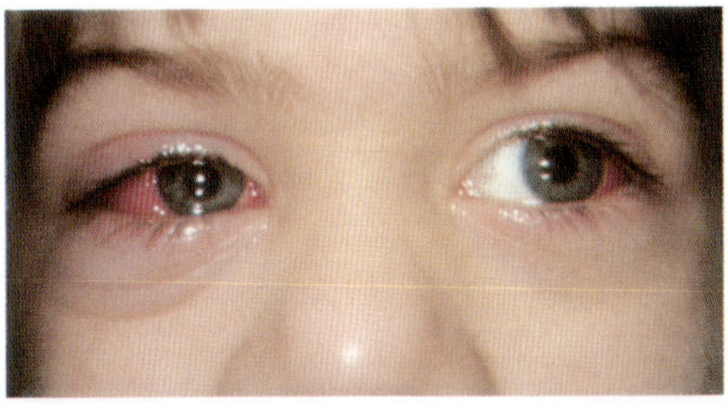

Figure 13-3 Orbital cellulitis, right eye, 2 days after bilateral recession of the lateral rectus muscles.

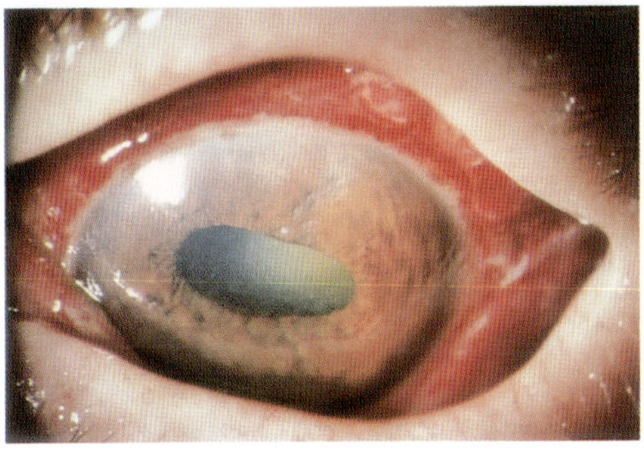

Figure 13-4 Superotemporal segmental anterior segment ischemia after simultaneous superior rectus muscle and lateral rectus muscle surgery following a scleral buckling procedure.

circulation through the limbal arcades, using fornix instead of limbal incisions may provide some protection against the development of ASI.

Delle

A *delle* (plural *dellen*) is a shallow area of corneal thinning near the limbus. Dellen occur when raised abnormal bulbar conjunctiva prevents adequate lubrication of the cornea adjacent to the raised conjunctiva (Fig 13-5). Dellen are more likely to occur when the limbal approach to EOM surgery is used. They usually heal with time. Artificial tears or lubricants may be used until the chemosis subsides.

Pyogenic Granuloma and Foreign-Body Granuloma

Pyogenic granuloma (lobular capillary hemangioma) consists of a lobular proliferation of capillaries with edema that can develop at the conjunctival incision site (Fig 13-6). It is prone to ulceration or bleeding but usually resolves spontaneously or responds to topical corticosteroid eyedrops. Persistent lesions may require surgical excision. In rare cases, sutures can cause foreign-body granulomas and allergic reactions (Fig 13-7).

Epithelial Cyst

A noninflamed, translucent subconjunctival mass may develop if conjunctival epithelium is buried during muscle reattachment or incision closure (Fig 13-8). Occasionally, the cyst

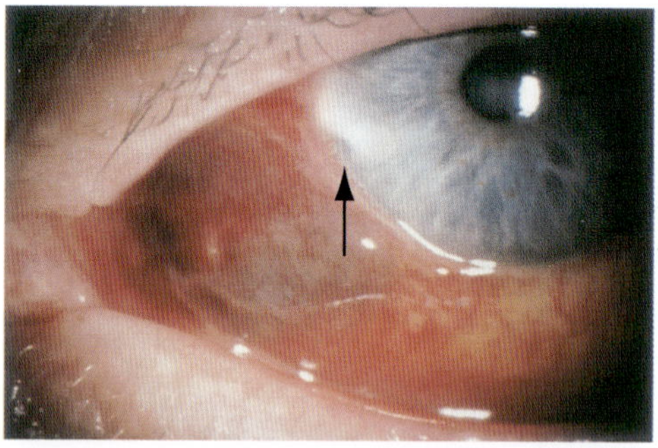

Figure 13-5 Corneal delle *(arrow)* following postoperative subconjunctival hemorrhage.

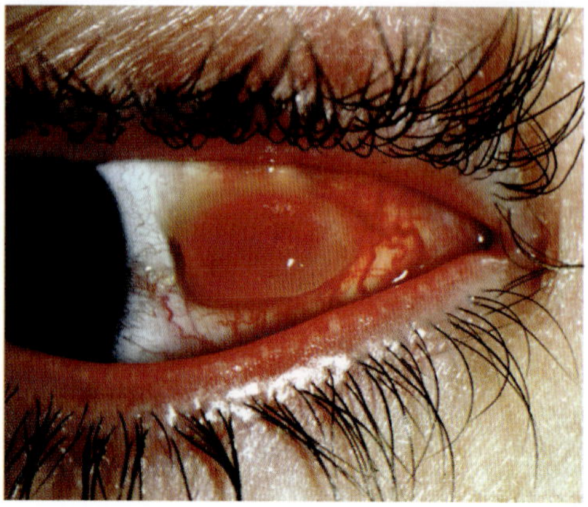

Figure 13-6 Postoperative pyogenic granuloma over the left lateral rectus muscle. *(Reprinted from Espinoza GM, Lueder GT. Conjunctival pyogenic granulomas after strabismus surgery.* Ophthalmology. *2005;112(7):1283–1286. With permission from Elsevier.)*

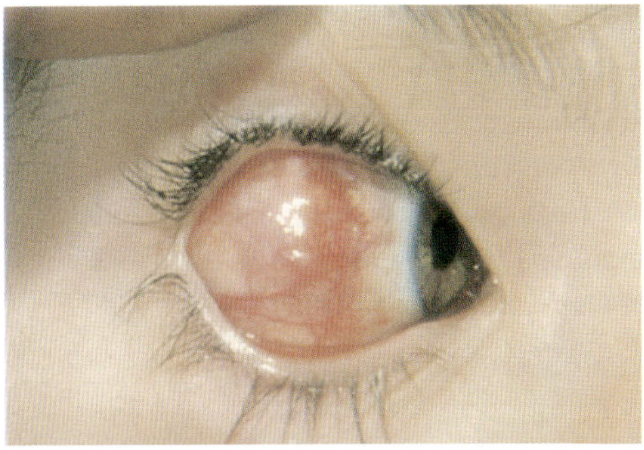

Figure 13-7 Allergic reaction to chromic gut suture. Allergic reactions are rare with modern synthetic suture material such as polyglactin.

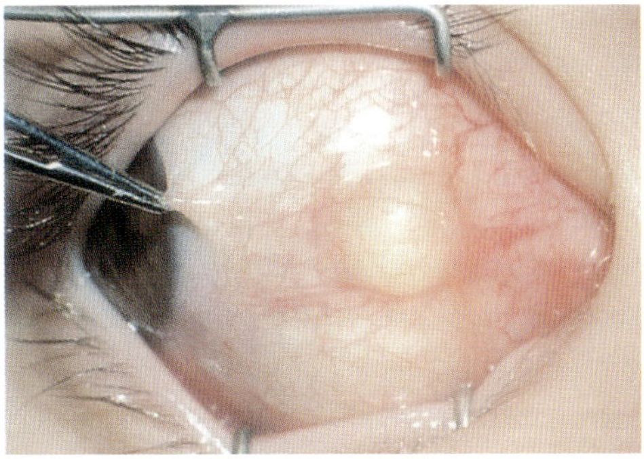

Figure 13-8 Postoperative epithelial cyst following right medial rectus muscle recession.

resolves spontaneously; persistent cases may require surgical intervention. In some cases, the cyst is incorporated into the muscle tendon, so careful exploration is necessary.

Conjunctival Changes

Satisfaction from improved alignment may occasionally be overshadowed by unsightly long-term changes to the conjunctiva and the Tenon capsule. The tissues may appear hyperemic and salmon pink. This complication may occur as a result of the following:

- *Advancement of thickened Tenon capsule too close to the limbus.* In resection procedures, pulling the muscle forward may advance the Tenon capsule. The undesirable result is exaggerated in reoperations, when the Tenon capsule may be hypertrophied.
- *Advancement of the plica semilunaris.* During surgery on the medial rectus muscle using the limbal approach, the surgeon may mistake the plica semilunaris for a conjunctival edge and incorporate it into the closure. The advanced plica, pulled forward and hypertrophied, retains its fleshy color (Fig 13-9).
- *Redundant and loose conjunctival fold.* Long-standing large-angle strabismus may result in excess conjunctival tissue over the muscle requiring resection. After alignment, this manifests as a conjunctival fold unless conjunctivoplasty is performed at the same time.

Treatment options include conjunctivoplasty with resection of scarred conjunctiva and transposition of adjacent conjunctiva, resection of subconjunctival fibrous tissue, recession of scarred conjunctiva, and amniotic membrane grafting.

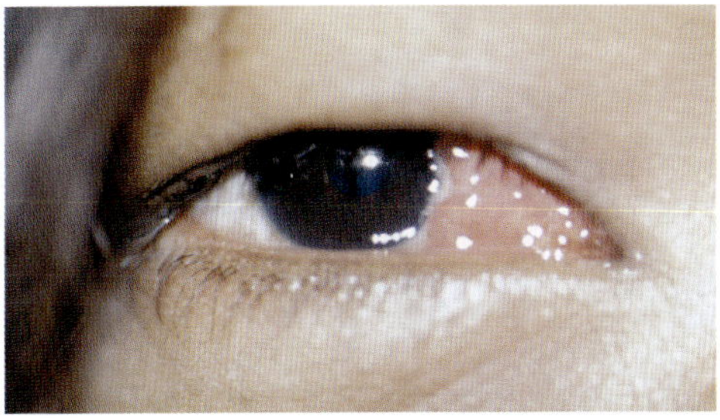

Figure 13-9 Fleshy medial conjunctiva resulting from a hypertrophic scar involving the plica semilunaris. *(Courtesy of Scott Olitsky, MD.)*

Adherence Syndrome

Tears in the Tenon capsule with prolapse of orbital fat into the sub-Tenon space can cause formation of a fibrofatty scar that may restrict ocular motility. Surgery involving the inferior oblique muscle is particularly prone to this complication because of the proximity of the fat space to the posterior border of the inferior oblique muscle. If recognized at the time of surgery, the prolapsed fat can be excised and the rent closed with absorbable sutures. Meticulous surgical technique usually prevents this serious complication.

Iatrogenic Brown Syndrome

Iatrogenic Brown syndrome (see Chapter 11) can result from superior oblique muscle tightening procedures. Taking care to avoid excessive tightening of the tendon when these procedures are performed minimizes the risk of this complication. A tuck can sometimes be reversed if reoperation is undertaken soon after the original surgery. Observation is also an option; superior oblique tucks tend to loosen with time.

Anti-Elevation Syndrome

Inferior oblique anteriorization can result in restricted elevation of the eye in abduction, known as *anti-elevation syndrome.* Reattaching the lateral corner of the muscle anterior to the spiral of Tillaux increases the risk of this syndrome; "bunching up" the insertion at the lateral border of the inferior rectus muscle may reduce the risk.

Change in Eyelid Position

Change in the position of the eyelids is most likely to occur with surgery on the vertical rectus muscles. Pulling the inferior rectus muscle forward, as in a resection, advances the lower eyelid upward; recessing this muscle pulls the lower eyelid down, exposing sclera below the lower limbus (Fig 13-10). Surgery on the superior rectus muscle is less likely to affect upper eyelid position.

Changes in eyelid position can be obviated somewhat by careful dissection. In general, all intermuscular septum and fascial connections of the vertical rectus muscle must be severed at least 12–15 mm posterior to the muscle insertion. Release of the lower

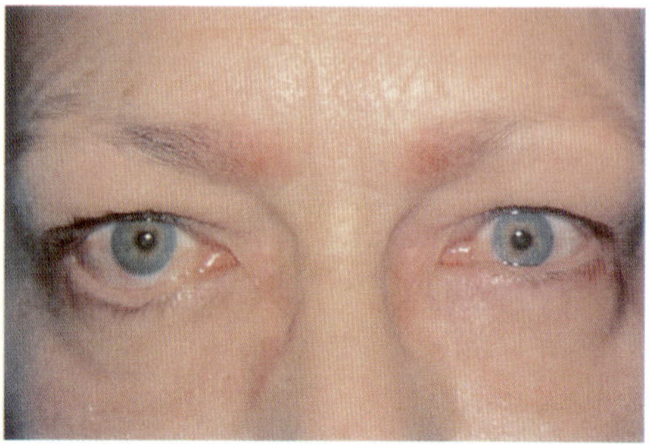

Figure 13-10 Patient treated for left hypertropia by recession of the right inferior rectus muscle, which pulled the right lower eyelid down, and resection of the left inferior rectus muscle, which pulled the left lower eyelid up.

eyelid retractors or advancement of the capsulopalpebral head is helpful to prevent lower eyelid retraction after inferior rectus muscle recession.

Refractive Changes

Changes in refractive error are most common when strabismus surgery is performed on 2 rectus muscles of an eye. An induced astigmatism of low magnitude usually resolves within a few months. Surgery on the oblique muscles can change the axis of preexisting astigmatism.

Kushner BJ. The effect of oblique muscle surgery on the axis of astigmatism. *J Pediatr Ophthalmol Strabismus.* 1986;23(6):277–280.

Diplopia

Diplopia occurs occasionally in older children but more often in adults. Preexisting diplopia may not be fully resolved after surgery. New diplopia can also develop after strabismus surgery due to overcorrection (in intermittent exotropia or unilateral superior oblique palsy), or paradoxically when the eyes are anatomically aligned in patients with anomalous retinal correspondence. In the weeks to months following surgery, various responses are possible:

- An initial overcorrection may resolve through postoperative drift and/or relaxation of habitual vergence that was used to control the preoperative deviation. This is especially true in cases of intermittent exotropia, in which immediate postoperative diplopia is common.
- Motor fusion may develop, controlling a residual phoria.
- A new suppression scotoma may form, corresponding to the new angle of alignment. If the initial strabismus was acquired before 10 years of age, the ability to suppress is generally well developed.
- Anomalous retinal correspondence may dissipate, along with the resulting paradoxical diplopia.
- Diplopia may persist.

Prolonged postoperative diplopia is uncommon. However, if strabismus was first acquired in adulthood, diplopia that was symptomatic before surgery is likely to persist unless comitant alignment and fusion are regained. Prisms that compensate for the deviation may be helpful during the preoperative evaluation to assess the fusion potential and the risk of bothersome postoperative diplopia.

A patient with unequal vision can often ignore the dimmer, more blurred image. Further treatment is indicated for patients whose symptomatic diplopia persists after surgery, especially if it is severe and present in the primary position. If vision in the eyes is equal or nearly so, temporary or permanent prisms can be tried to address any residual diplopia. If this approach fails, additional surgery or botulinum toxin injection may be considered. In some cases, intractable diplopia can be controlled only by occluding or blurring the less-preferred eye.

CLINICAL PEARL

In patients with intractable diplopia, Scotch Magic Tape (3M) placed on the inside of 1 spectacle lens can provide symptomatic relief.

Unsatisfactory Alignment

Unsatisfactory postoperative alignment—overcorrection, undercorrection, or development of an entirely new strabismus problem—is perhaps better characterized as a disappointing outcome of strabismus surgery, rather than as a complication. Postoperative drift may occur in the weeks after surgery, so the immediate postoperative result, whether satisfactory or not, may differ from the alignment seen a couple of months after surgery. Even with the achievement of satisfactory alignment a few months after surgery, strabismus may recur over the long term, especially in patients with poor fusion, poor vision, contracture of scar tissue, or intermittent exotropia. Reoperations are often necessary.

CLINICAL PEARL

Delayed development of limited rotation in the field of an operated muscle several weeks to months postoperatively may indicate *pseudotendon* or *stretched scar* formation. This must be excised and the "muscle" securely reattached in order to restore its function (Video 13-12).

VIDEO 13-12 Strabismus reoperation for a suspected pseudotendon.
Courtesy of Kamiar Mireskandari, MBChB, PhD.

Chemodenervation Using Botulinum Toxin

Pharmacology and Mechanism of Action

Botulinum toxin type A paralyzes muscles by blocking the release of acetylcholine at the neuromuscular junction. This agent, which now has a number of uses, was originally developed as a treatment for strabismus. Within 24–48 hours of injection, botulinum toxin is bound and internalized within local motor nerve terminals, where it remains active for many weeks. Paralysis of the injected EOM begins within 2–4 days of injection and lasts clinically for at least 5–8 weeks. This produces, in effect, a pharmacologic recession: the EOM lengthens while it is paralyzed by botulinum toxin, and its antagonist contracts. Due to muscle length adaptation, there may be long-term improvement in the alignment of the eyes even after the pharmacologic effect has worn off. Bupivacaine injection into an EOM causes fibrosis and may be a pharmacologic alternative to surgical tightening, used on its own or to enhance the effect of chemodenervation.

Debert I, Miller JM, Danh KK, Scott AB. Pharmacologic injection treatment of comitant strabismus. *J AAPOS*. 2016;20(2):106–111.

Indications, Techniques, and Results

Chemodenervation is an alternative for some patients with strabismus. Clinical trials in which botulinum toxin was used for the treatment of strabismus have shown this agent to be most effective in the following conditions:

- small- to moderate-angle esotropia and exotropia (<40Δ)
- postoperative residual strabismus (2–8 weeks following surgery or later)
- acute paralytic strabismus (especially CN VI palsy; sometimes CN IV palsy), to eliminate diplopia while the palsy resolves. The long-term recovery rate for acute CN VI palsy managed with observation alone is similar to that for cases treated with botulinum toxin.
- active thyroid eye disease (Graves disease) or inflamed or pre-phthisical eyes, when surgery is inappropriate
- as a supplement to medial rectus muscle recession for large-angle infantile esotropia or lateral rectus muscle recession for large-angle exotropia

When used to treat patients with strabismus, the toxin is injected directly, with a small-gauge needle, into selected EOMs. Injections into the EOMs may be performed with the use of a portable electromyographic device, although experienced practitioners often dispense with electromyography. In adults, injections are performed with topical anesthetic; in children, general anesthesia is usually necessary (Videos 13-13, 13-14).

VIDEO 13-13 Strabismus surgery: botulinum medial rectus under general anesthetic.
Courtesy of John D. Ferris, MBChB, and Peter E.J. Davies, MBBS, MPH.

VIDEO 13-14 Strabismus surgery: botulinum medial rectus.
Courtesy of John D. Ferris, MBChB, and Peter E.J. Davies, MBBS, MPH.

Multiple injections may be required, particularly in adults. As with surgery, results are best when there is fusion to stabilize the alignment. Botulinum toxin injection is usually not effective in patients with large deviations, restrictive or mechanical strabismus (eg, from trauma, chronic thyroid eye disease), or secondary strabismus wherein a muscle has been overly recessed. Chemodenervation is ineffective for treatment of A and V patterns, DVDs, and chronic paralytic strabismus.

Holmes JM, Beck RW, Kip KE, Droste PJ, Leske DA. Botulinum toxin treatment versus conservative management in acute traumatic sixth nerve palsy or paresis. *J AAPOS.* 2000;4(3):145–149.

Complications

Common adverse effects of ocular botulinum toxin treatment include ptosis, lagophthalmos, dry eye, and induced vertical strabismus after horizontal muscle injection. These are usually temporary, resolving after several weeks. Rare complications include scleral perforation, retrobulbar hemorrhage, pupillary dilation, and permanent diplopia. Systemic botulism has been reported following massive injections of large muscle groups, but this has not been encountered in ophthalmologic use of botulinum toxin.

PART II
Pediatric Ophthalmology

CHAPTER 14

Growth and Development of the Eye

Highlights

- Axial length increases by approximately 3 mm between birth and 1 year of age.
- The eye becomes slightly more hyperopic until 6–8 years of age, followed by a myopic shift toward emmetropia.
- Childhood myopia is increasingly prevalent; increased outdoor activities and low-dose atropine can decrease myopic progression in some children.

Normal Growth and Development

The human eye undergoes dramatic anatomic and physiologic development throughout infancy and early childhood (Table 14-1). Ophthalmologists caring for pediatric patients should be familiar with the normal growth and development of the child's eye because departures from the norm may indicate pathology. See also BCSC Section 2, *Fundamentals and Principles of Ophthalmology.*

Dimensions of the Eye

Most of the growth of the eye takes place in the first year of life. Change in the eye's axial length occurs in 3 phases. The first phase (birth to age 2 years) is a period of rapid growth: the axial length increases by approximately 1.8 mm in the first 6 months of life and by an additional 1 mm during the next 6 months. During the second (age 2 to 5 years) and third (age 5 to 13 years) phases, growth slows, with axial length increasing by about 1 mm per phase (Fig 14-1).

Similarly, with growth of the globe, the corneal diameter increases rapidly during the first year of life. The average horizontal diameter of the cornea is 9.5–10.5 mm in newborns and increases to 12.0 mm in adults. The cornea also flattens in the first year so that keratometry values change markedly, from approximately 52.00 diopters (D) at birth, to 46.00 D by age 6 months, to adult measurements of 42.00–44.00 D by age 12 months. The cornea gradually becomes thinner, decreasing from an average central thickness of 691 µm at 30–32 weeks of gestational age to 564 µm at full term.

The power of the pediatric lens decreases dramatically over the first several years of life—an important consideration when intraocular lens implantation is planned for

Table 14-1 Dimensions of Newborn and Adult Eyes

	Newborn	Adult
Axial length, mm	14.5–15.5	23.0–24.0
Corneal horizontal diameter, mm	9.5–10.5	12.0
K value, diopters	52.00	42.00–44.00

K = keratometry.

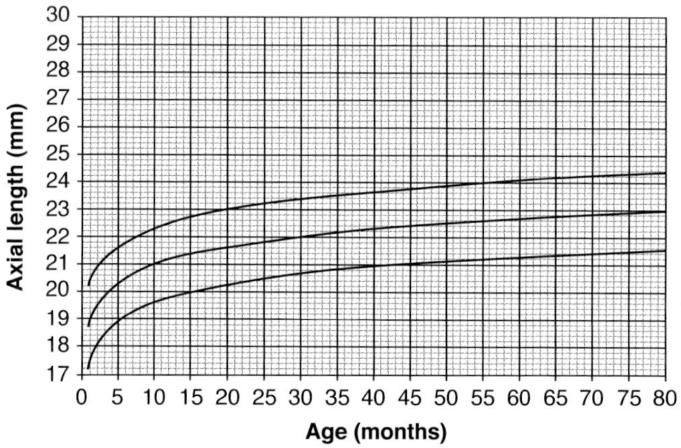

Figure 14-1 Change in mean axial length as a function of age. *(Courtesy of Bascom Palmer Eye Institute, adapted from data from Sampaolesi R, Caruso R. Ocular echometry in the diagnosis of congenital glaucoma.* Arch Ophthalmol. *1982;100(4):574–577.)*

infants and young children after cataract extraction. Lens power decreases from approximately 35.00 D at birth to about 23.00 D at age 2 years due to decrease in the anterior–posterior lens thickness. Subsequently, the change is more gradual: lens power decreases to approximately 19.00 D by age 11 years, with little or no change thereafter.

Gordon RA, Donzis PB. Refractive development of the human eye. *Arch Ophthalmol.* 1985;103(6):785–789.

Kirwan C, O'Keefe M, Fitzsimon S. Central corneal thickness and corneal diameter in premature infants. *Acta Ophthalmol Scand.* 2005;83(6):751–753.

Refractive State

The refractive state of the eye changes as the eye's axial length increases and the cornea and lens flatten. In general, eyes are hyperopic at birth, become slightly more hyperopic until approximately 6–8 years of age, and then experience a myopic shift until reaching adult dimensions, usually by about 16 years of age (Fig 14-2). *Emmetropization* in the developing eye refers to the combination of changes in the refractive power of the anterior segment and in axial length that drive the eye toward emmetropia. The reduction in astigmatism that occurs in many infant eyes and the decreasing hyperopia that occurs after 6–8 years of age are examples of emmetropization.

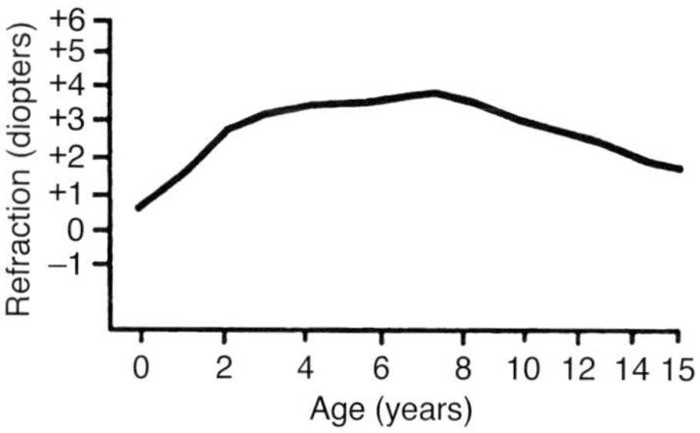

Figure 14-2 Change in mean refractive error as a function of age. *(Modified with permission from Eustis HS, Guthrie ME. Postnatal development. In: Wright KW, Strube YNJ, eds.* Pediatric Ophthalmology and Strabismus. *2nd ed. Springer-Verlag; 2003:49.)*

Race, ethnicity, and heredity play a role in the risk of particular types of refractive error. For example, myopia is highly prevalent among Asian children. Hyperopia is more common among non-Hispanic White children compared with African American and Hispanic children. Astigmatism is more common among Hispanic children and African American children than non-Hispanic White children.

Myopia is increasingly prevalent worldwide, and it is estimated that by 2050, 50% of the world population will have myopia. If myopia develops before age 10 years, there is a higher risk of eventual progression to myopia of 6.00 D or more. The etiology of increased myopia prevalence is unclear, but urbanization, increased near work, and decreased exposure to ultraviolet light are suggested influences. Increased outdoor activities may prevent or delay the onset of myopia, and topical low-dose atropine therapy has been shown to significantly decrease myopic progression in Asian children. Other strategies of mitigating myopia progression include the use of orthokeratology or multifocal contact lenses that cause myopic defocus in the peripheral retina.

Holden BA, Fricke TR, Wilson DA, et al. Global prevalence of myopia and high myopia and temporal trends from 2000 through 2050. *Ophthalmology.* 2016;123(5):1036–1042.

Vagge A, Ferro Desideri L, Nucci P, Serafino M, Giannaccare G, Traverso CE. Prevention of progression in myopia: A systematic review. *Diseases.* 2018;6(4):92.

Yam JC, Jiang Y, Tang SM, et al. Low-Concentration Atropine for Myopia Progression (LAMP) Study: A randomized, double-blinded, placebo-controlled trial of 0.05%, 0.025%, and 0.01% atropine eye drops in myopia control. *Ophthalmology.* 2019;126(1):113–124.

Orbit and Ocular Adnexa

During infancy and childhood, orbital volume increases, and the orbital opening becomes less circular, resembling a horizontal oval. The lacrimal fossa becomes more superficial and the angle formed by the axes of the 2 orbits less divergent.

The palpebral fissure measures approximately 18 mm horizontally and 8 mm vertically at birth. Growth of the palpebral fissure is greater horizontally than vertically, resulting in the eyelid opening becoming less round and acquiring its elliptical adult shape. Most of the horizontal growth occurs in the first 2 years of life.

Cornea, Iris, Pupil, and Anterior Chamber

Central corneal thickness (CCT) decreases during the first 6–12 months of life (see the section Dimensions of the Eye). It then increases from approximately 553 µm at age 1 year to about 573 μm by age 12 years and stabilizes thereafter. CCT is similar in White and Hispanic children, whereas African American children tend to have thinner corneas. The corneal endothelial cell density (ECD) is high at birth and decreases proportional to the increase in corneal diameter as cells migrate to cover a larger surface area. Pathological increases in corneal diameter, like those seen in cases of congenital glaucoma, will therefore result in greater ECD reduction.

Most changes in iris color occur over the first 6–12 months of life, as pigment accumulates in the iris stroma and melanocytes. Compared with the adult pupil, the infant pupil is relatively small. A pupil diameter less than 1.8 mm or greater than 5.4 mm is suggestive of an abnormality. The pupillary light reflex is normally present after 31 weeks of gestational age. At birth, the iris appears to insert at the level of the scleral spur, but during the first year of life, the lens and ciliary body move posteriorly, resulting in formation of the angle recess.

Elbaz U, Mireskandari K, Tehrani N, et al. Corneal endothelial cell density in children: normative data from birth to 5 years old. *Am J Ophthalmol.* 2017;173:134–138.

Pediatric Eye Disease Investigator Group; Bradfield YS, Melia BM, Repka MX, et al. Central corneal thickness in children. *Arch Ophthalmol.* 2011;129(9):1132–1138.

Intraocular Pressure

Measurement of intraocular pressure (IOP) in infants can be difficult; results may vary depending on the method used and may not accurately represent the actual IOP. Nevertheless, normal IOP is lower in infants than in adults, and a pressure higher than 21 mm Hg should be considered abnormal. CCT influences the measurement of IOP, but this effect is not well understood in children. See Chapter 21 in this volume and BCSC Section 10, *Glaucoma,* for further discussion.

Extraocular Muscles

The rectus muscles of infants are smaller than those of adults; muscle insertions, on average, are 2.3–3.0 mm narrower, and the tendons are thinner in infants than in adults. In newborns, the distance from the rectus muscle insertion to the limbus is roughly 2 mm less than that in adults; by age 6 months, this distance is 1 mm less; and at 20 months, it is similar to that in adults.

Extraocular muscle function continues to develop after birth. Eye movements driven by the vestibular-ocular system are present as early as 34 weeks of gestational age. Conjugate horizontal gaze is present at birth, but vertical gaze may not be fully functional until 6 months of age. Intermittent strabismus occurs in approximately two-thirds of young infants but resolves in most by 2–3 months of age. Accommodation and fusional convergence are usually present by age 3 months.

Retina

The macula is poorly developed at birth but changes rapidly during the first 4 years of life. Most significant are changes in macular pigmentation, development of the annular ring

Table 14-2 Types of Congenital Anomalies

Anomaly	Defect	Ocular Example
Agenesis	Developmental failure	Anophthalmia
Hypoplasia	Developmental arrest	Optic nerve hypoplasia
Hyperplasia	Developmental excess	Distichiasis
Dysraphism	Failure to fuse	Choroidal coloboma
	Failure to divide or canalize	Congenital nasolacrimal duct obstruction
	Persistence of vestigial structures	Persistent fetal vasculature

and foveal light reflex, and differentiation of cone photoreceptors. Improvement in visual acuity with age is due in part to development of the macula, specifically, differentiation of cone photoreceptors, narrowing of the rod-free zone, and an increase in foveal cone density (see Chapter 4). Retinal vascularization begins at the optic nerve head at 16 weeks of gestational age and proceeds to the peripheral retina, reaching the temporal ora serrata by 40 weeks of gestational age.

Hendrickson A, Possin D, Lejla V, Toth CA. Histologic development of the human fovea from midgestation to maturity. *Am J Ophthalmol.* 2012;154(5):767–778.

Abnormal Growth and Development

Major congenital anomalies, many of which involve the eyes, occur in 2%–3% of live births. Causes include chromosomal abnormalities, multifactorial disorders, and environmental agents, but many cases are idiopathic. Regardless of etiology, congenital anomalies may be categorized as shown in Table 14-2.

Select Abnormal Growth and Development Terminology

Association Defects that are known to occur together in a statistically significant number of patients, eg, VACTERL (vertebral, anorectal, cardiovascular, tracheoesophageal, renal, limb abnormalities) association.

Malformation A morphologic defect present from the onset of development or from a very early stage, eg, Chiari malformation.

Sequence A single structural defect or factor that leads to a cascade (domino effect) of secondary anomalies, eg, Pierre Robin sequence.

Syndrome A recognizable and consistent pattern of multiple malformations, eg, Sturge-Weber syndrome.

CHAPTER 15

Decreased Vision in Infants

This chapter includes a related video. Go to www.aao.org/bcscvideo_section06 or scan the QR code in the text to access this content.

Highlights

- Strabismus can be variable in children with cerebral visual impairment and may improve spontaneously as visual attention improves.
- Uncrowding the visual environment improves the visual behavior of children with cerebral visual impairment.
- In infants with poor vision, nystagmus raises suspicion for a pregeniculate disorder.

Introduction

When an infant has not developed good visual attention or the ability to fixate on and follow objects by 3–4 months of age, the clinician must determine whether the decreased vision is due to an ocular or optic nerve (pregeniculate) condition, cerebral (retrogeniculate) visual impairment, or delayed visual maturation. This chapter discusses the classification of visual impairment in infants and children, as well as the evaluation of these patients. Vision rehabilitation is discussed in Chapter 28 of this volume.

Visual Development in Young Infants

Visual development is a highly complex maturational process. Anterior segment maturation allows focus of visual input onto the retina. The fovea and central photoreceptors, which are structurally immature at birth, differentiate quickly in the first 6 months of life and continue to mature until 3–4 years of age (Fig 15-1). In the brain, myelination of the optic radiations occurs rapidly in the first year of life. Hubel and Weisel's seminal work showed that visual deprivation during this critical period of visual maturation leads to maldevelopment in the cerebral cortex.

A blink reflex to bright light should be present within a few days of birth, even in very premature infants, and it can often be detected through closed eyelids. The pupillary light reflex is usually present after 31 weeks of gestational age but can be difficult to evaluate in the early neonatal period because the newborn's pupils are miotic. Horizontal optokinetic nystagmus can also be intermittently triggered at birth.

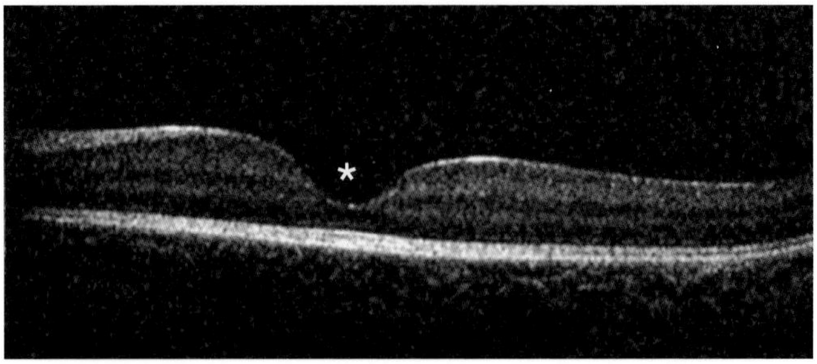

Figure 15-1 Normal fovea in a 2-month-old infant. Note lack of elongation of the cones under the foveal center *(asterisk)*. *(Courtesy of Mays El-Dairi, MD.)*

At approximately 6–8 weeks of age, a healthy full-term infant is able to make and maintain eye contact with other humans and react with facial expressions. Infants aged 2–3 months are interested in bright objects. By age 3–4 months, the nasal bias for smooth pursuit has resolved, the eyes are orthotropic, and fix-and-follow responses to a small (2–4 inches in diameter) toy are present. Premature infants can be expected to reach these landmarks later, but there is not an exact week-for-week correlation for the attainment of these milestones.

Dysconjugate eye movements, skew deviation, and *sunsetting* (tonic downward deviation of both eyes) may be noted in healthy newborns but typically do not persist beyond approximately 3–4 months of age. Signs of poor visual development include searching eye movements, lack of response to familiar faces and objects, and nystagmus. Staring at bright lights and forceful rubbing or poking of the eyes *(oculodigital reflex)* in a visually disinterested infant are signs of poor vision and suggest an ocular cause for the deficiency.

Classification of Visual Impairment in Infants and Children

The distinction between pregeniculate and cerebral visual impairment can be helpful in infants who present with poor vision, although some disorders cause both pregeniculate and retrogeniculate pathology. In addition, in some children, poor visual behavior normalizes over time, a phenomenon known as *delayed visual maturation.*

Pregeniculate Visual Impairment

Pregeniculate visual impairment results from pathology anterior to the lateral geniculate nucleus (the pregeniculate visual pathways). Causes of pregeniculate visual impairment in infants include corneal and lens opacities, glaucoma, retinal disorders, and optic nerve or optic tract abnormalities; results of the ocular examination will frequently be abnormal in patients with these pathologies. Strabismus is often present. If the pathology is bilateral, nystagmus is frequently present.

Cerebral Visual Impairment

Cortical or cerebral visual impairment (CVI) is defined as a decrease in visual function due to an insult to the cerebral cortex. The ocular examination results may be normal if CVI is isolated. Optic atrophy, refractive errors, ocular motor apraxia, and strabismus can coexist in patients with CVI but do not explain the extent of the poor visual behavior. Although the neurological damage in CVI is usually permanent and is stable on neuroimaging, children with CVI often show improvement in their visual behavior with increasing age; this improvement parallels their overall development. As visual attention improves, associated strabismus can improve spontaneously. It is important to treat any coexisting ophthalmic disease in children with CVI.

CVI can be congenital or acquired. The most common cause of CVI is periventricular leukomalacia due to perinatal hypoxia and/or prematurity, but CVI can be caused by any pediatric neurologic disease. Examples include intrauterine infection, structural central nervous system abnormalities, intracranial hemorrhage, seizures, hydrocephalus, meningitis, encephalitis, and accidental and nonaccidental trauma.

Visual characteristics associated with CVI include fluctuations in visual behavior, poor visual attention, and a delay in response to a novel or complex visual stimulus. Children with severe CVI will exhibit improved visual function in familiar settings and with familiar objects. They prefer looking at bright high-contrast objects at close range and odd angles, and they react better to moving objects than to stationary ones. Isolating the visual stimulus improves the visual behavior. Although older children with a history of CVI may appear to have normal visual behavior, they often perform better on isolated optotype acuity testing compared to crowded or Snellen acuity testing. This has implications for functional rehabilitation; see Chapter 28 for further discussion.

Chang MY, Borchert MS. Advances in the evaluation and management of cortical/cerebral visual impairment in children. *Surv Ophthalmol.* 2020;65(6):708–724.

Delayed Visual Maturation

If normal visual fixation and tracking do not develop within the first 3–4 months of life, visual behavior may still normalize subsequently; this condition is termed *delayed visual maturation (DVM),* or *cortical inattention.*

When DVM is suspected in an otherwise healthy infant, the following findings suggest a good visual and neurologic prognosis: normal ocular structures, some reaction to light, normal pupillary responses, and absence of nystagmus. If the visual behavior does not progress toward normal by 4–6 months of age, further investigation is warranted to assess for other causes of persistent visual impairment. DVM is a diagnosis made in retrospect in a neurologically normal child.

Azmeh R, Lueder GT. Delayed visual maturation in otherwise normal infants. *Graefes Arch Clin Exp Ophthalmol.* 2013;251(3):941–944.

Evaluation of the Infant With Decreased Vision

Obtaining a thorough history is very important in the evaluation of an infant with abnormal visual behavior. Important history details are listed in Table 15-1; Figure 15-2 presents a flowchart of steps for evaluation of an infant with decreased vision.

Table 15-1 Important History to Obtain in Infants With Decreased Visual Behavior

Details of the pregnancy (optic nerve hypoplasia and congenital brain malformations)
Gestational diabetes, in utero exposure to infection, drugs (including fertility and antidepressant medications), smoking, alcohol use, radiation, intrauterine growth retardation

Perinatal problems (optic atrophy and brain injury)
Fetal distress, bradycardia, meconium staining, oxygen deprivation

Prematurity (retinopathy of prematurity, intraventricular hemorrhage causing optic atrophy and brain injury, optic nerve hypoplasia)

Systemic abnormalities (optic atrophy and brain injury)
Prolonged jaundice, hypoxic ischemic encephalopathy

Delayed developmental milestones

Postnatal causes of brain injury
Trauma, infections, seizures

Family history
Any inherited retinal, optic nerve, or neurologic diseases

It is important to note parental impressions of the child's visual behavior. Vision in the infant is assessed qualitatively by observing the infant's visual behavior. A good stare response and eyelid retraction when the light is turned off are usually indicative of good vision (Video 15-1). To assess vision in a preverbal child, motor behavioral response tests can be used, such as Teller Acuity Cards II (Precision Vision) or optokinetic nystagmus tests (see Chapter 1 for a discussion of these quantitative tests). When needed, a visual evoked potential test can be used to quantify a sensory response.

VIDEO 15-1 Stare reflex.
Courtesy of Mays El-Dairi, MD. Narrated by Robert Clay, COT.

Infants and children with ocular motor apraxia (see Chapter 11) may falsely appear to have poor vision due to impaired horizontal eye movements. Vertical movements are usually spared (note that vertical movements are commonly absent before 3–4 months of age). The impression of poor vision may be exaggerated if ocular motor apraxia is paired with neck weakness.

Pupillary responses are sluggish or paradoxical in patients with severe pregeniculate causes of visual impairment such as optic nerve abnormalities or retinal dystrophies. In infants with poor vision, nystagmus should raise suspicion for a pregeniculate disorder (see Chapter 12).

Anterior segment and fundus examinations may reveal a pregeniculate cause of the visual impairment, such as bilateral cataracts, bilateral macular colobomas or scars, bilateral optic nerve hypoplasia, bilateral optic atrophy, or foveal hypoplasia with or without albinism or aniridia. However, some retinal causes of pregeniculate visual impairment may not be associated with any visible abnormalities on fundus examination.

If the ocular examination is unrevealing yet suspicion is high for a pregeniculate cause of visual impairment (eg, when poor vision is accompanied by nystagmus), then optical coherence tomography (OCT) and/or electroretinography (ERG) may be indicated to diagnose optic atrophy, foveal hypoplasia, or retinal dystrophy.

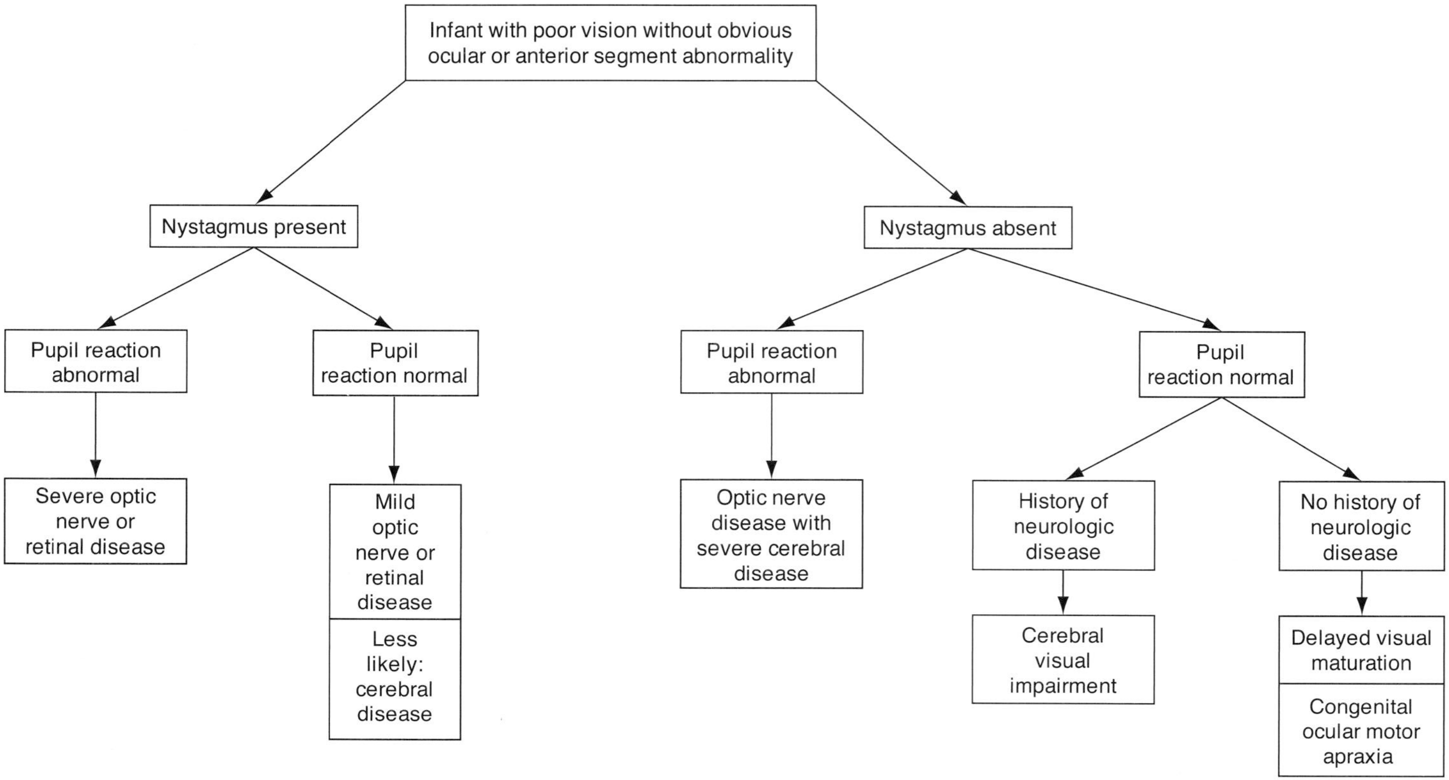

Figure 15-2 Evaluation of an infant with decreased vision. *(Adapted by Mays El-Dairi, MD, from Edmond JC. Why Can't My Baby See?* Focal Points: Clinical Modules for Ophthalmologists. *American Academy of Ophthalmology; 2014, module 1.)*

If the results of the ophthalmic examination of the anterior segment, pupils, and posterior segment with OCT and ERG are normal, but the infant has poor or variable visual behavior with no nystagmus by 3 months of age, the diagnosis is most likely CVI (or delayed visual maturation, if visual behavior normalizes by 6 months of age).

CHAPTER 16

Eyelid Disorders

This chapter includes a related video. Go to www.aao.org/bcscvideo_section06 or scan the QR code in the text to access this content.

Highlights

- Epiblepharon is best managed conservatively because it usually resolves as facial features mature.
- Ptosis can be accompanied by an ipsilateral deficit of upward eye movement.
- Congenital ptosis that requires surgical intervention early in infancy is rare.
- An eyelid blinking tic in childhood usually resolves spontaneously.

Congenital Eyelid Disorders

Eyelid anatomy is described in BCSC Section 2, *Fundamentals and Principles of Ophthalmology,* and Section 7, *Oculofacial Plastic and Orbital Surgery.* Section 7 also discusses many of the eyelid disorders covered in this chapter.

Eyelid malformations can be isolated or associated with orbital malformations; they can also represent features of a syndrome. Because of these possibilities, systematic evaluation of the eyelids and ocular adnexa may be an important part of the clinical evaluation of a dysmorphic infant.

Morphologic measurements of the eyelids and orbit can be compared with reference measurements and may have clinical significance (Fig 16-1; see also Chapter 17). The *Farkas canthal index,* defined as the ratio of inner canthal distance to outer canthal distance, can also be used. A canthal index lower than 38 signifies *ocular hypotelorism* (smaller-than-average distance between the eyes), and a canthal index greater than 42 indicates *ocular hypertelorism* (greater-than-average distance between the eyes).

Hall BD, Graham JM Jr, Cassidy SB, Opitz JM. Elements of morphology: standard terminology for the periorbital region. *Am J Med Genet A.* 2009;149A(1):29–39.

Dystopia Canthorum

Dystopia canthorum is lateral displacement of both the inner canthi and the lacrimal puncta so that an imaginary vertical line connecting the upper and lower puncta crosses the cornea (Fig 16-2). The displacement is a characteristic feature of Waardenburg syndrome type 1.

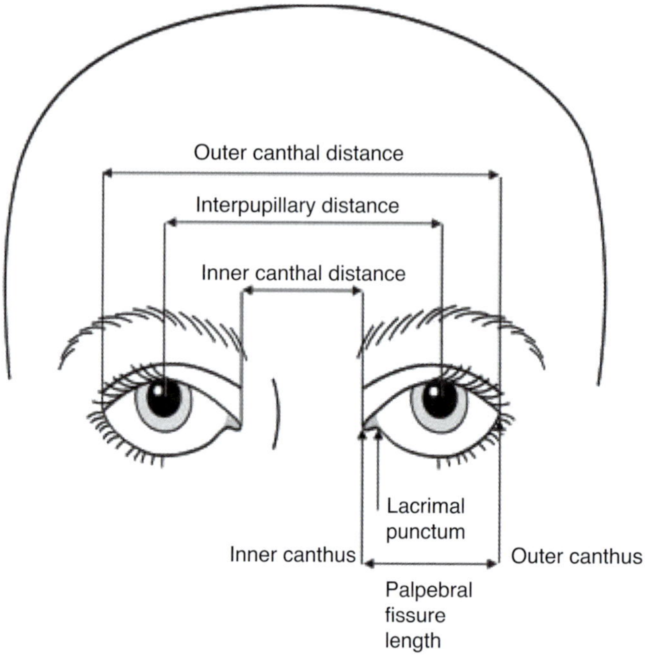

Figure 16-1 Schematic representation of measurements and physical landmarks involved in the evaluation of the orbital region. *(Reprinted with permission from Hall BD, Graham JM Jr, Cassidy SB, Opitz JM. Elements of morphology: standard terminology for the periorbital region.* Am J Med Genet A. *2009;149A(1):29–39. With permission from John Wiley and Sons.)*

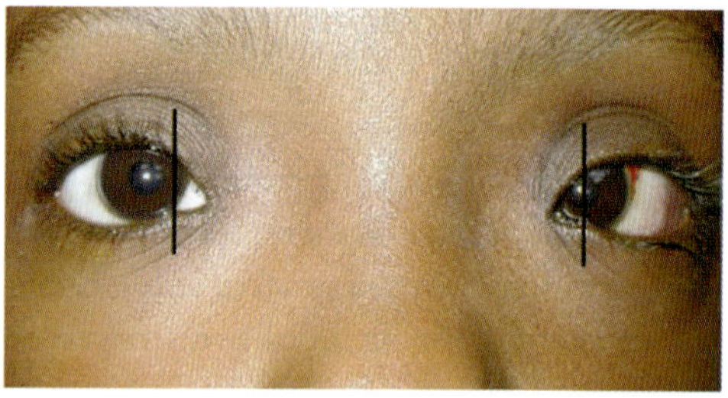

Figure 16-2 Dystopia canthorum in a patient with Waardenburg syndrome. The vertical lines drawn through the puncta intersect the cornea. *(Courtesy of Amy Hutchinson, MD.)*

Cryptophthalmos

Cryptophthalmos is a rare condition resulting from failed differentiation of eyelid structures. There is partial or complete absence of the palpebral fissure, as the skin extends uninterrupted from the forehead to the cheek, covering the eye (Fig 16-3). The adnexa are partially developed and fused to the anterior segment; the cornea is usually malformed. *Fraser syndrome,* an autosomal recessive disorder characterized by partial syndactyly and genitourinary anomalies, may include unilateral or bilateral cryptophthalmos and other ocular malformations.

Ablepharon

Ablepharon, absence or severe hypoplasia of the eyelids, is very rare. Affected patients are at high risk for exposure keratopathy. Ablepharon is a characteristic feature of ablepharon-macrostomia syndrome.

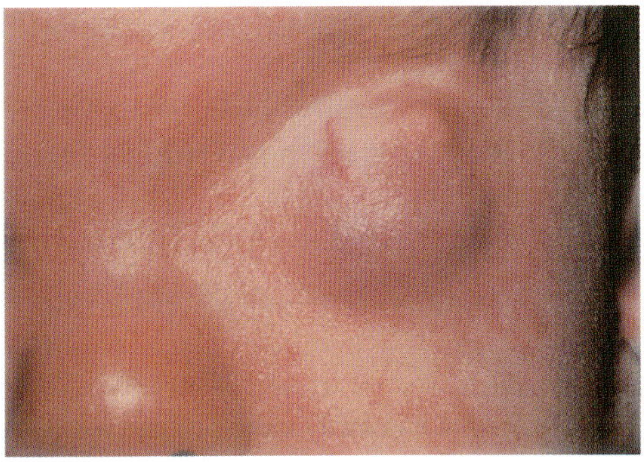

Figure 16-3 Cryptophthalmos, left eye.

Congenital Coloboma of the Eyelid

Congenital eyelid coloboma (eyelid cleft or notch) usually involves the upper eyelid and can range in size from a small notch to a defect that encompasses the horizontal length of the eyelid. The eyelid may be fused to the globe (Fig 16-4). Eyelid colobomas are unrelated to other ocular colobomas and are commonly associated with Goldenhar syndrome or amniotic band syndrome. The eye of an infant with a congenital eyelid coloboma should be monitored for exposure keratopathy. Surgical closure of the eyelid defect is required in most cases.

Ankyloblepharon

Fusion of part or all of the eyelid margins is termed *ankyloblepharon.* This condition may be dominantly inherited. Treatment is surgical. In *ankyloblepharon filiforme adnatum,* a variant of ankyloblepharon, the margins of the upper and lower eyelids are joined by fine strands of tissue (Fig 16-5). This variant is seen in Hay-Wells syndrome (also known as *ankyloblepharon–ectodermal dysplasia–clefting syndrome*), a form of ectodermal dysplasia that includes cleft lip or palate. The eyelid adhesions in children with ankyloblepharon filiforme adnatum can often be easily separated in the office with blunt scissors or a muscle hook, with topical anesthesia.

Congenital Ectropion

Congenital ectropion is a rare abnormality characterized by eversion of the eyelid margin. It usually involves the lower eyelid and is secondary to a vertical deficiency of the skin.

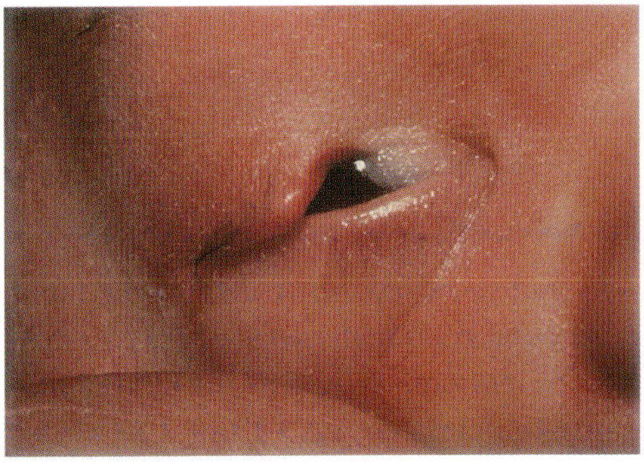

Figure 16-4 Congenital eyelid coloboma (cleft), right eye. The eyelid is fused to the globe.

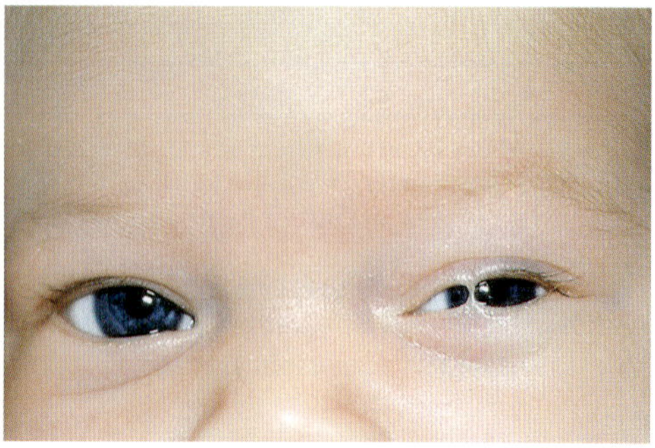

Figure 16-5 Ankyloblepharon filiforme adnatum. The eyelid margins are fused by a fine strand of tissue. *(Courtesy of Amy Hutchinson, MD.)*

Lateral tarsorrhaphy may be effective in mild cases. More severe cases may require a skin flap or graft.

Congenital Entropion

Congenital entropion is a rare abnormality characterized by eyelid margin inversion. It does not resolve spontaneously. Surgery is performed when corneal integrity is threatened.

Epiblepharon

Epiblepharon is a common congenital anomaly characterized by a horizontal fold of skin adjacent to the eyelid margin (most commonly the lower eyelid) that may turn the eyelashes inward, against the cornea (Fig 16-6). Infants' corneas often tolerate this condition surprisingly well. Unlike congenital entropion, epiblepharon often resolves spontaneously. Ocular lubricants may be beneficial. Surgical repair is required when the condition does not resolve, or when it causes chronic corneal irritation.

Congenital Tarsal Kink

In congenital tarsal kink, the tarsal plate of the upper eyelid is folded at birth, resulting in entropion. The cornea may be exposed and traumatized, leading to ulceration. The clinician can manage minor defects by manually unfolding the tarsus and taping the eyelid shut with a pressure dressing for 1–2 days. More severe cases require surgical incision of the tarsal plate or excision of a V-shaped wedge from the inner surface to permit unfolding.

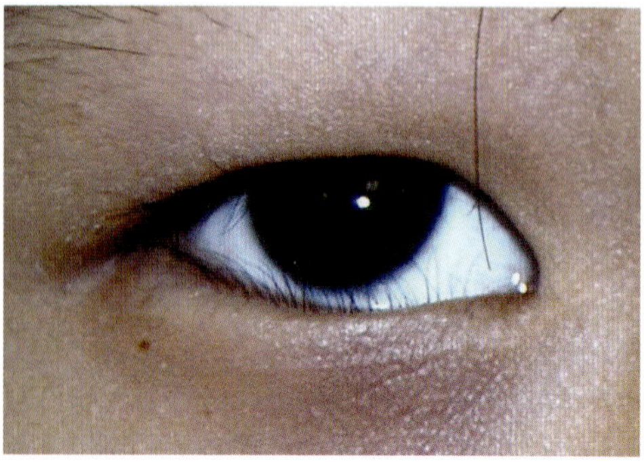

Figure 16-6 Epiblepharon, right eye. The lower eyelid eyelashes are turned inward, causing corneal irritation. *(© 2021 American Academy of Ophthalmology.)*

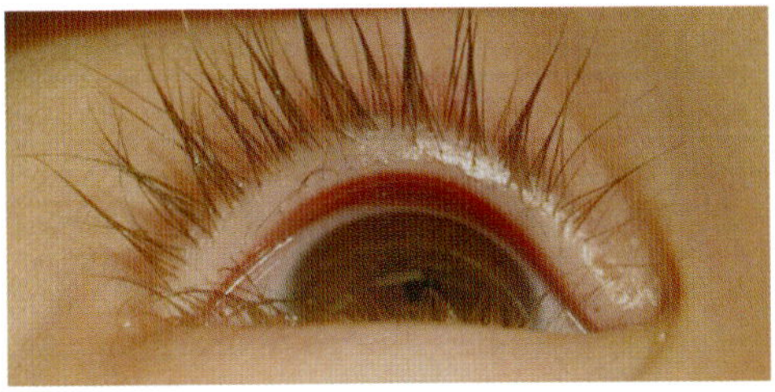

Figure 16-7 Distichiasis. An accessory row of eyelashes exits from the meibomian gland orifices. *(Courtesy of Jill Foster, MD.)*

Distichiasis

In distichiasis, an extra (partial or complete) row of eyelashes arises from or slightly posterior to the meibomian gland orifices (Fig 16-7). The abnormal eyelashes tend to be thinner, shorter, softer, and less pigmented than normal cilia and are therefore often well tolerated. Removal of the abnormal eyelashes with electrolysis, cryotherapy, or eyelid surgery may be indicated if chronic corneal irritation is present.

Euryblepharon

In euryblepharon, the lateral aspect of the palpebral aperture is enlarged, with downward displacement of the temporal half of the lower eyelid. This condition gives the appearance of a very wide palpebral fissure or a droopy lower eyelid. Euryblepharon may occur in Kabuki syndrome. Most patients do not require treatment.

Epicanthus

Epicanthus refers to a crescent-shaped fold of skin running vertically between the eyelids and overlying the inner canthus (Fig 16-8). There are 4 types:

- *epicanthus tarsalis:* The fold is most prominent in the upper eyelid.
- *epicanthus palpebralis:* The fold is equally distributed between the upper and lower eyelids.
- *epicanthus supraciliaris:* The fold arises from the eyebrow and terminates over the lacrimal sac.
- *epicanthus inversus:* The fold is most prominent in the lower eyelid.

Epicanthus inversus may be isolated or associated with ptosis or blepharophimosis–ptosis–epicanthus inversus syndrome. Surgical correction is only occasionally required.

Palpebral Fissure Slants

Most eyelids are generally positioned so that the lateral canthus is approximately 1 mm higher than the medial canthus. Slight upward or downward slanting of palpebral fissures normally occurs on a familial basis or in certain racial and ethnic groups (eg, in Asian individuals). An upward or downward slant is a characteristic feature of some craniofacial syndromes (eg, downward slant in Treacher Collins syndrome; see Chapter 17, Fig 17-7). Slanting of the palpebral fissures may be associated with A- or V-pattern strabismus (see Chapter 9).

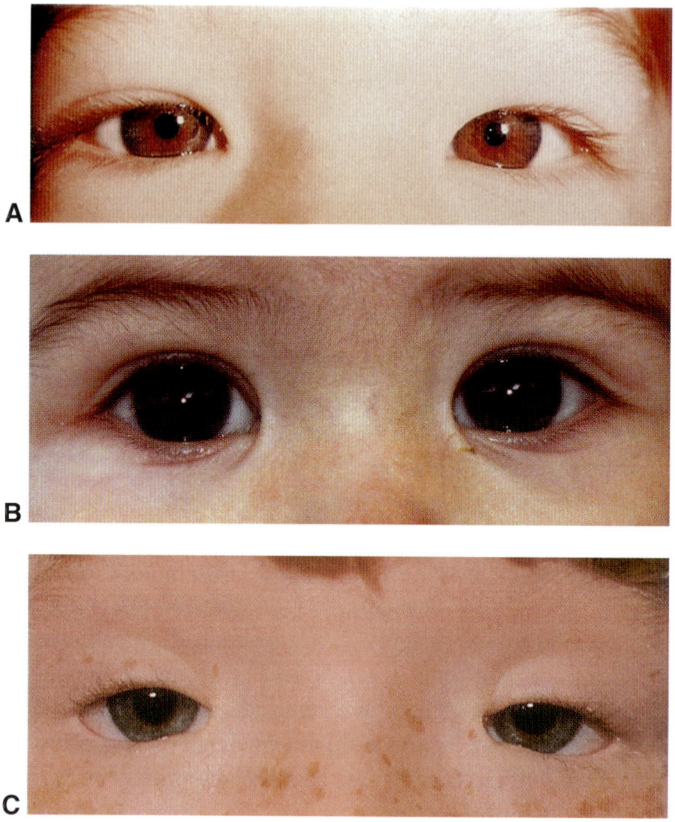

Figure 16-8 Epicanthus, bilateral. **A,** Epicanthus tarsalis. **B,** Epicanthus palpebralis. **C,** Epicanthus inversus in a patient with blepharophimosis–ptosis–epicanthus inversus syndrome. *(Part A reproduced with permission from Crouch E.* The Child's Eye: Strabismus and Amblyopia. *Slide script. American Academy of Ophthalmology; 1982. Part B courtesy of Robert W. Hered, MD.)*

Congenital Ptosis

Ptosis (ie, blepharoptosis) can be congenital or acquired. It is important to differentiate congenital ptosis from acquired cases with systemic associations (see the section Other Causes of Ptosis in Children, later in this chapter). Congenital ptosis is usually caused by decreased levator muscle function. It may be familial. Anisometropic amblyopia and strabismus are common associations.

Evaluation of ptosis requires assessment of

1. *the upper eyelid crease:* In severe congenital ptosis, it is usually absent.
2. *the palpebral fissure height:* The clinician can determine the amount of ptosis by measuring the distance between the upper and lower eyelids and the margin–reflex distances (MRD_1 and MRD_2). See Figure 16-9.
3. *levator muscle function:* This is assessed by measuring the distance that the upper eyelid moves when the patient shifts from downgaze to upgaze; during measurement, the examiner holds the brow to block recruitment of the frontalis muscle.

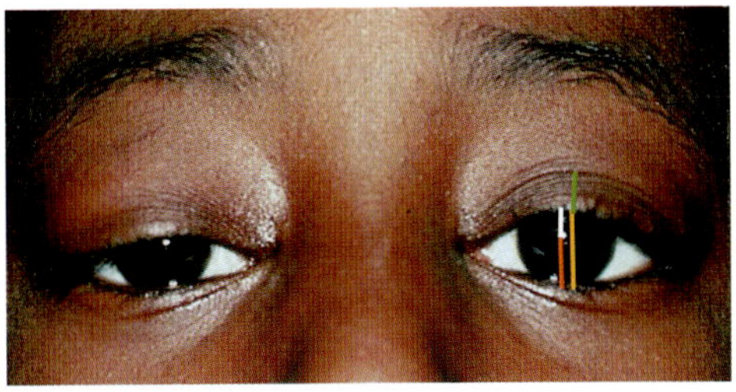

Figure 16-9 Child with right upper eyelid ptosis. Comparison of the ptotic right upper eyelid with the unaffected left upper eyelid shows a less distinct eyelid crease on the right, making the eyelid crease height *(green line)* on the right difficult to determine. The palpebral fissure height *(yellow line)* and margin–reflex distance 1 *(white line)* are reduced on the right. Margin–reflex distance 2 *(orange line)* appears similar in right and left eyes. *(© 2021 American Academy of Ophthalmology.)*

It is important to also evaluate tear function, corneal sensitivity, and the Bell phenomenon because corneal exposure may occur after surgical repair, should it be necessary. Tear function can be assessed by evaluating the tear lake and tear breakup time, as well as checking for the presence of punctate keratitis. Corneal sensitivity can be assessed by the presence of a blink reflex when the cornea is touched with a small thread pulled from the tip of a cotton swab. In addition, it is important to determine whether the globe is microphthalmic or whether a hypotropia is present, because either of these may produce pseudoptosis.

CLINICAL PEARL

If a hypotropia is also present and needs surgical correction, the strabismus surgery is performed first, because a change in globe position may affect eyelid position.

Marked congenital ptosis that obstructs vision is rare and must be corrected early in infancy to prevent deprivation amblyopia. Correction of severe ptosis usually requires frontalis suspension because of the lack of levator muscle function. Autologous or allogeneic fascia lata and synthetic material such as silicone rods can be used. Autologous fascia, however, cannot be obtained until the patient is 3 or 4 years old. Use of synthetic material or allogeneic fascia lata may lead to higher recurrence rates.

Repair of mild or moderate ptosis can usually be performed when the patient is older, although the presence of a compensatory chin-up head position may justify earlier surgery. External levator muscle resection is typically performed for mild or moderate congenital ptosis.

Blepharophimosis–ptosis–epicanthus inversus syndrome

Blepharophimosis–ptosis–epicanthus inversus syndrome (BPES; also referred to as *blepharophimosis syndrome*) may occur as a sporadic or autosomal dominant disorder with features of blepharophimosis, epicanthus inversus, telecanthus, and ptosis. Both of the 2 types of BPES include abnormalities of the eyelid; type I also includes premature ovarian failure. Mutations in the *FOXL2* gene have been found in both types. The palpebral fissures are shortened horizontally and vertically (blepharophimosis), levator muscle function is poor, and no upper eyelid fold is present (see Fig 16-8C). The length of the horizontal palpebral fissure, normally 25–30 mm, is only 18–22 mm in these patients. Repair of the ptosis, usually with frontalis suspension procedures, may be necessary early in life. Because the epicanthus and telecanthus may improve with age, repair of these defects is often delayed.

Marcus Gunn jaw-winking syndrome

Marcus Gunn jaw-winking syndrome, a congenital cranial dysinnervation disorder (CCDD), is a synkinetic syndrome in which the eyelid elevates with movement of the jaw (Video 16-1); it may present with ptosis. The synkinesis is thought to be caused by aberrant connections between the motor division of cranial nerve (CN) V and the levator muscle. The clinician may test an infant for this condition by having the child suck on a bottle or pacifier. Many patients do not require treatment. If the ptosis is amblyogenic or a chin-up head position develops, ptosis surgery may be indicated.

VIDEO 16-1 Marcus Gunn jaw-winking ptosis.
Courtesy of Katherine A. Lee, MD, PhD.

Other Causes of Ptosis in Children

Ptosis may occur in children as a result of several other disorders, including CN III palsy, monocular elevation deficiency, myasthenia gravis, congenital fibrosis of the extraocular muscles, chronic progressive external ophthalmoplegia, Horner syndrome, and mechanical causes. It may also be associated with several systemic disorders, including Turner, Cornelia de Lange, and fetal alcohol syndromes.

See Chapters 10 and 11 in this book and BCSC Section 5, *Neuro-Ophthalmology,* and Section 7, *Oculofacial Plastic and Orbital Surgery.*

Infectious and Inflammatory Eyelid Disorders

Inflammatory masses of the eyelids are common in children. *Chalazia* are caused by blockage of the meibomian glands, with secondary irritation due to lipid extravasation. *Hordeola* are localized infections of eyelid glands. Treatment of both disorders includes warm compresses and management of associated blepharitis (see Chapter 19). Omega-3 fatty acid dietary supplementation may be beneficial in some patients. Surgical treatment is reserved for large, painful, or chronic lesions. See BCSC Section 8, *External Disease and Cornea.*

Pyogenic granuloma (lobular capillary hemangioma)—a pedunculated, fleshy pink hemangiomatous growth—can develop on the tarsal conjunctiva, overlying a chalazion or trauma site (Fig 16-10). Patients with *molluscum contagiosum* may present with characteristic lesions of the eyelids and secondary follicular conjunctivitis (see Chapter 19).

Vascular Eyelid Disorders

Port-Wine Birthmark

Port-wine birthmark (PWB; also known as *port-wine stain, port-wine nevus,* or *nevus flammeus*) is a congenital vascular malformation that manifests as a flat red or pink cutaneous lesion. It may lighten during the first year of life but then tends to become darker, thicker,

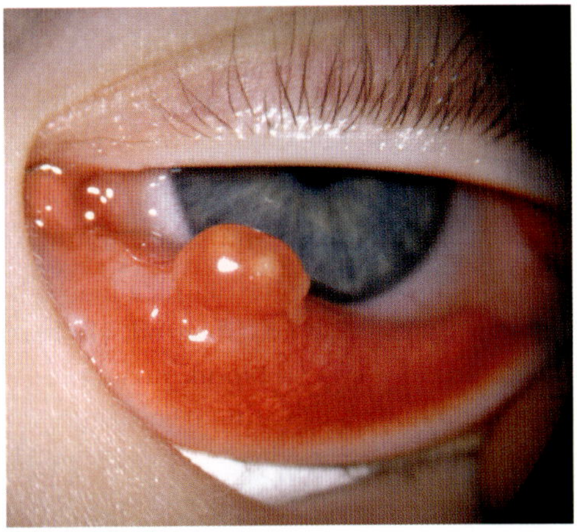

Figure 16-10 Pyogenic granuloma on tarsal conjunctiva at the site of a chalazion. *(Reproduced with permission from Lueder GT.* Pediatric Practice Ophthalmology. *McGraw-Hill Medical; 2010:178. Permission conveyed through Copyright Clearance Center, Inc.)*

and more nodular over time. PWB is associated with Sturge-Weber syndrome (encephalofacial angiomatosis) and *PIK3CA*-spectrum syndromes (eg, Klippel-Trénaunay-Weber syndrome) (see Chapter 27) and is seen in combination with ocular melanosis in phakomatosis pigmentovascularis. Glaucoma can occur in affected eyes (see Chapter 21). Lasers can be used to lighten the affected areas. Isolated PWB may result from somatic *GNAQ* mutation.

Eyelid Hemangioma

Hemangiomas are common vascular lesions that may involve the eyelid or orbit. They are discussed in Chapter 17.

Neoplasms and Other Noninflammatory Eyelid Lesions

Malignant tumors arising from eyelid skin or palpebral conjunctiva are extremely rare in children. Pediatric cases are likely to be associated with underlying systemic disorders that predispose to malignancy, such as basal cell nevus syndrome (Gorlin syndrome) or xeroderma pigmentosum. Rhabdomyosarcoma infrequently presents as an eyelid or conjunctival mass (see Chapter 17). Eyelid and epibulbar lesions can develop in juvenile xanthogranuloma (see Chapter 20).

Pilomatricoma

Pilomatricomas (sometimes spelled *pilomatrixomas* or called *Malherbe calcifying epitheliomas*) are benign tumors that arise from hair matrix. They may present as solid, noninflamed lesions, often with a whitish appearance (Fig 16-11). Surgical excision is curative.

Epithelial Lesions

Numerous types of benign superficial lesions may arise on the eyelids, including squamous papillomas, epidermal inclusion cysts, verruca vulgaris, and milia. These are discussed in BCSC Section 7, *Oculofacial Plastic and Orbital Surgery.*

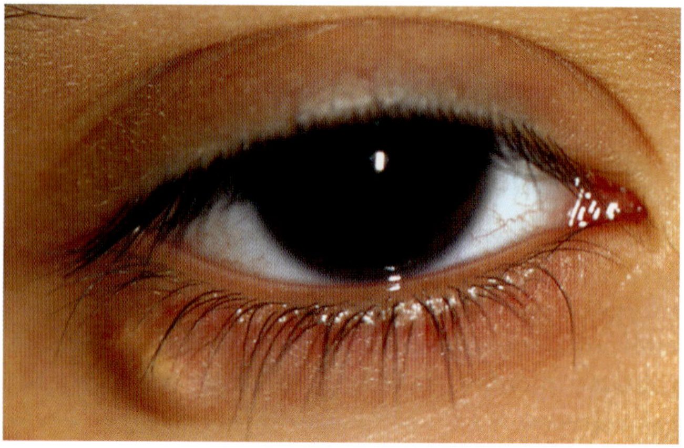

Figure 16-11 Pilomatricoma, right lower eyelid. Note the whitish center. *(Reproduced with permission from Lueder GT. Pediatric Practice Ophthalmology. McGraw-Hill Medical; 2010:84. Permission conveyed through Copyright Clearance Center, Inc.)*

Eyelid Nevi

Nevi arise from nevus cells, incompletely differentiated melanocytes in the epidermis and dermis and in the junction zone between these 2 layers; they are the third most common benign lesions encountered in the periocular region (after papillomas and epidermal inclusion cysts). The management of simple eyelid nevi in children is similar to that in adults (see BCSC Section 7, *Oculofacial Plastic and Orbital Surgery*).

Congenital nevocellular nevi

Congenital nevocellular (also called melanocytic) nevi can occur on the eyelids (Fig 16-12) and may cause visual deprivation amblyopia. They may undergo malignant transformation, the risk of which increases with the size of the lesion; large lesions (>20 cm) have a 5%–20% risk of malignant transformation. Observation is often recommended for small (<1.5 cm) and medium-sized (1.5–20.0 cm) lesions.

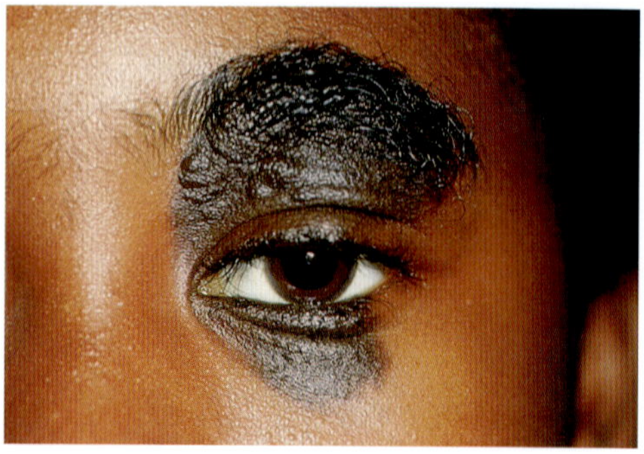

Figure 16-12 Congenital nevocellular nevus of the eyelid. *(Courtesy of Amy Hutchinson, MD.)*

Other Eyelid Conditions

Trichotillomania

Trichotillomania is characterized by the pulling out of one's hair, often including the eyebrows and eyelashes. It may be associated with obsessive-compulsive disorder or anxiety. The characteristic appearance includes madarosis, broken hairs, and regrowth of hairs of varying lengths (Fig 16-13).

Excessive Blinking

Excessive blinking is common in children. Causes include corneal and eyelid abnormalities, stress reactions, and tics. Ocular tics are usually benign and self-limited. Neurologic consultation may be indicated for patients with multiple tics to evaluate for Tourette syndrome. *Hemifacial spasm* causes unilateral forceful blinking and facial muscle contraction. Imaging is indicated in hemifacial spasm because the disorder may be caused by central nervous system lesions. See BCSC Section 7, *Oculofacial Plastic and Orbital Surgery,* for additional discussion of hemifacial spasm. Squinting may occur in patients with strabismus or uncorrected refractive errors.

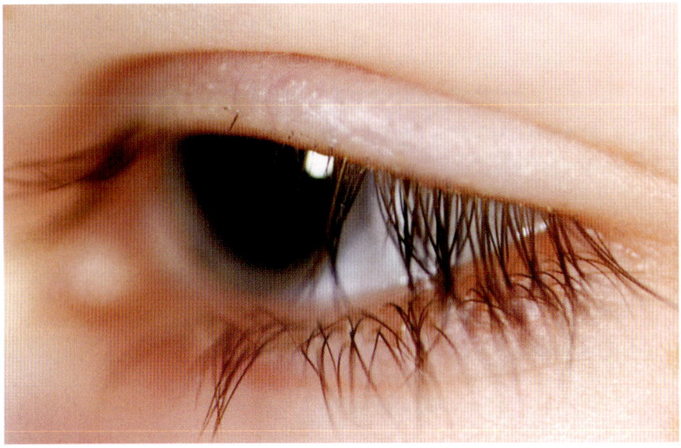

Figure 16-13 Trichotillomania. Note the segmental loss and irregular lengths of the eyelashes. *(Reproduced with permission from Lueder GT.* Pediatric Practice Ophthalmology. *McGraw-Hill Medical; 2010;155. Permission conveyed through Copyright Clearance Center, Inc.)*

CHAPTER 17

Orbital Disorders

Highlights

- Ophthalmic complications of craniofacial abnormalities include proptosis, strabismus, corneal exposure, and optic neuropathy.
- If untreated, orbital cellulitis and subperiosteal abscess can progress to cavernous sinus thrombosis.
- Rapidly progressing painless proptosis is suggestive of orbital rhabdomyosarcoma.

Introduction

Orbital disorders in children can be congenital or acquired and are often associated with ocular and intracranial abnormalities. Orbital anatomy is described in BCSC Section 2, *Fundamentals and Principles of Ophthalmology,* and Section 7, *Oculofacial Plastic and Orbital Surgery.* Many pediatric orbital disorders are also discussed in Section 7.

Abnormal Interocular Distance: Terminology and Associations

Telecanthus is common in many syndromes and is characterized by a greater-than-normal distance between the inner canthi; it is distinct from, but may accompany, orbital hypertelorism (excessive distance between the medial orbital walls). In primary telecanthus, the abnormality is confined to the soft tissue, occurring without hypertelorism: the interpupillary distance is normal (see also Chapter 16 and Fig 16-1). When telecanthus is secondary to hypertelorism, the interpupillary distance is greater than normal.

Orbital hypotelorism is a smaller-than-normal distance between the medial orbital walls, with reduced inner and outer canthal distances. This finding can be the result of skull malformation or a failure in brain development.

Exorbitism is variously defined as prominent eyes due to shallow orbits or as an increased angle of divergence of the orbital walls.

Congenital and Developmental Disorders: Craniofacial Malformations

Craniosynostosis

The skull is divided into 2 parts, the *calvarium* and the *skull base,* via an imaginary line drawn from the supraorbital rims to the base of the occiput (Fig 17-1). Cranial sutures are present throughout the skull and normally fuse during the first 2 years of life. *Craniosynostosis* is the premature closure of 1 or more cranial sutures during the embryonic period or early childhood.

Bony growth of the skull occurs in osteoblastic centers located at the suture sites. Bone is laid down parallel and perpendicular to the direction of the suture. Premature suture closure prevents perpendicular growth but allows parallel growth. This growth pattern, called *Virchow's law,* results in clinically recognizable cranial bone deformations. An abnormal head shape in a child raises suspicion for craniosynostosis, which is important to recognize because of the risk for hydrocephalus and ocular complications (see the section "Ocular complications of craniosynostosis").

Types of abnormal head shapes

See eTable 17-1 at www.aao.org/bcscsupplement_section06 for illustrations.

Plagiocephaly This shape often is deformational due to external compressive forces (either prenatally or during infancy). Deformational plagiocephaly due to intrauterine constraint (eg, oligohydramnios) is characterized by ipsilateral occipital flattening with contralateral forehead flattening. It may also be caused by unilateral coronal suture synostosis. Ipsilateral to the synostosis, there is occipitoparietal bone flattening, frontal bossing, and anterior ear displacement. On the affected side, the interpalpebral fissure is wider and the orbit is often higher.

Brachycephaly Brachycephaly (literally, "short head") is frequently the result of bilateral closure of both coronal sutures. Limited growth along the anterior-posterior axis results in a comparatively short head. Most often, the forehead is wide and flat.

Scaphocephaly/dolichocephaly Scaphocephaly ("boat head") and dolichocephaly ("long head") usually result from premature closure of the sagittal suture. There is anteroposterior elongation of the skull, along with bitemporal narrowing.

Trigonocephaly Metopic synostosis results in a triangle-shaped head with hypotelorism and pseudoesotropia.

Acrocephaly/kleeblattschädel The skull shape is trilobar. Kleeblattschädel ("cloverleaf skull") is typically the result of synostosis of the coronal, lambdoidal, and sagittal sutures.

Etiology of craniosynostosis

Early suture fusion can be sporadic and occur as an isolated abnormality (eg, sagittal suture synostosis and most cases of unilateral coronal suture synostosis), or it can be part of a genetic syndrome, associated with other abnormalities. Craniosynostosis syndromes are

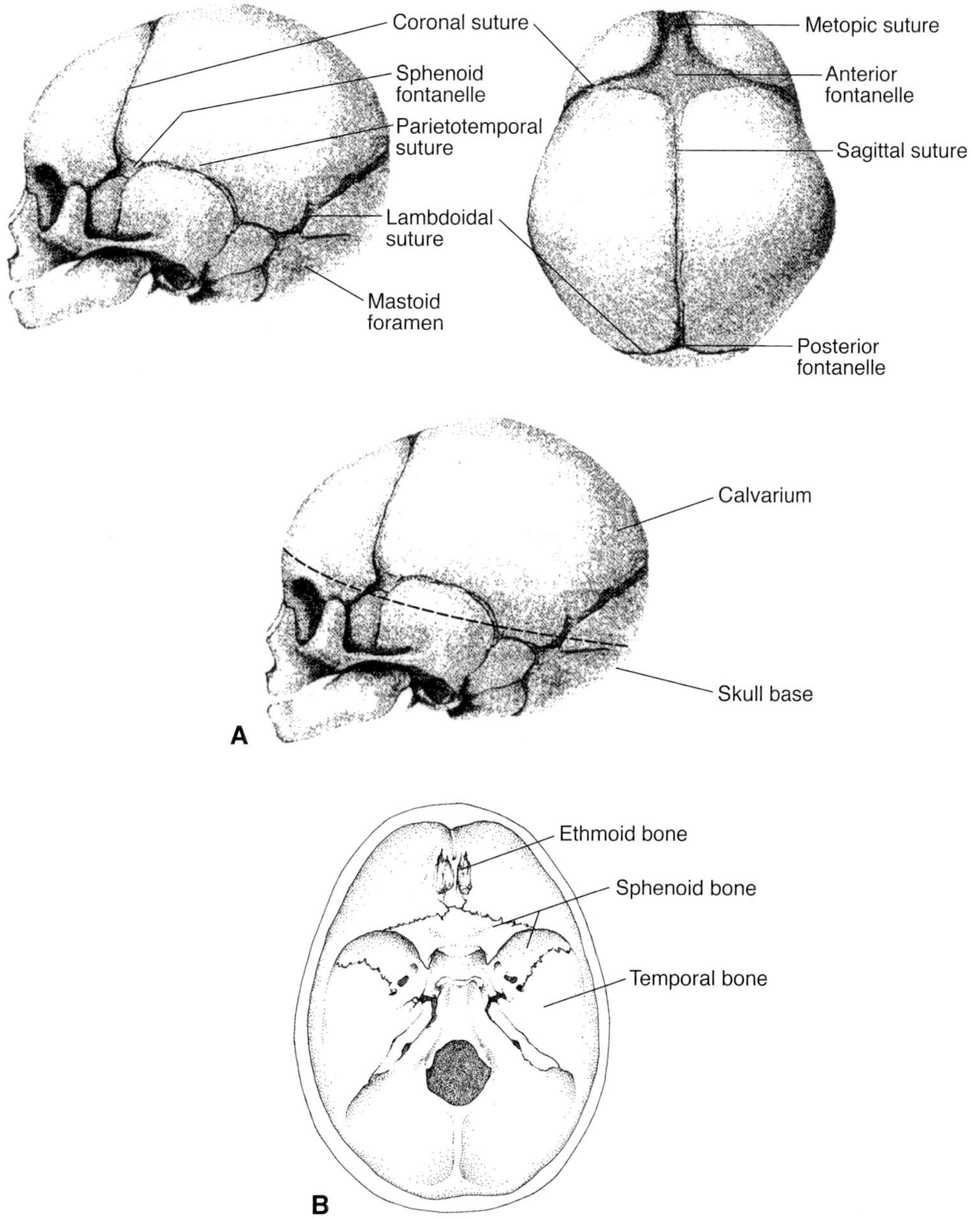

Figure 17-1 Major sutures of the skull. **A,** Normal sutures and fontanelles of the fetal skull. **B,** Adult cranial base, complete with sutures. *(Illustration by C.H. Wooley.)*

usually autosomal dominant conditions, often with associated limb abnormalities. Many of these syndromes have overlapping features, making accurate diagnosis based on clinical findings difficult. Identification of specific mutations may be diagnostic. Mutations in the fibroblast growth factor receptor genes (*FGFRs*) or in the *TWIST* gene are found in most patients with syndromic craniosynostosis.

Table 17-1 Craniosynostosis Syndromes

Syndrome	Potential Complications	Pathophysiology	Head Shape	Nonocular Cranial Findings	Extracranial Manifestations	External Ophthalmic Examination	Additional Signs and Symptoms
Crouzon syndrome (Fig 17-2; see also BCSC Section 7, Fig 3-4B[a])	Most common craniosynostosis syndrome Varying degree of deformity Mild cases can be missed	Calvarial bone synostosis often includes both coronal sutures Skull base sutures are also involved	Broad, retruded forehead Brachycephaly or scaphocephaly Tower-shaped skull Midfacial retrusion	Hydrocephalus (common) Normal intelligence	Usually none	Hypertelorism Proptosis Inferior scleral show Shallow orbits	Proptosis Corneal exposure Strabismus Papilledema Optic atrophy
Apert syndrome (eFig 17-1[b]; see also BCSC Section 7, Fig 3-5[a])	Can appear similar to Crouzon syndrome but has more cranial and extracranial manifestations	Fusion of multiple calvarial sutures, most often both coronal sutures Fusion of skull base sutures	Brachycephaly and acrocephaly Midface hypoplasia	Hydrocephalus Intellectual disability Conductive hearing loss Beak-shaped nose Cleft palate	Polydactyly Severe syndactyly ("mitten" deformity) Hyperhidrosis Vertebral fusion Visceral abnormalities	Hypertelorism Shallow orbits	Proptosis Corneal exposure Strabismus Papilledema Optic atrophy
Pfeiffer syndrome	Very severe craniofacial abnormalities	Fusion of both coronal sutures Possible fusion of the sagittal suture	Cloverleaf skull, more severe than in those with Apert syndrome Brachycephaly and acrocephaly Midface hypoplasia Tracheal abnormalities	Normal intelligence High risk of hydrocephalus Conductive hearing loss Hypoplastic maxilla, prominent upper jaw Dental abnormalities Beak-shaped nose	Syndactyly Short, broad thumbs and toes Visceral abnormalities Ankylosis of elbow	Hypertelorism Proptosis Inferior scleral show Shallow orbits	Proptosis Corneal exposure Strabismus Papilledema Optic atrophy
Saethre-Chotzen syndrome (Fig 17-3)	Features can easily be missed	Typically 1 coronal suture	Plagiocephaly	Normal intelligence Low hairline Ear abnormalities	Brachydactyly Mild syndactyly Short stature Cardiac defects	Ptosis Shallow orbits	Proptosis Corneal exposure Strabismus

[a] In BCSC Section 7, *Oculofacial Plastic and Orbital Surgery.*
[b] At www.aao.org/bcscsupplement_section06.

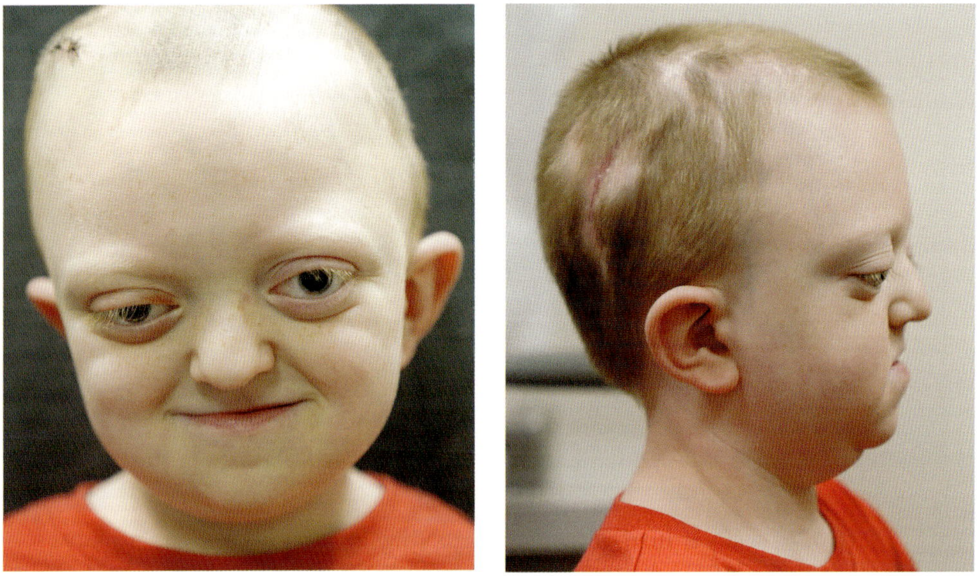

Figure 17-2 Crouzon syndrome. This patient exhibits brachycephaly and a tower-shaped skull with forehead retrusion, proptosis, inferior scleral show, midface hypoplasia, and a small, beak-like nose. He also had hydrocephalus and papilledema. Note the shunt scar on the scalp. *(Courtesy of Mays El-Dairi, MD.)*

Craniosynostosis syndromes

Common systemic features of the craniosynostosis syndromes include fusion of multiple calvarial sutures and skull base sutures. Syndactyly (partial fusion of the digits) and brachydactyly (short digits), ranging in severity, are hallmarks of these syndromes, the exception being Crouzon syndrome. Table 17-1 lists the common types of craniosynostosis syndromes that may be encountered by the ophthalmologist; all syndromes listed are autosomal dominant. (There are many other syndromes that have not been listed.)

Ocular complications of craniosynostosis

Proptosis Proptosis (or exorbitism) results from the reduced volume of the bony orbit. The severity of the proptosis in patients with craniosynostosis is not uniform and frequently increases with age because of the impaired growth of the bony orbit.

Corneal exposure Because the eyelids may not close completely over the proptotic globes, corneal exposure may occur, with possible development of exposure keratitis. Aggressive lubrication may be necessary to prevent corneal drying. Tarsorrhaphy can reduce the exposure. Surgically expanding the orbital volume, thereby eliminating the proptosis, may be indicated in extreme cases.

Globe luxation In patients with extremely shallow orbits, globe luxation may occur when the eyelids are manipulated or when there is increased pressure in the orbits, such as occurs with a Valsalva maneuver. The globe is luxated forward, the eyelids closing behind

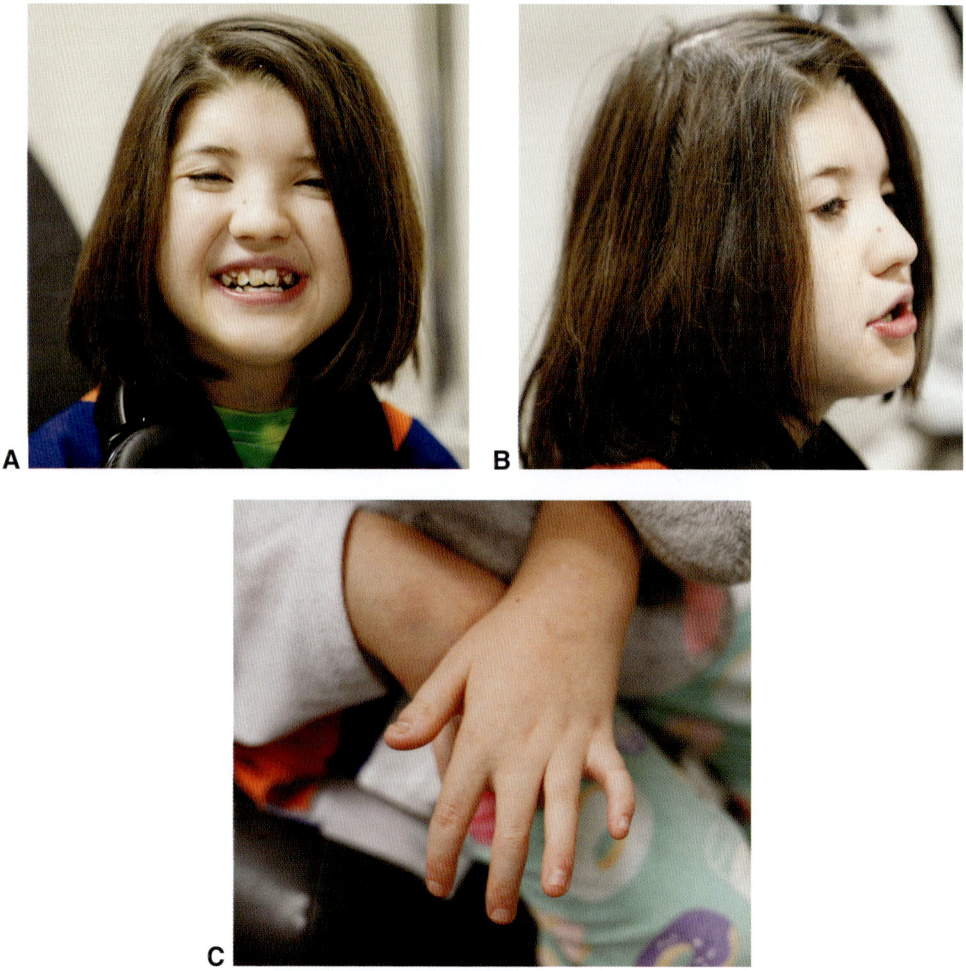

Figure 17-3 Saethre-Chotzen syndrome. Note the facial asymmetry, flat forehead, low hairline, dental abnormalities, bilateral ptosis (post frontalis sling) **(A, B)**, and partial syndactyly of fingers 2 and 3 **(C)**. (*Not shown here:* This patient also has syndactyly of toes, nasolacrimal duct obstruction, and hydrocephalus post shunt.) *(Courtesy of Mays El-Dairi, MD.)*

the equator of the globe. The condition is very painful and can cause corneal exposure. It may also compromise the blood supply to the globe, which is a medical emergency. Physicians and patients (or their caregivers) should quickly reposition the globe behind the eyelids. The best technique for doing this is to place a finger and thumb over the conjunctiva within the interpalpebral fissure and exert gentle but firm pressure; this technique does not damage the cornea. For recurrent luxation, the short-term solution is tarsorrhaphy; the long-term solution is orbital volume expansion.

Strabismus Patients with craniosynostosis show a variety of deviations. Exotropia is the most frequent horizontal deviation in the primary position. Marked V-pattern strabismus is very common (see Chapter 10) and is often accompanied by a marked overelevation

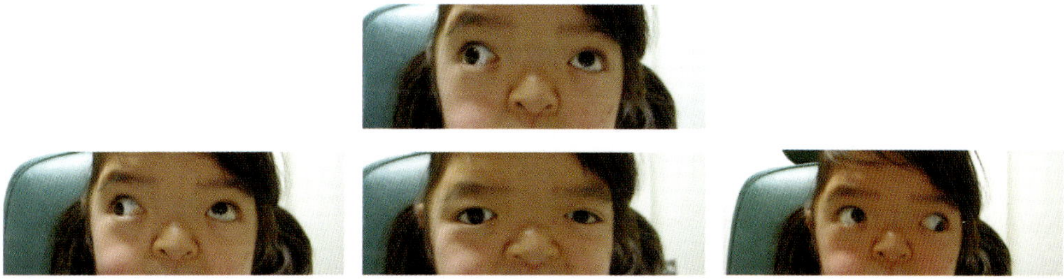

Figure 17-4 Strabismus in a patient with Apert syndrome. Note the good alignment in primary position with marked overelevation in adduction and exotropia in upgaze (V pattern). *(Courtesy of John Simon, MD.)*

in adduction, especially when 1 or both coronal sutures are fused, as occurs in Apert (Fig 17-4) and Crouzon syndromes. The apparent overaction of the inferior oblique muscle on the side of the coronal suture fusion may be due to 1 of the following:

- orbital and globe excyclorotation, which converts the medial rectus muscle into an elevator when the eye is in adduction (pseudo-overaction)
- superior oblique trochlear retrusion (because of superior orbital rim retrusion), which induces superior oblique underaction and secondary true inferior oblique overaction
- anomalous extraocular muscle insertions or agenesis, most commonly absence of the superior oblique
- orbital pulley abnormalities (see Chapter 2)

Optic nerve abnormalities Optic nerve damage may occur for several reasons in patients with craniosynostosis. Optic nerve function may deteriorate in patients with chronically elevated intracranial pressure (ICP), which may result from hydrocephalus or be caused by crowding of the intracranial contents due to synostosis. In patients with midfacial retrusion, sleep apnea may develop and can cause idiopathic intracranial hypertension. In rare cases, optic nerve damage can occur secondary to compression stemming from synostosis of the optic foramina. Optic atrophy may occur with or without antecedent papilledema.

Ocular adnexal abnormalities Common ocular adnexal abnormalities include orbital hypertelorism, telecanthus, abnormal slant of the palpebral fissures secondary to superior displacement of the medial canthi, ptosis, and nasolacrimal abnormalities. Epiphora is common and may be secondary to nasolacrimal duct obstruction, poor blink secondary to proptosis, obliquity of the palpebral fissures, or ocular irritation from corneal exposure.

Surgical management of craniosynostosis

Reconstructive surgery for severe craniofacial malformation is frequently extensive and involves en bloc movement of the facial structures. It is important to document the status of the visual system preoperatively and monitor it postoperatively, with appropriate treatment as indicated. Procedures that involve moving the orbits may significantly change the degree or type of strabismus. Because of this, deferring treatment of strabismus until craniofacial surgery is completed may be appropriate. Papilledema from increased ICP can still occur after cranial surgery.

Proctor MR, Meara JG. A review of the management of single-suture craniosynostosis, past, present, and future. *J Neurosurg Pediatr.* 2019;24(6):622–631.

Nonsynostotic Craniofacial Conditions

Many craniofacial syndromes do not involve synostosis. Nonsynostotic syndromes and conditions of particular importance to the ophthalmologist are discussed in the following sections.

Anophthalmia

Anophthalmia (anophthalmos), the absence of tissues of the eye (Fig 17-5), is the most severe and rare phenotypic expression of a spectrum of abnormalities that includes typical coloboma and microphthalmia (see also Chapter 20). These conditions may be isolated, but they are frequently associated with other congenital anomalies. Anophthalmia and severe microphthalmia are associated with hypoplastic orbits and eyelids. Various techniques have been utilized for orbital expansion. The best results are achieved with early treatment.

Branchial arch syndromes

Branchial arch syndromes are caused by disruptions in the embryonic development of the first 2 branchial arches, which are responsible for formation of the maxillary and mandibular bones, the ear, and facial musculature. The best-known branchial arch syndromes include Treacher Collins syndrome and the *oculoauriculovertebral spectrum (OAVS),* which includes hemifacial microsomia and Goldenhar syndrome. Hemifacial microsomia is a milder form of OAVS. Patients with OAVS may have vertebral abnormalities such as hemivertebrae and vertebral hypoplasia. They may also have neurologic, cardiovascular, and genitourinary abnormalities. Most cases are sporadic.

Goldenhar syndrome Patients with Goldenhar syndrome have hemifacial microsomia (unilateral or bilateral) and characteristic ophthalmic abnormalities (Fig 17-6). Most cases are sporadic.

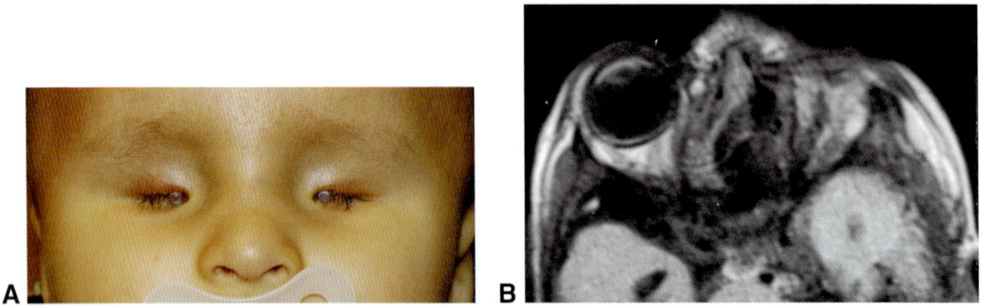

Figure 17-5 Anophthalmia. **A,** Clinical photo of a patient with anophthalmia, both eyes. **B,** Magnetic resonance imaging from a patient with unilateral anophthalmia shows absence of ocular structures. *(Part A courtesy of Steven Couch, MD; part B courtesy of Alice Bashinsky, MD.)*

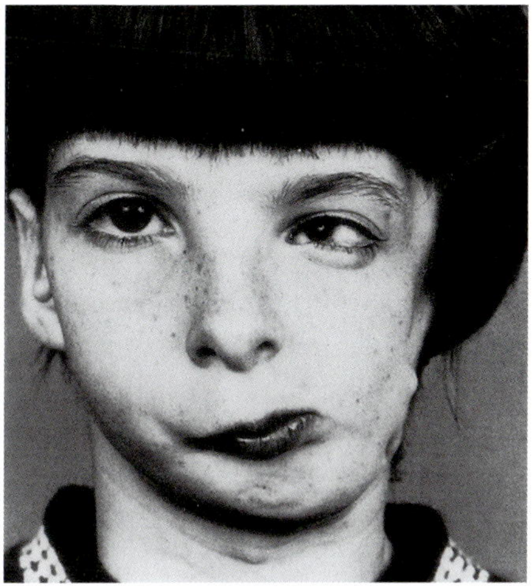

Figure 17-6 Goldenhar syndrome with hemifacial microsomia. The patient has facial asymmetry, a hypoplastic left ear (microtia), an ear tag near the right ear, epibulbar dermolipoma in the left eye, and esotropia. The patient also has Duane syndrome in the left eye.

Epibulbar (limbal) dermoids and dermolipomas are characteristic ocular signs. Dermolipomas (also termed *lipodermoids*) usually occur in the temporal quadrant, covered by conjunctiva and often hidden by the lateral upper and lower eyelids. Epibulbar limbal dermoids occur more frequently than dermolipomas and can be bilateral (approximately 25% of cases). They occasionally impinge on the visual axis but more commonly interfere with vision by causing astigmatism and anisometropic amblyopia. Eyelid colobomas may occur. Other ocular conditions include microphthalmia, cataract, and iris abnormalities. Duane syndrome is more common in patients with Goldenhar syndrome.

Treacher Collins syndrome Treacher Collins syndrome (mandibulofacial dysostosis) is caused by abnormal growth of the first and second branchial arches, with underdevelopment and even agenesis of the zygoma and malar eminences. The lateral orbital rims are depressed and the palpebral fissures slant downward because of lateral canthal dystopia (Fig 17-7). Pseudocolobomas (uncommonly, true colobomas) occur in the outer third of

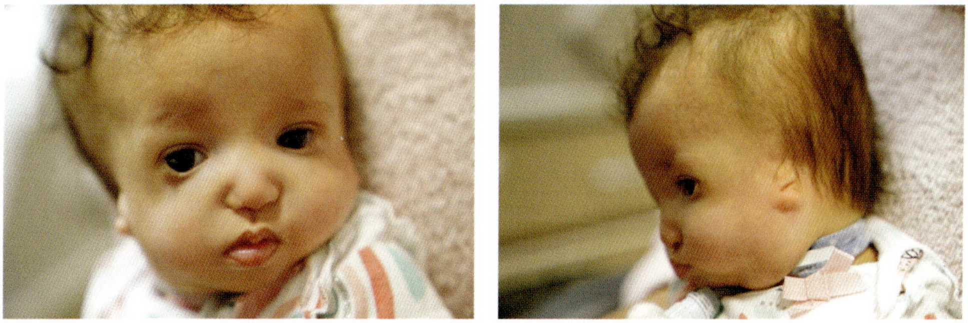

Figure 17-7 Treacher Collins syndrome (mandibulofacial dysostosis). Note the downward slant of the palpebral fissure (pseudocoloboma, because there is partial continuation of the meibomian glands and cilia), notch or curving of the inferotemporal eyelid margin, low-set abnormal ears, and maxillary and mandibular hypoplasia. *(Courtesy of Mays El-Dairi, MD.)*

the lower eyelids. Meibomian glands may be absent. The cilia of the lower eyelid medial to the pseudocoloboma may also be absent. The ears are malformed and hearing loss is common. The mandible is typically hypoplastic, leading to micrognathia. Intelligence is normal. The syndrome has an autosomal dominant pattern of inheritance. Most affected patients have a mutation in the *TCOF1* gene.

Pierre Robin sequence

The Pierre Robin sequence (also *anomaly, deformity*) is characterized by micrognathia, glossoptosis, and cleft palate. The sequence is a frequent finding in Stickler syndrome. Associated ocular anomalies include retinal detachment, microphthalmia, childhood glaucoma, cataracts, and high myopia.

Fetal alcohol syndrome

Fetal alcohol syndrome is caused by in utero exposure to ethanol. It is characterized by prenatal and postnatal growth retardation, central nervous system and craniofacial abnormalities, and intellectual disability.

The classic ocular features of fetal alcohol syndrome are short palpebral fissures, telecanthus, epicanthus, ptosis, microphthalmia, and esotropia (Fig 17-8). Anterior segment dysgenesis, optic nerve hypoplasia, and high refractive errors have been reported. Fifty percent of children with this underdiagnosed syndrome have some form of visual impairment.

Nonsynostotic disorders of bone growth

Infantile malignant osteopetrosis In this rare and severe autosomal recessive form of osteopetrosis, proliferation of bone results in narrowing of the foramina of the skull. Stenosis of the optic canal increases the risk of compressive optic neuropathy. Bone marrow

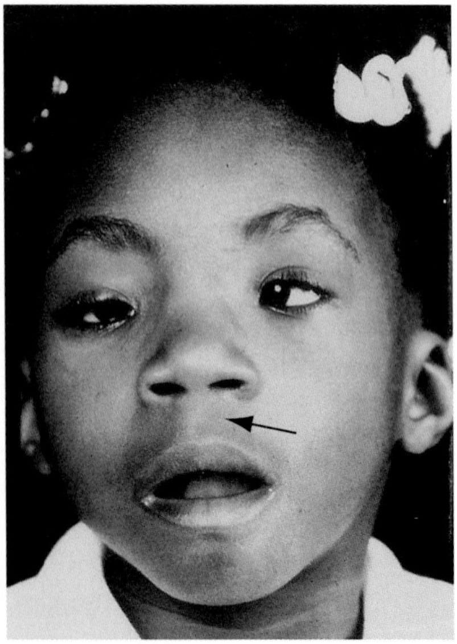

Figure 17-8 Fetal alcohol syndrome. Asymmetric ptosis; telecanthus; strabismus; long, flat philtrum *(arrow);* anteverted nostrils. This child also had Peters anomaly, left eye, and myopia, right eye. *(Reproduced with permission from Miller MT, Israel J, Cuttone J. Fetal alcohol syndrome.* J Pediatr Ophthalmol Strabismus. *1981;18(4):6–15.)*

transplant at approximately 12 months of age is associated with improved long-term survival and decreased disability, but there is a high rate of graft failure and hepatic and pulmonary toxicity.

Craniometaphyseal dysplasia Craniometaphyseal dysplasia is a rare disorder of osteoclast resorption that causes hyperostosis of the cranial bones. The typical facial appearance includes frontal and paranasal bossing. Progressive stenosis of cranial nerve foramina can result in compressive optic neuropathy.

Infectious and Inflammatory Conditions

Preseptal and orbital cellulitis usually progress more rapidly and are more severe in children than in adults. See also BCSC Section 7, *Oculofacial Plastic and Orbital Surgery.*

Preseptal Cellulitis

Preseptal cellulitis, a common infection in children, is an inflammatory process involving the tissues anterior to the orbital septum. Eyelid edema may extend into the forehead. The periorbital skin becomes taut and inflamed, and edema of the contralateral eyelids may appear. Proptosis is not a feature of preseptal cellulitis, and the globe remains uninvolved. Full ocular motility and absence of pain on eye movement help distinguish preseptal cellulitis from orbital cellulitis.

Preseptal cellulitis typically develops in 1 of 3 ways:

- following puncture, insect bite, or laceration of the eyelid skin (posttraumatic cellulitis): In these cases, organisms found on the skin, such as *Staphylococcus* or *Streptococcus* species, are most commonly responsible for the infection.
- in conjunction with severe conjunctivitis such as epidemic keratoconjunctivitis or methicillin-resistant *Staphylococcus aureus* (MRSA) conjunctivitis, or with skin infection such as impetigo or herpes zoster.
- secondary to upper respiratory tract or sinus infection: The most common causative organisms are *S aureus* and *Streptococcus pneumoniae* and other streptococcal species.

Children with mild preseptal infections (eyelid swelling without chemosis, fever, proptosis, ophthalmoplegia, or optic neuropathy) can be treated with oral antibiotics as outpatients. Broad-spectrum drugs effective against the most common pathogens, such as cephalosporins or an ampicillin–clavulanic acid combination, are usually effective. Particularly with eyelid abscesses, clindamycin may be an appropriate choice because of the increasing prevalence of MRSA, which should also be considered in patients who do not improve with treatment. Eyelid abscesses may require urgent incision and drainage.

For young infants or patients with signs of systemic illness such as sepsis or meningeal involvement, hospital admission may be indicated for appropriate cultures, imaging of the sinuses and orbits, and intravenous (IV) antibiotics. In newborns, dacryocystocele should be considered in the differential diagnosis (see Chapter 18).

Orbital Cellulitis

Orbital cellulitis involves the tissues posterior to the orbital septum. It is most commonly associated with ethmoid or frontal sinusitis but can also occur following penetrating injuries of the orbit.

Most young children with orbital cellulitis have infections caused by a single aerobic pathogen. In the neonate, *S aureus* and gram-negative bacilli are most common. In older children and adults, *S aureus, Streptococcus pyogenes,* and *Streptococcus pneumoniae* are common etiologic agents. Concurrent infections with multiple pathogens, including gram-negative and anaerobic organisms, can occur in older or immunosuppressed patients.

Early signs and symptoms of orbital cellulitis include lethargy, fever, eyelid edema, rhinorrhea, headache, orbital pain, and tenderness on palpation. The nasal mucosa becomes hyperemic, with a purulent nasal discharge. Increased venous congestion may cause elevated intraocular pressure. Proptosis, chemosis, and limited ocular movement suggest orbital involvement.

The differential diagnosis of orbital cellulitis includes nonspecific orbital inflammation, benign orbital tumors such as lymphatic malformation and hemangioma, and malignant tumors such as rhabdomyosarcoma, leukemia, and metastases.

Paranasal sinusitis is the most common cause of bacterial orbital cellulitis (Fig 17-9). In children younger than 10 years, the ethmoid sinuses are most frequently involved. If orbital cellulitis is suspected, orbital imaging is indicated to confirm orbital involvement, to document the presence and extent of sinusitis and a subperiosteal abscess (Fig 17-10), and to rule out a foreign body in a patient with a history of trauma.

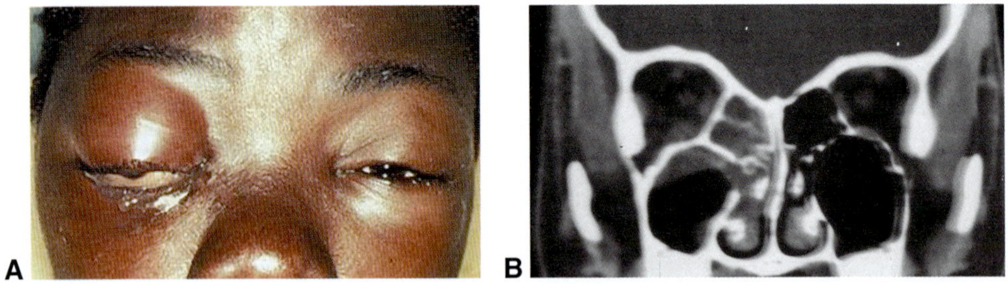

Figure 17-9 Bacterial orbital cellulitis with proptosis **(A)** secondary to sinusitis **(B).** *(Courtesy of Jane Edmond, MD.)*

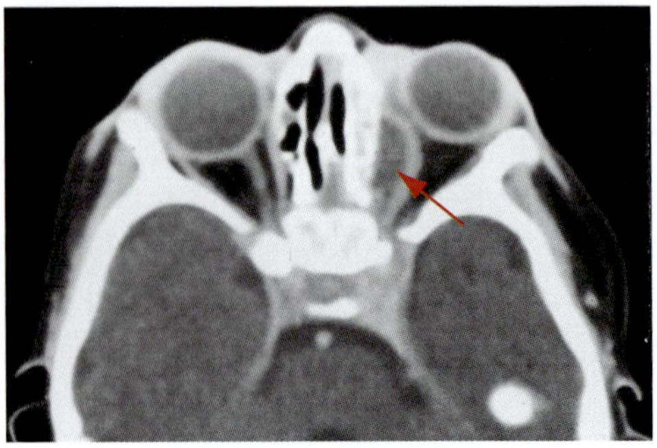

Figure 17-10 Axial computed tomography (CT) image shows a medial subperiosteal abscess *(arrow)* of the left orbit associated with ethmoid sinusitis. *(Courtesy of Jane Edmond, MD.)*

It is crucial to distinguish orbital cellulitis from preseptal cellulitis because the former requires hospital admission and treatment with IV broad-spectrum antibiotics. The choice of IV antibiotic is based on the most likely pathogens until results from cultures are known. If associated sinusitis or subperiosteal abscess is present, pediatric otolaryngologists should be consulted. Radiographic findings suggestive of an abscess are listed in Table 17-2.

It is important to closely observe the patient for signs of visual compromise. Many subperiosteal abscesses in children younger than 9 years resolve with medical management. Emergency drainage of a subperiosteal abscess is indicated for a patient of any age with *any* of the following:

- evidence of optic nerve compromise (decreasing vision, relative afferent pupillary defect)
- enlarging subperiosteal abscess
- an abscess that does not resolve within 48–72 hours of administration of antibiotics
- presence of intraconal orbital abscesses; these are much less common than subperiosteal abscesses in children and require urgent surgical drainage
- suspicion for anaerobic infection (gas in abscess on computed tomography [CT])

Abscess drainage is usually performed by an orbital surgeon in collaboration with an otolaryngologist or neurosurgeon. CT-guided percutaneous drainage is controversial because of its low success and high recurrence rates (because the sinus cannot be drained). Trying the percutaneous approach first might help avoid a more invasive surgery but is more likely to subject the child to general anesthesia twice. Surgical drainage can be done via a transnasal endoscopic approach (for a medially located abscess) or an external approach (for a superiorly located abscess). A combination approach can be used for a larger abscess.

Complications of orbital cellulitis include cavernous sinus thrombosis and intracranial extension (subdural or brain abscesses, meningitis, periosteal abscess), which may result in death. Cavernous sinus thrombosis can be difficult to distinguish from simple orbital cellulitis.

Table 17-2 Computed Tomography Findings of Preseptal and Orbital Cellulitis and Subperiosteal Abscess

Preseptal Cellulitis	Orbital Cellulitis	Subperiosteal Abscess
Periorbital soft tissue swelling and stranding anterior to the orbital septum	Diffuse soft tissue stranding posterior to the orbital septum (exophthalmos)	Lenticular rim–enhancing fluid collection along the orbital wall with adjacent sinusitis
Obliteration of the adjacent fat planes	Proptosis	Air-fluid level in the extraconal space
Pertinent negatives:		Acute ethmoid sinusitis (common in children)
No exophthalmos		If proptosis is severe, globe deformity ("guitar pick" sign) may be present
No retrobulbar inflammation		Displacement of adjacent rectus muscle
No evidence of ethmoid sinusitis		Osteomyelitis of the orbital wall (very severe cases)
No displacement or enlargement of extraocular muscles		

Paralysis of eye movement in individuals with cavernous sinus thrombosis is often out of proportion to the degree of proptosis. Pain on motion and tenderness on palpation are absent. Decreased sensation along the maxillary division of cranial nerve V (trigeminal nerve) supports the diagnosis. Bilateral ophthalmoplegia is virtually diagnostic of cavernous sinus thrombosis.

Other complications of orbital cellulitis include corneal exposure with secondary ulcerative keratitis, neurotrophic keratitis, secondary glaucoma, septic uveitis or retinitis, exudative retinal detachment, optic nerve edema, inflammatory neuritis, infectious neuritis, central retinal artery occlusion, and panophthalmitis.

Liao JC, Harris GJ. Subperiosteal abscess of the orbit: evolving pathogens and the therapeutic protocol. *Ophthalmology.* 2015;122(3):639–647.

Related conditions

Fungal orbital cellulitis (mucormycosis) occurs most frequently in patients with ketoacidosis or severe immunosuppression. The infection causes thrombosing vasculitis with ischemic necrosis of involved tissue (Fig 17-11). Cranial nerves often are involved, and extension into the central nervous system is common. Smears and biopsy of the involved tissues reveal the fungal organisms. Treatment includes debridement and systemic administration of antifungal medication. *Allergic fungal sinusitis* is a less fulminant condition that frequently presents with orbital signs, including proptosis from remodeling of the bony orbit. See BCSC Section 7, *Oculofacial Plastic and Orbital Surgery,* for further discussion.

Childhood Orbital Inflammation

Several noninfectious, nontraumatic disorders can cause orbital inflammation in children that may simulate infection or an orbital mass lesion. Thyroid eye disease, the most common cause of proptosis in adults, rarely occurs in prepubescent children but occasionally affects adolescents. Bilateral orbital inflammation may occur with sarcoidosis.

Nonspecific orbital inflammation

Nonspecific orbital inflammation (NSOI) (also known as *orbital pseudotumor, idiopathic orbital inflammatory syndrome*) is an inflammatory cause of proptosis in childhood that differs significantly from the adult form. The typical pediatric presentation is acute and painful; it more closely resembles orbital cellulitis, with decreased vision, red eye,

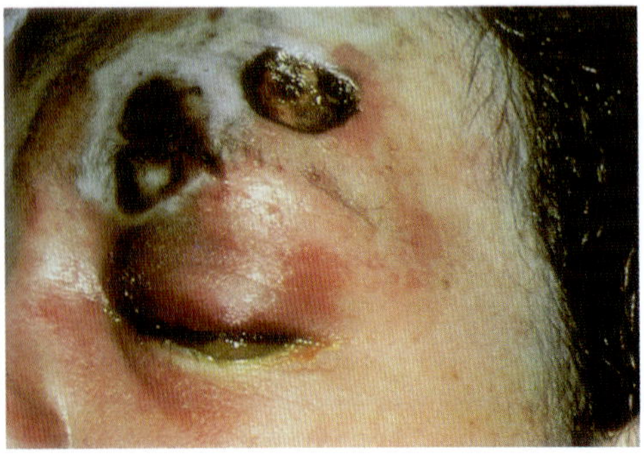

Figure 17-11 Mucormycosis, left orbit.

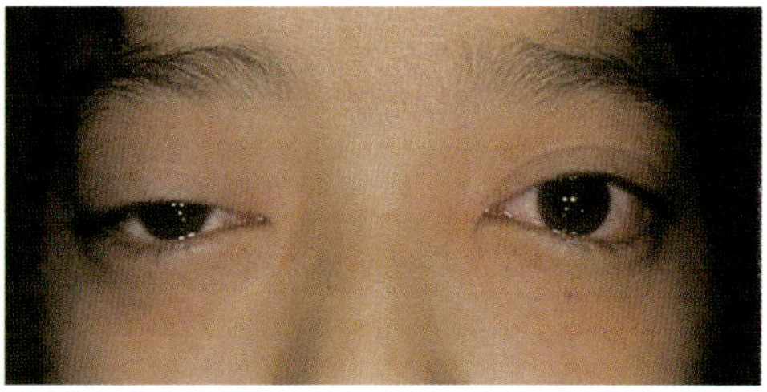

Figure 17-12 Bilateral nonspecific orbital inflammation (orbital pseudotumor) in an 11-year-old boy with a 1-week history of eye pain. Ocular rotation was markedly limited in all directions. CT confirmed proptosis and showed enlargement of all extraocular muscles. Laboratory workup was negative for thyroid disease and rheumatologic disorders. Complete resolution occurred after 1 month of corticosteroid treatment.

proptosis, periorbital edema, ophthalmoplegia, and pain/anesthesia, than it does tumor or thyroid eye disease (Fig 17-12). However, unlike orbital cellulitis, fever is usually absent, and the complete blood cell count is usually normal. Iritis and scleritis are rare. NSOI is often bilateral and may be associated with systemic manifestations such as headache, nausea, vomiting, and lethargy. Imaging studies may show increased density of orbital fat, thickening of posterior sclera and the Tenon layer, or enlargement of extraocular muscles. The lacrimal gland is often involved. Sinusitis is typically not present.

Orbital myositis Orbital myositis describes NSOI that is confined to 1 or more extraocular muscles. The clinical presentation depends on the amount of inflammation. Diplopia, conjunctival chemosis, and orbital pain are common. Symptoms can be subacute or progress rapidly. Vision is rarely impaired unless massive muscle enlargement is present. Imaging studies show diffusely enlarged muscles with the enlargement extending all the way to the insertion (unlike in thyroid myopathy, which mainly involves the muscle belly).

Both NSOI and orbital myositis are a diagnosis of exclusion. Evaluation for infectious (including viral) and systemic inflammatory or infiltrative causes are mandatory. Corticosteroid treatment usually produces rapid relief of symptoms for NSOI and orbital myositis. Prolonged treatment is often necessary, and recurrence is common.

Neoplasms

Several pediatric malignancies may occur in the orbit. Benign adnexal masses, which may threaten vision, are common in the pediatric population.

Differential Diagnosis

Diagnosis of space-occupying lesions in the orbit is particularly challenging because the clinical manifestations are both nonspecific and relatively limited:

- proptosis or other displacement of the globe
- swelling or discoloration of the eyelids
- palpable subcutaneous mass
- ptosis
- strabismus

Many orbital processes may cause rapid onset of symptoms. These include trauma, which may occur without a reliable history. Mild or moderate proptosis can be difficult to detect in an uncooperative child with associated eyelid swelling. Nevertheless, typical presentations of the more common benign orbital and periorbital masses in infants and children (eg, hemangioma and dermoid cyst, discussed later) are sufficiently distinctive to permit confident clinical diagnosis in most cases. A malignant process is suspected when proptosis and eyelid swelling suggestive of cellulitis are not accompanied by signs of inflammation or when periorbital ecchymosis or hematoma develops in the absence of a history of trauma. Pseudoproptosis can result when the volume of the globe exceeds the capacity of the orbit (eg, in patients with primary congenital glaucoma or high myopia).

High-quality imaging allows orbital masses to be differentiated noninvasively in many cases. Magnetic resonance imaging (MRI) is the preferred modality for most patients. CT is superior at detecting bone abnormalities but exposes the child to radiation and thus should be avoided unless necessary, especially repeatedly. Ultrasonography may be useful.

Definitive diagnosis often requires biopsy. A pediatric oncologist is consulted when appropriate. A metastatic workup can be considered prior to orbital surgery, because other, more easily accessible sites can sometimes be biopsied.

Primary Malignant Neoplasms

Malignant diseases of the orbit include primary and metastatic tumors. Most primary malignant tumors of the orbit in childhood are sarcomas. Tumors of epithelial origin are extremely rare.

Rhabdomyosarcoma

The most common primary orbital malignant tumor in children is rhabdomyosarcoma, which is thought to originate from undifferentiated mesenchymal cells. The incidence of this disease (which is found in approximately 5% of pediatric orbital biopsies) exceeds that of all other sarcomas combined. The orbit is the origin of 10% of rhabdomyosarcomas; 25% of these tumors arise elsewhere in the head and neck, occasionally involving the orbit secondarily. The average age at onset is 5–7 years, but rhabdomyosarcoma can occur at any age. Rhabdomyosarcoma in infancy is more aggressive and carries a poorer prognosis.

Although ocular rhabdomyosarcoma usually originates in the orbit, it occasionally arises in the conjunctiva, eyelid, or anterior uveal tract. Presenting signs and symptoms include proptosis (80%–100% of cases), globe displacement (80%), blepharoptosis (30%–50%) (Fig 17-13), conjunctival and eyelid swelling (60%), palpable mass (25%), and pain (10%). Onset of symptoms and signs is usually rapid. Acute, rapidly progressive proptosis with an absence of pain is suggestive of orbital rhabdomyosarcoma. Imaging shows an irregular but well-circumscribed mass of uniform density.

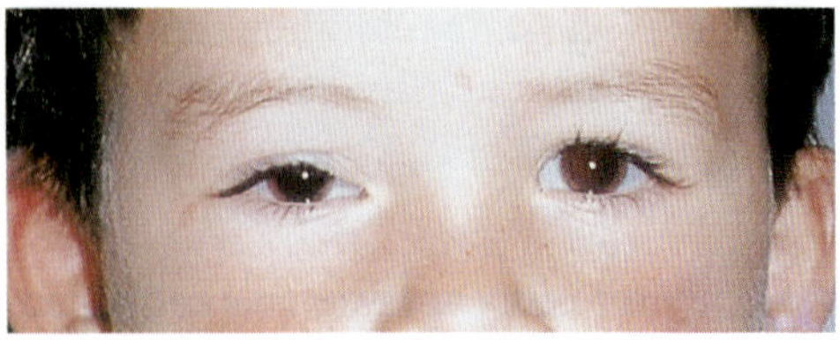

Figure 17-13 Rhabdomyosarcoma in a 4-year-old boy who presented with right upper eyelid ptosis of 3 weeks' duration and a palpable subcutaneous mass.

A biopsy is required for confirmation of the diagnosis whenever rhabdomyosarcoma is suspected. The most common histologic type is embryonal, which shows few cells containing characteristic cross-striations. Second in frequency is the prognostically unfavorable alveolar pattern, showing poorly differentiated tumor cells compartmentalized by orderly connective tissue septa. Botryoid (grapelike) or well-differentiated pleomorphic tumors are rarely found in the orbit but may originate in the conjunctiva (see also BCSC Section 4, *Ophthalmic Pathology and Intraocular Tumors,* Fig 14-15).

Small encapsulated or otherwise well-localized rhabdomyosarcomas should be totally excised when possible. Usually, chemotherapy and radiation are used in conjunction with surgery. Exenteration of the orbit is seldom indicated. Primary orbital rhabdomyosarcoma has a relatively good prognosis. The 5-year survival rates are 74% and 94% for patients with alveolar cell type and those with embryonal cell type, respectively.

Other sarcomas

Osteosarcoma, chondrosarcoma, and fibrosarcoma can develop in the orbit during childhood. The risk of sarcoma is increased in children with a history of heritable retinoblastoma, particularly when external-beam radiation treatment has been given.

Metastatic Tumors

The orbit is the most common site of ocular metastasis in children, in contrast to adults, in whom the uvea is the most frequent site.

Neuroblastoma

Neuroblastoma is the most frequent source of orbital metastasis in childhood. This disorder is discussed in Chapter 27.

Ewing sarcoma

Ewing sarcoma is composed of small round cells and usually originates in the long bones of the extremities or in the axial skeleton. Among solid tumors, Ewing sarcoma is the second most frequent source of orbital metastasis. Treatment regimens involving surgery, radiation, and chemotherapy allow long-term survival in many patients with disseminated disease.

Hematopoietic, Lymphoproliferative, and Histiocytic Neoplasms

Leukemia

Leukemic infiltration of the orbit is relatively uncommon and more characteristic of acute myelogenous leukemia. Orbital involvement may be difficult to distinguish from bacterial or fungal orbital cellulitis, but on radiologic examination, the infiltrates in leukemia are usually bilateral and do not destroy bone. Orbital infiltration can cause proptosis, eyelid swelling, ecchymosis, ophthalmoplegia, and optic neuropathy. It may be best managed by radiation therapy. *Granulocytic sarcoma,* or *chloroma* (a reference to the greenish color of involved tissue), is a localized accumulation of myeloid leukemic cells; the tumor may occur anywhere in the body, including in the orbit. This lesion may develop several months before leukemia becomes evident hematologically. Leukemia is discussed in Chapter 27.

Lymphoma

In contrast to lymphoma in adults, lymphoma in children very rarely involves the orbit. Burkitt lymphoma, endemic to East Africa and uncommon in North America, is the most likely form to involve the orbit.

Langerhans cell histiocytosis

Langerhans cell histiocytosis (*LCH;* formerly called *histiocytosis X*) is the collective term for a group of disorders, usually arising in childhood, that involve abnormal proliferation of histiocytes, often within bone. The disorders are classified as unifocal eosinophilic granuloma of the bone, multifocal eosinophilic granuloma of the bone, and diffuse soft-tissue histiocytosis.

Unifocal eosinophilic granuloma of the bone, the most localized and benign form of LCH, produces a bone lesion that involves the orbit, skull, ribs, or long bones in childhood or adolescence. Signs and symptoms may include proptosis, ptosis, and periorbital swelling; localized pain and tenderness are relatively common. CT characteristically shows sharply demarcated osteolytic lesions without surrounding sclerosis (Fig 17-14). Treatment consists of observation of isolated asymptomatic lesions, excision or curettage, systemic or intralesional corticosteroid administration, or low-dose radiation therapy. All modalities have a high rate of success.

Multifocal eosinophilic granuloma of the bone is a disseminated and aggressive form of LCH. It usually presents between 2 and 5 years of age and may produce proptosis from involvement of the bony orbit. Pituitary dysfunction is common. Chemotherapy is often required, but the prognosis is generally good.

Diffuse soft-tissue histiocytosis, the most severe form, usually affects infants younger than 2 years. It is characterized by soft-tissue lesions of multiple viscera (liver, spleen) but rarely involves the eye.

Benign Tumors

Vascular lesions: hamartomas

The current classification of vascular lesions establishes clinical, histologic, and prognostic differences between hemangiomas (hamartomatous growths) and vascular malformations. The older terms *capillary* and *strawberry hemangioma* have been replaced by the

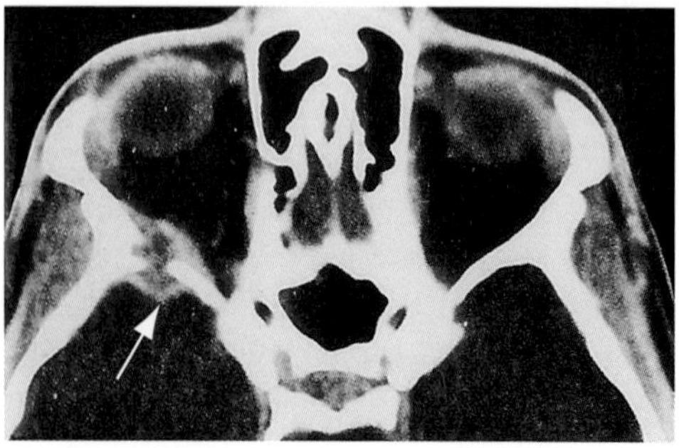

Figure 17-14 Axial CT image shows unifocal eosinophilic granuloma with partial destruction of the right posterior lateral orbital wall *(arrow)* in a 15-year-old boy, who presented with retrobulbar pain and mild edema and erythema of the right upper eyelid.

single term *hemangioma.* Cavernous hemangiomas, port-wine birthmarks, and lymphangiomas are classified as "malformations." This nomenclature has not been used consistently in ophthalmic literature.

Hemangiomas are composed of proliferating capillary endothelial cells. Periocular hemangiomas can be classified as follows:

- *preseptal:* involving the skin and preseptal orbit
- *intraorbital:* involving the postseptal orbit
- *compound/mixed:* involving the preseptal and postseptal orbit

Hemangiomas occur in 1%–3% of term newborns and are more common in premature infants, in females, and after chorionic villus sampling. Most hemangiomas are clinically insignificant at birth. They can be inapparent or can appear as an erythematous macule or a telangiectasia. The natural history is one of rapid proliferation and growth over the first several months of life, rarely lasting beyond 1 year. Periocular lesions may cause amblyopia by inducing astigmatism or obstructing the visual axis. After the first year of life, the lesions usually begin to regress, although the rate and degree of involution vary.

Systemic disease associated with hemangiomas *PHACE* is an acronym for *p*osterior fossa malformations, *h*emangiomas, *a*rterial lesions, and *c*ardiac and *e*ye anomalies. The eye abnormalities include increased retinal vascularity, microphthalmia, optic nerve hypoplasia, proptosis, choroidal hemangiomas, strabismus, colobomas, cataracts, and glaucoma. The PHACE syndrome should be considered in any infant presenting with a large, segmental, plaquelike facial hemangioma involving 1 or more dermatomes (Fig 17-15).

Kasabach-Merritt syndrome is a thrombocytopenic coagulopathy with a high mortality rate. It is caused by sequestration of platelets within a vascular lesion.

Diffuse neonatal hemangiomatosis is a potentially lethal condition that occurs in infants, with multiple small cutaneous hemangiomas associated with visceral lesions affecting the liver, gastrointestinal tract, and brain. These hemangiomas are initially asymptomatic but can lead to cardiac failure and death within weeks. Evaluation for visceral lesions is indicated in infants with more than 3 cutaneous lesions.

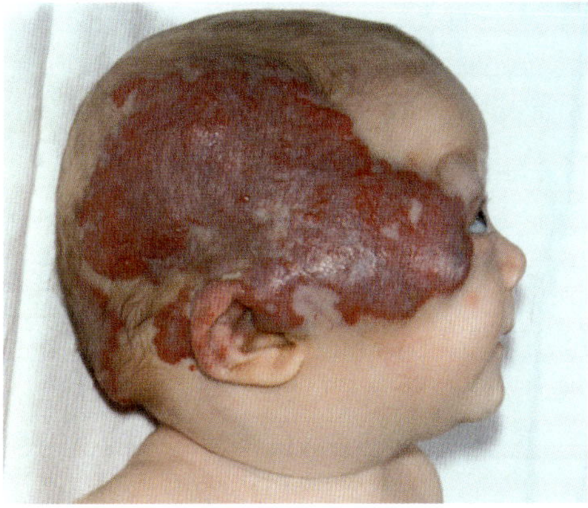

Figure 17-15 Plaque hemangioma in a child with PHACE (posterior fossa malformations, hemangiomas, arterial lesions, and cardiac and eye anomalies) syndrome. *(Courtesy of Ken K. Nischal, MD.)*

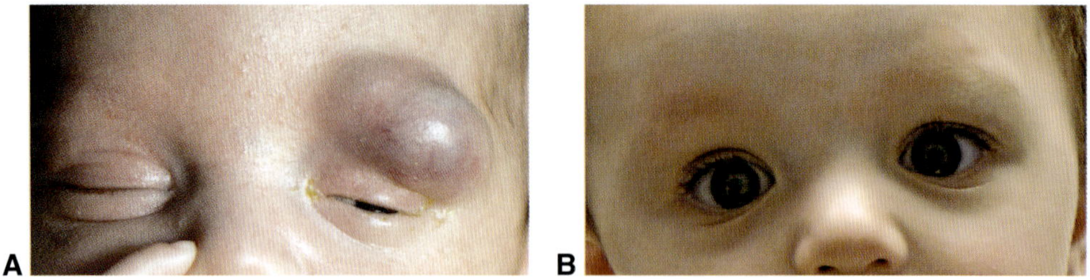

Figure 17-16 Hemangioma response to treatment. **A,** Two-month-old infant with a large hemangioma above the left eye. **B,** Resolution of the lesion following treatment with propranolol. *(Courtesy of Gregg T. Lueder, MD.)*

Treatment of hemangiomas The diagnosis of hemangiomas is usually obvious from the clinical presentation. MRI or ultrasonography is sometimes helpful in establishing the diagnosis and delineating the posterior extent of the lesion.

Observation is indicated when hemangiomas are small and there is no risk of amblyopia.

Propranolol, a nonselective β-adrenergic blocking agent, induces involution of most hemangiomas (Fig 17-16). The risks of systemic treatment with β-blockers in infants include bradycardia, hypotension, hypoglycemia, and bronchospasm, but the medication is usually well tolerated. It is important to be cautious when using propranolol in children with PHACE syndrome, because this drug may increase their risk of stroke. Timolol maleate solution applied topically may be effective in treating superficial hemangiomas. Pulsed dye laser can treat superficial hemangiomas and is associated with few complications, but it has little effect on deeper components of the tumor.

Surgical excision of periocular hemangiomas is feasible for some well-localized lesions or for lesions that do not respond to propranolol.

Drolet BA, Frommelt PC, Chamlin SL, et al. Initiation and use of propranolol for infantile hemangioma: report of a consensus conference. *Pediatrics.* 2013;131(1):128–140.

Vascular lesions: malformations

Vascular malformations are developmental anomalies derived from capillary venous, arterial, or lymphatic vessels. In contrast to hemangiomas, vascular malformations remain relatively static. The age at onset and mode of clinical presentation vary. Cutaneous vascular malformations such as port-wine birthmarks are evident from birth, but many vascular malformations do not manifest until later in life.

Orbital lymphatic malformation Orbital lymphatic malformation, previously known as *lymphangioma,* may produce proptosis in infancy, but usually does not until the second decade of life or later. Unilateral smaller cornea, anomalous anterior segment vessels, and abnormal retinal vessel branching in association with orbital lymphatic malformation represent a unique malformation syndrome. Lymphatic malformation of the orbit is best managed conservatively. Exacerbations tend to occur during upper respiratory tract infections and may be managed with a short course of systemic corticosteroids. Rapid expansion may be seen in cases of intralesional hemorrhage (Fig 17-17). Partial resection

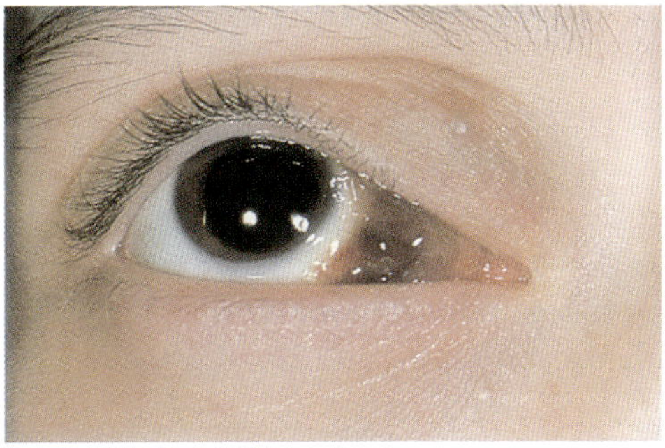

Figure 17-17 Lymphatic malformation with hemorrhage involving the right orbit, upper eyelid, and conjunctiva in a 15-year-old girl.

and drainage may be required if vision is threatened. Because of the infiltrative character of this malformation, complete removal is usually impossible; the risks of intraoperative hemorrhage and recurrence are high. Newer treatments include oral sildenafil and intralesional injection of sclerosing agents. There have been no clinical trials comparing the outcomes of medical and surgical treatments.

Patel SR, Rosenberg JB, Barmettler A. Interventions for orbital lymphangioma. *Cochrane Database Syst Rev.* 2019;5(5):CD013000. Epub 2019 May 15.

Orbital venous malformations Orbital venous malformations, or varices, can be divided into 2 types. The *primary* type is confined to the orbit and is not associated with arteriovenous malformations (AVMs). *Secondary* orbital varices occur as a result of intracranial AVM shunts that cause dilation of the orbital veins. Orbital venous malformations usually become symptomatic after years of progressive congestion; they manifest before the second decade of life only in rare cases. Treatment is reserved for highly symptomatic lesions.

Orbital arteriovenous malformations AVMs isolated within the orbit are extremely rare. Patients with congenital AVMs of the retina and midbrain (*racemose angioma* or *Wyburn-Mason syndrome;* see Chapter 27) may have orbital involvement. AVMs of the bony orbit manifest in childhood only in rare cases; when present, they are characterized by pulsatile proptosis, chemosis, congested conjunctival vessels, and elevated intraocular pressure. AVMs may be treated by embolization, surgical resection, or both.

Tumors of bony origin

A variety of uncommon benign orbital tumors of bony origin can present with gradually increasing proptosis in children during the early years of life. *Fibrous dysplasia* and *juvenile ossifying fibroma* are similar disorders in which normal bone is replaced by fibro-osseous tissue. In both conditions, orbital CT shows varying degrees of lucency and sclerosis (see BCSC Section 7, *Oculofacial Plastic and Orbital Surgery,* Fig 5-15).

Fibrous dysplasia has a slow progression that ceases when skeletal maturation is complete. The most serious complication is vision loss caused by optic nerve compression, which may occur acutely. Periodic assessment of vision, pupil function, and optic nerve head appearance is indicated. Surgical treatment is indicated for functional deterioration or disfigurement. In cases of continuous vision deterioration due to optic nerve compression, therapeutic optic canal decompression is performed by a neurosurgeon in collaboration with a plastic surgeon.

Juvenile ossifying fibroma is distinguished on histologic examination by the presence of osteoblasts. It tends to be more locally invasive than fibrous dysplasia; some authorities recommend early excision.

Brown tumor of bone is an osteoclastic giant cell reaction resulting from hyperparathyroidism. *Aneurysmal bone cyst* is a degenerative process in which normal bone is replaced by cystic cavities containing fibrous tissue, inflammatory cells, and blood, producing a characteristic radiographic appearance.

Tumors of connective tissue origin

Benign orbital tumors originating from connective tissue are rare in childhood. *Juvenile fibromatosis* may present as a mass in the inferoanterior part of the orbit. These tumors, sometimes called *myofibromas* or *desmoid tumors,* are composed of relatively mature fibroblasts. They tend to recur locally after excision and can be difficult to control, but they do not metastasize.

Tumors of neural origin

Optic pathway glioma is the most common orbital tumor of neural origin in childhood. Optic pathway gliomas are usually low-grade pilocytic astrocytomas, but the rate of growth with or without therapeutic intervention is unpredictable. Management of these tumors is controversial and depends largely on visual function. Frequent visual acuity checks are warranted. Serial visual field tests and optical coherence tomography should be used when possible. Approximately 50% of optic pathway gliomas are associated with neurofibromatosis type 1. *Plexiform neurofibroma* nearly always occurs in individuals with neurofibromatosis and frequently involves the eyelid and orbit. See Chapter 27 for further discussion of plexiform neurofibroma and optic pathway glioma. Orbital *meningioma* and *schwannoma* (neurilemoma, neurinoma) are rare in childhood.

Ectopic Tissue Masses

The term *choristoma* is applied to growths consisting of tissue that is histologically normal but is present in an abnormal location. The growths may result from abnormal sequestration of germ layer tissue during embryonic development or from faulty differentiation of pluripotential cells. Masses composed of such ectopic tissue that are growing in the orbit can also be a consequence of herniation of tissue from adjacent structures.

Cystic Lesions

Dermoid and epidermoid cysts

Dermoid cysts are the most common space-occupying orbital lesions of childhood. They are benign developmental choristomas that arise from primitive dermal and epidermal elements sequestered in fetal skull suture lines. The tissue forms a cyst lined with keratinized epithelium and dermal appendages, including hair follicles, sweat glands, and sebaceous glands. Cysts containing squamous epithelium without dermal appendages are called *epidermoid cysts* (see BCSC Section 4, *Ophthalmic Pathology and Intraocular Tumors,* Fig 5-2).

Orbital dermoid cysts in childhood most commonly arise in the superotemporal and superonasal quadrants (Fig 17-18) but sometimes extend into the bony suture line. Clinically, they present as painless, smooth masses that are mobile and unattached to overlying skin. Inflammation may occur with ruptures of the cyst and extrusion of cyst contents. Most patients have no visual symptoms. Clinical examination is often sufficient for diagnosis. In some cases, imaging is indicated to identify and delineate the extent of the cyst. Imaging reveals a well-circumscribed lesion with a low-density lumen and often bony remodeling (Fig 17-19).

Management of dermoid cysts is surgical. Early excision can reduce the risk of traumatic rupture and subsequent inflammation. An infrabrow or eyelid crease incision is used, and the cyst is carefully dissected. If possible, rupture of the cyst at the time of surgery is avoided to limit lipogranulomatous inflammation and scarring. If the cyst is entered, it is important to thoroughly remove the intraluminal material. Sutural cysts sometimes cannot be removed intact because of their extension into or through bone. To limit the possibility of recurrence, the surgeon should attempt removal of all remaining cyst lining.

Microphthalmia with cyst

Microphthalmia with cyst (also known as *colobomatous cyst*) is characterized by a small, malformed globe with posterior segment coloboma and a cyst composed of tissues originating from the eye wall of the globe. Most fundus colobomas show some degree of scleral

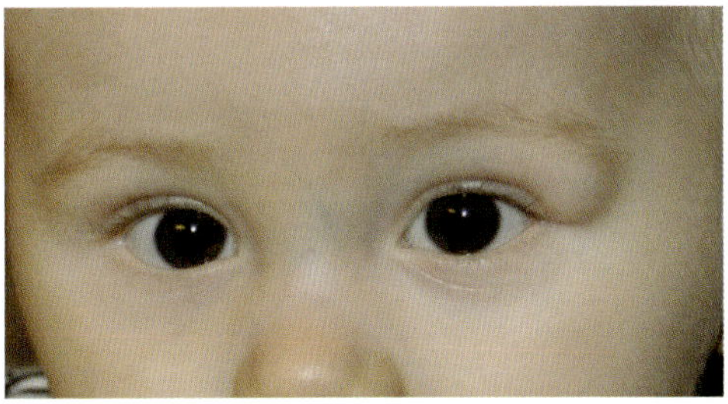

Figure 17-18 Eight-month-old boy with a periorbital dermoid cyst in the left eye, with typical superotemporal location. *(Courtesy of Robert W. Hered, MD.)*

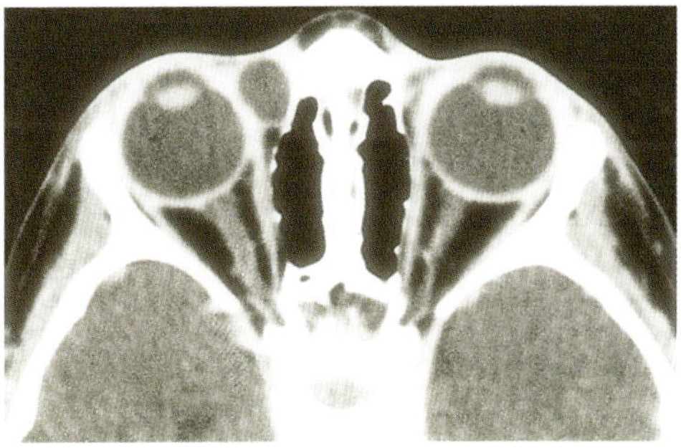

Figure 17-19 Axial CT image shows a dermoid cyst of the superonasal anterior orbit in the right eye, in a 6-year-old boy.

ectasia. In extreme cases, a bulging globular appendage grows to become as large as or larger than the globe itself, which is invariably microphthalmic, sometimes to a marked degree.

Microphthalmia with cyst may occur either as an isolated congenital defect or in association with a variety of intracranial or systemic anomalies. Frequently, the fellow eye shows evidence of coloboma as well. The usual location of the cyst is inferior or posterior to the globe, with which the cyst is always in contact.

Whether posteriorly located cysts cause proptosis depends on the size of the globe and the cyst. Inferiorly located cysts present as a bulging of the lower eyelid or a bluish subconjunctival mass (Fig 17-20). If fundus examination does not make the diagnosis obvious, orbital imaging may reveal a cystic lesion that is attached to the globe and has the uniform internal density of vitreous (see BCSC Section 7, *Oculofacial Plastic and Orbital Surgery,* Fig 3-3). The goal of treatment is to promote normal growth of the orbit; methods include aspiration or surgical excision of the cyst and use of orbital expanders and conformers.

Mucocele

Mucoceles are cystic lesions that originate from obstructed paranasal sinus drainage. They may expand over time, potentially causing destruction of bone and eroding into the orbit or intracranial space. These lesions most commonly arise from the frontal or anterior ethmoid sinuses, resulting in inferior or medial displacement of the globe. The differential diagnosis includes encephalocele with skull base deformity. Treatment involves reestablishing normal sinus drainage and removing the cyst wall.

Encephalocele and meningocele

Encephaloceles and meningoceles in the orbital region may result from a congenital bony defect that allows herniation of intracranial tissue, or they may develop after trauma that disrupts the bone and dura mater of the anterior cranial fossa. An intraorbital location leads to proptosis or downward displacement of the globe. Anterior presentation takes the

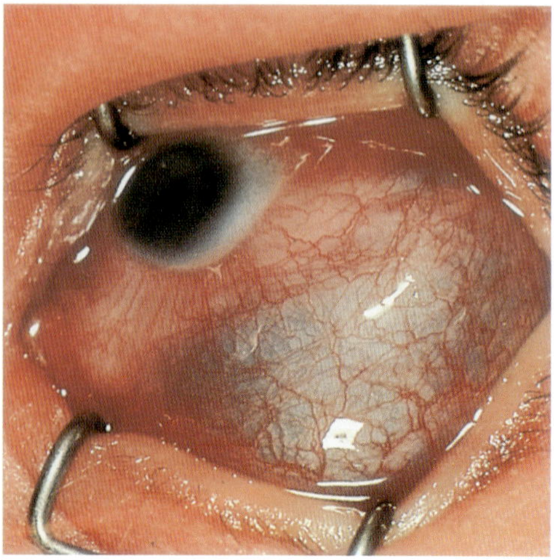

Figure 17-20 Microphthalmia with cyst (colobomatous cyst), left eye.

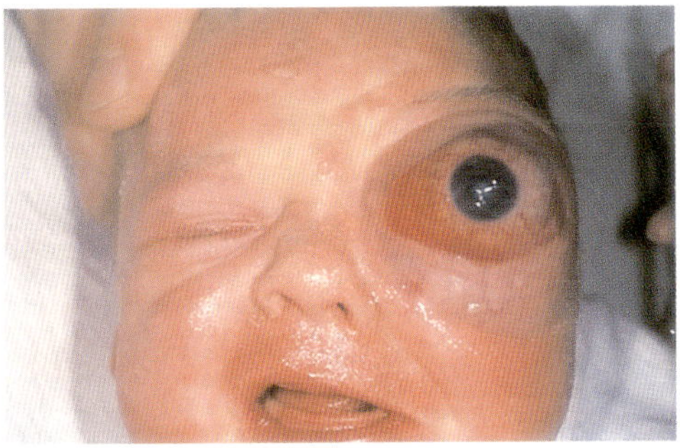

Figure 17-21 Congenital cystic teratoma originating in the left orbit of a 1-day-old girl.

form of a subcutaneous mass that can be misdiagnosed as a dacryocystocele. However, encephaloceles and meningoceles are typically located above the medial canthal tendon; dacryocystoceles are typically located below it (see Chapter 18). Pulsation of the globe or the mass from the transmission of intracranial pulse pressure is characteristic. Neuroimaging confirms the diagnosis. Surgical repair is usually performed by neurosurgeons.

Teratoma

Choristomatous tumors that contain multiple tissues derived from all 3 germinal layers (ectoderm, mesoderm, and endoderm) are referred to as *teratomas.* Most teratomas are partially cystic, with varying fluid content. Orbital teratomas account for a very small fraction of both orbital tumors and teratomas in general. The clinical presentation of orbital teratomas may be particularly dramatic, with massive proptosis evident at birth (Fig 17-21). In contrast to teratomas in other locations, which tend to show malignant growth, most orbital lesions are benign. Surgical excision, facilitated by prior aspiration of fluid, can often be accomplished without sacrificing the globe. Permanent optic nerve damage from stretching and compression may cause poor vision in the involved eye.

Ectopic Lacrimal Gland

These are rare choristomatous lesions that may present with proptosis in childhood. Cystic enlargement and chronic inflammation sometimes aggravate the condition.

CHAPTER 18

Lacrimal Drainage System Abnormalities

This chapter includes related videos. Go to www.aao.org/bcscvideo_section06 or scan the QR codes in the text to access this content.

Highlights

- A dacryocystocele (mucocele) presents at or soon after birth as a bluish lump below the medial canthus and can become infected, leading to cellulitis and sepsis if not managed promptly.
- Congenital nasolacrimal duct obstruction (CNLDO) affects up to 5% of newborns; most cases resolve with conservative management.
- Nasolacrimal duct probing is often performed if CNLDO does not resolve spontaneously; the success rate of properly performed initial probing before 15 months of age exceeds 80%.

Introduction

Nasolacrimal duct obstruction (NLDO) can be congenital or acquired. This chapter discusses congenital NLDO (CNLDO), including nonsurgical and surgical management, as well as other congenital and developmental anomalies of the lacrimal drainage system. Acquired NLDO is discussed in BCSC Section 7, *Oculofacial Plastic and Orbital Surgery.*

Figure 18-1 shows the anatomy of the lacrimal drainage system and common sites of CNLDO. Anatomical features of the lacrimal drainage system and their development are further discussed in BCSC Section 2, *Fundamentals and Principles of Ophthalmology,* and Section 7, *Oculofacial Plastic and Orbital Surgery.*

Congenital and Developmental Anomalies

Atresia of the Lacrimal Puncta or Canaliculi

Obstruction of the upper lacrimal drainage system may result from a thin membrane obstructing an otherwise normal lacrimal punctum; this can be treated with a simple puncture of the membrane using a punctal dilator. Obstruction may also result from more

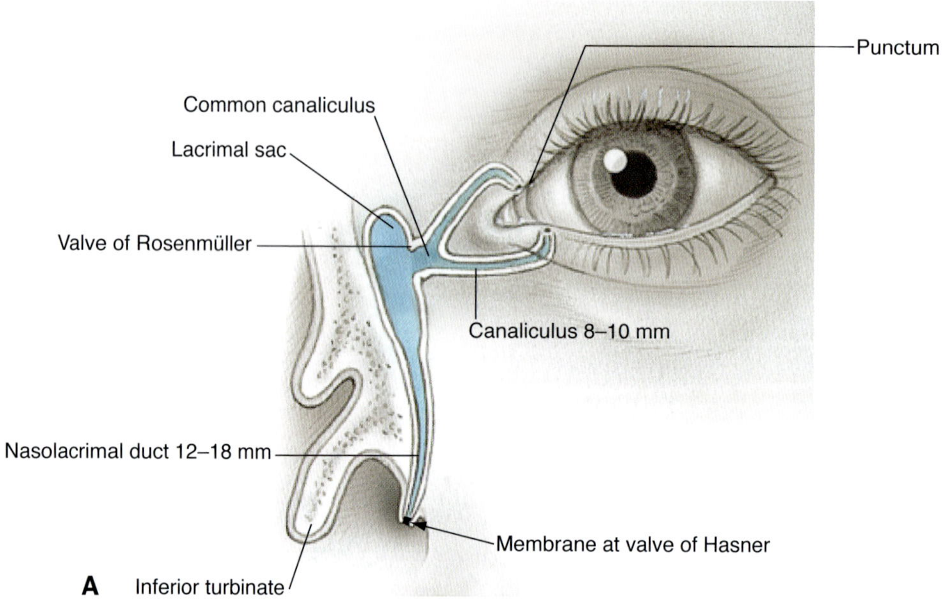

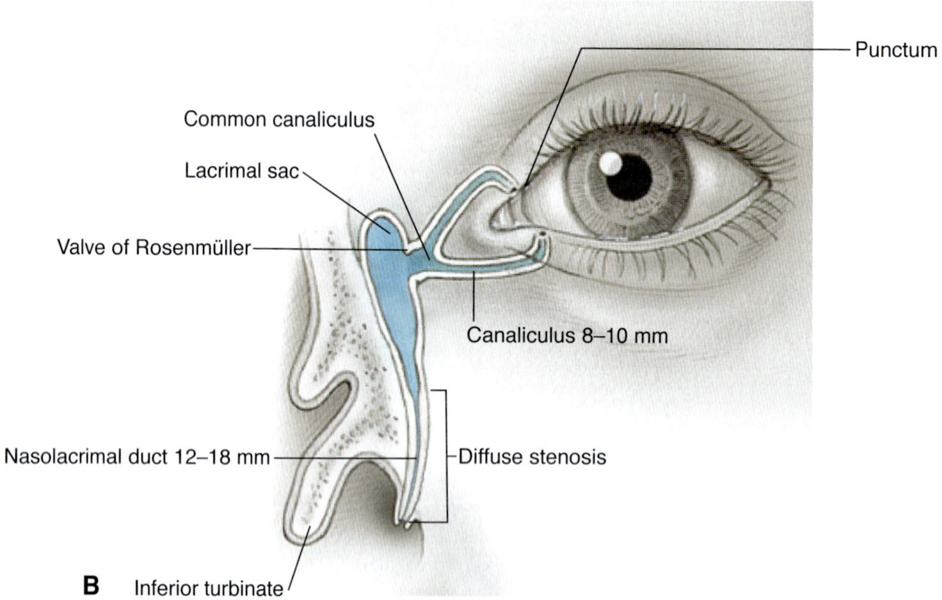

Figure 18-1 Lacrimal drainage system. **A,** Anatomy of the lacrimal system and typical location of the membrane causing simple nasolacrimal duct obstruction (NLDO) *(arrow).* **B,** Diffuse stenosis of the distal NLD. *(Adapted from an illustration by Christine Gralapp.)*

severe *atresia,* or failure of canalization, of the lacrimal punctum and/or canaliculus during fetal development. In patients with atresia, no punctum can be seen (Fig 18-2).

Patients with isolated upper lacrimal drainage system obstruction usually present with overflow of clear tears. In a patient with obstruction of only 1 canaliculus, reflux of

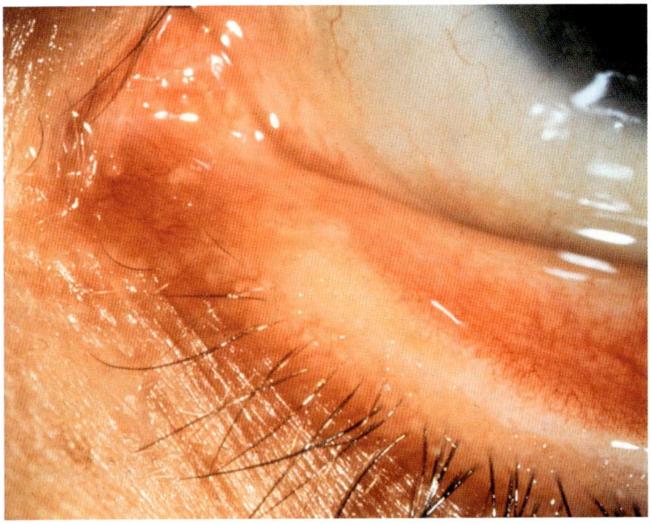

Figure 18-2 Atresia of the lacrimal puncta. No indentation is visible at the expected site of normal punctal opening. *(Reproduced with permission from Lueder GT. Neonatal lacrimal system anomalies.* Semin Ophthalmol. *1997;12(2):109.)*

mucopurulent discharge from the normal canaliculus usually indicates concomitant distal NLDO, probing of which may be curative.

If both the upper and the lower canaliculi are absent, an incision through the eyelid margin at the expected location of the canaliculi may reveal structures that can be cannulated. However, many patients ultimately require conjunctivodacryocystorhinostomy (CDCR), a procedure that creates a complete bypass of the lacrimal drainage system. CDCR is usually deferred until patients are older. See BCSC Section 7, *Oculofacial Plastic and Orbital Surgery,* for a discussion of this procedure.

Congenital Lacrimal Fistula

A congenital lacrimal fistula (lacrimal–cutaneous fistula) is an epithelium-lined tract that extends from the common canaliculus or lacrimal sac to the overlying skin surface. It usually presents as a small dimple medial to the eyelids and may be difficult to detect in the absence of symptoms (Fig 18-3). It is not always patent. If the patient is asymptomatic, no treatment is necessary. Discharge from the fistula is often associated with distal NLDO and may cease after probing of the distal obstruction. If discharge persists despite a patent lacrimal duct, the fistula between the skin and normal lacrimal structures can be surgically excised.

Dacryocystocele

Dacryocystocele (dacryocele, mucocele, amniotocele) is present in approximately 3% of infants with NLDO. It develops when a distal blockage causes distention of the lacrimal sac. The valve of Rosenmüller (see Fig 18-1) can act as a one-way valve, thereby preventing

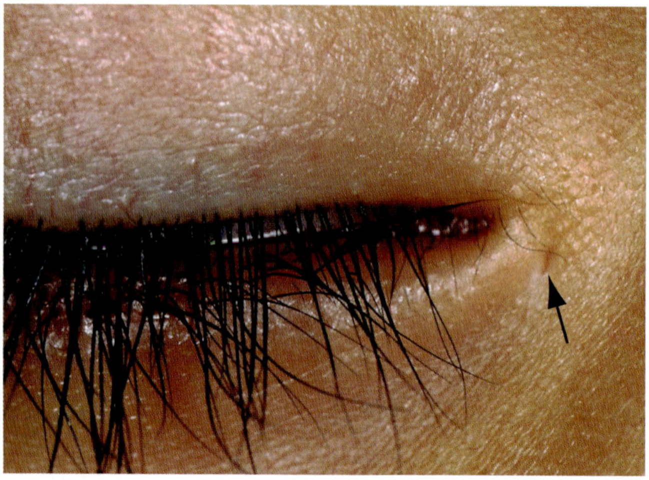

Figure 18-3 Lacrimal fistula. *(Reproduced with permission from Lueder GT. Neonatal lacrimal system anomalies.* Semin Ophthalmol. *1997;12(2):109.)*

decompression of the lacrimal sac. Most patients with dacryocystoceles have associated cysts of the distal nasolacrimal duct (NLD), which may be seen beneath the inferior turbinate. Involvement is bilateral in 20%–30% of cases.

Clinical features and diagnosis

Dacryocystocele presents at birth or within the first few days of life as a bluish swelling just below and nasal to the medial canthus (Fig 18-4A). The differential diagnosis includes hemangioma, dermoid cyst, and encephalocele. Hemangiomas are not typically present at birth, have a vascular appearance, and are generally less firm than dacryocystoceles. Dermoid cysts and encephaloceles present most often above the medial canthal tendon. The diagnosis is clinically apparent when a newborn has a nasal mass beneath the medial canthus that is associated with symptoms of NLDO (discussed later in the chapter); imaging is usually not required in this case.

Dacryocystoceles are prone to infection, and acute dacryocystitis often develops. The skin over the distended lacrimal sac becomes erythematous (Fig 18-4B), and pressure applied on the sac may produce reflux of purulent material.

Infants who have large intranasal cysts may present with respiratory symptoms. Respiratory difficulty may occur during feeding (when the infant cannot breathe through the mouth), because infants tend to be nasal breathers.

Management

In patients experiencing acute respiratory distress from nasal cysts associated with a dacryocystocele, immediate surgical intervention with nasal endoscopy is required. Early treatment of dacryocystoceles is advised even in the absence of respiratory distress, to prevent complications related to infection. Infants are relatively immunocompromised and are therefore at risk for local or systemic spread of infection. Digital massage may be attempted to decompress the dacryocystocele; this can resolve the condition without surgery.

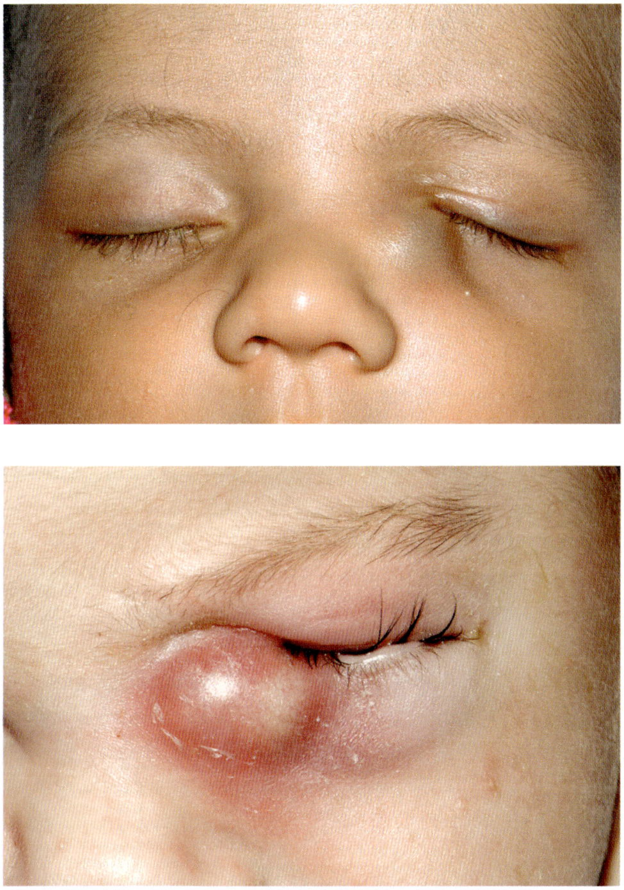

A

B

Figure 18-4 Dacryocystocele. **A,** Congenital dacryocystocele in a newborn, left eye. Note the typical location below the medial canthus and the bluish color of the distended lacrimal sac. **B,** Dacryocystitis in a newborn, left eye. Note the erythema overlying the pus-filled lacrimal sac. *(Courtesy of Kamiar Mireskandari, MBChB, PhD.)*

If the lesions do not resolve within the first 1–2 weeks of life or if there is acute infection of the dacryocystocele, surgery is necessary. NLD probing alone may be curative, but in approximately 25% of patients, the condition persists after probing. NLD probing in combination with nasal endoscopy and intranasal cyst removal is effective in more than 95% of infants. Because approximately 20%–30% of patients have bilateral nasal cysts, sometimes without visible dacryocystoceles, bilateral endoscopy is appropriate. Systemic antibiotics should be used perioperatively if acute dacryocystitis is present. Surgical treatment of an infected dacryocystocele via a skin incision should be avoided because of the risk of creating a persistent fistulous tract.

Lueder GT. The association of neonatal dacryocystoceles and infantile dacryocystitis with nasolacrimal duct cysts (an American Ophthalmological Society thesis). *Trans Am Ophthalmol Soc.* 2012;110:74–93.

Congenital Nasolacrimal Duct Obstruction

Congenital nasolacrimal duct obstruction (CNLDO) (dacryostenosis) is the most common lacrimal drainage system disorder encountered in pediatric ophthalmology. It occurs in approximately 5% of infants and is more common in patients with Down syndrome (22%) and in those with midfacial abnormalities.

CNLDO can be classified as simple or complex. Simple CNLDO is caused by a thin mucosal membrane at the distal end of the NLD, at the valve of Hasner (see Fig 18-1). Complex CNLDO results from diffuse obstruction or bony obstruction, which is frequently found in patients with midfacial abnormalities.

Clinical Features and Examination

Infants with CNLDO usually present within the first month of life with epiphora, recurrent periocular crusting, or both (Fig 18-5). They do not have photophobia or blepharospasm. Symptoms are usually chronic and worsen with nasal congestion; bilateral involvement is common. Applying digital pressure to the lacrimal sac usually results in retrograde discharge of mucoid or mucopurulent material.

Excessive tearing due to CNLDO must be differentiated from epiphora due to primary congenital glaucoma, which has additional characteristics, including photophobia, blepharospasm, ocular hypertension, corneal clouding with or without enlargement, and breaks in Descemet membrane (see Chapter 21). The differential diagnosis of CNLDO also includes conjunctivitis and epiblepharon with irritation due to trichiasis. A thorough examination is necessary to rule out other ocular abnormalities. A cycloplegic refraction should be performed; some studies suggest an increased rate of anisometropia and amblyopia in patients with CNLDO.

Nonsurgical Management

There is a high rate of spontaneous resolution of CNLDO; approximately 90% of patients improve within the first 9–12 months of life. Thus, conservative treatment is recommended initially for these patients.

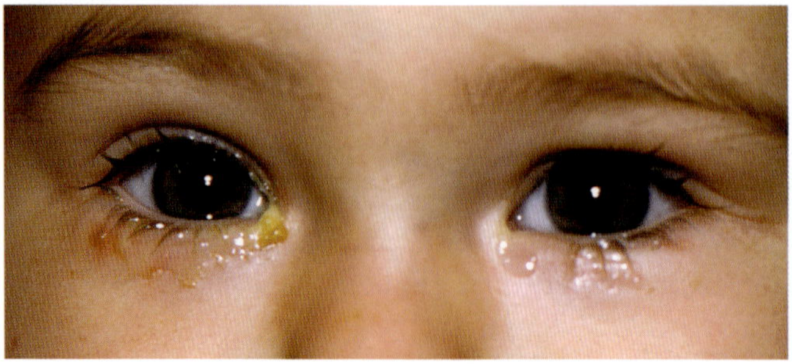

Figure 18-5 Bilateral NLDO. Note epiphora and periocular crusting without evidence of inflammation. *(Reproduced with permission from Lueder GT.* Pediatric Practice Ophthalmology. *McGraw-Hill Medical; 2011:55. Permission conveyed through Copyright Clearance Center, Inc.)*

Conservative treatment includes lacrimal sac massage and, if needed, use of topical antibiotics. Massage serves 2 purposes: it empties the sac, thereby reducing the opportunity for bacterial growth, and it applies hydrostatic pressure to the obstruction, which may open the duct and resolve the condition. Massage is performed by applying pressure to the lacrimal sac, at the medial canthus, a few times per day. This is the only location where application of external pressure on the lacrimal sac can be effective. Passing the finger along the nares, which is often recommended by primary care providers, is not effective because the NLD is covered by bone at this site.

In patients with significant mucopurulent discharge, topical antibiotics may reduce the amount of the discharge; however, they will not cure the obstruction. Bacterial growth in CNLDO is due to stasis of fluid within the lacrimal sac, so almost any bacteria, including normal flora, may contribute. Most broad-spectrum antibiotics are effective in reducing discharge, so culturing is usually not necessary. A few days of treatment often produce improvement, and prolonged courses are not necessary. Parents may be instructed to administer the antibiotics periodically when the amount of discharge is significantly increased.

Surgical Management

Surgical procedures for CNLDO are also discussed in BCSC Section 7, *Oculofacial Plastic and Orbital Surgery.*

Probing

Nasolacrimal probing is one of the most common procedures performed by pediatric ophthalmologists and is very effective in treating CNLDO. Some ophthalmologists recommend in-office probing of young infants, whereas others prefer to delay treatment and perform surgery in the operating room on older infants whose symptoms do not resolve over time with conservative treatment. The advantages of early in-office probing are that it avoids the use of general anesthesia, resolves symptoms earlier, and is typically more cost effective. The disadvantages are that a painful procedure is performed on an awake infant and that surgery is performed on many infants who would have spontaneously improved without surgery. The advantages of waiting to perform the surgery until the child is older and performing it in an operating room are that fewer infants require treatment, and the procedure is performed in a more controlled environment in which additional procedures can be performed concurrently. Either of these approaches is acceptable.

When probing is performed in the operating room, placing oxymetazoline-soaked pledgets beneath the inferior turbinate before surgery may decrease intraoperative bleeding. The initial step in nasolacrimal probing is dilation of the puncta and proximal canaliculi. Punctal membranes and atretic canaliculi are sometimes not recognized until surgery. Their management is discussed earlier in this chapter. Because the lacrimal drainage system cannot be visualized beyond the puncta, knowledge of the anatomy and normal course of the lacrimal excretory system is essential for passing lacrimal probes properly. The probes are initially inserted in the puncta, perpendicular to the eyelid. Within 1–2 mm of the eyelid margin, the canaliculi turn approximately 90°; the probes are therefore turned almost immediately and passed along the course of the canaliculi until the nasal bone is encountered on the medial side of the lacrimal sac. The probes are held flat on the patient's face and rotated and passed gently into the distal duct (Video 18-1). In patients with simple CNLDO, most surgeons feel a slight popping sensation as the probe passes through the membrane causing the obstruction. In complex CNLDO (see the following section), the surgeon's probe may encounter a firmer obstruction or a tight passage throughout the length of the NLD. A submucosal or false passage may occur during NLDO probing in patients with inflamed or fragile mucosal membranes and/or unusual anatomy (Video 18-2).

VIDEO 18-1 Probing of the nasolacrimal duct.
Courtesy of Kamiar Mireskandari, MBChB, PhD.

VIDEO 18-2 Demonstration of how a submucosal (false) passage can occur with nasolacrimal duct probing.
Courtesy of Kamiar Mireskandari, MBChB, PhD.

A wide variety of techniques are used for probing in cases of NLDO. Most surgeons begin with a size 0 or 1 Bowman probe, and some pass successively larger probes to enlarge the distal duct. Introducing a second metal probe into the nares and making direct contact with the previously placed lacrimal probe verify the position of the latter. Alternatively, direct inspection with a nasal speculum and headlamp or with a nasal endoscope can precisely determine the position of the probe. Irrigation may be performed following probing in order to verify that the system is patent. It is important to discuss this with the anesthetist beforehand to ensure the airway is protected and/or suction is performed. Infracture of the inferior turbinate may be used to widen the area where fluid drains beneath the inferior turbinate. The surgeon accomplishes this by placing a small periosteal elevator beneath the turbinate or by grasping it with a hemostat and then rotating the instrument.

Postoperatively, minor bleeding from the nose or into the tear film commonly occurs and usually requires no treatment. Optional postoperative medications include antibiotic eyedrops, corticosteroid eyedrops, or both instilled 1–4 times daily for 1–2 weeks. Phenylephrine or oxymetazoline nasal spray may be used to control nasal bleeding or congestion. Because transient bacteremia can occur after probing, systemic antibiotic prophylaxis should be considered for patients with cardiac disease.

Resolution of signs after probing may not occur until 1 week or more postoperatively. Recurrence after unsuccessful probing is usually evident within 1–2 months. The success rate of properly performed initial probing for CNLDO before 15 months of age exceeds 80%. In some patients, mild epiphora still occurs occasionally, particularly outdoors in cold weather or in conjunction with an upper respiratory tract infection. This epiphora is probably attributable to a patent but narrow lacrimal drainage channel. Usually no additional treatment is required. Significant complications of probing are rare.

Pediatric Eye Disease Investigator Group. A randomized trial comparing the cost-effectiveness of 2 approaches for treating unilateral nasolacrimal duct obstruction. *Arch Ophthalmol.* 2012;130(12):1525–1533.

Surgery in patients with complex CNLDO or persistent symptoms after initial probing

A variety of treatment options are available for patients with complex CNLDO (which is usually discovered at the time of initial surgery) or for those with symptoms that persist following initial probing. Some surgeons may choose to perform balloon dacryoplasty or NLD stenting as the initial procedure in patients they believe are at risk for recurrence of NLDO. NLDO is more likely to recur in persons with chronic rhinitis, those older than 36 months, or those with complex CNLDO. Balloon dacryoplasty or intubation is more successful than probing alone for persistent NLDO after initial probing. The selection of intubation or balloon dacryoplasty is based on surgeon preference. Routine infracture of the inferior turbinate has not been shown to improve surgical outcomes, but infracture may facilitate stent passage in some cases. Perioperative systemic antibiotics and corticosteroids may be beneficial in children at risk for recurrence.

Repka MX, Chandler DL, Holmes JM, et al; Pediatric Eye Disease Investigator Group. Balloon catheter dilation and nasolacrimal duct intubation for treatment of nasolacrimal duct obstruction after failed probing. *Arch Ophthalmol.* 2009;127(5):633–639.

Silbert DI, Matta N. Congenital nasolacrimal duct obstruction. *Focal Points: Clinical Practice Perspectives.* American Academy of Ophthalmology; 2016, module 6.

Balloon dacryoplasty Balloon dacryoplasty (balloon catheter dilation) is performed by passing a catheter into the distal NLD and inflating a balloon at the site of obstruction (Fig 18-6). This procedure is particularly useful for patients with diffuse, rather than localized, obstruction of the distal duct.

Intubation Intubation of the lacrimal drainage system is recommended when probing or balloon dacryoplasty has failed, or as the primary procedure in patients with complex CNLDO or in those older than 36 months. One of several methods of intubation may be used. Bicanalicular intubation is performed by passing stents through the upper and lower canaliculi and recovering them in the nares. Most surgeons secure the stents in the nares by using a bolster or by suturing the stents to the nasal mucosa. Monocanalicular stents may be placed in 1 or both canaliculi.

Complications associated with stents include elongation of the lacrimal puncta, dislodging and protrusion of the stents, and corneal abrasions. In some cases, the stent can be repositioned, but early removal may be necessary.

Stents are usually left in place for 2–6 months, but shorter durations can be successful. The technique used for stent removal depends on the age of the patient, the measure employed to secure the stent, and the position of the stent (in place or partially dislodged).

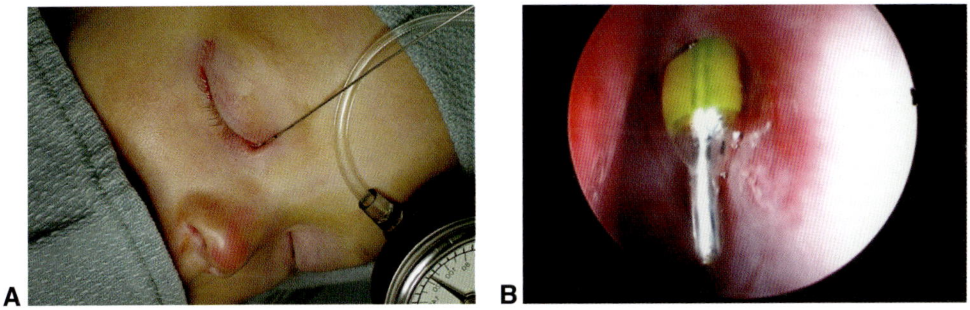

Figure 18-6 Balloon dacryoplasty. **A,** Passing the balloon into the NLD. **B,** Endoscopic view of the inflated balloon. *(Part B courtesy of Eric Paul Purdy, MD.)*

Nasal endoscopy Initial probing may fail in patients with anatomical abnormalities of the distal NLD, such as cysts in infants with dacryocystoceles and flaccid mucosal membranes obstructing the distal duct. In these cases, probing may be repeated, with removal of abnormal structures under endoscopic guidance, either by the ophthalmologist alone or in conjunction with an otolaryngologist.

Surgery in older children with NLDO

There is some controversy in the literature regarding success rates for NLD surgery in older children. The Pediatric Eye Disease Investigator Group (PEDIG) found a high success rate for simple probing in children up to 36 months of age. Many older children have simple NLDO; they have the same membranous obstruction of the distal duct found in younger children with NLDO (see Fig 18-1A). Probing in older patients with this finding has a success rate similar to that in younger children. Because probing is less likely to be successful in those with complex NLDO, particularly older children, balloon dacryoplasty or stent placement can be considered as the initial surgical procedure.

Pediatric Eye Disease Investigator Group; Repka MX, Chandler DL, Beck RW, et al. Primary treatment of nasolacrimal duct obstruction with probing in children younger than 4 years. *Ophthalmology.* 2008;115(3):577–584.

Dacryocystorhinostomy

In dacryocystorhinostomy, a new opening is created between the lacrimal sac and the nasal cavity. It is an option when the procedures described in the preceding sections are unsuccessful and NLDO persists or recurs. See BCSC Section 7, *Oculofacial Plastic and Orbital Surgery,* for further discussion of this procedure.

CHAPTER 19

External Diseases of the Eye

This chapter includes related videos. Go to www.aao.org/bcscvideo_section06 or scan the QR codes in the text to access this content.

Highlights

- Dry eye disease is uncommon in children and thus raises suspicion for secondary causes such as dietary vitamin A deficiency.
- Blepharokeratoconjunctivitis in children can be severe and may cause permanent vision loss. It can be mistaken for bacterial or herpetic infection, delaying appropriate management.
- Children with uncontrolled allergies are chronic eye rubbers; this increases their risk for developing keratoconus.
- Amniotic membrane grafting with symblepharon ring, conformer, or forniceal sutures on bolsters can significantly reduce long-term complications from Stevens-Johnson syndrome or toxic epidermal necrolysis.

This chapter focuses on external diseases of the eye that are seen in the pediatric population. Many of the topics covered in this chapter are also discussed in BCSC Section 8, *External Disease and Cornea.*

Infectious Conjunctivitis

Bacterial and viral infections are common causes of infectious conjunctivitis in children. Presenting symptoms of infectious conjunctivitis commonly include burning, stinging, and foreign-body sensation; signs include conjunctival hyperemia, ocular discharge, and matting of the eyelids. Symptoms and signs may be present unilaterally or bilaterally. The characteristics of the discharge are diagnostically helpful:

- *Purulent* discharge suggests a polymorphonuclear response to a bacterial infection.
- *Mucopurulent* discharge suggests a viral or chlamydial infection.
- *Serous* or watery discharge suggests a viral or allergic reaction.

Membrane or pseudomembrane formation may occur in severe viral or bacterial conjunctivitis, Stevens-Johnson syndrome, ligneous conjunctivitis, and chemical burns. Other potential causes of conjunctival hyperemia, or *red eye,* in infants and children include trauma, reaction to a foreign body or chemical, eyelash malposition (eg, in epiblepharon), allergy, dry eye, and uveitis.

Ophthalmia Neonatorum

Ophthalmia neonatorum refers to conjunctivitis that occurs in the first month of life. This condition can be caused by bacterial, viral, or chemical agents (Table 19-1). Widespread effective prophylaxis has diminished its occurrence to very low levels in high-income countries, but ophthalmia neonatorum remains a significant cause of ocular infection, blindness, and even death in medically underserved areas around the world.

Epidemiology and etiology

Worldwide, the incidence of ophthalmia neonatorum is greater in areas with high rates of sexually transmitted infections and poor access to health care. The prevalence ranges from 0.1% in countries with effective prenatal and perinatal care to 10% in areas such as East Africa. Because a mother may have multiple sexually transmitted infections, it is important to screen infants with 1 type of ophthalmia neonatorum for other such diseases. Public health authorities should be contacted to initiate evaluation and treatment of other maternal contacts in cases of sexually transmitted infections.

The causative organism usually infects the infant through direct contact during passage through the birth canal. Infection can ascend to the uterus, especially if there is prolonged rupture of membranes, so even with caesarean delivery, infants can be infected.

Neisseria gonorrhoeae Ophthalmia neonatorum caused by *Neisseria gonorrhoeae* typically presents in the first 3–4 days of life. Patients may present with mild conjunctival hyperemia and ocular discharge. In severe cases, there is marked chemosis, copious discharge, and potentially rapid corneal ulceration and perforation (Fig 19-1). Systemic infection can cause sepsis, meningitis, and arthritis.

Table 19-1 Common Causes of Ophthalmia Neonatorum

Presentation Timeline	Cause/Organism	Clinical Characteristics	Treatment
1 day	Silver nitrate	Mild irritation and redness	Self-limiting
3–4 days	*Neisseria gonorrhoeae*	Moderate injection to chemosis Copious purulent discharge in severe cases Corneal ulceration/perforation	Systemic ceftriaxone Regular eye irrigation Topical antibiotic (if corneal involvement)
5–10 days	*Chlamydia trachomatis*	Moderate injection to chemosis Copious mucopurulent discharge in severe cases Pseudomembranes	Systemic erythromycin or azithromycin Topical erythromycin
7–14 days	Herpes simplex virus	Injection and watery discharge Eyelid vesicular rash	Systemic acyclovir

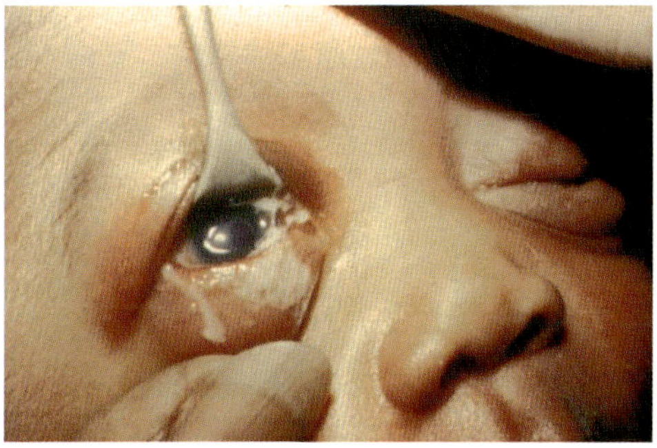

Figure 19-1 *Neisseria gonorrhoeae* conjunctivitis. *(Courtesy of Jane C. Edmond, MD.)*

Gram stain of the conjunctival exudate that shows gram-negative intracellular diplococci allows a presumptive diagnosis of *N gonorrhoeae* infection; treatment should be started immediately. Ophthalmia neonatorum caused by *Neisseria meningitidis* has also been reported. Definitive diagnosis is based on culture of the conjunctival discharge. Treatment of gonococcal ophthalmia neonatorum includes systemic ceftriaxone and topical irrigation with saline. Topical antibiotics may also be indicated if there is corneal involvement.

Chlamydia trachomatis *Chlamydia trachomatis* is an obligate intracellular bacterium that can cause neonatal inclusion conjunctivitis. Onset of conjunctivitis usually occurs around 1 week of age, although it may be earlier, especially in cases with premature rupture of membranes. Eye infection is characterized by minimal to moderate filmy discharge, mild swelling of the eyelids, and hyperemia with a papillary reaction of the conjunctiva (Fig 19-2). Severe chlamydial infection in infants differs from that in adults in several ways: in infants, pseudomembrane formation may occur, the amount of mucopurulent discharge is greater, and there is no follicular response.

Chlamydial infections can be diagnosed by culture of conjunctival scrapings, polymerase chain reaction (PCR), direct fluorescent antibody tests, and enzyme immunoassays. Systemic treatment of neonatal chlamydial disease is indicated because of the risk of pneumonitis and otitis media. The treatment of choice is oral erythromycin for 14 days or

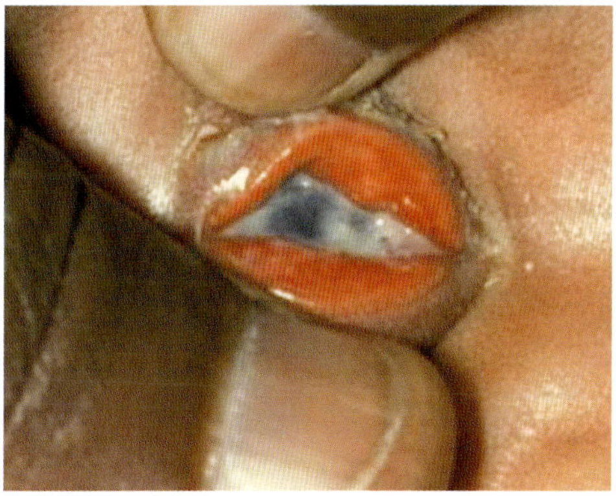

Figure 19-2 Chlamydial ophthalmia neonatorum. *(Courtesy of Jane C. Edmond, MD.)*

azithromycin for 3 days. Topical erythromycin ointment may be used in addition to but not as a replacement for oral therapy.

Herpes simplex virus Infection with herpes simplex virus (HSV) is usually secondary to HSV type 2 and typically presents later than does infection with *N gonorrhoeae* or *C trachomatis,* frequently in the second week of life. See the discussion of congenital HSV infection in Chapter 27.

Chemical conjunctivitis

Chemical conjunctivitis refers to a mild, self-limited irritation and redness of the conjunctiva occurring in the first 24 hours after instillation of silver nitrate, a preparation used for ophthalmia neonatorum prophylaxis. This condition improves spontaneously by the second day of life.

Ophthalmia neonatorum prophylaxis

Originally, 2% silver nitrate was used as prophylactic treatment of gonorrheal ophthalmia neonatorum. However, it is not effective against *C trachomatis* and has largely been supplanted by agents that are effective against both *N gonorrhoeae* and *C trachomatis,* such as erythromycin and tetracycline ointments and 2.5% povidone-iodine solution. Silver nitrate is still used in some parts of the world.

Bacterial Conjunctivitis in Children and Adolescents

The most common causes of bacterial conjunctivitis in school-aged children are *Streptococcus pneumoniae, Haemophilus* species, *Staphylococcus aureus,* and *Moraxella.* The incidence of infection from *Haemophilus* has decreased because of widespread immunization, whereas the incidence of methicillin-resistant *S aureus* (MRSA) conjunctivitis has increased. More severe forms of bacterial conjunctivitis accompanied by copious discharge suggest infection with more virulent organisms, including *N gonorrhoeae* and *N meningitidis.*

Diagnosis is made based on clinical presentation. Culture to identify the offending agent is usually not necessary in mild cases but is typically performed in severe cases. If the infection is untreated, symptoms are self-limited but may last up to 2 weeks. A broad-spectrum topical ophthalmic drop or ointment typically shortens the course to a few days. Topical treatment options include polymyxin combinations, aminoglycosides, erythromycin, bacitracin, fluoroquinolones, and azithromycin. Patients with *N meningitidis* conjunctivitis, and others exposed to these patients, require systemic treatment because of the high risk of meningitis.

Parinaud oculoglandular syndrome

Parinaud oculoglandular syndrome (POS) manifests as unilateral granulomatous conjunctivitis associated with preauricular and submandibular lymphadenopathy that can be very pronounced (Fig 19-3). MRSA conjunctivitis can have a similar presentation. The most common cause of POS is *Bartonella henselae,* a pleomorphic gram-negative bacillus that is endemic in cats and causes cat-scratch disease. Other causative organisms include *Mycobacterium tuberculosis, Mycobacterium leprae, Francisella tularensis, Yersinia*

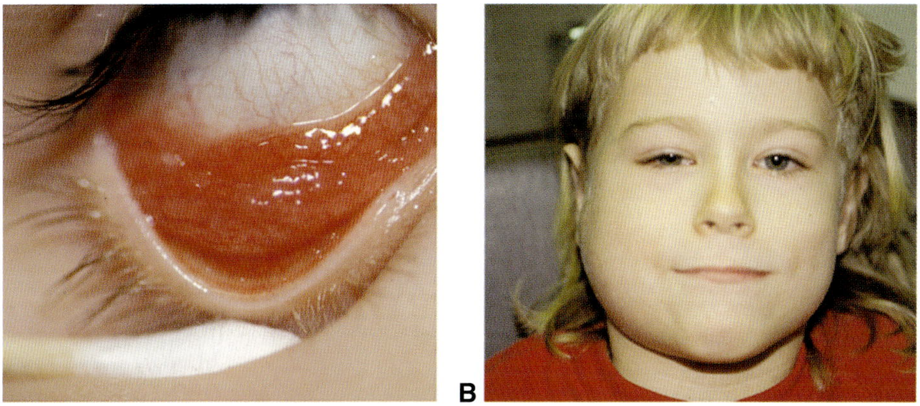

Figure 19-3 Parinaud oculoglandular syndrome. **A,** Marked follicular reaction in the lower fornix. **B,** Massive enlargement of submandibular lymph node on the affected right side. *(Courtesy of David A. Plager, MD.)*

pseudotuberculosis, Treponema pallidum, and *C trachomatis.* Cat-scratch disease is usually associated with a scratch from a kitten, but the disease can also be caused by a bite from a cat or even by touching the eye with a hand that has been licked by an infected kitten.

Serologic testing is an effective means of diagnosing POS. Treatment can be supportive in mild cases of cat-scratch disease because the disease is self-limited. In more severe cases, systemic treatment, usually with azithromycin, may be indicated. Appropriate systemic antibiotics are used to treat the other organisms that cause POS.

Chlamydial infections

Two different diseases can be caused by *C trachomatis* in children and adolescents: trachoma (serotypes A–C) and adult inclusion conjunctivitis (serotypes D–K).

Trachoma Trachoma is the most common cause of preventable blindness in the world. This disease is uncommon in Europe and the United States, except in areas of the southern United States and on American Indian reservations. It is caused by poor hygiene and inadequate sanitation and is spread from eye to eye or by flies or fomites. Clinical manifestations include acute purulent conjunctivitis, a follicular reaction, papillary hypertrophy, vascularization of the cornea, and progressive cicatricial changes of the cornea and conjunctiva. Diagnosis is made based on Giemsa stain, cell culture, or PCR. Treatment includes both topical and systemic erythromycin. Tetracycline can be used in children 8 years of age and older.

Adult inclusion conjunctivitis Adult inclusion conjunctivitis is a sexually transmitted infection that can be found in sexually active adolescents in association with chlamydial urethritis or cervicitis. However, there are nonsexual modes of transmission, including shared eye cosmetics and contaminated swimming pools. Patients present with follicular conjunctivitis, scant mucopurulent discharge, and preauricular lymphadenopathy. There is no membrane formation. The recommended treatment is oral tetracycline, doxycycline, azithromycin, or erythromycin. The clinician should consider whether the patient has been sexually abused, especially if adult inclusion conjunctivitis is found in a young child.

Viral Conjunctivitis in Infants and Children

Adenovirus

Viral conjunctivitis is most often caused by an adenovirus, a DNA virus that can cause a range of human diseases, including upper respiratory tract infection and gastroenteritis. The following are adenoviral diseases, listed with their associated serotypes:

- epidemic keratoconjunctivitis: serotypes 8, 19, and 37, subgroup D
- pharyngoconjunctival fever: serotypes 3 and 7
- acute hemorrhagic conjunctivitis: serotypes 11 and 21
- acute follicular conjunctivitis: serotypes 1, 2, 3, 4, 7, and 10

Contact precautions are especially important during the examination of infants. Outbreaks of adenoviral conjunctivitis have been associated with retinopathy of prematurity examinations in neonatal intensive care units. In neonates, adenoviral pneumonia can be fatal or lead to serious morbidity.

Epidemic keratoconjunctivitis Epidemic keratoconjunctivitis (EKC) is a highly contagious conjunctivitis that tends to occur in epidemic outbreaks. This infection is an acute bilateral follicular conjunctivitis that is usually unilateral at onset and is associated with preauricular lymphadenopathy. Initial symptoms are foreign-body sensation and periorbital pain. A diffuse superficial keratitis is followed by focal epithelial lesions that stain with fluorescein. After 11–15 days, subepithelial opacities begin to form beneath the focal epithelial infiltrates. The epithelial component fades by day 30, but the subepithelial opacities may remain for up to 2 years. In severe infections, particularly in infants, a conjunctival membrane forms and marked swelling of the eyelids occurs; these signs must be differentiated from those of orbital or preseptal cellulitis. In severe cases, complications include persistent subepithelial opacities and conjunctival scar formation.

Because EKC is easily transmitted, contact precautions must be maintained for up to 2 weeks. Isolation areas should be designated for examination of patients known or suspected to have adenoviral infections.

Diagnosis is usually based on clinical presentation but can be confirmed in the office by a rapid immunodetection assay. The organism can be recovered from the eyes and throat for 2 weeks after onset, demonstrating that patients are infectious during this period. Treatment is supportive in most cases. Artificial tears and cold compresses can provide symptomatic relief. Topical corticosteroids may be used judiciously to decrease symptoms in severe cases and in cases of decreased vision secondary to subepithelial opacities; such agents may prolong the time to full recovery. Corticosteroid use in adenoviral infection is seldom indicated in children.

Herpes simplex virus

Conjunctivitis caused by HSV type 1 is covered in BCSC Section 8, *External Disease and Cornea*.

Varicella-zoster virus

Varicella-zoster virus (VZV) is a herpesvirus that can cause varicella and herpes zoster, both of which are covered in BCSC Section 8, *External Disease and Cornea.*

Epstein-Barr virus

Epstein-Barr virus is a herpesvirus that can cause infectious mononucleosis, conjunctivitis, and nummular keratitis. See BCSC Section 8, *External Disease and Cornea.*

Molluscum contagiosum

Molluscum contagiosum is caused by a DNA poxvirus and usually presents as numerous umbilicated skin lesions (Fig 19-4A). Lesions on or near the eyelid margin can release viral particles onto the conjunctival surface, resulting in a follicular conjunctivitis (Fig 19-4B). Most lesions do not require treatment because they tend to resolve spontaneously; however, resolution can take months or years. Lesions causing conjunctivitis can be treated by incising each lesion and debriding the central core; in young children, such treatment usually requires general anesthesia.

Dry Eye Disease

The assessment and treatment of dry eye disease (DED) in children are similar to those in adults and are covered in BCSC Section 8, *External Disease and Cornea.* DED is not common in children and is generally less symptomatic in children than in adults, even in children with significant punctate epitheliopathy. True aqueous deficiency is rare, but evaporative dry eye signs can be seen in patients with pediatric blepharitis. Furthermore, when children are engrossed in an activity such as playing video games, they may have a markedly reduced blink rate, which can exacerbate dry eye signs. Incomplete blink, lid lag during sleep, and air conditioning also contribute to DED symptoms. Of all clinical testing for DED, only corneal fluorescein staining correlates well with symptoms of DED in children.

An important consideration in children with malabsorption syndromes or who have a restricted diet, such as those with severe autism, is potential vitamin A deficiency. Xerophthalmia

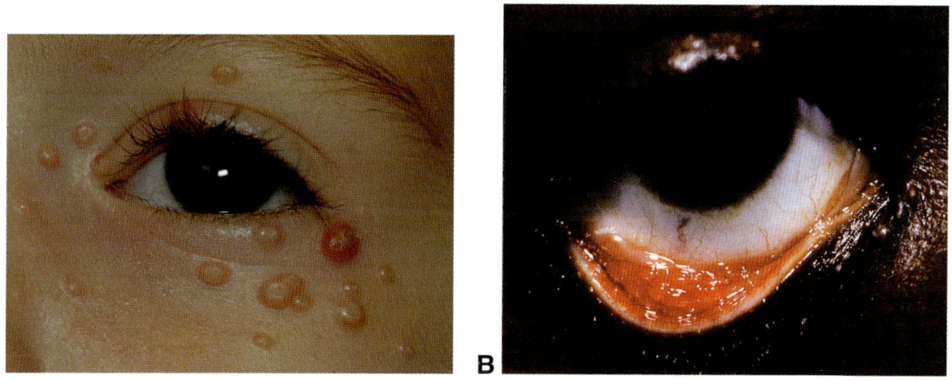

A B

Figure 19-4 Molluscum contagiosum. **A,** Eyelid lesions. **B,** Secondary follicular conjunctivitis. *(Part A courtesy of Edward L. Raab, MD; part B courtesy of Gregg T. Lueder, MD.)*

and/or Bitôt spots may be the presenting features of vitamin A deficiency. Nyctalopia may not be volunteered in the history unless the clinician specifically inquires. Vision loss from photoreceptor dysfunction as well as severe DED are preventable in these children.

Ong Tone S, Elbaz U, Silverman E, et al. Evaluation of dry eye disease in children with systemic lupus erythematosus and healthy controls. *Cornea.* 2019;38(5):581–586.

Inflammatory Disease

Blepharitis

Blepharitis is a common cause of chronic conjunctivitis in children. The signs and symptoms of blepharitis in children are similar to those in adults and include ocular irritation, conjunctival hyperemia, morning eyelid crusting, eyelid margin erythema, and meibomian gland dysfunction. Intermittent blurred vision may occur because of tear film instability. Blepharokeratoconjunctivitis (BKC) represents more severe ocular surface inflammation and can cause phlyctenules, keratitis, corneal vascularization, scarring, perforation, and permanent vision loss (Figs 19-5, 19-6). BKC in children can be misdiagnosed and treated as herpetic or bacterial infection because the keratitis can affect the central cornea without previous signs of marginal keratitis or severe meibomian gland disease. A history of chalazia, active or in earlier childhood, is closely associated with BKC.

Acne rosacea in children may be manifested by chronic blepharitis and facial telangiectasias, papules, and pustules. *Demodex* (mites that inhabit human hair follicles) may play a role in the pathogenesis of blepharitis and need to be considered when blepharitis does not respond to treatment. Patients with demodicosis typically present with a waxy, sleevelike buildup at the base of the eyelashes. Demodicosis may respond to a dilute tea tree oil solution applied to the base of the eyelashes.

Initial treatment of blepharitis includes the application of warm compresses, cleaning of the eyelids with baby shampoo, and the application of topical erythromycin or bacitracin ophthalmic ointment or azithromycin ophthalmic solution, 1%. Severe cases may benefit from oral antibiotic use. Macrolides (erythromycin, azithromycin) or doxycycline

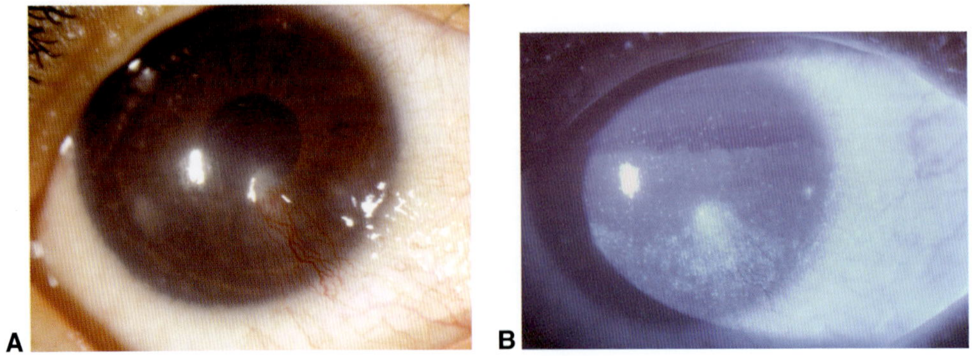

Figure 19-5 Blepharokeratoconjunctivitis **A,** Inferior keratitis secondary to severe blepharitis. **B,** Fluorescein staining of keratitis (same patient as in **A**). *(Courtesy of Robert W. Hered, MD.)*

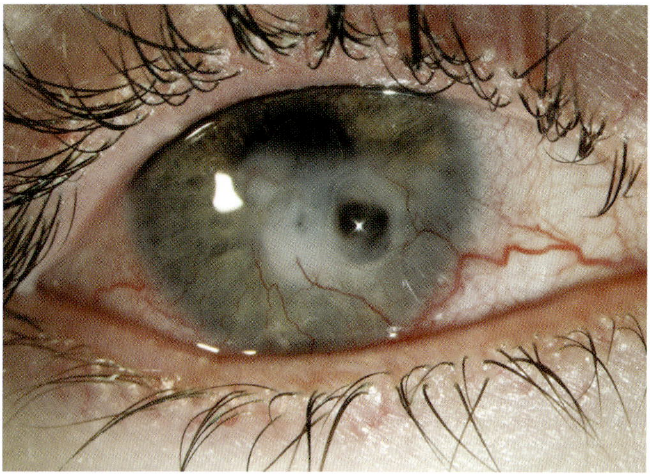

Figure 19-6 Blepharitis with meibomian gland dysfunction, scurf, and telangiectasia. Chronic inflammation has led to corneal thinning and perforation. *(Courtesy of Kamiar Mireskandari, MBChB, PhD.)*

may be helpful in severe cases of BKC. Macrolides are typically used in children younger than 12 years to avoid the potential dental staining associated with use of doxycycline. Judicious use of topical corticosteroids is indicated in patients with corneal disease. Dietary supplementation with omega-3 fatty acids may benefit some patients.

Hammersmith KM. Blepharoconjunctivitis in children. *Curr Opin Ophthalmol.* 2015;26(4): 301–305.

Ocular Allergy

Allergies are thought to affect approximately 20% of the US and European populations; more than 50% of patients who seek treatment for allergies have ocular symptoms. Allergic ocular disease is a common problem in children and is often associated with asthma, allergic rhinitis, and atopic dermatitis. The cascade of biochemical events involved in allergic response is covered in BCSC Section 8, *External Disease and Cornea.*

Marked itching and bilateral conjunctival inflammation of a chronic, recurrent, and possibly seasonal nature are hallmarks of allergic eye disease. Other signs and symptoms may be nonspecific and include tearing, mucoid discharge, stinging, burning, and photophobia.

Seasonal and perennial allergic conjunctivitis

Seasonal and perennial allergic conjunctivitis are due to type I hypersensitivity reaction. Seasonal allergy is a common clinical entity that affects approximately 40 million people in the United States, including many children. It occurs in the spring and fall and is triggered by environmental contact with specific airborne allergens such as pollens from grasses, flowers, weeds, and trees. Patients typically present with red and watery eyes, boggy-appearing conjunctiva, and ocular itching (Fig 19-7). Blue-gray to purple discoloration of the lower eyelids, termed *allergic shiners,* can occur secondary to venous stasis from nasal congestion.

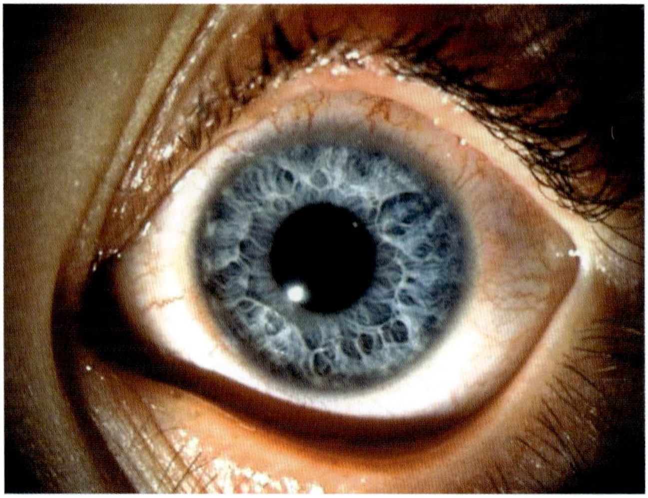

Figure 19-7 Seasonal allergic conjunctivitis showing red, watery eye with mild conjunctival edema. *(Courtesy of Albert W. Biglan, MD.)*

Perennial allergic conjunctivitis has similar signs and symptoms to those of seasonal allergic conjunctivitis. However, the type I hypersensitivity reaction occurs after contact with ubiquitous household allergens, such as dust mites and dander from domestic pets, and hence is present all year long. This condition is diagnosed based on the history and clinical presentation.

Vernal keratoconjunctivitis

Vernal keratoconjunctivitis (VKC) is caused by type I and type IV hypersensitivity reactions. This condition most commonly affects males in the first 2 decades of life and, similar to seasonal allergic conjunctivitis, usually occurs in the spring and fall. VKC has 2 forms: palpebral and limbal (bulbar). Both types manifest with severe itching and photosensitivity.

The palpebral form of VKC preferentially affects the tarsal conjunctiva of the upper eyelid. In the early stages, the eye may be diffusely injected, with little discharge. However, tarsal papillae may increase and coalesce, forming characteristic giant papillary conjunctivitis (Fig 19-8). A thick, ropy, whitish mucoid discharge is often present.

The limbal form of VKC manifests with thickening and opacification of the conjunctiva at the limbus, usually most pronounced at the upper margin of the cornea. The discrete limbal nodules that appear are gray, jellylike, elevated lumps with vascular cores. A whitish center filled with eosinophils and epithelioid cells may appear in the raised lesion. This complex is called a *Horner-Trantas dot.* Limbal nodules may increase in number and become confluent (Fig 19-9). They persist as long as the seasonal exacerbation of the disease lasts. The limbal form is more common in patients of African or Asian descent and is more prevalent in warm, subtropical climates.

The cornea may become involved in VKC, with punctate epithelial erosions. Corneal involvement may progress to a large, confluent epithelial defect, typically in the upper half of the cornea, called a *shield ulcer.* This ulcer is sterile and clinically resembles an ovoid corneal abrasion (Fig 19-10). If untreated, mucoid and epithelial debris accumulates in the base of the ulcer, forming a *corneal plaque* (Fig 19-11). This plaque forms a physical barrier to reepithelialization and requires removal to allow epithelial healing.

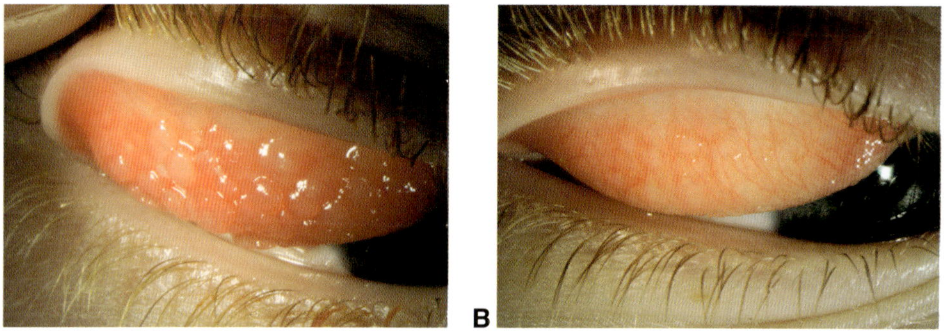

A B

Figure 19-8 Vernal keratoconjunctivitis (VKC). **A,** Palpebral VKC, showing characteristic dome-shaped giant papillary conjunctivitis (GPC) on the upper eyelid. **B,** Same patient as in **(A)** showing resolution of GPC following 6 weeks of topical treatment. *(Courtesy of Kamiar Mireskandari, MBChB, PhD.)*

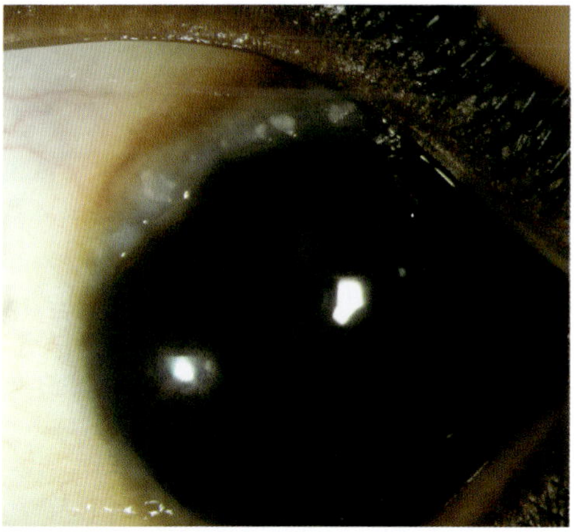

Figure 19-9 Limbal VKC with Horner-Trantas dots. *(Courtesy of Kamiar Mireskandari, MBChB, PhD.)*

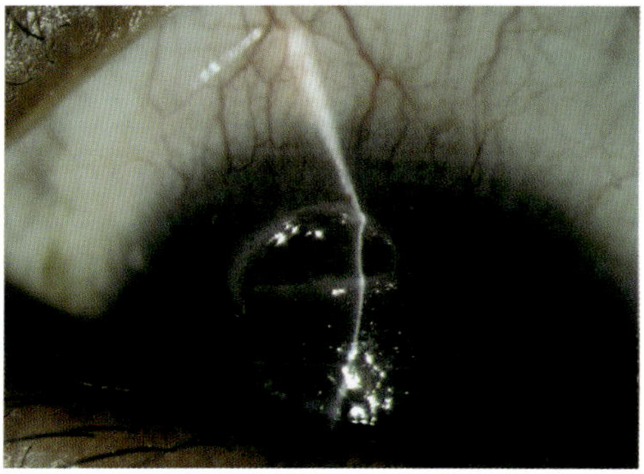

Figure 19-10 Shield ulcer in VKC. Note the epithelial defect with clear base. *(Courtesy of Kamiar Mireskandari, MBChB, PhD.)*

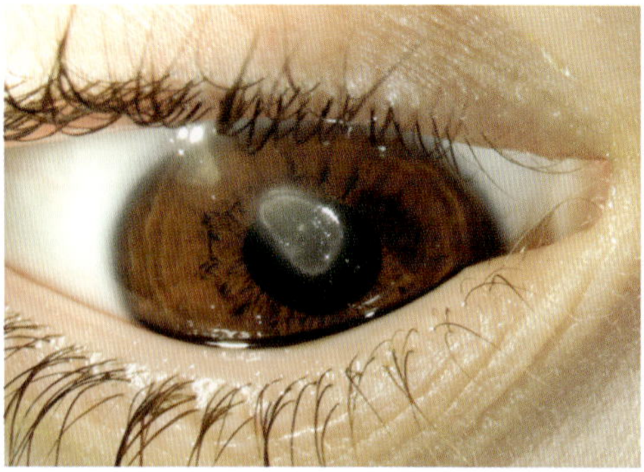

Figure 19-11 Corneal plaque in VKC. Note the epithelial and mucoid debris at the base of the ulcer. *(Courtesy of Kamiar Mireskandari, MBChB, PhD.)*

Atopic keratoconjunctivitis

Atopic keratoconjunctivitis is a nonseasonal disorder that occurs in patients with atopic disease. It is relatively rare in young children. See BCSC Section 8, *External Disease and Cornea,* for further discussion.

Management of allergic eye disease

Treatment of all ocular allergy disorders is fundamentally similar to that of other allergy-related disorders. The most effective treatment is to avoid offending allergens or remove them from the patient's environment. Unfortunately, avoidance may not be possible or adequate to alleviate the patient's symptoms. Simple measures to help patient symptoms include cold compresses, artificial tear eyedrops, and topical vasoconstrictors. These measures may be adequate in the mildest cases.

Topical medication is often required and can be tailored to disease severity. Treatments include mast-cell stabilizers, H_1-receptor antagonists, antihistamines, corticosteroids, and calcineurin inhibitors, or a combination of these drugs. Mast-cell stabilizers should be used continuously through the allergy season to build and maximize their effectiveness. H_1-receptor antagonists and antihistamines can be used as needed in patients with mild allergies; however, these medications are often required to be (and work better if) taken regularly. Nonsteroidal anti-inflammatory eyedrops should be used with caution; cases of corneal perforation, though rare, have been reported.

Topical corticosteroid eyedrops used in pulsed doses can effectively reduce the signs and symptoms of severe allergic eye disease. Patients must be closely monitored for adverse effects, including glaucoma and cataracts, and parents must be educated to not self-medicate with corticosteroids. The aim of corticosteroid eyedrops is to bring the disease under control, while initiating other agents for maintenance of good control. Calcineurin inhibitors, cyclosporin 0.1%–2.0% or tacrolimus 0.02%–0.1%, have been effective when used to maintain remission or minimize reliance on corticosteroids. These treatments are off-label, but clinical experience has shown them to be efficacious and safe.

Systemic treatment is sometimes required in ocular allergy. Although oral antihistamines may be less effective at relieving specific ocular symptoms, they can be a helpful adjunct and are typically tolerated well in children, especially as they alleviate other allergic symptoms such as itching and rhinitis. In children with severe ocular allergy and other atopic disease, discussion with their dermatologist or immunologist is warranted to consider allergen immunotherapy or immunomodulatory drugs. Allergen immunotherapy involves IgE sensitization to relevant allergens to increase the patient's sensitivity threshold to the allergen. Immunomodulatory drugs such as methotrexate and cyclosporin may be used if indicated. It is important to note that systemic agents are rarely warranted for treatment of eye disease alone. Finally, the interleukin 4 and 13 inhibitor, dupilumab, is increasingly used to treat severe atopic dermatitis. This drug is associated with severe ocular surface disease and may be confused with worsening of the patient's ocular allergy.

Allergy is a "medical condition," and surgical intervention is required only in rare cases. Even severe giant papillae typically do not require excision as they are very responsive to medical therapy (see Fig-19-8). One notable exception is when a corneal plaque has developed after a shield ulcer. As previously noted, such plaques need to be removed to allow epithelial healing (Videos 19-1, 19-2). Supratarsal injection of triamcinolone (4 mg in 0.1 mL) may be used to aid recovery in patients with refractory palpebral VKC. Because many pediatric patients require anesthesia for this procedure, it is usually reserved for cases in which a superficial keratectomy is required for a corneal plaque at the same time.

VIDEO 19-1 Removal of fresh corneal plaque due to severe allergy.
Courtesy of Kamiar Mireskandari, MBChB, PhD.

VIDEO 19-2 Removal of long-standing corneal plaque due to severe allergy.
Courtesy of Kamiar Mireskandari, MBChB, PhD.

Children with allergies, especially if the allergies are not fully controlled, are chronic eye rubbers and are therefore at risk of developing keratoconus. These children and their caretakers must be counseled about this association. Good disease control is doubly important, and monitoring for keratoconus, through serial corneal topography or tomography, should be considered. Atopic patients have poor contact lens tolerance and have very poor prognosis with keratoplasty. Therefore, preventing keratoconus, or at least identifying it at an early stage to allow corneal collagen crosslinking, is an important aspect of managing children with ocular allergy.

Roumeau I, Coutu A, Navel V, et al. Efficacy of medical treatments for vernal keratoconjunctivitis: a systematic review and meta-analysis. *J Allergy Clin Immunol.* 2021;148(3):822–834.

Stevens-Johnson Syndrome and Toxic Epidermal Necrolysis

Stevens-Johnson syndrome (SJS) and toxic epidermal necrolysis (TEN) are rare hypersensitivity reactions that affect skin and mucous membranes. The most common etiologies of SJS and TEN in children are medications (usually anticonvulsants and sulfonamides) and infections (usually due to *Mycoplasma* species or herpes simplex virus). The pathogenesis of SJS and TEN is discussed further in BCSC Section 8, *External Disease and Cornea.*

Systemic manifestations range from mild to severe. A prodrome of fever, malaise, and upper respiratory tract infection is followed by bullous mucosal and skin lesions. These lesions rupture, ulcerate, and become covered by gray-white membranes and a hemorrhagic

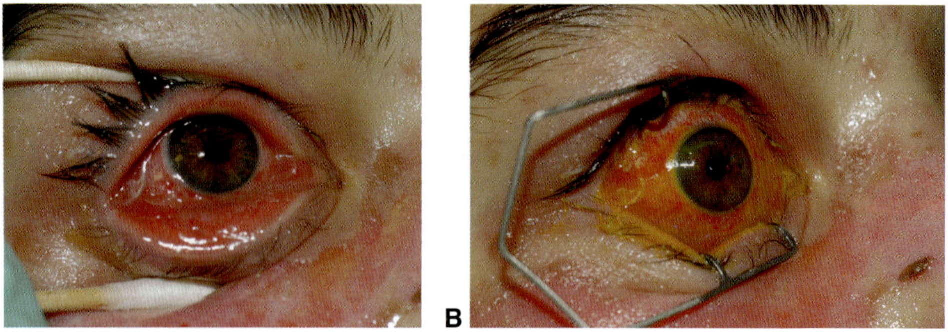

A B

Figure 19-12 Stevens-Johnson syndrome. **A,** Early, severe involvement showing injection and petechial hemorrhages of the conjunctiva and membrane formation laterally. **B,** Extensive conjunctival epithelial defect stained with fluorescein. *(Courtesy of Kamiar Mireskandari, MBChB, PhD.)*

crust. Severe cases require supportive medical treatment akin to severe burns and are often seen in intensive care or burn units. The mortality rates for SJS and TEN are lower in children: 0% in SJS and 16% in TEN, compared to 1%–5% in SJS and 25%–35% in TEN for adults.

Ocular involvement occurs in 80% of pediatric patients acutely. Initially edema, erythema, and crusting of the eyelids as well conjunctivitis may be seen. In many instances, membranous or pseudomembranous conjunctivitis (Fig 19-12) and tarsal and palpebral epithelial defects may occur, leading to symblepharon formation. Corneal epithelial defects, thinning, ulceration, bacterial superinfection, and perforation may develop. Late ocular complications occur in approximately 27% of pediatric patients; these complications include conjunctival scarring, including symblepharon formation and cicatricial entropion; DED; trichiasis; corneal scarring and vascularization; and limbal stem cell deficiency.

The most important prognostic factor for ocular complications is the severity of the initial disease, followed by how quickly the ophthalmology team is consulted. Early intervention is important for preventing late ocular complications. Frequent ocular lubrication with artificial tears and ointments (preferably preservative-free) may be adequate for mild cases. In patients with more severe disease, topical corticosteroids to control local inflammation are often required. The fornices may be swept to lyse adhesions, although some ophthalmologists believe that doing so may stimulate inflammation and cause further scarring. In severe cases, amniotic membrane grafting in conjunction with a symblepharon ring, conformer, or forniceal sutures on bolsters should be considered early to decrease the risk of late ocular complications (Video 19-3).

VIDEO 19-3 Amniotic membrane graft at the bedside for Stevens-Johnson syndrome.
Courtesy of Kamiar Mireskandari, MBChB, PhD.

Catt CJ, Hamilton GM, Fish J, Mireskandari K, Ali A. Ocular manifestations of Stevens-Johnson syndrome and toxic epidermal necrolysis in children. *Am J Ophthalmol.* 2016;166:68–75.

Yang Y, Fung SSM, Chew H, Mireskandari K, Ali A. Amniotic membrane transplantation for Stevens-Johnson syndrome/toxic epidermal necrolysis: the Toronto experience. *Br J Ophthalmol.* 2021;105(9):1238–1243.

Other Conjunctival and Subconjunctival Disorders

Papillomas

Papillomas are benign epithelial proliferations that usually appear as sessile masses at the limbus or as pedunculated lesions of the caruncle, fornix, or palpebral conjunctiva. They may be transparent, pale yellow, or salmon colored and are sometimes speckled with red dots. Papillomas in children usually result from viral infection and often resolve spontaneously. Oral cimetidine can induce papilloma regression. Surgical excision is indicated when symptoms are severe or if new lesions continue to appear.

Conjunctival Epithelial Inclusion Cysts

Conjunctival inclusion cysts are clear, fluid-filled cysts on the conjunctiva. These cysts are often noted in patients who had ocular surgery or trauma. Excision is indicated if the cyst causes irritation.

Conjunctival Nevi

Conjunctival nevi are relatively common in children. Nevi of the conjunctiva consist of nests or more diffuse infiltrations of benign melanocytes. On histologic examination, most of these nevi are compound (nevus cells found in both epithelium and substantia propria); others are junctional (nevus cells confined to the interface between epithelium and substantia propria). The lesions are occasionally noted at birth. More commonly, they develop and/or enlarge during later childhood or adolescence. The lesions may be flat or elevated. Nevi are typically brown, but approximately one-third are nonpigmented (amelanotic) and have a pinkish appearance with microcyst (Fig 19-13). Removal may be indicated if significant irritation, redness, or growth occurs, although transformation to malignant melanoma is extremely rare in childhood (Videos 19-4, 19-5).

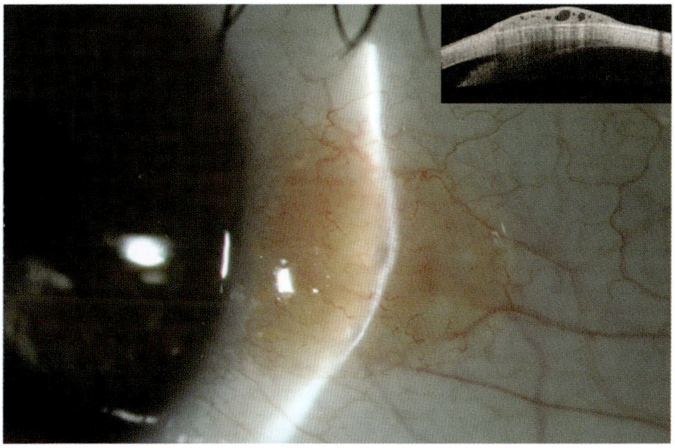

Figure 19-13 Amelanotic nevus of the bulbar conjunctiva, left eye. Note typical cysts within the creamy pink lesion. *Inset:* Optical coherence tomography of same lesion. Note the cysts within the lesion and normal corneal epithelium. *(Courtesy of Kamiar Mireskandari, MBChB, PhD.)*

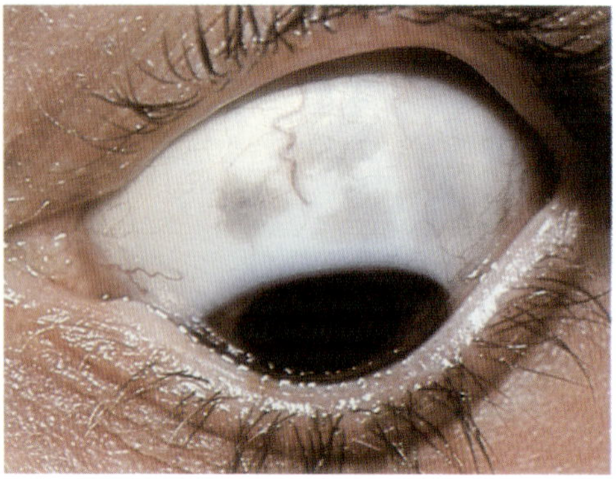

Figure 19-14 Ocular melanocytosis.

VIDEO 19-4 Excision of small conjunctival nevus and direct closure.
Courtesy of Kamiar Mireskandari, MBChB, PhD.

VIDEO 19-5 Excision of large conjunctival nevus and closure with free conjunctival autograft.
Courtesy of Kamiar Mireskandari, MBChB, PhD.

Ocular Melanocytosis

Ocular melanocytosis *(melanosis oculi)* is a congenital focal proliferation of subepithelial melanocytes characterized by unilateral patchy but extensive slate-gray or bluish discoloration of the episclera (Fig 19-14). Intraocular pigmentation is also increased and is associated with a higher incidence of glaucoma and risk of malignant melanoma. Some patients, particularly persons of Asian ancestry, may have associated involvement of eyelid and adjacent skin with dermal hyperpigmentation that produces brown, bluish, or black discoloration without thickening *(oculodermal melanocytosis, nevus of Ota)*. Small patches of slate-gray scleral pigmentation, typically bilateral and without clinical significance, are common in Black and Asian children. Melanosis of skin and sclera is occasionally associated with encephalofacial angiomatosis (Sturge-Weber syndrome) and Klippel-Trénaunay-Weber syndrome.

Ligneous Conjunctivitis

Ligneous conjunctivitis is a rare bilateral chronic disorder characterized by firm ("woody"), yellowish, fibrinous pseudomembranes on the conjunctiva. It is secondary to severe deficiency in type I plasminogen and can affect persons of all ages. Although treatment with plasminogen eyedrops has shown promising results, these eyedrops are not readily available. Other treatment options include fresh frozen plasma and heparin eyedrops. Surgical removal with amniotic membrane transplantation has a high recurrence rate without preventative eyedrops.

CHAPTER 20

Disorders of the Anterior Segment

Highlights

- In congenital corneal opacities, the density and location of the opacity guide management.
- Congenital glaucoma must always be considered in an infant with corneal edema but is not the only possible cause for the finding.
- Keratoconus has a more aggressive clinical course in children than in adults.

Introduction

Disorders of the anterior segment represent a wide spectrum of conditions involving the cornea, iris, anterior chamber angle, and lens. Childhood glaucoma and lens disorders are discussed in Chapters 21 and 22, respectively, in this volume. Anatomy of the anterior segment and its development are discussed in BCSC Section 2, *Fundamentals and Principles of Ophthalmology.* See also BCSC Section 8, *External Disease and Cornea,* for detailed discussions of some of the disorders covered in this chapter.

Congenital Abnormalities of Corneal Size or Shape

Megalocornea

Megalocornea is characterized by bilateral congenitally enlarged corneas, with an increased horizontal corneal diameter and a deep anterior chamber (Fig 20-1); it is often associated with iris transillumination. On biometry, the ratio of anterior chamber depth to total axial length is typically 0.19 or greater, a feature that is useful for distinguishing this anomaly from buphthalmos, which results in axial length growth from increased intraocular pressure (IOP). Late changes include corneal mosaic degeneration (shagreen), arcus juvenilis, early adult-onset cataracts, and glaucoma. The phenotype is often caused by X-linked recessive mutation in *CHRDL1*.

Davidson AE, Cheong SS, Hysi PG, et al. Association of *CHRDL1* mutations and variants with X-linked megalocornea, Neuhäuser syndrome and central corneal thickness. *PLoS One.* 2014;9(8):e104163.

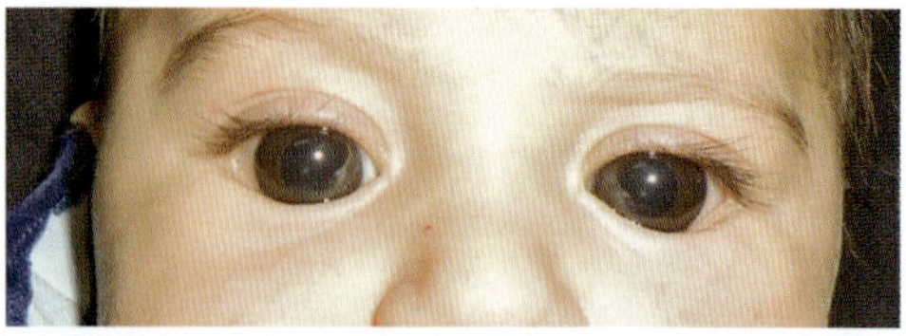

Figure 20-1 Megalocornea. The depth of the anterior chamber in this male infant was >19% of total axial length, a feature that is useful for distinguishing the anomaly from buphthalmos. *(Courtesy of Arif O. Khan, MD.)*

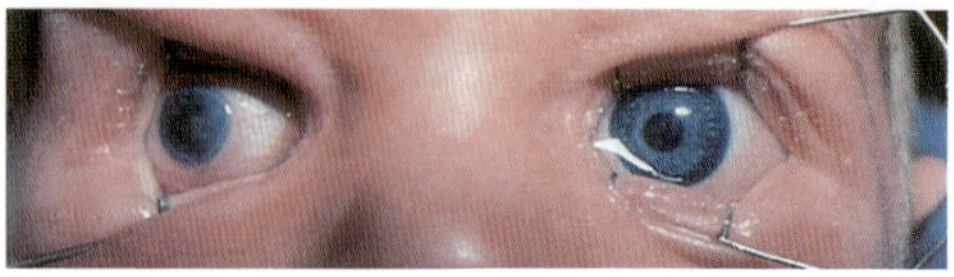

Figure 20-2 Microcornea, right eye.

Microcornea

Microcornea is characterized by a horizontal corneal diameter of 9 mm or less at birth and 10 mm or less after 2 years of age (Fig 20-2). It is often a component of ocular malformations such as microphthalmia and persistent fetal vasculature and of oculodentodigital, Nance-Horan, Lenz, and other syndromes.

Keratoglobus

Keratoglobus is characterized by a steep corneal curvature, peripheral corneal thinning, and a very deep anterior chamber. The phenotype may be due to brittle cornea syndrome, which often results from biallelic mutations in *ZNF469* or *PRDM5.* Spontaneous breaks in Descemet membrane may produce acute corneal edema. Because the cornea can be ruptured by minor blunt trauma, full-time use of protective spectacles is appropriate.

Congenital Abnormalities of Peripheral Corneal Transparency

Posterior Embryotoxon

Posterior embryotoxon (prominent Schwalbe line) represents thickening and anterior displacement of the Schwalbe line, causing the anomaly to appear as an irregular white line just concentric with and anterior to the limbus (Fig 20-3). Although this is a common isolated finding (occurring in 15% of healthy patients), it is often seen in Axenfeld-Rieger syndrome, arteriohepatic dysplasia (Alagille syndrome), and velocardiofacial syndrome (22q11 deletion syndrome).

Cornea Plana

The pathognomonic phenotype of *cornea plana* includes a flat cornea, indistinct limbus, shallow anterior chamber, hyperopia, and associated accommodative esotropia (Fig 20-4); it is specific for biallelic *KERA* mutations. Refractive correction and monitoring for glaucoma, which may develop later in life, are the mainstays of treatment.

Khan AO, Aldahmesh M, Meyer B. Recessive cornea plana in the Kingdom of Saudi Arabia. *Ophthalmology.* 2006;113(10):1773–1778.

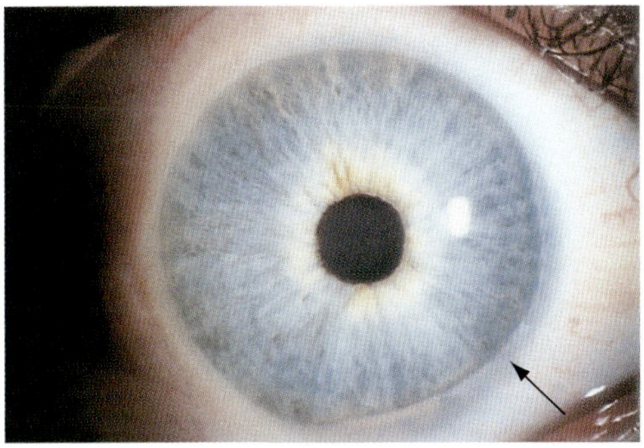

Figure 20-3 Posterior embryotoxon *(arrow)* in a patient with Axenfeld-Rieger syndrome.

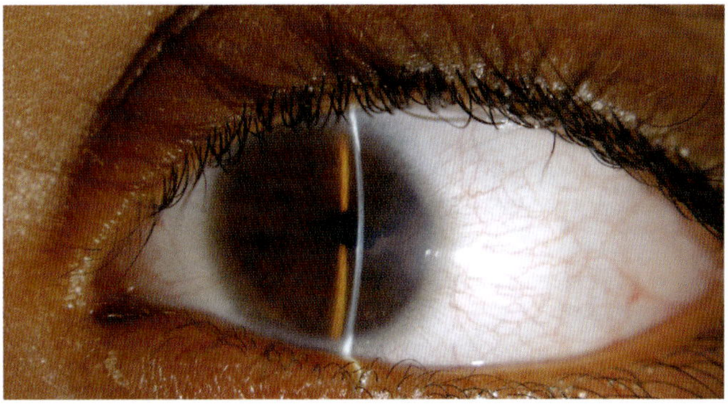

Figure 20-4 An extremely flat cornea is apparent in this child with cornea plana. Also note the indistinct limbus. In this case, the pupil was also irregular. *(Reproduced with permission from Khan AO. Ocular genetic disease in the Middle East.* Curr Opin Ophthalmol. *2013;24(5):369–378.)*

Epibulbar Dermoid

An *epibulbar (limbal) dermoid* is a choristoma composed of fibrofatty tissue covered by keratinized epithelium; it may contain hair follicles, sebaceous glands, or sweat glands. The dermoid often straddles the limbus (typically inferotemporally) or, less frequently, resides more centrally in the cornea (Fig 20-5). It is typically less than 10 mm in diameter, with minimal postnatal growth. The dermoid may extend into the corneal stroma and adjacent sclera but seldom encompasses the full thickness. Often, a lipoid infiltration of the corneal stroma is noted at the leading edge. Sometimes the lesion is continuous with epibulbar dermolipomas that involve the lateral quadrant of the eye.

Epibulbar dermoids may be seen in Goldenhar syndrome (see also Chapter 17). Patients with Goldenhar syndrome may have 1 or more of a variety of anomalies, including ear deformities or periauricular tags, maxillary or mandibular hypoplasia, vertebral deformities, eyelid colobomas, or Duane syndrome.

Epibulbar dermoids can produce astigmatism with secondary anisometropic amblyopia, which is managed with refractive correction and amblyopia treatment. It is important that parents understand that excision will not eliminate the preexisting astigmatism. Occasionally, scarring and astigmatism are increased when the edge of the dermoid is close to the visual axis. Surgical excision may be indicated when the dermoid causes ocular

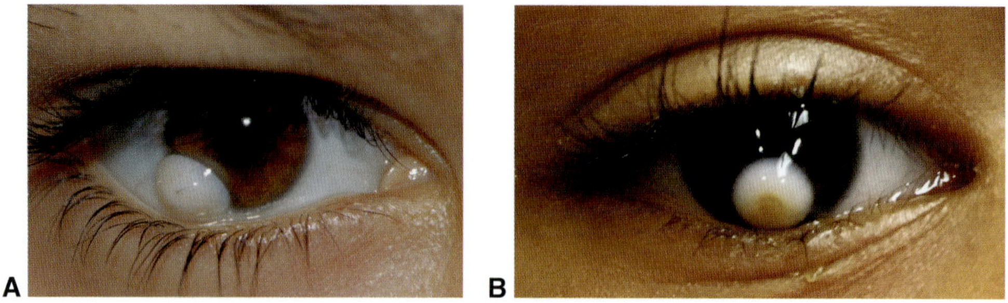

Figure 20-5 Dermoids. A, Epibulbar (limbal) dermoid with hair growing in the center. B, Corneal dermoid. *(Part A courtesy of Kamiar Mireskandari, MBChB, PhD; part B courtesy of Robert W. Hered, MD.)*

irritation, is very elevated, is large enough to block the visual axis, or is aesthetically troublesome in older children. Surgery involves excising the lesion flush with the plane of the surrounding tissue. In general, the surgeon need not remove underlying clear corneal tissue, mobilize surrounding tissue, or apply a patch graft over the resulting surface defect. However, when the lesion is deep or is thought to extend into the anterior chamber, tissue should be available in the event a patch graft is required. The cornea and conjunctiva heal within a few days to several weeks, generally with some scarring and imperfect corneal transparency; nevertheless, the appearance can be improved considerably.

Dermolipoma

A *dermolipoma* is an epibulbar choristoma composed of adipose and dense connective tissue (Fig 20-6). Often, dermal tissue, including hairs, has replaced a portion of the overlying conjunctiva. Dermolipomas may be extensive, involving orbital tissue, the lacrimal gland, extraocular muscle, or a combination of these. Like limbal dermoids, dermolipomas may be associated with Goldenhar syndrome (see Chapter 17).

In rare instances, dermolipomas require excision. When surgery is undertaken, the surgeon should attempt to remove only the portion of the lesion that is visible within the palpebral fissure, disturbing the conjunctiva and the Tenon layer as little as possible to minimize scarring and the risks of strabismus and dry eye. Cicatrization may occur even with a conservative operative approach.

Congenital Abnormalities of Central and Diffuse Corneal Transparency

The mnemonic *STUMPED* refers to *s*clerocornea, *t*ears in Descemet membrane (usually owing to forceps trauma or congenital glaucoma), *u*lcers (infection; see Chapter 27), *m*etabolic disorders (eg, mucopolysaccharidosis), *P*eters anomaly, *e*dema (eg, in congenital hereditary endothelial dystrophy [CHED], posterior polymorphous corneal dystrophy [PPCD], congenital hereditary stromal dystrophy [CHSD], and glaucoma), and *d*ermoid. Although this mnemonic has been used when the differential diagnosis of corneal opacity in young patients is considered (Table 20-1), it is not a classification system. In some

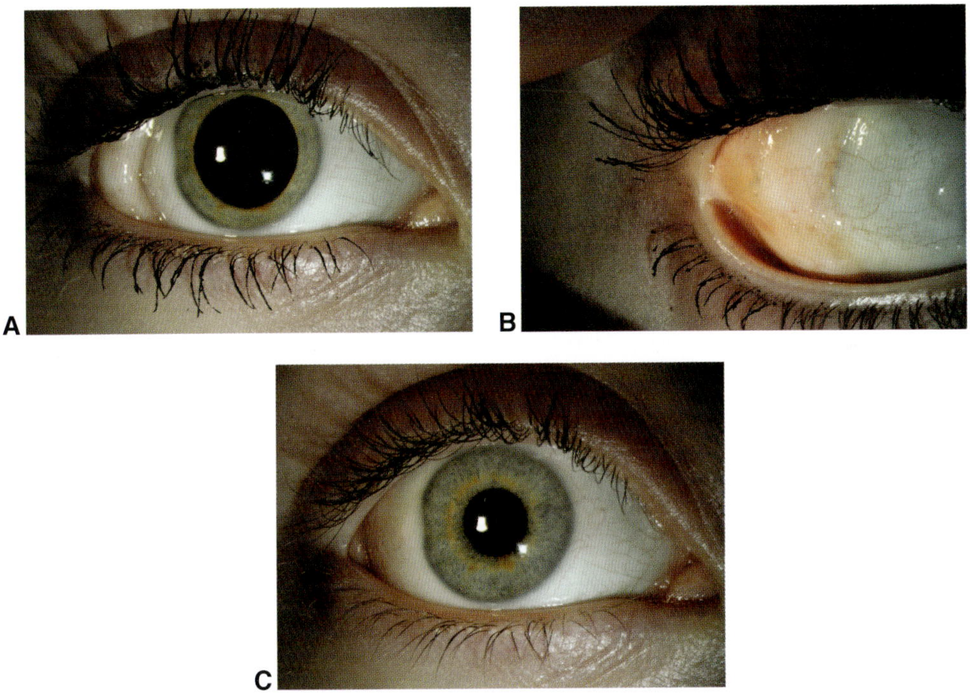

Figure 20-6 Dermolipoma before and after treatment. **A,** Dermolipoma in the right lateral canthal area. Note the incidental flat limbal dermoid temporally. **B,** Same patient looking to the left. Note the fibrofatty appearance and tethering to the lateral canthus. **C,** Same patient after anterior excision and conjunctival autograft. Note that the orbital component of the dermolipoma was not excised and can be seen deep in the lateral canthal area. *(Courtesy of Kamiar Mireskandari, MBChB, PhD.)*

congenital corneal opacifications, the embryological processes are disrupted—notably, the separation of the lens (surface ectoderm) from the cornea and the migration of neural crest cells, which form corneal stroma and endothelium, iris stroma, and trabecular meshwork (See BCSC Section 2, *Fundamentals and Principles of Ophthalmology*, Part II: Embryology, and BCSC Section 8, *External Disease and Cornea,* Video 6-2).

Congenital Hereditary Endothelial Dystrophy

In CHED, the cornea is diffusely and uniformly edematous (ie, thick) with bluish discoloration, often with a mosaic haze (Fig 20-7). The phenotype is specific for biallelic *SLC4A11* mutations. IOP is sometimes falsely elevated, which can lead to the misdiagnosis of glaucoma. Deafness presents later in some cases (Harboyan syndrome).

Posterior Polymorphous Corneal Dystrophy

This condition typically causes polymorphic vesicular changes in the endothelium with thickened Descemet membrane. Patients present in adolescence with good vision and incidental finding of PPCD, which may slowly progress over many years. In rare instances,

Table 20-1 Differential Diagnosis of Infantile Corneal Opacities

Diagnosis	Location and Description of Opacity	Other Signs	Method of Diagnosis
"Sclerocornea"[a]	Total corneal opacification; may be more dense in periphery; unilateral or bilateral; often vascularized	Flat cornea	Inspection; UBM, AS-OCT
Forceps injury	Central edema; unilateral	Breaks in Descemet membrane	History; inspection
Peters anomaly (type 1 or 2)	Spectrum of disease from mild to severe corneal opacity (peripheral, paraxial, central, or total); unilateral or bilateral	Iris adherence to cornea; posterior corneal defect, also involves the lens in type 2; keratolenticular adhesions and/or cataract	Inspection; UBM, AS-OCT
Infection	Localized or diffuse opacity; unilateral or bilateral	Dendrites; infiltrate; ulceration; late scarring	Culture; polymerase chain reaction; serologic tests
Mucopolysaccharidosis	Diffuse stromal opacity; bilateral	Smooth epithelium	Biochemical testing
Congenital hereditary stromal dystrophy (CHSD)	Diffuse stromal opacity; bilateral	Normal thickness; normal epithelium	Inspection, examination of family members for autosomal dominance
Congenital hereditary endothelial dystrophy (CHED)	Diffuse corneal edema; bilateral	Thickened cornea, corneal diameter, and optic nerves; axial length normal	Inspection, examination of family members for autosomal dominance
Posterior polymorphous corneal dystrophy (PPCD)	Diffuse corneal edema; bilateral	Thickened cornea; normal corneal diameter, optic nerves, and axial length	Inspection, examination of family members for autosomal dominance
Primary congenital glaucoma	Diffuse corneal edema; unilateral or bilateral	Enlarged cornea; breaks in Descemet membrane; optic nerve cupping and increased axial length	Tonometry, A-scan axial length measures
Dermoid	Inferotemporal opacity; unilateral; elevated; surface hair; keratinized; usually limbal	Associated with Goldenhar syndrome	Inspection

AS-OCT = anterior segment optical coherence tomography; UBM = ultrasound biomicroscopy.
[a]A description rather than a diagnosis; better to use "severe congenital corneal opacification."

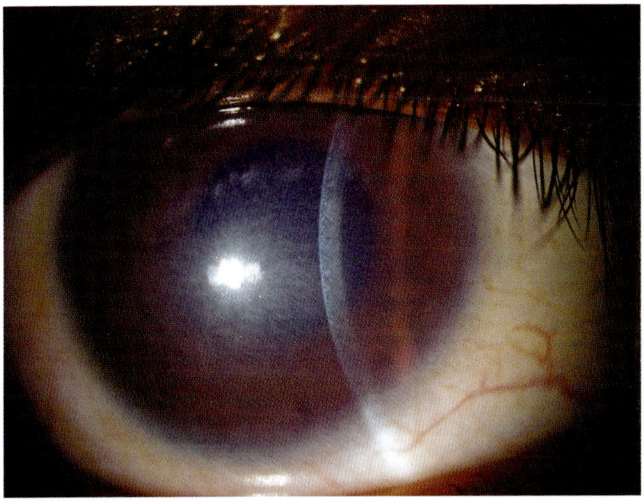

Figure 20-7 Congenital hereditary endothelial dystrophy. Note the diffuse mosaic haze, bluish discoloration, and thickness of the cornea. *(Courtesy of Arif O. Khan, MD.)*

PPCD manifests in infancy with diffuse corneal edema. As with CHED, penetrating keratoplasty and endothelial keratoplasty carry a very good prognosis.

Congenital Hereditary Stromal Dystrophy

An autosomal dominant condition, CHSD is extremely rare. It is characterized by a smooth, normal epithelium with flaky or feathery clouding of the stroma, which has increased thickness.

> **CLINICAL PEARL**
>
> In premature infants, transient corneal haze and edema may be encountered during retinopathy of prematurity screening.

Weiss JS, Møller HU, Aldave AJ, et al. IC3D classification of corneal dystrophies—edition 2. *Cornea.* 2015;34(2):117–159. Published correction appears in *Cornea.* 2015;34(10):e32.

Peters Anomaly

Peters anomaly is characterized by a posterior corneal defect with an overlying stromal opacity, often accompanied by adherent iris strands (Peters anomaly type 1; Fig 20-8A, B). Peters anomaly type 2 has a more severe phenotype involving adherence of the lens to the cornea at the site of the central defect and/or a cataract (Fig 20-8C). The corneal opacity ranges from a dense to mild central leukoma. In severe cases, the central leukoma may be vascularized and may protrude above the level of the cornea (anterior staphyloma). In rare cases, a membrane may form posterior to the posterior corneal defect, causing the appearance of a central cyst in an opacified cornea (Fig 20-8D). The stromal opacity

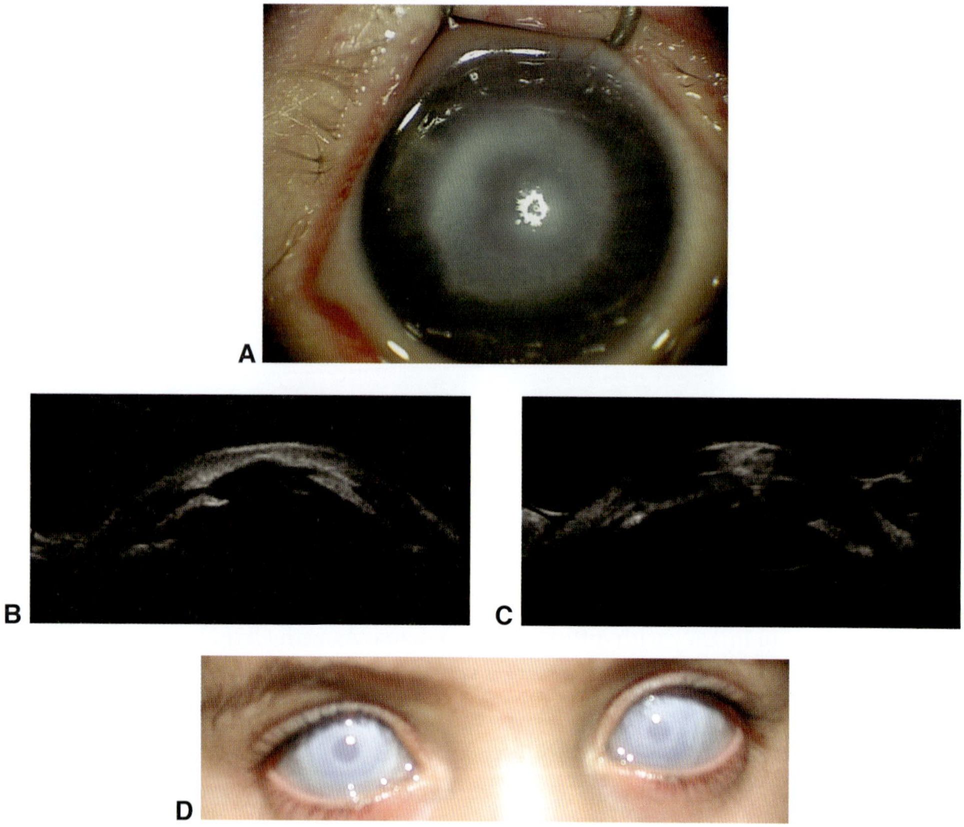

Figure 20-8 Peters anomaly. **A,** Corneal opacity due to Peters anomaly type 1. **B,** Ultrasound biomicroscopy (UBM) image from the same patient as in **(A)** showing iris adhesions to the cornea, a posterior corneal defect, and opacity. **C,** UBM image from a patient with Peters anomaly type 2 showing a cataract and keratolenticular adhesion to dense corneal opacity. **D,** Bilateral posterior corneal defect with a thin posterior membrane, causing the appearance of a central cyst in an opacified cornea. *(Parts A–C courtesy of Kamiar Mireskandari, MBChB, PhD; part D courtesy of Arif O. Khan, MD.)*

may decrease with time in some cases. Lysis of adherent iris strands has been reported to improve corneal clarity in some cases.

Peters anomaly may arise from a variety of gene mutations (eg, heterozygous *PAX6* mutation, biallelic *CYP1B1* mutations) or from in utero insult (eg, congenital rubella). One Peters anomaly syndrome, *Peters-plus syndrome,* is caused by biallelic *B3GLCT* mutations. It is associated with short stature, a distinct craniofacial appearance, shortened fingers and toes, and intellectual disability. Even in mild and unilateral cases, Peters anomaly may be associated with other systemic abnormalities in a third of patients, warranting referral to pediatrics for workup.

Elbaz U, Ali A, Strungaru H, Mireskandari K. Phenotypic spectrum of Peters anomaly: implications for management. *Cornea.* 2022;41(2):192–200.

Khan AO, Al-Katan H, Al-Gehedan S, Al-Rashed W. Bilateral congenital stromal cyst of the cornea. *J AAPOS.* 2007;11(4):400–401.

Sclerocornea

Sclerocornea (total corneal opacification) is a descriptive term for a congenitally opaque cornea resembling sclera (Fig 20-9). Because *sclerocornea* is a vague term that fails to suggest causation, its use should be avoided.

Congenital or Primary Congenital Glaucoma

In young children, glaucoma can cause the cornea to become edematous, cloudy, and enlarged (Fig 20-10). Breaks in Descemet membrane from glaucomatous enlargement are termed *Haab striae* (Fig 20-11A). See Chapter 21 in this volume and Chapter 11 of BCSC Section 10, *Glaucoma,* for further discussion.

Traumatic Breaks in Descemet Membrane

Breaks in Descemet membrane may be caused by forceps trauma during delivery. Other signs of trauma are frequently apparent on the neonate's head. Traumatic breaks are usually

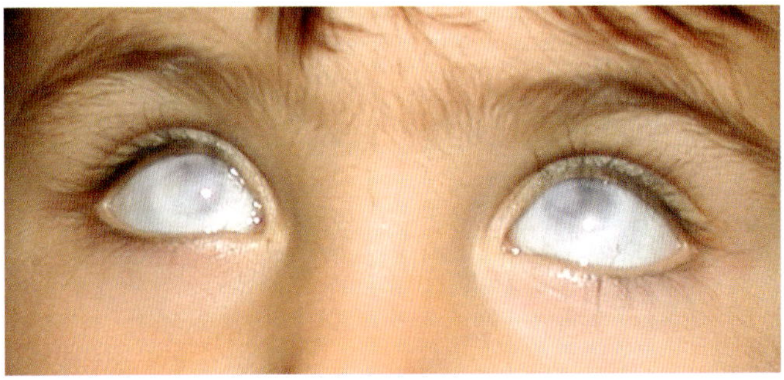

Figure 20-9 Bilateral severe congenital corneal opacity (terminology preferable to "sclerocornea"). *(Courtesy of Arif O. Khan, MD.)*

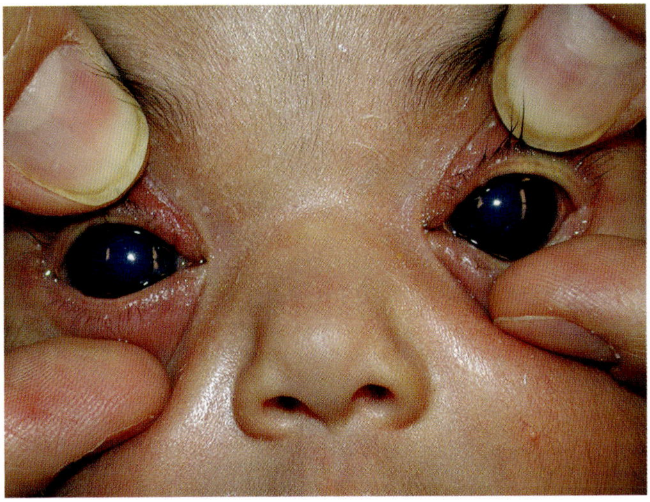

Figure 20-10 Primary congenital glaucoma. *(Reproduced with permission from Khan AO. Genetics of primary glaucoma.* Curr Opin Ophthalmol. *2011;22(5):347–355.)*

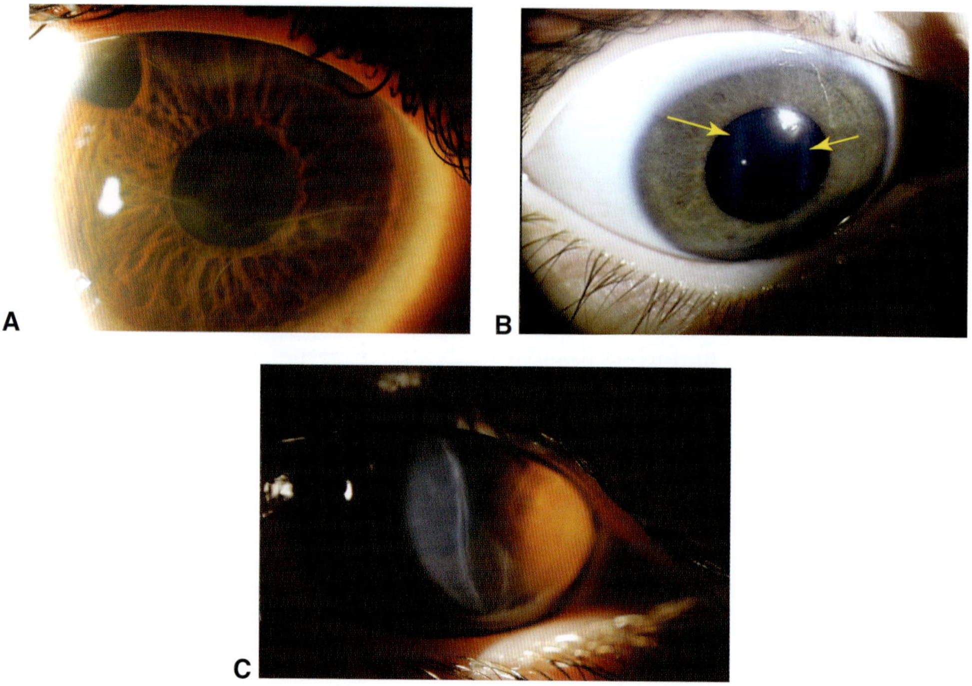

Figure 20-11 Breaks in Descemet membrane. **A,** Haab striae in an eye with congenital glaucoma. Note the curvilinear and horizontal orientation of the breaks in Descemet membrane. **B,** In contrast, the breaks in forceps injury are usually vertically oriented *(arrows).* **C,** Descemet tears resulting from minor trauma in a child with brittle cornea syndrome. *(Parts A and C courtesy of Arif O. Khan, MD; part B courtesy of Kamiar Mireskandari, MBChB, PhD.)*

vertical and linear (Fig 20-11B), unlike the curvilinear and often horizontal Haab striae of congenital glaucoma. Acute rupture leads to stromal and sometimes epithelial edema. Once edema regresses, the edges of the broken Descemet membrane are visible as ridges protruding slightly from the posterior corneal surface. Amblyopia may result from prolonged corneal opacity or, more commonly, from induced anisometropic astigmatism. In patients with brittle cornea syndrome, a disorder of corneal fragility (see previous discussion in this chapter), minor trauma may also cause traumatic breaks in Descemet membrane (Fig 20-11C).

Khan AO. Conditions that can be mistaken as early childhood glaucoma. *Ophthalmic Genet.* 2011;32(3):129–137.

Corneal Ulcers

Congenital corneal ulcers are rare and may be caused by herpes simplex keratitis or other infection (see Chapter 27).

Management of Corneal Opacities

When management options for corneal opacities are considered, the underlying pathology for the corneal opacities should be taken into account and the status of the posterior segment assessed. Important factors influencing management include the age of the child, location and density of the opacity, corneal diameter, IOP, refraction and status of the lens, and the iris. For dense corneal opacities, ultrasound biomicroscopy (UBM), anterior segment optical coherence tomography (AS-OCT), and A- and B-scan ultrasonography are needed to assess lens status, possible glaucoma, and the presence of posterior segment pathology.

The density and location of corneal opacity are critical in determining management options. A small central or paraxial opacity may potentially be managed using pupillary dilation (either pharmacologic or optical iridectomy) to create a new visual axis through an area of clear cornea (Fig 20-12). These patients generally do quite well, and the risks of transplantation are avoided. Similarly, pupillary management can bypass an associated small nuclear cataract or may be combined with lensectomy in patients with a dense cataract. See eFigure 20-1 online at www.aao.org/bcscsupplement_section06 for a management algorithm flowchart for corneal opacities.

When large dense opacities are present, early keratoplasty may be considered depending on the underlying cause:

- *Stromal opacity with endothelial dysfunction* (eg, severe Peters anomaly) requires penetrating keratoplasty (PKP).
- *Endothelial disease only* (eg, CHED, PPCD) requires selective replacement of endothelium. In younger children, Descemet stripping automated endothelial keratoplasty (DSAEK) and, in older children, Descemet membrane endothelial keratoplasty (DMEK) have been successful.
- *Stromal disease with healthy endothelium* (eg, mucopolysaccharidosis) requires deep anterior lamellar keratoplasty (DALK).
- *In unilateral cases of large dense opacities in children with poor prognosis for vision or many ocular and systemic comorbidities,* parents should be counseled regarding surgical intervention and potential for complications and multiple anesthesia exposures.

A

B

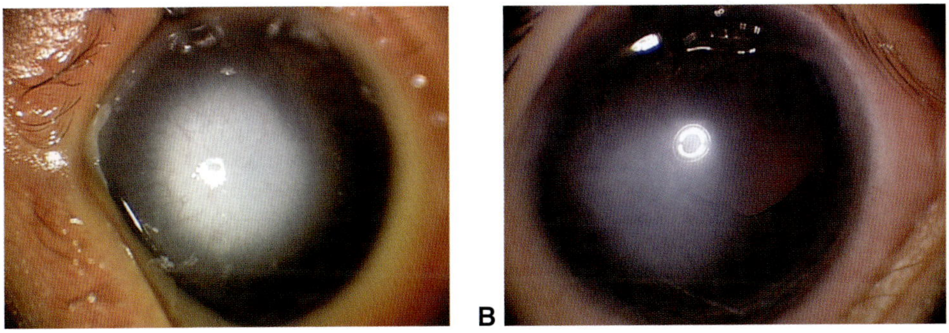

Figure 20-12 Corneal opacity managed with optical iridectomy. **A,** Peters anomaly type 1 in a 1-week-old neonate. A dense central and temporal opacity is surrounded by edema. Note the superficial vascularization, which is common. **B,** Same patient at 16 weeks old after optical iridectomy and division of iris adhesions at 10 weeks of age. Note that the density and extent of the opacity have decreased significantly, creating a paraxial area of clear cornea nasally to allow vision rehabilitation. *(Courtesy of Kamiar Mireskandari, MBChB, PhD.)*

Keratoplasty should be undertaken only when the family and the ophthalmologists involved in the child's care are prepared for the significant time commitment and effort needed to deal with complex postoperative management, which includes suture management, frequent eyedrop use, hospital visits (including examinations under anesthesia as needed), and the potential for corneal graft rejection, as well as with amblyopia management. The team should include ophthalmologists skilled in pediatric corneal surgery, pediatric glaucoma, and amblyopia. Contact lens expertise is also important for the care of infants with small eyes and large refractive errors.

Ashar JN, Ramappa M, Vaddavalli PK. Paired-eye comparison of Descemet's stripping endothelial keratoplasty and penetrating keratoplasty in children with congenital hereditary endothelial dystrophy. *Br J Ophthalmol.* 2013;97(10):1247–1249.

Elbaz U, Kirwan C, Shen C, Ali A. Avoiding big bubble complications: outcomes of layer-by-layer deep anterior lamellar keratoplasty in children. *Br J Ophthalmol.* 2018;102(8):1103–1108.

Elbaz U, Strungaru H, Mireskandari K, Stephens D, Ali A. Long-term visual outcomes and clinical course of patients with Peters anomaly. *Cornea.* 2021;40(7):822–830.

Mireskandari K, Tehrani NN, Vandenhoven C, Ali A. Anterior segment imaging in pediatric ophthalmology. *J Cataract Refract Surg.* 2011;37(12):2201–2210.

Congenital and Developmental Anomalies of the Globe

Microphthalmia, Anophthalmia, and Coloboma

Microphthalmia, anophthalmia, and coloboma (MAC) represent a spectrum of diseases that may be isolated or syndromic. They have been associated with mutations in numerous genes, including *CHX10, MAF, PAX6, PAX2, RAX, SHH, SIX3,* and *SOX2.*

In affected patients, early prosthetic fitting may induce orbital growth (volume deficiency may limit growth), prevent forniceal shrinkage, and improve cosmesis.

Microphthalmia

Microphthalmia is a small, disorganized globe that may be associated with cystic outpouching of the posteroinferior sclera.

Anophthalmia

Anophthalmia is the absence of any ocular globe tissue (see Chapter 17). It is very rare; often, when anophthalmia is clinically suspected, the child actually has severe microphthalmia.

Coloboma

Coloboma is the most common of the MAC spectrum disorders and results from failure of the embryonic fissure to close in the fifth week of gestation. In its least severe manifestation, coloboma typically presents as an inferonasal gap in the iris (Fig 20-13A). Chorioretinal and/or optic nerve involvement is seen in more severe forms (Fig 20-13B).

Nanophthalmos

Nanophthalmos is a small eye, typically with an axial length of 18 mm or less and with associated high hyperopia. The cornea is abnormally steep in the recessive form, distinguishing

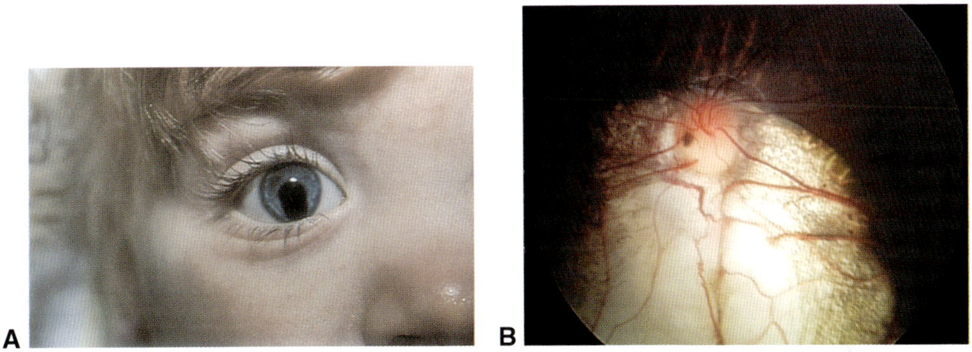

Figure 20-13 Coloboma. **A,** Typical iris coloboma, right eye. **B,** Large chorioretinal coloboma of the left eye. Note involvement of the optic nerve head; however, superior neuroretinal rim is usually present. *(Part B courtesy of Kamiar Mireskandari, MBChB, PhD.)*

it from ordinary hyperopia. The lens-to-eye ratio is high, with a shallow anterior chamber and risk for later angle-closure glaucoma. Another distinguishing feature is a characteristic papillomacular fold. The phenotype may result from biallelic mutations in *PRSS56* or *MFRP* or from heterozygous mutations in *TMEM98*. When the anterior segment is of grossly normal depth, the phenotype is termed *posterior microphthalmos*.

Nowilaty SR, Khan AO, Aldahmesh MA, Tabbara KF, Al-Amri A, Alkuraya FS. Biometric and molecular characterization of clinically diagnosed posterior microphthalmos. *Am J Ophthalmol.* 2013;155(2):361–372.e7.

Congenital and Developmental Anomalies of the Iris or Pupil

Persistent Pupillary Membrane

Persistent pupillary membrane (Fig 20-14) is the most common developmental abnormality of the iris. Persistent pupillary membranes are visually significant only in rare cases. If especially prominent, they can adhere to the anterior lens capsule, causing a small anterior polar cataract. They may also be associated with other anterior segment abnormalities.

Iris Hypoplasia

Iris hypoplasia refers to an underdeveloped iris stroma. It may be focal (iris coloboma) or diffuse (aniridia). If only the posterior pigment epithelium is underdeveloped, iris transillumination occurs.

Iris transillumination

Iris transillumination is a clinical sign due to reduced pigment in the posterior epithelial layers or from iris hypoplasia. It may be seen in albinism, Axenfeld-Rieger syndrome, Marfan syndrome, Prader-Willi syndrome, ectopia lentis et pupillae, and X-linked megalocornea. Patchy areas of transillumination may also be seen after trauma, surgery, or

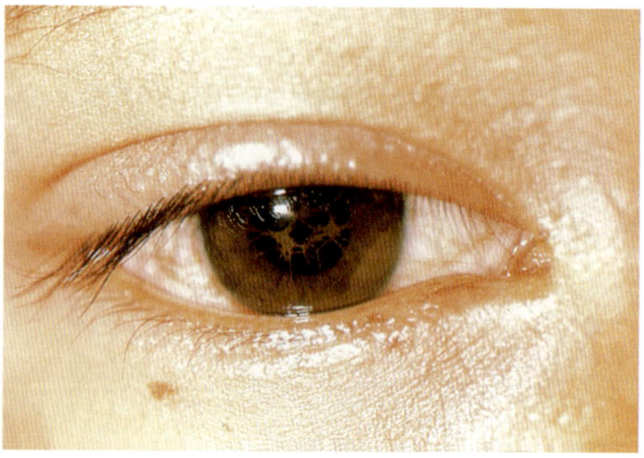

Figure 20-14 Persistent pupillary membrane. The patient's uncorrected visual acuity was 20/40.

uveitis. Scattered iris transillumination defects may be a normal variant in individuals with very lightly pigmented irides.

Axenfeld-Rieger syndrome

Axenfeld-Rieger syndrome (ARS) is the most common cause of iris (stromal) hypoplasia. ARS is a spectrum disorder that shows phenotypic and genetic heterogeneity. Conditions previously considered distinct—such as Axenfeld anomaly, Rieger anomaly or syndrome, iridogoniodysgenesis anomaly or syndrome, iris hypoplasia, and familial glaucoma iridogoniodysplasia—are now recognized as part of the spectrum of ARS.

Characteristic findings of ARS include posterior embryotoxon with attached iris strands and iris hypoplasia (Fig 20-15). Patients with ARS have a 50% lifetime risk of glaucoma. The features of ARS range from a smooth, cryptless iris surface to a phenotype that mimics aniridia. Examples include mild stromal thinning, marked atrophy with hole formation, corectopia, and ectropion uveae. Buphthalmos (secondary to glaucoma) or microcornea may also be present. Associated nonocular abnormalities include abnormal teeth, distinct facies, redundant periumbilical skin, hypospadias, cardiac valve abnormalities, and pituitary abnormalities. Heterozygous mutations in *PITX2* or *FOXC1*, homeobox genes that regulate other ocular developmental genes, are the most common identifiable cause of this syndrome.

Iris coloboma

In patients with a typical inferonasal iris coloboma, the pupil is shaped like a classic incandescent light bulb, keyhole, or inverted teardrop (see Fig 20-13A). Typical colobomas may also involve the ciliary body, choroid, retina, or optic nerve and are part of the MAC spectrum (discussed previously in this chapter). Parents of an affected child may have small, previously undetected chorioretinal or iris defects in an inferonasal location; thus, careful examination of family members is indicated.

Atypical iris colobomas occur in areas other than the inferonasal quadrant and are not usually associated with posterior uveal colobomas. Lens colobomas have been described; however, this is a misnomer, as these abnormalities represent loss of zonules in an area of a ciliary body coloboma, causing flattening of the lens equator in that area.

A 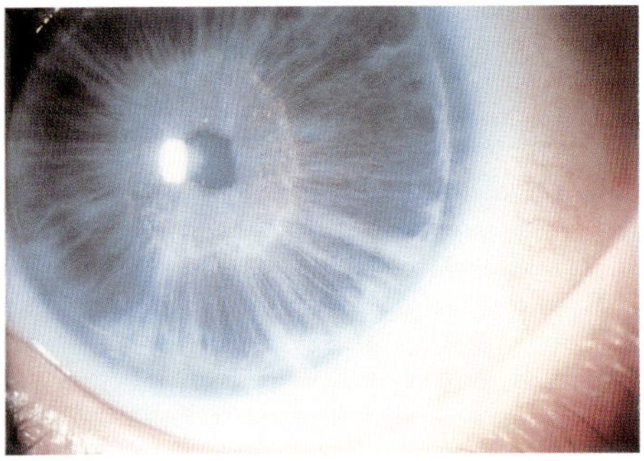 B 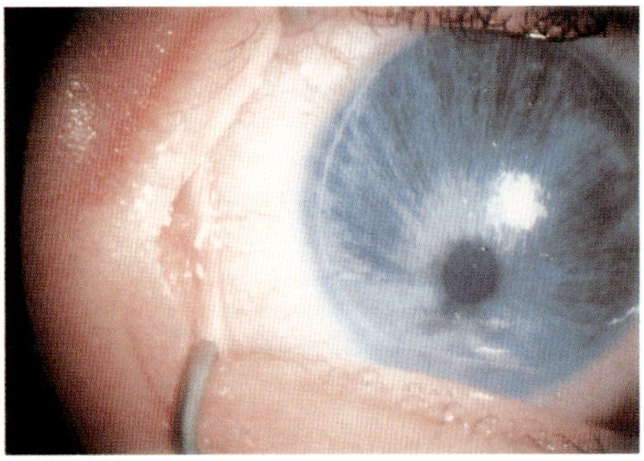

C 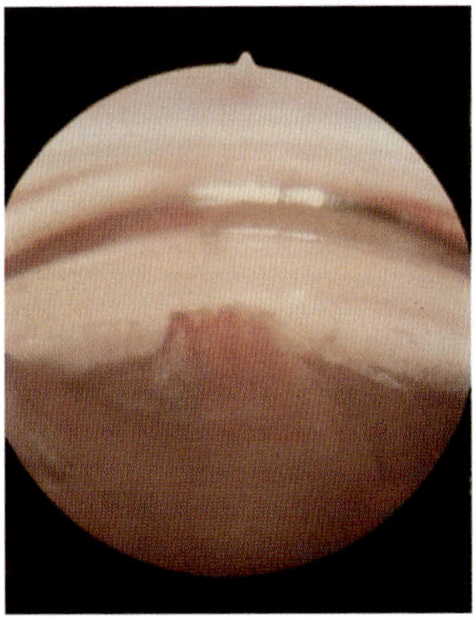

Figure 20-15 Axenfeld-Rieger syndrome (ARS). **A,** Iris hypoplasia and posterior embryotoxon. **B,** Note that the pupil may be displaced or distorted in ARS owing to adhesions to posterior embryotoxon. **C,** Gonioscopic view in ARS shows iris adhesions to posterior embryotoxon. *(Part A courtesy of Jane D. Kivlin, MD.)*

Aniridia

Classic *aniridia* is a panocular bilateral disorder. The degree of iris formation ranges from almost total absence to only mild hypoplasia, overlapping with ARS. The abnormality typically presents with nystagmus in infants, who appear to have absent irides or dilated, unresponsive pupils (Fig 20-16). Examination findings commonly include anterior polar or pyramidal lens opacities, at times with attached strands of persistent pupillary membranes. Foveal hypoplasia is usually present, with visual acuity often less than 20/100. Glaucoma, typically juvenile, and optic nerve hypoplasia are also common. Keratopathy often develops later in childhood and may lead to progressive deterioration of visual acuity. The corneal abnormality is due to a stem cell deficiency; therefore, keratolimbal allograft stem cell transplantation may be required in severe cases.

Heterozygous *PAX6* gene mutations (11p13) cause classic aniridia, particularly nonsense mutations (haploinsufficiency). Missense mutations are more likely associated with variable expressivity and partial phenotypes. Most children with aniridia (approximately two-thirds) have the familial form of the disorder. The *PAX6* gene is a homeotic gene

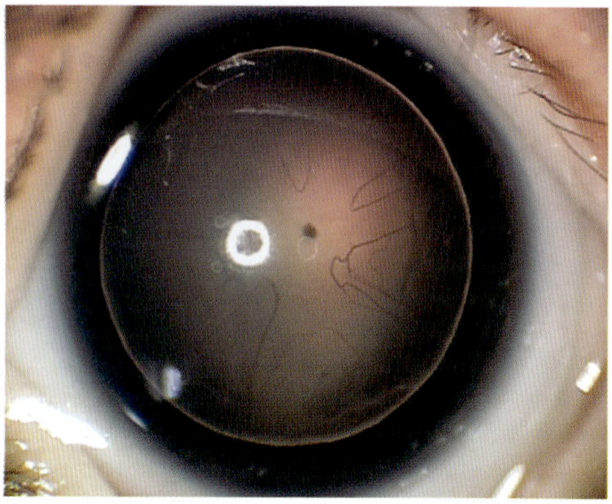

Figure 20-16 Clinical photograph of aniridia in a newborn girl shows minimal iris stump nasally, an anterior polar cataract, and residual vessels from tunica vasculosa lentis. The vessels regressed over a few months. *(Courtesy of Kamiar Mireskandari, MBChB, PhD.)*

controlling eye morphogenesis; it is involved in complex interactions among the optic cup, surface ectoderm, and neural crest during formation of the iris and other ocular structures.

Approximately one-third of aniridia cases result from new deletions that, if large enough, may also affect the contiguous *WT1* gene (a contiguous gene syndrome); affected patients are therefore at risk for Wilms tumor (nephroblastoma) before 5 years of age. This phenotype represents part of WAGR syndrome (ie, *W*ilms tumor, *a*niridia, *g*enitourinary malformations, and mental *r*etardation). All children with sporadic aniridia should undergo chromosomal deletion analysis of 11p13 to exclude increased risk of Wilms tumor. Abdominal ultrasonography is performed to look for kidney tumors while waiting for genetic results. Familial aniridia does not carry a significant risk, although there have been rare reports of Wilms tumor associated with familial aniridia.

Congenital Iris Ectropion

Ectropion of the posterior pigment epithelium onto the anterior surface of the iris is referred to as *ectropion uveae,* but this is a misnomer because posterior iris epithelium is derived from neural ectoderm and is not considered part of the uvea. Congenital iris ectropion may occur as an acquired tractional abnormality, often associated with rubeosis iridis, or as a congenital nonprogressive abnormality, which may be associated with later glaucoma. It may occur in patients with neurofibromatosis, facial hemihypertrophy, or Prader-Willi syndrome. *Congenital iris ectropion syndrome* is a constellation of unilateral congenital iris ectropion, a glassy-smooth cryptless iris surface, a high iris insertion, dysgenesis of the drainage angle, and glaucoma risk, often with ptosis.

Dyscoria

Dyscoria is an abnormal pupil shape, typically resulting from congenital malformation such as Axenfeld-Rieger syndrome.

Congenital Miosis

Congenital miosis (microcoria) may represent an absence or malformation of the dilator pupillae muscle. It can also occur secondary to contracture of fibrous material on the pupil margin owing to remnants of the tunica vasculosa lentis or neural crest cell anomalies. In affected patients, the pupil rarely exceeds 2 mm in diameter, is often eccentric, and reacts poorly to mydriatic drops. Severe cases require pupilloplasty. *Ectopia lentis et pupillae* refers to eccentric microcoria with lens subluxation (see the section Corectopia).

Congenital Mydriasis

Many cases of *congenital mydriasis (iridoplegia)* fall within the aniridia spectrum, especially if the central iris structures—from the collarette to the pupillary sphincter—are absent. The disorder may also be associated with congenital cardiovascular defects in patients with heterozygous *ACTA2* mutation, which sometimes causes an alternate phenotype of prominent iris flocculi (discussed in the section "Cysts," later in this chapter), rather than iridoplegia. Other causes include iris sphincter trauma, pharmacologic mydriasis, and acquired neurologic disease that affects parasympathetic innervation.

Corectopia

Normally, the pupil is located approximately 0.5 mm inferonasally from the center of the iris. Minor deviations of up to 1.0 mm are usually cosmetically insignificant and are not considered abnormal; displacement greater than this is considered *corectopia.* Sector iris hypoplasia or other colobomatous lesions can lead to corectopia. Vision can be good despite corectopia.

Isolated noncolobomatous, autosomal dominant corectopia has been reported. Progressive corectopia may be associated with ARS or, in adults, with iridocorneal endothelial (ICE) syndrome.

Ectopia lentis et pupillae is corectopia associated with lens subluxation. It is often due to biallelic *ADAMTS4* mutations. With this disorder, pupils and lenses are displaced in opposite directions. The pupils may be very small and misshapen, and they often dilate poorly (see Chapter 22).

Polycoria and Pseudopolycoria

True *polycoria* (in which each pupil has a sphincter mechanism) is very rare. Most accessory iris openings are *pseudopolycoria.* These iris holes may be congenital or may develop in response to progressive corectopia and iris hypoplasia in ARS (Fig 20-17) or, in adults, in ICE syndrome. Pseudopolycoria may also result from trauma, surgery, or persistent pupillary membranes.

Acquired Corneal Conditions

Keratitis

Keratitis may be epithelial, stromal, peripheral, or, in rare cases, endothelial. See BCSC Section 8, *External Disease and Cornea,* for further details.

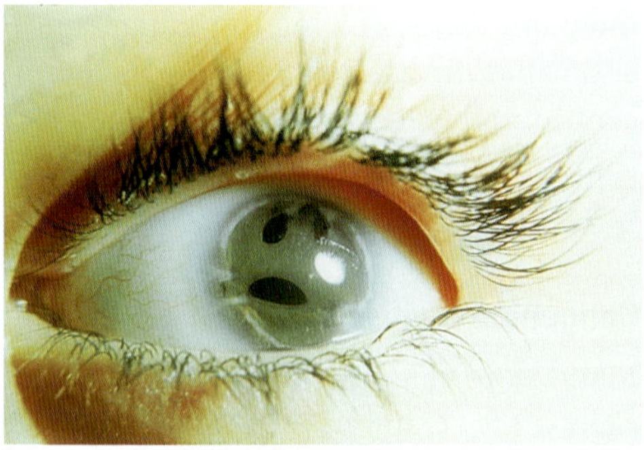

Figure 20-17 Pseudopolycoria secondary to ARS. *(Courtesy of John W. Simon, MD.)*

Infectious causes

Syphilis Interstitial keratitis may occur in the first decade of life secondary to congenital syphilis (discussed in Chapter 27). The keratitis presents as a rapidly progressive corneal edema followed by abnormal vascularization in the deep stroma adjacent to Descemet membrane. Intense vascularization may give the cornea a salmon-pink color—hence the term *salmon patch.* Blood flow through these vessels gradually ceases over several weeks to several months, leaving empty "ghost" vessels in the corneal stroma. Immune-mediated uveitis, arthritis, and hearing loss may also develop and may recur even after treatment of syphilis. Immunosuppression may be necessary to diminish sequelae.

Herpes simplex infection Herpes simplex virus (HSV) infections of the cornea are discussed in BCSC Section 8, *External Disease and Cornea.* Congenital HSV infection is discussed in Chapter 27.

Adenovirus infection Punctate epithelial keratitis is most often seen after adenoviral infection; it is due to subepithelial immune complex deposition. See BCSC Section 8, *External Disease and Cornea,* for further discussion.

Noninfectious causes

Punctate epithelial erosions are most commonly seen in patients with lagophthalmos or dry eye disease. Peripheral (marginal) keratitis is usually associated with blepharokeratoconjunctivitis secondary to meibomian gland disease; however, in children central involvement may occur with resultant visual impairment (see Chapter 19).

Thygeson superficial punctate keratitis The etiology of *Thygeson superficial punctate keratitis* is unclear, but it is thought to be immune mediated. It can occur in children and presents with tearing, photophobia, and reduced vision. The condition is bilateral but often asymmetric. Characteristic features include slightly elevated white-gray corneal epithelial lesions with negative staining. It is treated with mild corticosteroids (eg, fluorometholone 0.1%) or topical cyclosporine.

Cogan syndrome This syndrome is a rare vasculitis that presents with ocular, audiovestibular, and systemic features. Interstitial keratitis, uveitis, conjunctivitis, episcleritis, or a combination of these features may be seen.

Keratoconus

Keratoconus is noninflammatory, progressive thinning and bulging of the central or paracentral cornea leading to increasing myopic astigmatism and abnormal retinoscopy reflex (ie, scissoring). It may present and progress during adolescence and is often familial. Keratoconus is more common with chronic eye rubbing and hence is seen in atopic diseases, Leber congenital amaurosis, and Down syndrome. Iron lines (Fleischer rings), stress lines (Vogt striae), and apical scarring are often noted. Tears in Descemet membrane may occur and cause acute corneal edema (hydrops).

Keratoconus is more aggressive with faster progression in children than in adults. However, keratoconus is amenable to preventive treatment using corneal collagen cross-linking (CXL). Therefore, early detection of at-risk populations and the CXL procedure may prevent progression and improve uncorrected and best corrected visual acuity. It will likely reduce the need for keratoplasty in the patient's lifetime as well. Therefore, children with increasing astigmatism and reduced best corrected visual acuity should be screened with corneal tomography to detect keratoconus early.

Fard AM, Reynolds AL, Lillvis JH, Nader ND. Corneal collagen cross-linking in pediatric keratoconus with three protocols: a systematic review and meta-analysis. *J AAPOS.* 2020;24(6):331–336.

Systemic Diseases Affecting the Cornea or Iris

Metabolic Disorders Affecting the Cornea or Iris

See also Chapter 27, Ocular Manifestations of Systemic Disease, and Table 27-2.

Mucopolysaccharidosis

Mucopolysaccharidosis (MPS) comprises a group of lysosomal storage diseases. MPS I is divided into 2 subtypes, severe MPS I and attenuated MPS I. Ocular manifestations may include corneal haze from incompletely degraded glycosaminoglycan. Corneal haze may be present in early life in both types of MPS I. Treatment options for significant opacities include DALK, as the endothelium is usually healthy, or PKP. Bone marrow transplant and enzyme replacement therapy are available for certain forms of these lysosomal storage diseases and can affect vision prognoses. See BCSC Section 8, *External Disease and Cornea,* for further discussion.

Cystinosis

Cystinosis is caused by biallelic *CTNS* mutations. The infantile form includes failure to thrive, rickets, and progressive renal failure, resulting in Fanconi syndrome.

Iridescent, elongated corneal crystals appear at approximately age 1 year, first in the peripheral cornea and the anterior stroma. Crystals also present in the uvea and on the surface of the iris. Corneal crystals result in severe photophobia. There are reports of angle-closure glaucoma secondary to crystal deposition in the ciliary body.

Oral cysteamine alleviates systemic problems but not the corneal crystal deposition. Topical cysteamine can reduce corneal crystal deposition but requires frequent application, may be difficult to obtain, and has an unpleasant odor. Newer, more viscous preparations with less frequent dosing may improve adherence.

Tyrosinemia type II

Tyrosinemia type II (Richner-Hanhart syndrome) results from biallelic *TAT* mutations and is associated with photophobia, pseudodendritic epitheliopathy on the cornea, and ulceration on the palms and soles. Systemic problems include liver and kidney dysfunction. Dietary restriction of phenylalanine and tyrosine is the mainstay of treatment.

Wilson disease

In *Wilson disease (hepatolenticular degeneration),* there is excess copper deposition in the liver, kidneys, and basal ganglia of the brain, leading to cirrhosis, renal tubular damage, and a Parkinson-like disorder of motor function. The phenotype results from biallelic *ATP7B* mutations. The characteristic Kayser-Fleischer ring—a golden-brown, ruby-red, or green pigment ring consisting of copper deposits—is limited to peripheral Descemet membrane, may be several millimeters in width, and may resolve with treatment. Laboratory tests for serum copper and ceruloplasmin are better than an eye examination for early diagnosis because the ring may develop late.

Fabry disease

Fabry disease is an X-linked lysosomal storage disease with variable systemic manifestations. It is due to α-galactosidase deficiency (hemizygous *GLA* mutations). Vortex keratopathy (verticillata) can be seen in affected males and in female carriers.

Schnyder corneal dystrophy

Schnyder corneal dystrophy is a predominantly local disorder of corneal lipid metabolism arising from biallelic *UBIAD1* mutations. Although crystalline keratopathy is characteristic, stromal haze without crystals is a common presentation.

Other Systemic Diseases Affecting the Cornea or Iris

Familial dysautonomia

Familial dysautonomia (Riley-Day syndrome) is a disorder of autonomic dysfunction characterized by relative insensitivity to pain, temperature instability, and absence of the fungiform papillae of the tongue. The phenotype occurs largely in children of Eastern European Jewish (Ashkenazi) descent and results from biallelic *IKBKAP* mutations. Failure to respond with a wheal and flare to intradermal injection of 1:1000 histamine solution is characteristic. Exposure keratopathy and neurotrophic corneal ulcers with secondary opacification are frequent. Treatment includes artificial tears and tarsorrhaphy.

Waardenburg syndrome

Waardenburg syndrome is a rare neurocristopathy characterized by Hirschsprung disease; deafness; and depigmentation of hair (a white forelock), skin, and iris. Other ophthalmic findings include telecanthus and dystopia canthorum (see Chapter 16).

Tumors of the Anterior Segment

Cornea

Tumors of the cornea are extremely rare in children, but squamous cell carcinomas have been reported in cases of xeroderma pigmentosum. See BCSC Section 8, *External Disease and Cornea,* for further details.

Iris

Nodules

Lisch nodules *Lisch nodules* occur in patients with neurofibromatosis and are discussed in Chapter 27.

Juvenile xanthogranuloma *Juvenile xanthogranuloma* is a nonneoplastic histiocytic proliferation that typically develops in infants younger than 2 years. It is characterized by the presence of Touton giant cells. Skin involvement—consisting of one or more small, round, orange or tan papules—is usually but not always present. Iris lesions are relatively rare and virtually always unilateral. The fleshy, yellow-brown masses may be small and localized or may diffusely infiltrate the entire iris, resulting in heterochromia. Spontaneous bleeding with hyphema is a characteristic clinical presentation. Secondary glaucoma may cause acute pain, photophobia, and vision loss. Those at greatest risk for ocular involvement are children with multiple skin lesions.

Juvenile xanthogranuloma is a self-limited condition that usually regresses spontaneously by age 5 years; however, to avoid complications, treatment is indicated for ocular involvement. Topical corticosteroids and pharmacologic agents to lower IOP, given as necessary, are generally sufficient to control the problem. Surgical excision or radiation may be considered when intractable glaucoma is present.

Iris mammillations *Iris mammillations* may be unilateral or bilateral. They appear as numerous tiny, diffuse, pigmented nodules on the surface of the iris (Fig 20-18). They are

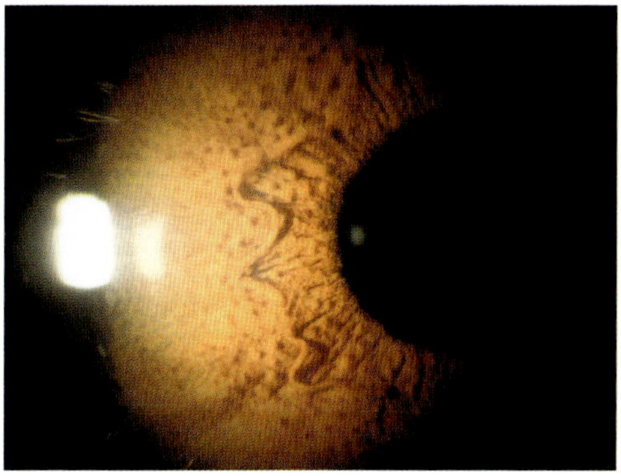

Figure 20-18 Iris mammillations. The nodules are diffuse and are the same color as the iris (Lisch nodules, by contrast, are lighter or darker than the surrounding iris). *(Courtesy of Arlene Drack, MD.)*

more common in darkly pigmented eyes and are usually the same color as the iris. These nodules may be bilateral, autosomal dominant, and isolated, or they may be associated with oculodermal melanocytosis or phakomatosis pigmentovascularis type IIb (nevus flammeus with persistent, aberrant mongolian spots). Iris mammillations have also been reported in cases of ciliary body tumor and choroidal melanoma. They can be differentiated from Lisch nodules, as mammillations are usually dark brown, smooth, uniformly distributed, and equal in size or slightly larger near the pupil. The incidence of iris mammillations is higher among patients with neurofibromatosis type 1.

Brushfield spots Focal areas of iris stromal hyperplasia surrounded by relative hypoplasia occur in up to 90% of patients with Down syndrome; these lesions are known as *Brushfield spots.* Similar lesions, known as *Wolfflin nodules,* occur in up to 24% of healthy individuals. Neither condition is visually significant.

Cysts

Primary iris cysts These cysts may originate from the iris pigment epithelium or the iris stroma.

CYSTS OF IRIS PIGMENT EPITHELIUM Spontaneous cysts of the iris pigment epithelium result from a separation of the 2 layers of epithelium anywhere between the pupil and ciliary body. These cysts tend to be stable and rarely cause ocular complications. They are usually not diagnosed until the teenage years.

CENTRAL CYSTS Pigment epithelial cysts at the pupillary border, also termed *iris flocculi,* are sometimes hereditary (Fig 20-19). In rare cases, they may be due to an *ACTA2* mutation (see the section Congenital Mydriasis). They are usually diagnosed in infancy. The cysts may enlarge slowly but generally remain asymptomatic and rarely require treatment. Cholinesterase-inhibiting eyedrops such as echothiophate may produce similar pupillary cysts, especially in young phakic eyes. Discontinuation of the drug or concomitant administration of phenylephrine generally results in improvement.

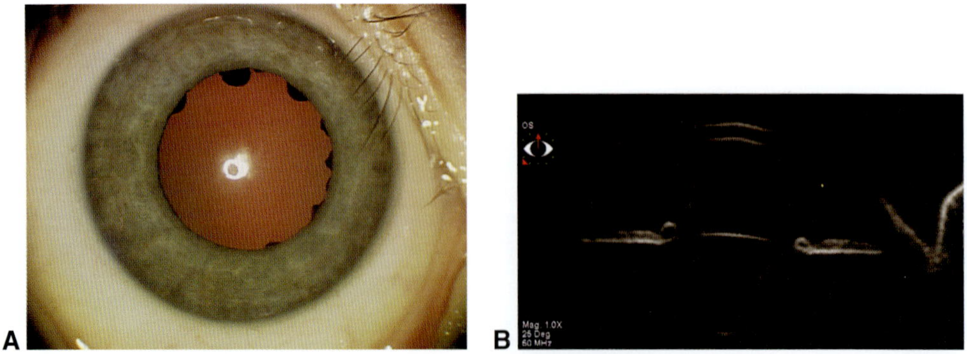

Figure 20-19 Pigment epithelial cysts at the pupillary border (flocculi). **A,** Multiple cysts are seen against the red reflex. **B,** UBM shows the cystic nature of the flocculi. *(Courtesy of Kamiar Mireskandari, MBChB, PhD.)*

CYSTS OF IRIS STROMA Primary iris stromal cysts are often diagnosed in infancy. They are most likely caused by sequestration of epithelium during embryologic development. The epithelium-lined stromal cysts usually contain goblet cells, and they may enlarge, causing obstruction of the visual axis, glaucoma, corneal decompensation, or anterior uveitis from cyst leakage.

Numerous treatments have been described, including cyst aspiration and photocoagulation or photodisruption, but the sudden release of cystic contents may result in transient anterior uveitis and glaucoma. Because of these potential complications and frequent cyst recurrence, surgical excision may be the preferred treatment method. Iris stromal cysts account for approximately 16% of childhood iris cysts. The visual prognosis may be guarded.

Secondary iris cysts Secondary iris cysts have been reported in childhood after trauma; they are also associated with tumors and iris nevi.

Ciliary Body

Medulloepithelioma

A *medulloepithelioma* originates from the nonpigmented epithelium of the ciliary body. It often presents in the first decade of life as secondary glaucoma, hyphema, ectopia lentis, sectoral cataract (Fig 20-20), or an iris mass. This rare lesion shows a spectrum of clinical and pathologic characteristics, ranging from benign to malignant. Teratoid elements are often present. Although distant metastasis is rare, local invasion may lead to death. Small lesions are amenable to cryotherapy, plaque radiotherapy, or partial lamellar sclerouviectomy. Use of intra-arterial and intravitreal chemotherapy has also been reported. Enucleation is required for larger lesions and is curative if extraocular spread has not occurred.

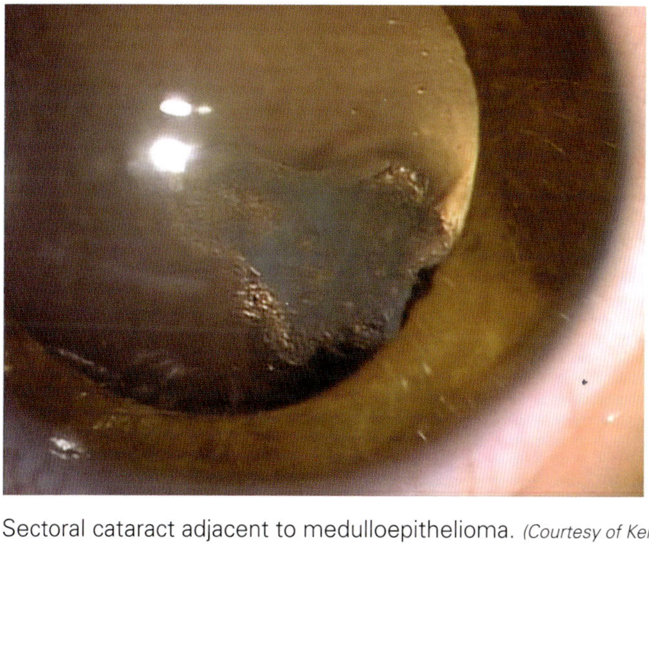

Figure 20-20 Sectoral cataract adjacent to medulloepithelioma. *(Courtesy of Ken K. Nischal, MD.)*

Miscellaneous Clinical Signs

Pediatric Iris Heterochromia

The differential diagnosis of pediatric iris heterochromia is extensive. Causes can be classified according to whether the condition is congenital or acquired and whether the affected eye is hypopigmented or hyperpigmented (Fig 20-21). Trauma, chronic iridocyclitis, intraocular surgery, and use of topical prostaglandin analogues are important causes of acquired hyperpigmented heterochromia. Whether congenital or acquired, hypopigmented heterochromia that is associated with a more miotic pupil and ptosis on the ipsilateral side should prompt a workup for Horner syndrome.

Anisocoria

Inequality in the diameters of the 2 pupils is called *anisocoria.* For a detailed discussion of anisocoria and a diagnostic flowchart for the following conditions, see BCSC Section 5, *Neuro-Ophthalmology.*

Physiologic anisocoria

Physiologic anisocoria is a common cause of a difference in size between the 2 pupils. This difference is usually less than 1 mm and may vary from day to day in an individual. The inequality does not change significantly when the patient is in dim light or bright light.

Tonic pupil

Features of a unilateral tonic pupil include anisocoria that is greater in bright light than in dim light and a pupil that is sluggishly and segmentally responsive to light and is more responsive to near effort. Greater-than-normal constriction in response to dilute pilocarpine is diagnostic. In children, possible causes include varicella-zoster virus infection and Adie syndrome with absence of deep tendon reflexes.

Horner syndrome

See BCSC Section 5, *Neuro-Ophthalmology,* for additional discussion of Horner syndrome.

A lesion at any location along the oculosympathetic pathway may lead to *Horner syndrome.* Affected patients have anisocoria that is greater in dim light and ptosis secondary to paralysis of the Müller muscle. Congenital cases may be associated with iris heterochromia

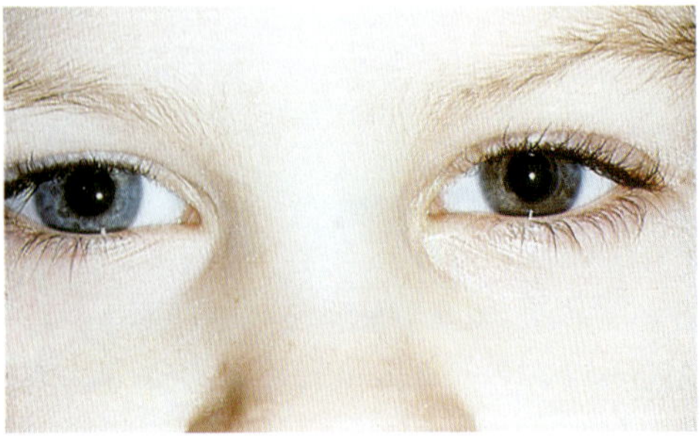

Figure 20-21 Iris heterochromia. The left iris has become darker as a result of trauma. *(Courtesy of John W. Simon, MD.)*

in which the affected iris is lighter in color. However, the heterochromia may not be present in infants because the normal iris needs time to acquire pigment.

The diagnosis of Horner syndrome can be confirmed with the use of topical cocaine or apraclonidine eyedrops. Apraclonidine reverses the anisocoria, causing dilation of the affected (smaller) pupil and having no effect on the normal pupil. However, this agent should be used with caution in young children, as it may cause excessive sedation owing to its central nervous system effects. Additional pharmacologic testing may not be necessary in the presence of typical clinical findings.

In children, Horner syndrome may be idiopathic or may be caused by trauma, surgery, or the presence of neuroblastoma affecting the sympathetic chain in the chest. For children with acquired Horner syndrome but no history of trauma or surgery that could explain the anisocoria, evaluation should include imaging studies of the brain, neck, and chest. The value of measuring catecholamine excretion has been questioned because some patients with normal catecholamine measurements have been found to have neuroblastomas.

CHAPTER 21

Childhood Glaucomas

This chapter includes related videos. Go to www.aao.org/bcscvideo_section06 or scan the QR codes in the text to access this content.

Highlights

- In neonates and infants, glaucoma is a panocular disease, whereas in older children, it is predominantly a chronic, progressive optic neuropathy.
- The diagnosis of childhood glaucoma is made based on many factors, not solely on increased measured intraocular pressure.
- Prompt surgery may be required in young patients, patients with severe glaucomatous damage on presentation, and those with unreliable adherence with medical therapy and/or long-term follow-up.

Introduction

Childhood glaucomas may result from an isolated developmental abnormality of the aqueous outflow pathways (primary glaucoma), or it may occur in individuals with other acquired or nonacquired conditions (secondary glaucoma). A variety of systemic conditions are associated with childhood glaucoma. See BCSC Section 10, *Glaucoma,* for additional discussion of topics covered in this chapter.

Classification and Natural History

In 2013, an international classification system for childhood glaucoma was established by the Childhood Glaucoma Research Network and the World Glaucoma Association. The classification system defined *childhood glaucoma* as intraocular pressure (IOP)–related damage to the eye, as opposed to adult-onset glaucoma, which results from IOP-related damage to the optic nerve. Table 21-1 summarizes this classification, and Figure 21-1 presents an algorithm for classifying a patient with childhood glaucoma using this system.

In cases of primary congenital glaucoma that result from gene mutation, the most common mutations found are biallelic *CYP1B1* mutations, particularly in certain regions of the Middle East. Many cases in the United States do not have an identifiable gene mutation.

Table 21-1 Classification of Childhood Glaucoma

Primary childhood glaucoma
Primary congenital glaucoma
Neonatal onset (age 0–1 month)
Infantile onset (age 1–24 months)
Late onset or late recognized (age ≥24 months)
Juvenile open-angle glaucoma
Secondary childhood glaucoma
Glaucoma associated with nonacquired ocular anomalies
Glaucoma associated with nonacquired systemic disease or syndrome
Glaucoma associated with acquired condition
Glaucoma following cataract surgery

Information from Beck AD, Chang TCP, Freedman SF. Definition, classification, differential diagnosis. In: Weinreb RN, Grajewski AL, Papadopoulos M, Grigg J, Freedman S, eds. *Childhood Glaucoma.* Kugler Publications; 2013:3–10. *World Glaucoma Association Consensus Series—9.*

A detailed discussion of the genetics, incidence, pathophysiology, and clinical features of both primary and secondary childhood glaucomas can be found in Chapter 11 of BCSC Section 10, *Glaucoma.*

Untreated childhood glaucoma almost always progresses to blindness, although there are rare reports of spontaneous resolution. In infants and neonates with immature and distensible globes, the cornea enlarges and opacifies, and it may vascularize. The entire globe enlarges, leading to an "ox eye" appearance (buphthalmos), scleral thinning, and myopic chorioretinal changes. Zonular weakness can occur in extreme cases. Optic nerve damage progresses, leading to complete blindness. In older children with mature globes, the natural history of untreated glaucoma is similar to that of adult-onset glaucoma. Progressive glaucomatous optic neuropathy is associated with visual field defects, fixation loss, and eventually loss of light perception vision without significant alteration of the rest of the globe. Amblyopia is the major cause of vision loss in children with glaucoma.

Beck AD, Chang TCP, Freedman SF. Definition, classification, differential diagnosis. In: Weinreb RN, Grajewski AL, Papadopoulos M, Grigg J, Freedman S, eds. *Childhood Glaucoma.* Kugler Publications; 2013:3–10. *World Glaucoma Association Consensus Series—9.*

Clinical Decisions in Childhood Glaucoma

Initial Evaluation

Children may present for a glaucoma evaluation due to signs/symptoms associated with glaucoma (Table 21-2), incidental findings suspicious of glaucoma (such as optic nerve head cupping in an asymptomatic child), a family history of primary childhood glaucoma, or a condition associated with a high risk of developing glaucoma (Table 21-3). The initial evaluation may involve 1 clinic visit, several clinic visits within a short period of time, or a combination of clinic visits and examinations under anesthesia

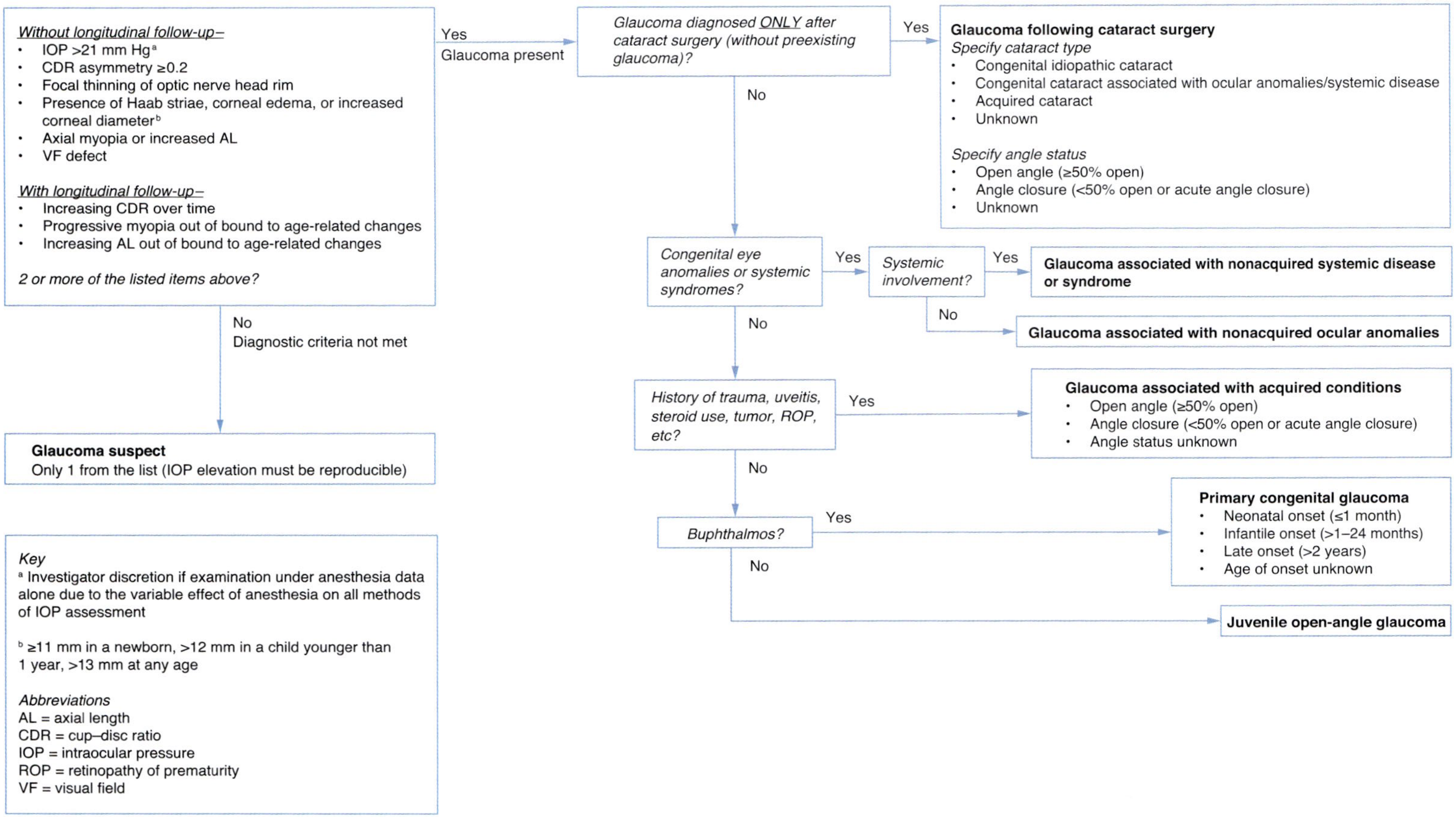

Figure 21-1 Modified Childhood Glaucoma Research Network/World Glaucoma Association algorithm for the classification of childhood glaucoma. *(Courtesy of Ta Chen Peter Chang, MD, on behalf of the Childhood Glaucoma Research Network (CGRN) and the Samuel & Ethel Balkan International Pediatric Glaucoma Center, Bascom Palmer Eye Institute, University of Miami.)*

Table 21-2 Differential Diagnosis of Signs in Childhood Glaucoma

Conditions sharing signs of epiphora and red eye
Conjunctivitis
Congenital nasolacrimal duct obstruction
Corneal epithelial defect/abrasion
Keratitis
Ocular inflammation (eg, due to uveitis, trauma, foreign body)
Epiblepharon with eyelash touch
Conditions sharing sign of corneal edema or opacification
Corneal dystrophies: congenital hereditary endothelial dystrophy, posterior polymorphous dystrophy
Obstetric birth trauma with Descemet tears
Storage diseases: mucopolysaccharidoses, cystinosis, sphingolipidosis
Congenital anomalies: congenital corneal opacification, Peters anomaly, choristomas
Keratitis (eg, secondary to maternal rubella, herpes, phlyctenules)
Keratomalacia (from vitamin A deficiency)
Skin disorders affecting the cornea: congenital ichthyosis, congenital dyskeratosis
Idiopathic (diagnosis of exclusion only)
Conditions sharing sign of corneal enlargement
Axial myopia
Megalocornea
Conditions sharing sign of optic nerve head cupping or rim thinning (real or apparent)
Physiologic optic nerve head cupping
Cupping associated with prematurity, periventricular leukomalacia
Optic nerve coloboma or pit
Optic atrophy
Optic nerve hypoplasia
Optic nerve malformation

Adapted with permission from Buckley EG. Primary congenital open-angle glaucoma. In: Epstein DL, Allingham RR, Schuman JS, eds. *Chandler and Grant's Glaucoma.* 4th ed. Lippincott Williams & Wilkins; 1987:598–608.

Table 21-3 Nonacquired Conditions Associated With Secondary Glaucoma

Ocular anomalies	Systemic disease or syndrome
Anterior segment abnormalities	Sturge-Weber syndrome (encephalofacial angiomatosis)
Aniridia	Neurofibromatosis type 1
Axenfeld-Rieger syndrome	Lowe (oculocerebrorenal) syndrome
Congenital corneal opacification	Lens-associated disorders
Congenital iris ectropion	Homocystinuria
Microcornea	Marfan syndrome
Microspherophakia	Weill-Marchesani syndrome
Primary congenital aphakia	
Peters anomaly	
Tumors of the iris	
Posterior segment abnormalities	
Familial exudative vitreoretinopathy	
Persistent fetal vasculature	
Retinopathy of prematurity	
Tumors of the retina or ciliary body	

(EUAs). During the initial evaluation for childhood glaucoma, the clinician's goals are as follows:

1. determine whether the child has manifest glaucoma or is a glaucoma suspect
2. decide on the appropriate therapy, if needed
3. obtain a comprehensive baseline assessment (including corneal diameter, IOP, central corneal thickness, axial lengths (ALs), and optic nerve head imaging) for future comparison
4. determine the interval and type of follow-up

Determine whether the child has manifest glaucoma or is a glaucoma suspect

In addition to the classification system, the Childhood Glaucoma Research Network and World Glaucoma Association have published a set of 9 diagnostic features for childhood glaucoma (see Fig 21-1):

1. IOP greater than 21 mm Hg (note: consider the variable effect of anesthesia if IOP was measured while patient was under anesthesia)
2. cup–disc ratio (CDR) asymmetry of 0.2 or greater
3. focal thinning of optic nerve head rim
4. presence of Haab striae (Fig 21-2), corneal edema, or an increased corneal diameter (≥11 mm in a newborn, >12 mm in a child younger than 1 year of age, >13 mm at any age; Fig 21-3)
5. axial myopia or increased AL compared to typical values for age group
6. reproducible visual field defect
7. increasing CDR over time
8. progressive myopia out of proportion to age-related changes over time
9. increasing AL out of proportion to age-related changes over time

If the patient has 2 or more of these features, a diagnosis of childhood glaucoma can be made. If the patient has only 1 of these features, the child is a glaucoma suspect. Because IOP may vary and is subject to measurement artifact, it is important to confirm IOP multiple times. Some diagnostic features, for example, elevated IOP and CDR asymmetry, can be determined

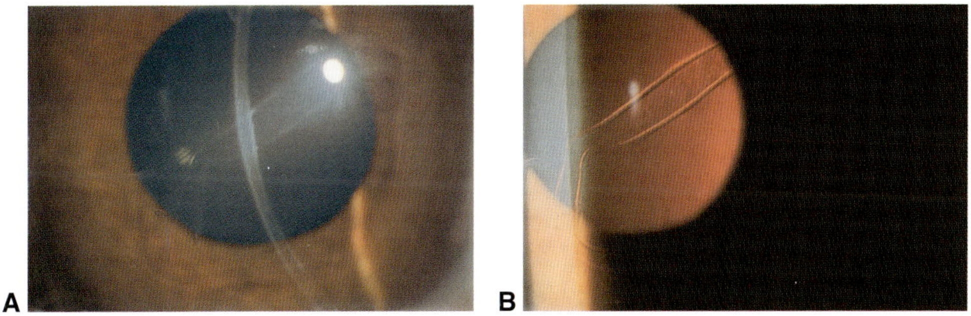

Figure 21-2 Haab striae in primary childhood glaucoma. **A,** Breaks in Descemet membrane (Haab striae), right eye. **B,** Retroillumination, same eye.

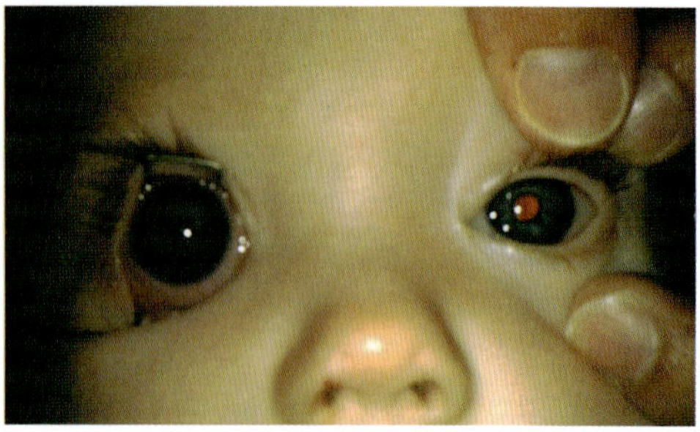

Figure 21-3 Unilateral congenital glaucoma, right eye. The cornea is enlarged compared to the unaffected left eye. *(Courtesy of Gregg T. Lueder, MD.)*

over 1 or 2 clinic visits. Others, such as increasing CDR, progressive myopia, and abnormally rapid globe growth (AL increase), require a longer follow-up interval to establish. If a child is not able to cooperate sufficiently for an office examination to confirm or rule out the diagnosis, an EUA should be considered. Techniques and details of examinations in the clinic and under anesthesia are discussed in detail in Chapter 11 of BCSC Section 10, *Glaucoma.*

Decide on the appropriate therapy, if needed

IOP-lowering therapy (medical and/or surgical) is warranted for all children with confirmed glaucoma. Therapy can also be considered for children who are high-risk glaucoma suspects.

Infants and young children with confirmed glaucoma Surgery is indicated in most cases of newly diagnosed primary congenital glaucoma. Topical and/or systemic IOP-lowering medication may be given prior to surgery to reduce corneal edema and facilitate visualization for ab interno angle surgery. In young children with confirmed secondary diagnoses and an open angle (eg, glaucoma associated with aniridia or with port-wine birthmark without blood in Schlemm canal, or glaucoma following cataract extraction), surgery is typically a first-line therapy. Medication may be the first choice for long-term therapy in patients in whom surgery is considered high risk due to ocular or systemic comorbidities (eg, a medically unstable child, a patient with glaucoma in a globe with severe malformations).

Older children and teenagers with confirmed glaucoma Most cases of newly diagnosed juvenile open-angle glaucoma can be managed medically, especially if the damage is mild and the IOP responds well to topical medical therapy. However, surgery may be required for definitive control in older children who present with advanced glaucoma, children with modest response to topical medical therapy, or children with poor adherence to medical therapy. Selection of an appropriate glaucoma medication is based on the medication's possible adverse effects and dosing schedule; medication selection is discussed in detail in Chapter 11 of BCSC Section 10, *Glaucoma.*

Children with suspected glaucoma If the child does not meet the diagnostic criteria for glaucoma, topical IOP-lowering medications may be given for diagnostic purposes. For example, if a newborn with bilateral corneal edema as the sole finding is given IOP-lowering medications unilaterally, and the cornea of the treated eye clears when compared to the untreated eye, then the probability of bilateral glaucoma increases. Because every therapy that lowers IOP has potential adverse effects, costs money, and may be stressful for the child and caretaker, only children at high risk of developing glaucoma should be offered medical therapy. Pediatric glaucoma suspects with confirmed elevated IOP (either isolated or as part of a syndrome/anomaly) have a high risk of developing glaucoma; in these patients, prophylactic treatment with IOP-lowering medication is warranted.

Greenberg MB, Osigian CJ, Cavuoto KM, Chang TC. Clinical management outcomes of childhood glaucoma suspects. *PLoS One.* 2017;12(9):e0185546.

Khan AO. Conditions that can be mistaken as early childhood glaucoma. *Ophthalmic Genet.* 2011;32(3):129–137.

Obtain a comprehensive baseline assessment for future comparison

Management of glaucoma depends on the ability to recognize change in disease status over time. Thus, establishing a comprehensive baseline by quantifying the structural and functional status of the eye is paramount; the more precise the baseline assessment is, the less ambiguous any future pathologic changes will be. The assessment may be accomplished in the clinic, during an examination under anesthesia, or via a combination of the 2, depending on the patient's ability to cooperate. Techniques for measuring corneal diameter, AL, and central corneal thickness and for obtaining optic nerve head imaging are outlined in Chapter 11 of BCSC Section 10, *Glaucoma.*

Determine the interval and type of follow-up

Confirmed glaucoma It is important to closely monitor children and teenagers with confirmed glaucoma after glaucoma surgery or initiating medical therapy, for both surgical complications and medication adherence. For children within the amblyogenic age range, aggressive amblyopia therapy should be initiated. Children with an established history of well-controlled IOP without medication can be monitored less frequently than children on IOP-lowering medication; a medically controlled IOP in the clinic or during EUA does not imply adequate medication adherence and glaucoma control between visits. Similarly, children who undergo glaucoma tube shunt surgery require frequent follow-up because hardware exposure and/or malfunction can present with minimal or no symptoms.

Glaucoma suspect Regardless of whether medical therapy has been initiated, glaucoma suspects should be monitored closely initially, with the interval of follow-up lengthened as the duration of stability increases. If the child cannot be adequately examined in the office, serial EUA may be considered to rule out progressive, pathologic changes. Up to 50% of childhood glaucoma suspects who eventually developed glaucoma had normal IOP on initial presentation.

Follow-Up Evaluation

During the follow-up evaluation for childhood glaucoma, the goals are to

1. determine whether the glaucoma has progressed
2. decide on whether the current therapy is appropriate as long-term management

Determine whether the glaucoma has progressed

In infants and children under 3 years of age, normal ocular growth (AL increase) and stable optic nerve head appearance on serial photos suggest the absence of progressive glaucomatous damage. Frequently, a reversal of optic nerve head cupping is observed in eyes with substantially lowered IOP (Fig 21-4). A stable cycloplegic refraction suggests stability, because a pathologic increase in AL often results in a myopic shift. However, in some instances, such as glaucoma associated with port-wine birthmark and choroidal hemangioma, a myopic shift may not result despite axial elongation of the sclera due to concurrent expansion of the choroidal hemangioma. The IOP should be considered not as an isolated finding but rather in conjunction with other measurements obtained from the examination. If the IOP is less than 20 mm Hg under anesthesia but clinical evidence shows persistent corneal edema or enlargement, progressive optic nerve head cupping, or axial elongation, further intervention should be pursued despite the IOP reading. In contrast, a young child who has a borderline or slightly elevated IOP but shows evidence of clinical improvement may be followed up with careful observation.

In older children, AL becomes a less informative tool in gauging glaucoma progression due to increased scleral rigidity; the absence of glaucoma progression is often made based on stable optic nerve head appearance. Most children aged 3 years and older are able to cooperate with optic nerve head imaging in the clinic, although some may require continued serial EUAs until older. Optical coherence tomography (OCT) imaging enables analysis of the optic nerve and retinal nerve fiber layer for follow-up of children with elevated IOP and glaucoma. Macular thickness, retinal nerve fiber layer thickness, and optic nerve topography have been shown to vary with race, AL, and age in children, but normative data are becoming more readily available, which should further increase the usefulness of OCT in the assessment of childhood glaucoma.

El-Dairi MA, Asrani SG, Enyedi LB, Freedman SF. Optical coherence tomography in the eyes of normal children. *Arch Ophthalmol.* 2009;127(1):50–58.

Prakalapakorn SG, Freedman SF, Lokhnygina Y, et al. Longitudinal reproducibility of optical coherence tomography measurements in children. *J AAPOS.* 2012;16(6):523–528.

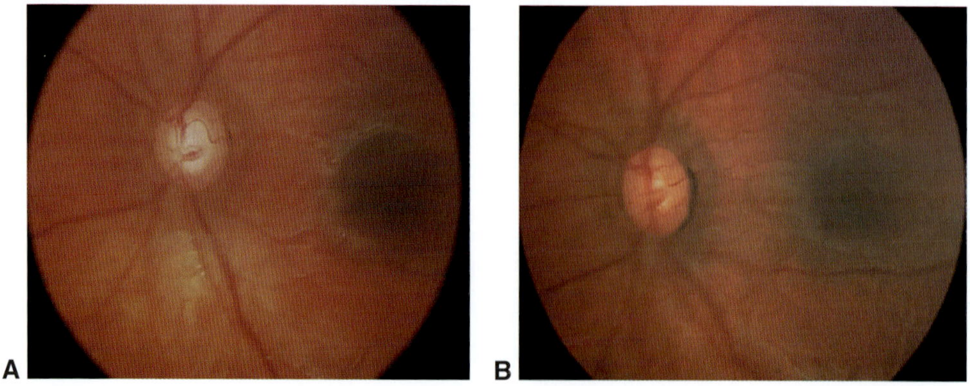

Figure 21-4 Optic nerve changes after treatment of congenital glaucoma. **A,** Preoperative enlarged optic nerve head cup. **B,** Reduction in optic nerve head cupping after intraocular pressure is reduced by goniotomy. *(Reprinted from Mochizuki H, Lesley AG, Brandt JD. Shrinkage of the scleral canal during cupping reversal in children.* Ophthalmology. *2011;118(10):2009. With permission from Elsevier.)*

Decide on whether the current therapy is appropriate as long-term management

Young children typically rely on parents and/or caretakers to administer glaucoma medications. It may be helpful to provide multiple copies of a clear and detailed medication schedule so that all the caretakers can share in the task of administering medications. Older children sometimes are asked to administer their own medications, and it is important to review the medication laterality, schedule, and dosages with these young patients at every visit. Although being able to describe medication laterality, schedule, and dosages correctly does not prove good adherence, the inability to do so strongly suggests poor adherence. It is also useful to ask the patients and/or caretakers to demonstrate how they administer the medications while in the clinic; the inability to do so correctly suggests poor adherence. See Chapter 28 for further discussion of issues regarding pediatric chronic eye disease care.

The use of glaucoma medications in children is discussed in Chapter 11 of BCSC Section 10, *Glaucoma*. Table 21-4 summarizes the common adverse effects associated with glaucoma medication use in children.

Surgical Decisions in Childhood Glaucoma

Surgical Principles and General Considerations

The goal of glaucoma surgery in children is to achieve IOP control while minimizing both complications and anesthetic exposure. As with glaucoma surgery in adults, the more aggressive procedures typically result in greater IOP reduction and also carry greater risks. In general:

- Conjunctiva-sparing procedures are preferred over conjunctiva-violating procedures.
- Hardware-free procedures are preferred over procedures that involve hardware implantation, due to the lifelong risks of hardware malfunction, malposition, and exposure.
- Blebless procedures are preferred over bleb-forming procedures, because complications related to an externally filtering bleb (eg, trabeculectomy, tube shunt surgery) are lifelong.
- Any risk of sympathetic ophthalmia in the unaffected fellow eye must be weighed against the utility of sight preservation in the glaucomatous eye.

There are special considerations when planning intraocular surgery in children. Pediatric eyes are distensible, with more elastic sclera compared to adult eyes. Thus, most wounds, including clear corneal incisions, paracentesis tracks, and sclerotomies, are prone to gaping. Furthermore, children are less likely to adhere to postoperative instructions to avoid eye rubbing, and corneal/perilimbal sutures are likely to result in large magnitudes of induced astigmatism, which may further contribute to amblyopia. Thus, it is important to suture all incisions, including some needle tracks. Dissolvable sutures are generally preferred over nondissolvable sutures to avoid long-term suture-induced astigmatism.

Typically, the status of the angle and the clarity of the corneal are the 2 major anatomic factors in deciding the surgical approach. The choice of procedure depends heavily on the presentation of the disease and the training and experience of the surgeon. In most

Table 21-4 **Systemic and Ocular Adverse Effects of Glaucoma Medications in Children**

Drug	Adverse Effects	Precautions
β-Adrenergic antagonists		
Betaxolol, carteolol, levobunolol, metipranolol, timolol hemihydrate, timolol maleate	Hypotension, bradycardia, bronchospasm, apnea Hallucinations Masking of hypoglycemia in children with diabetes	Avoid in premature or small neonates or infants Use with caution in infants, children with asthma, or children with cardiac disease Select lower concentrations Use punctal occlusion Consider cardioselective β-blocker to reduce risk of bronchospasm
Prostaglandin analogues		
Bimatoprost, latanoprost, latanoprostene bunod, tafluprost, travoprost	May exacerbate uveitis Risk of retinal detachment in patients with Sturge-Weber syndrome Low systemic risk; possible sleep disturbance or exacerbation of asthma Eyelash growth; iris and periocular skin pigmentation Redness, epiphora	Avoid in patients with uveitis Use with caution following intraocular surgery
α_2-Adrenergic agonists		
Apraclonidine, brimonidine	Apraclonidine: tachyphylaxis, allergy Apraclonidine and brimonidine: hypotension, bradycardia, hypothermia, CNS depression, coma Risks are greater with brimonidine	Brimonidine is contraindicated in children <2 years of age Caution in children <6 years of age or with weight <20 kg Use low dosage Avoid in patients with cardiovascular disease or hepatic or renal impairment
Topical CAIs		
Brinzolamide, dorzolamide	Metabolic acidosis (rare) Toxic epidermal necrolysis Corneal edema	Contraindicated in infants with renal insufficiency Contraindicated in patients with sulfonamide hypersensitivity Monitor infant feeding, weight gain Caution in patients with corneal disease
Oral CAIs		
Acetazolamide, methazolamide	Metabolic acidosis Stevens-Johnson syndrome Headache, nausea, dizziness, paresthesia Growth suppression, failure to thrive, weight loss Bed-wetting	Contraindicated in patients with renal insufficiency, hypokalemia, hyponatremia Contraindicated in patients with sulfonamide hypersensitivity Monitor for metabolic acidosis Monitor infant feeding, weight gain
Parasympathomimetic agents (miotics)		
Echothiophate, pilocarpine	Risk of pupillary block Paradoxical rise in IOP Echothiophate: diarrhea, urinary incontinence, cardiac arrhythmia, weakness, headache, fatigue, iris pigment cysts Pilocarpine: bronchospasm, hypertension, vomiting, diarrhea, dizziness, weakness, headache	Avoid in patients with uveitis Use with caution in patients with cardiac disease, asthma, or urinary tract obstruction Limit dosage and use lower concentrations Echothiophate: avoid succinylcholine Consider stopping before general anesthesia

CAIs = carbonic anhydrase inhibitors; CNS = central nervous system; IOP = intraocular pressure.

cases of primary glaucoma, the angle is presumed to be open. However, the angle may be either open or closed if 1 or more of the following is present:

- history of prior surgeries (eg, cataract extraction, vitreoretinal procedures, corneal procedures)
- history of chronic uveitis
- history of retinal ablation (laser or cryotherapy) for proliferative retinopathies (eg, retinopathy of prematurity)
- history of anterior segment dysgenesis (eg, Peters anomaly, Axenfeld-Rieger syndrome)
- presence of iris/ciliary body mass (eg, iris stroma cysts)

If the angle status is uncertain, ultrasound biomicroscopy images can be used to assess the anterior segment. A clear cornea with adequate gonioscopic visualization of angle landmarks is key to successful ab interno angle surgery. If the cornea is edematous, preoperative administration of aqueous suppressant medication and intraoperative topical glycerin and/or epithelial debridement may improve visualization.

Angle open, cornea clear

When the angle is open and the cornea is clear, the preferred procedure is an *ab interno* angle surgery, such as goniotomy or gonioscopy-assisted transluminal trabeculotomy (GATT). Some evidence shows that the greater extent of angle treated, the greater the IOP reduction, suggesting that circumferential angle treatment with GATT (Video 21-1) or multiple-site goniotomy may be more beneficial than single-site goniotomy (Video 21-2). The therapeutic effect of laser trabeculoplasty in childhood glaucoma is unclear, although some case reports suggest a favorable outcome in both primary and secondary open-angle childhood glaucomas. See Chapter 13 of BCSC Section 10, *Glaucoma,* for a detailed discussion of laser and surgical treatments for glaucoma. Some pediatric glaucoma surgeons advocate against angle surgery in glaucoma associated with elevated episcleral venous pressure evidenced by blood in the Schlemm canal (eg, encephalofacial angiomatosis/Sturge-Weber syndrome, Radius-Maumenee syndrome) despite the presence of an open angle.

VIDEO 21-1 Gonioscopy-assisted transluminal trabeculotomy using a blunted 5-0 polypropylene suture.
Courtesy of Ta Chen Peter Chang, MD.

VIDEO 21-2 Goniotomy using a 25-gauge needle.
Courtesy of Elizabeth Hodapp, MD.

Grover DS, Smith O, Fellman RL, et al. Gonioscopy assisted transluminal trabeculotomy: an ab interno circumferential trabeculotomy for the treatment of primary congenital glaucoma and juvenile open angle glaucoma. *Br J Ophthalmol.* 2015;99(8):1092–1096.

Neustein RF, Beck AD. Circumferential trabeculotomy versus conventional angle surgery: comparing long-term surgical success and clinical outcomes in children with primary congenital glaucoma. *Am J Ophthalmol.* 2017;183:17–24.

Angle open, cornea opaque

When the angle is open but the cornea is opaque despite aqueous suppressant, angle surgery may be performed using an *ab externo* technique. A rigid probe technique is used in a sector trabeculotomy; a blunted polyproplene suture or an illuminated microcatheter can enable a circumferential trabeculotomy (Video 21-3). Some pediatric glaucoma surgeons advocate for combining an ab externo trabeculotomy with trabeculectomy, although the efficacy and bleb-related risk of the combined procedure have not been compared to those of trabeculotomy alone in a clinical trial. Deep sclerectomy is another approach used in some regions of the Middle East where *CYP1B1* mutations are common and the response to conventional angle surgery is less favorable.

VIDEO 21-3 Circumferential ab externo trabeculotomy using an illuminated microcatheter.
Courtesy of Ta Chen Peter Chang, MD.

Al-Shahrani NO, Khan AO. Observations regarding gender and response to initial angle surgery in *CYP1B1*-related primary congenital glaucoma. *Ophthalmic Genet.* 2017;38(3):294.

Angle closed, cornea clear

Angle closure with or without glaucoma is an unusual finding in children. Primary angle closure in children is most often due to plateau iris syndrome and nanophthalmos, whereas secondary angle closure is usually associated with iridociliary cysts, uveitis, lens disorders, and retinopathy of prematurity (both with attached retina following retinal ablation and with detached retina as end-stage disease). Angle closure that results in high IOP is also a common finding following intraocular procedures. The efficacy of laser iridotomy in appositional primary or secondary pediatric angle closure is uncertain, although the risks are acceptable in some cooperative older children. Lensectomy with goniosynechialysis (Video 21-4) may achieve adequate IOP control in some cases. Certain types of pediatric angle closure mechanisms, such as synechial closure in patients with aniridia, Axenfeld-Rieger syndrome, and synechial angle closure in patients with active uveitis are not likely to respond to goniosynechialysis without additional glaucoma procedures.

VIDEO 21-4 Lensectomy and goniosynechialysis in a child with angle closure glaucoma.
Courtesy of Ta Chen Peter Chang, MD.

Acute or subacute angle closure with iris bombé is a rare form of glaucoma that develops following cataract surgery. Although it usually occurs soon after surgery, onset can be delayed by a year or more. The diagnosis should be apparent with a slit-lamp examination, but this type of examination may be difficult in young children. Treatment consists of anterior vitrectomy to relieve the pupillary block, often with surgical iridectomy and goniosynechialysis.

In rare cases, acute angle closure occurs following the ingestion of certain medications, including topiramate, acetazolamide, methazolamide, bupropion, 3,4-methylenedioxymethamphetamine (MDMA, also known as "ecstasy"). Drug-induced secondary angle closure is typically treated by cessation of the offending agent, aggressive cycloplegia, and topical medications for IOP control.

Freedman SF, Lynn MJ, Beck AD, Bothun ED, Örge FH, Lambert SR; Infant Aphakia Treatment Study Group. Glaucoma-related adverse events in the first 5 years after unilateral cataract removal in the Infant Aphakia Treatment Study. *JAMA Ophthalmol.* 2015;133(8):907–914.

Lee JY, Berrocal AM, Grajewski AL, Chang TC. Juvenile angle closure management: The role of lens extraction and goniosynechialysis. *Am J Ophthalmol Case Rep.* 2020;19:100080.

Angle closed, cornea opaque

Pediatric eyes with angle closure glaucoma and corneal opacity are amongst the most challenging surgically. If corneal clarity can be improved with medical therapy to allow intraocular visualization, lensectomy and goniosynechialysis may be performed. If the corneal opacity is refractory to medical treatment, such as in eyes with Peters anomaly or severe ocular surface disease (eg, Stevens-Johnson syndrome or prior chemical burn), the choice of procedure depends on the specific anatomy (including conjunctival mobility), the long-term visual prognosis, and the experience of the surgeon. The full spectrum of glaucoma surgical procedures is discussed in detail in Chapter 13 of BCSC Section 10, *Glaucoma.*

Prognosis and Long-Term Follow-Up

The prognosis for control of IOP and preservation of vision is poor for patients who present with primary congenital glaucoma at birth; at least half of these patients eventually become legally blind. If the horizontal diameter of the cornea is greater than 14 mm at diagnosis, the visual prognosis is similarly poor. In up to 90% of cases in the "favorable prognostic group" (onset at 3–12 months of age), the glaucoma can be controlled with angle surgery and medications. In the remaining 10%, and in many of the remaining cases of primary and secondary glaucomas, glaucoma presents a lifelong challenge.

Vision loss in childhood glaucoma is multifactorial. It may result from corneal scarring and opacification, optic nerve damage, myopic astigmatism, and anisometropic and strabismic amblyopia. Myopia results from axial enlargement of the eye in patients with high IOP; astigmatism may result from unequal expansion of the anterior segment or from corneal scarring. Careful treatment of refractive errors and amblyopia is necessary to optimize outcomes.

Long-term follow-up of children with glaucoma is important. Relapse can occur years later, with elevated IOP and subsequent vision loss. Parents, and patients themselves as they become older, should be educated about the need for lifelong monitoring and management. In particular, regimen adherence can be problematic during the teenage years.

CHAPTER 22

Childhood Cataracts and Other Pediatric Lens Disorders

This chapter includes related videos. Go to www.aao.org/bcscvideo_section06 or scan the QR codes in the text to access this content.

Highlights

- For infants with visually significant congenital cataract, surgery is urgent; however, it should be deferred to soon after 4 weeks of age to decrease glaucoma risk without affecting vision potential.
- In young children undergoing cataract surgery, primary posterior capsulectomy with anterior vitrectomy is needed if postoperative capsulotomy is not likely to be readily available or feasible.
- The possibility of an undiagnosed syndrome should be considered in all children with ectopia lentis, particularly the diagnoses Marfan syndrome and homocystinuria.

Introduction

Disorders of the pediatric lens include cataract and abnormalities in lens shape, size, and location. Such abnormalities constitute a significant source of visual impairment in children. The incidence of lens abnormalities ranges from 1:4000 to 1:10,000 live births per year worldwide. See BCSC Section 11, *Lens and Cataract,* for additional discussion of many of the topics covered in this chapter.

Pediatric Cataracts

General Features

Cataracts are responsible for nearly 10% of vision loss in children worldwide. They can be isolated or associated with a number of conditions, including chromosomal abnormalities, systemic syndromes and diseases, infection, trauma, and radiation exposure. In almost all cases of cataract associated with systemic disease, the cataracts are bilateral (Table 22-1); however, not all bilateral cataracts are associated with systemic disease. In addition, bilateral cases may be associated with significant asymmetry.

Table 22-1 Etiology of Pediatric Cataracts

Bilateral cataracts	
Familial (hereditary), often autosomal dominant but also X-linked and autosomal recessive	
Chromosomal abnormality	Trisomy 21 (Down syndrome), 13, 18; other translocations, deletions, and duplications
Craniofacial syndromes	Hallermann-Streiff, Rubinstein-Taybi, Smith-Lemli-Opitz, and others
Musculoskeletal disorders	Albright syndrome, Conradi-Hünermann syndrome, myotonic dystrophy
Renal syndromes	Alport syndrome, Lowe syndrome
Metabolic diseases	Cerebrotendinous xanthomatosis, diabetes, Fabry disease, galactosemia, mannosidosis, Wilson disease
Intrauterine infections	Cytomegalovirus, rubella, syphilis, toxoplasmosis, varicella
Ocular anomalies	Aniridia, anterior segment dysgenesis
Iatrogenic origin	Corticosteroid use, radiation exposure
Idiopathic origin	
Unilateral cataract	
Ocular anomalies	Persistent fetal vasculature, posterior lenticonus or lentiglobus, posterior segment tumor, retinal detachment (from any cause) or coloboma, uveitis
Trauma (including child abuse)	
Radiation exposure	
Idiopathic origin	

Cataracts may also be associated with other ocular anomalies, including persistent fetal vasculature (PFV), anterior segment dysgenesis, aniridia, and retinal disorders (eg, coloboma, detachment).

In addition to congenital causes, pediatric cataracts may have acquired causes. Congenital cataracts are present at birth, although they may not be identified until later. Infantile cataracts are present during the first year of life. The terms *congenital* and *infantile cataract* are typically used synonymously. In general, the earlier the onset, the more amblyogenic the cataract will be, particularly in unilateral cases. Lens opacities that are visually significant before 2–3 months of age are most likely to harm vision.

Most hereditary cataracts show an autosomal dominant mode of transmission, and they are almost always bilateral. X-linked and autosomal recessive inheritance may occur; the latter is more common in consanguineous populations. *OMIM* (*Online Mendelian Inheritance in Man;* www.omim.org) includes the most up-to-date information on genetic disorders with lens involvement.

Morphology

Cataracts may involve the entire lens (*total,* or *complete,* cataract) or only part of the lens structure. In certain circumstances, the location of the opacity in the lens and the morphology of the cataract may provide information about etiology (Table 22-2) and prognosis. However, precise characterization of the cataract morphology may not be possible on

Table 22-2 Morphology and Etiology of Select Cataracts With Systemic Findings

Cataract Morphology	Etiology	Other Possible Findings
Spokelike	Fabry disease	Corneal whorls
	Mannosidosis	Hepatosplenomegaly
Vacuolar	Diabetes	Elevated blood glucose level
	Prematurity	Not related to severity of retinopathy; may resolve spontaneously
Multicolored flecks	Hypoparathyroidism	Low serum calcium level
	Myotonic dystrophy	Characteristic facial features, tonic "grip"
Green "sunflower"	Wilson disease	Kayser-Fleischer ring, liver failure due to abnormal copper metabolism
Thin disciform	Lowe syndrome	Hypotonia, glaucoma, kidney disease (proximal tubular acidosis, aminoaciduria)

initial evaluation in a young/uncooperative patient. Important types and causes of cataract in children are discussed in Chapter 4 of BCSC Section 11, *Lens and Cataract.*

Evaluation of Pediatric Cataracts

All newborns should have a screening eye examination performed by their primary care provider, including an evaluation of the red reflex. In a preverbal child, retinoscopy through an undilated pupil is helpful for assessing the potential visual significance of an axial lens opacity. Table 22-3 summarizes the evaluation of pediatric cataracts.

History

It is important to obtain a detailed history of the child's growth, development, and systemic disorders, in addition to a family history, as this information can help guide the evaluation. For example, a patient with acquired cataract and a history of intractable diarrhea (even years before) should be evaluated for the treatable metabolic disorder cerebrotendinous xanthomatosis (see Chapter 27). A slit-lamp examination of immediate family members may reveal previously undiagnosed lens opacities that are visually insignificant but may support an inherited cause for a child's cataracts. An important example is the female carrier state for Lowe, Nance-Horan, and other X-linked cataract syndromes (Fig 22-1).

Visual function

The mere presence of a lens opacity does not mean surgical removal is necessary. That determination requires assessment of the cataract's visual significance.

In healthy infants aged 2 months or younger, the fixation reflex may not be fully developed; thus, its absence in these patients is not necessarily abnormal. In preverbal children older than 2 months, standard clinical assessment of fixation behavior, fixation preference, and objection to occlusion provides additional evidence of the visual significance of the cataract. For bilateral cataracts, assessment of the child's visual behavior and the family's observations of the child at home help determine the level of visual function. Preferential looking tests and visual evoked potentials can provide quantitative information (see Chapter 1). In older children, particularly those with lamellar or posterior subcapsular cataracts, glare testing may be useful for assessing decreased vision.

Table 22-3 Evaluation of Pediatric Cataracts

History

- Family history (autosomal dominant, X-linked, autosomal recessive, reduced penetrance, variable expressivity; associated anomalies may be indicative of chromosomal translocation, balanced in the parent, unbalanced in the child)
- Detailed history of the child's growth, development, and systemic disorders
- Pediatric physical examination, including assessment for evidence of perinatal infection (toxoplasmosis, rubella, cytomegalovirus, herpes simplex virus [TORCH]; varicella; syphilis)
- Genetic evaluation

Examination

- Visual function
- Corneal diameter
- Iris configuration
- Anterior chamber depth
- Lens position
- Cataract morphology
- Posterior segment
  - Rule out posterior mass
  - Rule out retinal detachment
  - Rule out persistent fetal vasculature
    - Stalk between optic nerve and lens
    - Vessels at the lens periphery or dragged/straightened ciliary processes
- Intraocular pressure

Ocular imaging

- B-scan ultrasonography if no posterior view is possible
- Ultrasound biomicroscopy if peripheral lesion (tumor) or retinal involvement in persistent fetal vasculature is suspected

Potential laboratory studies (for bilateral cataracts of unknown etiology)

- Disorders of galactose metabolism: urine for reducing substances; galactose-1-phosphate uridyltransferase; galactokinase
- Metabolic diseases: urine amino acids test (Lowe syndrome); serum calcium level (low in hypoparathyroidism), phosphorus level (high in hypoparathyroidism), glucose level (high in diabetes), and ferritin level (high in hyperferritinemia)
- Genetic testing: next-generation sequencing

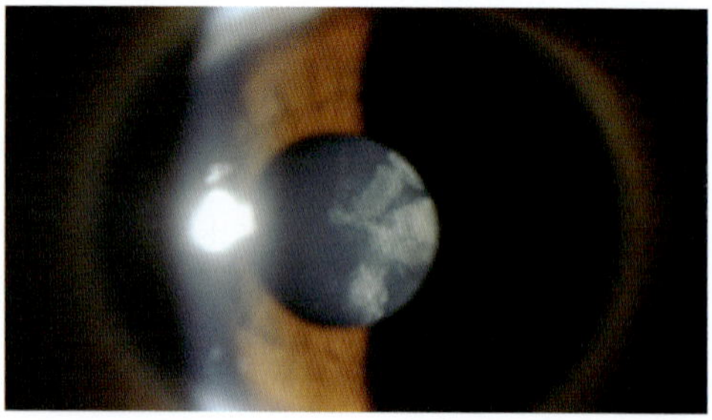

Figure 22-1 The asymptomatic sister of a boy with suspected Nance-Horan syndrome was examined for potential female carrier signs. Both of her eyes showed partial sutural lens opacity (left eye shown). Genetic testing confirmed the boy's diagnosis and his sister's carrier state. *(Courtesy of Arif O. Khan, MD.)*

Ocular examination

Slit-lamp examination can help classify the morphology of the cataract and reveal associated abnormalities of the anterior segment. In general, anterior capsule opacities are not visually significant unless they occlude a large portion of the undilated pupil. In contrast, central or posterior lens opacities of sufficient density that are greater than

3 mm in diameter are often visually significant. Opacities surrounded by a large area of normal red reflex or that contain clear areas may allow good visual development, whereas strabismus associated with a unilateral cataract and nystagmus associated with bilateral cataracts indicate that the opacities are visually significant. Although these signs may also indicate that the optimal time for treatment has passed, cataract surgery may still improve visual function. If the cataract allows some view of the posterior segment, the optic nerve and fovea should be examined. If no such view is possible, B-scan ultrasonography should be performed to assess for anatomical abnormalities of the posterior segment. Retinal or optic nerve abnormalities cannot be definitively ruled out, however, until the posterior pole can be visualized directly. See Table 22-3 for additional information. Uncorrected high refractive error should always be ruled out as the cause of poor vision and dim red reflex.

Workup

Unilateral cataracts are not usually associated with systemic disease; laboratory tests are therefore not warranted in these cases. Similarly, laboratory tests and systemic evaluation are unnecessary in cases of bilateral cataracts with a positive family history of isolated congenital or childhood cataract. If an examination of the parents reveals previously undiagnosed lens opacities with no associated systemic diseases, systemic evaluation is unnecessary, although genetic testing may be considered. Otherwise, bilateral cataracts may be associated with many metabolic or other systemic diseases. A potential basic laboratory evaluation for bilateral cataracts of unknown etiology is outlined in Table 22-3.

Further workup is directed by the presence of other systemic abnormalities. Evaluation by a geneticist may be helpful for determining whether there are associated disorders and for counseling the patient's family regarding recurrence risks. Next-generation gene sequencing, which analyzes large portions of the genome, is of increasing utility, even in cases without evidence of systemic disease.

Cataract Surgery in Pediatric Patients

Timing of the Procedure

In general, the younger the child at the time of diagnosis, the greater the urgency to remove the cataract because of the potential for reversing deprivation amblyopia. However, surgery before the age of 4 weeks increases the risk of anesthetic complications and glaucoma after cataract surgery. Thus, for optimal visual development, a visually significant unilateral cataract should be removed between the ages of 4 and 6 weeks and visually significant bilateral cataracts removed before age 10 weeks.

For older children with bilateral cataracts, surgery is indicated when the level of visual function interferes with the child's visual needs. Although children with best-corrected visual acuity of approximately 20/70 may function relatively well in early grade school, their participation in activities such as driving may be restricted later. Surgery should be considered when visual acuity decreases to 20/40 or worse. Glare may also significantly affect participation in outdoor play, sports, and driving in some patients, warranting surgery.

Intraocular Lens Use in Children

The choice of optical device for correction of aphakia depends primarily on the age of the patient and the laterality of the cataract. As of 2021, no intraocular lenses (IOLs) had been approved by the US Food and Drug Administration for use in children, although IOL implantation is widely accepted and considered the standard of care in children aged 1–2 years and older. However, in younger infants the use of IOLs is associated with a higher rate of complications and larger shifts in refractive error with age, without clear visual benefit over aphakia. Early surgical intervention followed by consistent aphakic correction and amblyopia therapy usually provides some useful vision in the affected eye. In most children who are left aphakic and unable to tolerate or cooperate with other types of aphakic correction, secondary IOL implantation may be performed after 1–2 years of age (see Clinical Trial 22-1).

CLINICAL TRIAL 22-1

Infant Aphakia Treatment Trial (IATS)

Study question: In infants with unilateral congenital cataracts, does primary intraocular lens (IOL) implantation improve visual outcome compared with postoperative aphakia with aphakic contact lens?

Enrollment: 114 patients with unilateral, visually significant congenital cataracts (≥3 mm central opacity) and median age of 1.8 months (range, 4 weeks to 6.7 months) at the time of surgery. Children who were preterm and had corneal diameter <9 mm, intraocular pressure ≥25 mm Hg, or persistent fetal vasculature with ciliary process stretching or tractional retinal detachment were excluded. Children with active uveitis, retinal diseases, prior intraocular surgery, optic nerve disease, or disease in the fellow eye were also excluded.

Study groups:

1. Control group: 57 eyes randomly assigned to postoperative aphakia with aphakic contact lens fitting.
2. Intervention group: 57 eyes randomly assigned to primary IOL with primary posterior capsulectomy and anterior vitrectomy.

Outcome variables: Optotype acuity, adverse events.

Results: At age 4.5 years, median logMAR visual acuity in the treated eyes did not differ significantly between the two groups (0.90 [20/159] for both groups, P=0.54). About 50% of treated eyes in both treatment groups had poor visual acuity (≤20/200), although more than twice as many treated eyes in the contact lens group had visual acuity ≥20/32 (contact lens, n=13 [23%]; IOL, n=6 [11%]). By age 5 years, at least 1 adverse event had occurred in 32 eyes (56%) in the contact lens group compared with 46 eyes (81%) in the IOL group (P=0.008), most commonly reopacification of the visual axes and/or corectopia.

Lambert SR, Cotsonis G, DuBois L, et al; Infant Aphakia Treatment Study Group. Long-term effect of intraocular lens vs contact lens correction on visual acuity after cataract surgery during infancy: a randomized clinical trial. *JAMA Ophthalmol.* 2020;138(4):365–372.

Management of the Anterior Capsule

To enable access to the lens nucleus and cortex during cataract surgery, a *capsulorrhexis* is performed. Because the tearing characteristics of the elastic pediatric capsule are quite different from those of the adult capsule, modified techniques are utilized for pediatric patients to minimize the risk of inadvertent extension of capsulorrhexis. The elasticity of the capsule is greatest in younger patients, especially infants, making continuous curvilinear capsulorrhexis more difficult. The pulling force is directed nearly perpendicular to the direction of intended tear, and the capsule is regrasped frequently to maintain optimal control over the direction of tear. Trypan blue ophthalmic solution 0.06% is often applied to the capsule, even in patients without dense cataracts, as it helps to reduce the elasticity of the capsule. In infants, an alternative to capsulorrhexis is *vitrectorrhexis,* the creation of an anterior capsule opening using a vitrectomy instrument.

Lensectomy Without Intraocular Lens Implantation

In children who will be left aphakic, lensectomy is done through a small peripheral corneal, limbal, or pars plana incision with a vitreous-cutting instrument (ie, vitrector). Irrigation may be provided by an integrated infusion sleeve or by a separate anterior chamber cannula. Ultrasonic phacoemulsification is not required, as the lens cortex and nucleus are generally soft in children of all ages. Removal of all cortical material is important because of the propensity for reproliferation of pediatric lens epithelial cells (Video 22-1).

VIDEO 22-1 Congenital cataract extraction with vitrectorrhexis.
Courtesy of Ta Chen Peter Chang, MD.

Management of the Posterior Capsule

Because posterior capsule opacification occurs rapidly in young children, a controlled posterior capsulectomy and anterior vitrectomy are performed at the time of cataract surgery. This technique allows rapid, permanent establishment of a clear visual axis for retinoscopy and prompt fitting and monitoring of the aphakic optical correction. If possible, sufficient peripheral lens capsule should be left anteriorly and posteriorly to facilitate secondary posterior chamber IOL implantation later. Tough, fibrotic plaques (eg, in severe PFV) may require manual excision with intraocular scissors and forceps.

When IOL implantation is performed (see the following section), the posterior capsulotomy may be created before implantation. However, there is a risk of IOL dislocation into the vitreous or tear out of the capsulotomy during implantation. Capsulotomy after IOL implantation may be performed through the anterior approach by going under the IOL to access the capsule (after wound suturing to avoid vitreous loss) or through a separate pars plana approach.

Lensectomy With Intraocular Lens Implantation

Single- and 3-piece foldable acrylic IOLs, which may be placed through a 3-mm clear corneal or scleral tunnel incision (Video 22-2), have become popular in pediatric cataract surgery, although larger single-piece polymethyl methacrylate lenses are also still used. Silicone lenses have not been well studied in children. Hydrophilic material is not recommended because of the potential for opacification in the long term.

VIDEO 22-2 Congenital cataract extraction, intraocular lens implantation, and posterior capsulotomy.
Courtesy of Ta Chen Peter Chang, MD.

Intraocular lens implantation issues

Because the eye continues to elongate throughout the first decade of life and beyond, selecting an appropriate IOL power is complicated. Power calculations in infants and young children may be unpredictable for several reasons, including

- widely variable growth of the eye
- difficulty obtaining accurate keratometry and axial length measurements
- use of power formulas that were developed for adults rather than children

Studies have shown that in aphakic pediatric eyes, a variable myopic shift in refractive error of approximately 7.00–8.00 D occurs from 1 year to 10 years of age, with a wide standard deviation. This suggests that if a child is made emmetropic with an IOL at 1 year of age, refractive error at 10 years of age may be –8.00 D or greater. Refractive change in children younger than 1 year is even more unpredictable. This assumes that the presence of an IOL does not alter the normal growth curve of the aphakic eye, an assumption that may not be valid according to results from both animal and early human studies.

Lens implantation in children requires consideration of the age of the child, the target refractive error at the time of surgery, and the refractive error of the contralateral eye. Some surgeons implant IOLs with powers that are expected to be required in adulthood, allowing the child to grow into the selected lens power. Thus, the child initially requires hyperopic correction. Other surgeons aim for emmetropia at the time of lens implantation, especially in unilateral cases, believing that this approach improves the treatment of amblyopia and facilitates development of binocular function by decreasing anisometropia in the early childhood years. These children usually become progressively more myopic and may eventually require a second procedure to address the increasing anisometropia.

Postoperative Care

Medical therapy

When all cortical material is adequately removed in a child undergoing cataract surgery without a lens implant, postoperative inflammation is usually mild. Topical antibiotics, corticosteroids, and cycloplegics are commonly applied for a few weeks after surgery. In children who have undergone IOL implantation, topical corticosteroids are used more aggressively. Some surgeons administer intracameral corticosteroids at the time of surgery, and others use oral corticosteroids postoperatively, especially in very young children and children with heavily pigmented irides. Some surgeons administer intracameral antibiotics in addition to topical antibiotics.

Optical correction and amblyopia management

Optical correction with contact lenses and/or glasses and amblyopia therapy should begin as soon after surgery as practically possible, taking into account postoperative recovery.

For infants with bilateral aphakia, glasses are the safest and simplest method of correction. They can be easily changed according to the refractive shifts that occur with growth of the eye. Until the child can use a bifocal lens properly, the power selected should make the eye myopic, because most of an infant's visual activity occurs at near. Contact lenses may also be used in bilaterally aphakic patients, but they require more effort on the part of both the caregiver and the physician than do glasses.

For infants with unilateral aphakia, contact lenses are the most common method of correction. Advantages of contact lenses include relatively easy power changes and the potential for extended wear with certain lenses. Disadvantages include easy displacement by eye rubbing, the expense of replacement, and the risk of microbial keratitis. In infants with unilateral aphakia who are unable to tolerate contact lenses, aphakic glasses are occasionally used; however, these glasses are suboptimal because of the amblyogenic effect of aniseikonia and the difficulty of wearing glasses that are much heavier on one side.

After optical correction of aphakia, amblyopia therapy is necessary in patients with unilateral cataract and in some patients with bilateral cataracts if visual acuity is asymmetric. The amount of therapy is based on the degree of amblyopia and the age of the child.

Complications After Pediatric Cataract Surgery

In the days and week after surgery, the eyes are examined to rule out shallow/flat chamber due to wound leaks, infection, or intraocular pressure spike. This can usually be accomplished in the clinic with meticulous anterior segment examination. Later on, the eyes are monitored for strabismus, secondary glaucoma, corneal decompensation, and retinal detachment. Strabismus is very common in children after surgery for either unilateral or bilateral cataracts. The risk of glaucoma is increased in children who have cataract surgery in infancy and in those with small eyes (see Chapter 21 in this volume and Chapter 11 in BCSC Section 10, *Glaucoma*), but glaucoma often does not develop until several years after surgery. Corneal decompensation is very rare in children. Retinal detachments are also rare; male sex, axial myopia, and intellectual disability are the main risk factors. The incidence of macular edema is unknown, as it is difficult to detect ophthalmoscopically in young children and optical coherence tomography is usually not possible.

Visual Outcome After Cataract Extraction

Visual outcome after cataract surgery depends on many factors, including age at onset and type of cataract, timing of surgery, choice of optical correction, and treatment of amblyopia.

Early surgery by itself does not ensure a good outcome. Optimal vision requires careful, long-term postoperative management, particularly regarding amblyopia. Even when congenital cataracts are detected late (ie, after 4 months of age), cataract removal combined with a strong postoperative vision rehabilitation program can achieve good vision in some eyes. In both infants and toddlers, unilateral congenital cataracts tend to have poorer visual outcome than the better-seeing eye of the child with bilateral congenital cataracts, regardless of IOL implantation, because of amblyopia.

Infants with PFV have a higher incidence of adverse events after lensectomy than children with other forms of unilateral cataract. Visual outcomes for mild, anterior PFV can be encouraging, with more than a third of patients achieving visual acuity of 20/200 or better.

Structural or Positional Lens Abnormalities

Congenital Aphakia

Congenital aphakia, the absence of the lens at birth, is rare. This condition is usually associated with a markedly abnormal eye.

Spherophakia

A lens that is spherical and smaller than normal is termed *spherophakic*. This condition is usually bilateral. The lens may cause secondary glaucoma.

Coloboma

A lens coloboma involves flattening or notching of the lens periphery (Fig 22-2). It may be associated with a coloboma of the iris, optic nerve, or retina, all of which are caused by abnormal closure of the embryonic fissure. The term *lens coloboma* is a misnomer because

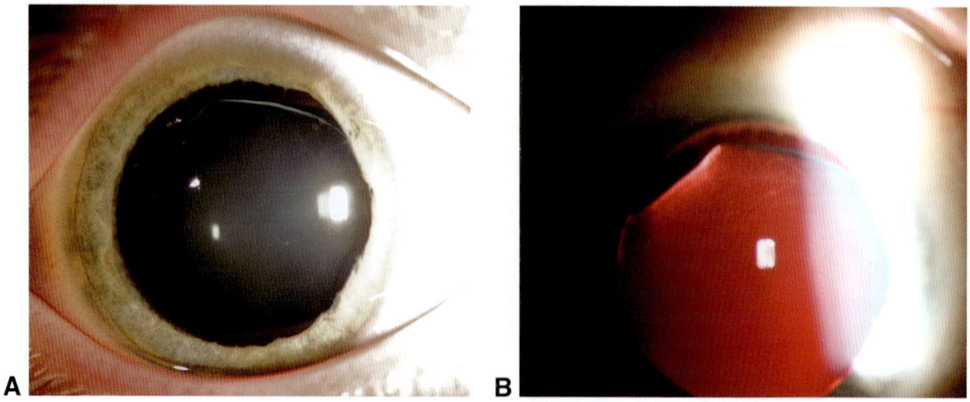

Figure 22-2 Lens coloboma viewed with slit-beam illumination **(A)** and retroillumination **(B)**. The lens is subluxated inferonasally, and there is a notch in the superotemporal portion of the lens where zonules are lacking. *(Courtesy of Gregg T. Lueder, MD.)*

the lens defect is caused by absence or stretching of the zonular fibers in the affected area (usually inferonasally) and is not directly due to embryonic fissure closure of the lens itself. In more significant colobomatous defects, lens dislocations may occur superiorly and temporally. Most colobomatous lenses do not progressively worsen.

Dislocated Lenses in Children

When the lens is not in its normal position, it is said to be *dislocated*. The amount of dislocation can vary, from slight displacement *(subluxation)* with minimal *iridodonesis* (ie, tremulousness of the iris) to severe displacement in which the lens periphery is not visible through the pupillary opening. *Luxated* (or *luxed*), or *ectopic*, lenses are completely detached from the ciliary body; they are free in the posterior chamber (Fig 22-3), or they have prolapsed into the anterior chamber. With 360° of zonular weakness, the result may be *spherophakia*.

Lens dislocation may be familial or sporadic. It may be associated with gene mutations that specifically affect the eye, with multisystem disease, and with inborn errors of metabolism (Table 22-4). Lens dislocation may occur with trauma, usually involving significant injury to the eye, but this is not common. Spontaneous lens dislocation has been reported in homocystinuria, aniridia, buphthalmos associated with congenital glaucoma, and congenital megalocornea with zonular weakness (due to mutations in latent transforming growth factor beta binding protein 2 [*LTBP2*]).

Khan AO, Aldahmesh MA, Alkuraya FS. Congenital megalocornea with zonular weakness and childhood lens-related secondary glaucoma—a distinct phenotype caused by recessive *LTBP2* mutations. *Mol Vis.* 2011;17:2570–2579.

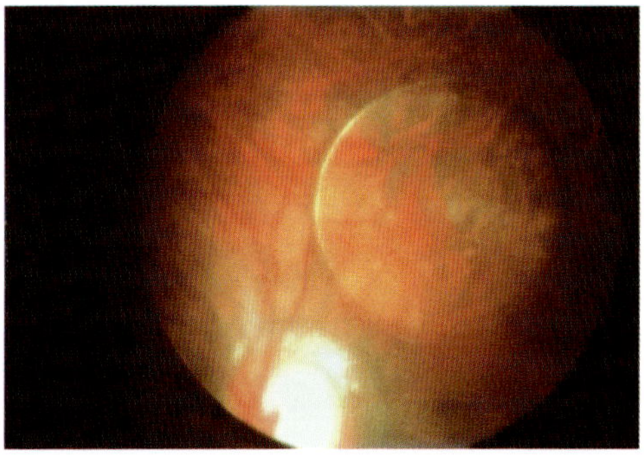

Figure 22-3 Lens dislocation into vitreous.

Table 22-4 Conditions Associated With Dislocated Lenses

Systemic Conditions	Ocular Conditions
Marfan syndrome	Aniridia
Homocystinuria	Iris coloboma
Weill-Marchesani syndrome	Trauma
Sulfite oxidase deficiency	Hereditary ectopia lentis
	Congenital megalocornea with zonular weakness
	Glaucomatous buphthalmos with zonular weakness

Isolated Ectopia Lentis

In simple ectopia lentis, the lens is displaced superiorly and temporally. The condition is usually bilateral and symmetric. Most commonly, it is inherited as an autosomal dominant trait. Onset may be at birth or later in life. Glaucoma is common in the late-onset type.

Some patients with heterozygous mutations in *FBN1,* which cause Marfan syndrome (discussed later in this chapter), have ectopia lentis without evidence for systemic findings in childhood. However, it is appropriate that such patients be considered lifelong Marfan syndrome suspects.

Ectopia Lentis et Pupillae

Ectopia lentis et pupillae is a rare autosomal recessive condition (*ADAMTSL4* mutations) in which the pupil is displaced bilaterally, usually inferotemporally, and the lens is dislocated in the opposite direction (Fig 22-4A). The condition is characterized by small, round lenses (ie, spherophakia); miosis; and poor pupillary dilation with mydriatics. Ectopia lentis et pupillae may be the result of a membrane extending from the posterior iris face and attaching to the proximal pupil margin (Fig 22-4B).

Marfan Syndrome

Marfan syndrome is the systemic disease most commonly associated with subluxated lenses. The syndrome consists of abnormalities of the cardiovascular, musculoskeletal, and ocular systems. It is inherited as an autosomal dominant trait, but family history is negative in 15% of cases. Marfan syndrome is caused by mutations in *FBN1,* which provides instructions for making the protein fibrillin-1, the major constituent of extracellular microfibrils. Affected patients are characteristically tall, with long limbs and fingers *(arachnodactyly)* (Fig 22-5); loose, flexible joints; scoliosis; and chest deformities. Cardiovascular abnormalities are a source of significant mortality and manifest as enlargement

A 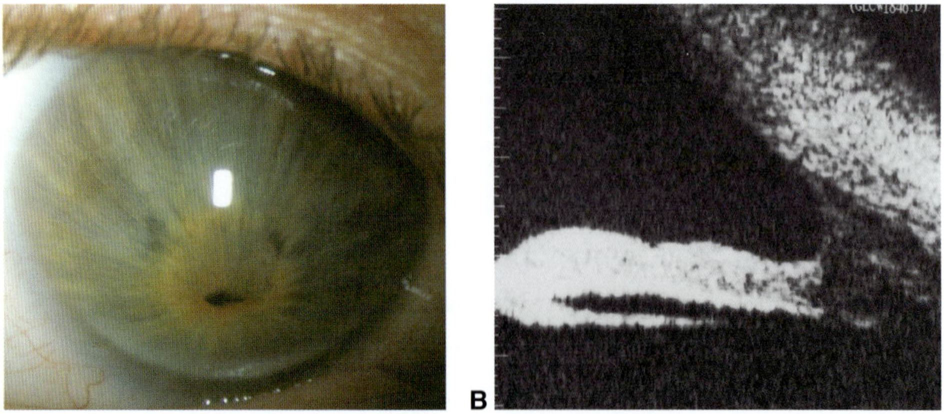 B

Figure 22-4 Ectopia lentis et pupillae. **A,** Miotic and displaced pupil. **B,** Ultrasonography shows a membrane posterior to the iris attaching at the pupil margin. *(Part A reproduced from Byles DB, Nischal KK, Cheng H. Ectopia lentis et pupillae: a hypothesis revisited.* Ophthalmology. *1998;105(7):1331–1336. Part B courtesy of Ken K. Nischal, MD.)*

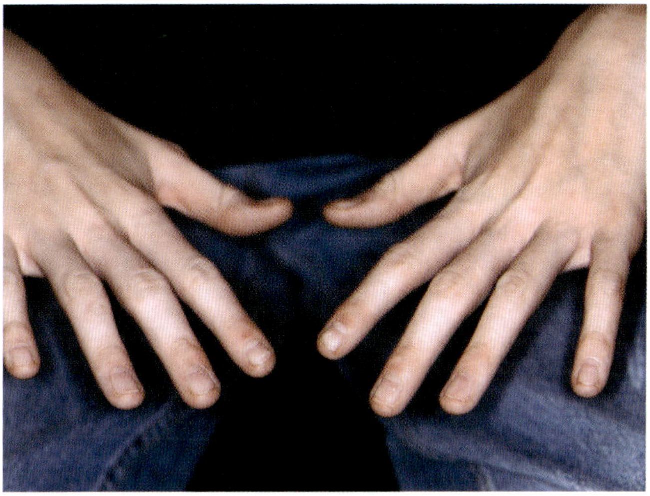

Figure 22-5 Long, slender digits in a patient with Marfan syndrome. *(Reproduced with permission from Lueder GT.* Pediatric Practice: Ophthalmology. *McGraw-Hill Medical; 2010:222. Permission conveyed through Copyright Clearance Center, Inc.)*

of the aortic root, dilation of the descending aorta, a dissecting aneurysm, and a floppy mitral valve. The life expectancy of patients with Marfan syndrome is about half that of the general population.

Ocular abnormalities occur in more than 80% of affected patients, with lens subluxation being the most common (Fig 22-6). In approximately 75% of cases, the lens is subluxated superiorly. Typically, the zonules that are visible are intact and unbroken. Examination of the iris usually shows iridodonesis and may reveal transillumination defects near the iris base. The pupil is small and dilates poorly. The corneal curvature is often decreased. The axial length is increased, and affected patients have myopic astigmatism due to refraction through the lens periphery. Retinal detachment may occur spontaneously, usually in the second and third decades of life, or as a complication after lensectomy.

Homocystinuria

Homocystinuria is a rare autosomal recessive condition occurring in approximately 1 in 100,000 births. The classic form is usually due to mutations in the gene encoding cystathionine

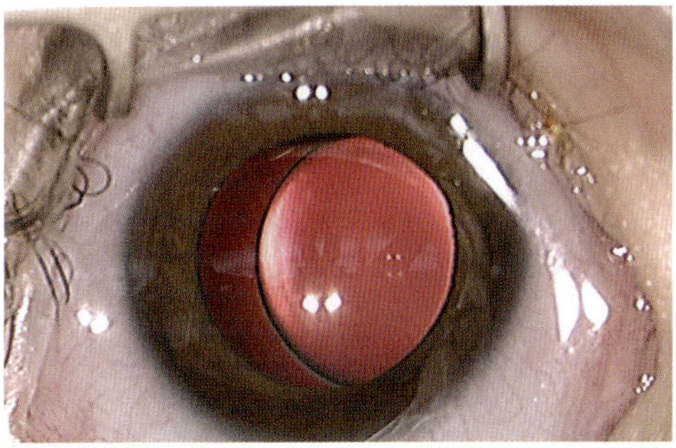

Figure 22-6 Lens subluxation in a patient with Marfan syndrome. *(Courtesy of Gregg T. Lueder, MD.)*

β-synthase, which causes homocysteine to accumulate in the plasma and be excreted in the urine.

The clinical manifestations of homocystinuria vary; the eye, skeletal system, central nervous system, and vascular system may be affected. Most of these abnormalities develop after birth and worsen with age. The skeletal features are similar to those of Marfan syndrome. Affected patients are usually tall and have osteoporosis, scoliosis, and chest deformities. Central nervous system abnormalities occur in approximately 50% of patients; intellectual disability and seizures are the most common.

Vascular complications are common and are secondary to thrombotic disease, which affects large or medium-sized arteries and veins anywhere in the body. Hypertension and cardiomegaly are also frequent. Anesthesia increases risk for patients with homocystinuria because of thromboembolic phenomena; thus, it is important to identify this disorder before patients undergo general anesthesia.

The ophthalmologist may see patients with this disorder before the systemic diagnosis is made. The main ocular finding in homocystinuria is lens subluxation, most frequently inferiorly; however, the direction of subluxation is not diagnostic. Subluxation typically begins between the ages of 3 and 10 years. The lens may luxate anteriorly into the anterior chamber (with or without pupillary block), a finding suggestive of homocystinuria (Fig 22-7). The zonular fibers are frequently broken, in contrast to Marfan syndrome, in which the fibers are stretched and intact.

The diagnosis is confirmed by the detection of disulfides, including homocysteine, in the urine. Medical management of homocystinuria is directed toward normalizing the biochemical abnormality. Dietary management (low-methionine diet and supplemental cysteine) early in life can prevent intellectual disability. Supplementation with the coenzyme pyridoxine (vitamin B_6) diminishes systemic problems in approximately 50% of cases.

Weill-Marchesani Syndrome

Patients with Weill-Marchesani syndrome can be thought of as clinical opposites of patients with Marfan syndrome in that the former are characteristically short, with brachydactyly and short limbs. Inheritance can be autosomal dominant or recessive. Mutations in the *ADAMTS10* gene have been identified in patients with this disorder. The lenses are spherophakic, and with time, they may dislocate into the anterior chamber and cause pupillary block glaucoma. For this reason, lensectomy may be indicated.

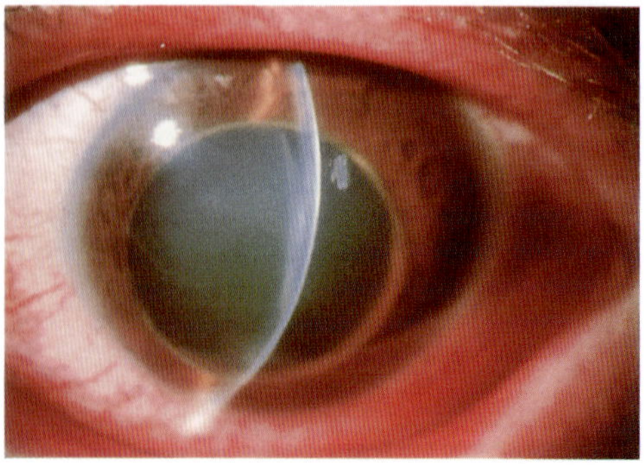

Figure 22-7 Homocystinuria. The lens may dislocate into the anterior chamber and cause acute pupillary block.

Sulfite Oxidase Deficiency

Sulfite oxidase deficiency (molybdenum cofactor deficiency) is a very rare hereditary disorder of sulfur metabolism manifested by severe neurologic disorders and ectopia lentis. The enzyme deficiency interferes with conversion of sulfite to sulfate, resulting in increased excretion of sulfite in the urine. The diagnosis can be confirmed by the absence of sulfite oxidase activity in skin fibroblasts. Neurologic abnormalities include infantile hemiplegia, choreoathetosis, and seizures. Irreversible brain damage and death usually occur by 5 years of age.

Treatment

Optical correction

Optical correction of the refractive error caused by lens dislocation is often difficult. With mild subluxation, the patient may be only myopic, and corrected visual function may be good. More severe dislocation causes optical distortion because the patient is looking through the far periphery of the lens. The resultant myopic astigmatism is difficult to measure accurately by retinoscopy or to correct with glasses. If the subluxated lens does not fill the pupil, use of the aphakic portion of the pupil (with or without optical pupillary dilation with daily topical cycloplegic agents) may improve the patient's vision. Refraction before and after pupil dilation is often helpful for selecting the best type of optical correction. When satisfactory visual function cannot be achieved with glasses or if visual function worsens, lens removal should be considered.

Surgery

Systemic comorbidities that may increase the risk of anesthetic complications should be evaluated and managed before surgery.

Subluxated lenses can be removed either from the anterior segment through a limbal incision or posteriorly through the pars plana. In most circumstances, complete lensectomy is indicated. In the United States, contact lenses or glasses are usually used for postoperative vision rehabilitation, with good visual results. Scleral-fixated IOL techniques are sometimes utilized with caution because of the high rate of suture breakage over the child's lifetime. Iris-claw lenses (Artisan; OPHTEC BV) are widely used in other countries and are currently under investigation in the United States.

CHAPTER 23

Optic Nerve Head Abnormalities

Highlights

- Optic nerve hypoplasia can be associated with undiagnosed endocrine abnormalities.
- Patients with tilted optic nerve heads may have amblyogenic astigmatism, often in the same direction of the nerve head tilt.
- Optic neuritis as a manifestation of myelin-oligodendrocyte glycoprotein (MOG)–associated disease is more common in children than in adults.

Developmental Anomalies

Developmental abnormalities of the optic nerve may or may not limit vision. To maximize vision potential in a child with an optic nerve head (ONH; also called *optic disc*) abnormality, treatment of possible superimposed amblyopia should always be considered.

Optic Nerve Hypoplasia

Optic nerve (ON) hypoplasia, the most common developmental ONH anomaly, is characterized by a small optic nerve associated with a decreased number of optic nerve axons. It can be unilateral, bilateral, or segmental and is often asymmetric if bilateral. The typical affected ONH can be pale, gray, and relatively small with vascular tortuosity (Fig 23-1A). A yellow-to-white ring around the ONH that corresponds to abnormal extension of retina over the lamina cribrosa may be present. This is known as the *double ring sign*; when it is present, the hypoplastic nerve head–ring complex can be mistaken for a normal-sized optic nerve with normal cup–disc ratio (Fig 23-1B, C). One rule of thumb is that the ratio (ONH-to-fovea)/(nerve head diameter) is often greater than 3 in patients with ON hypoplasia.

Visual acuity can range from 20/20 to no light perception. The extent of papillomacular fiber involvement and any associated amblyopia determines visual acuity. Visual field defects are common.

ON hypoplasia is usually idiopathic and sporadic. It is more prevalent in children with fetal alcohol syndrome and can be associated with central nervous system (CNS) abnormalities. Segmental ON hypoplasia may be associated with maternal diabetes mellitus. ON hypoplasia may be associated with pituitary gland dysfunction. Magnetic resonance imaging (MRI) in affected children reveals an ectopic posterior pituitary bright spot at the upper infundibulum. This finding is associated with pituitary hormone deficiencies,

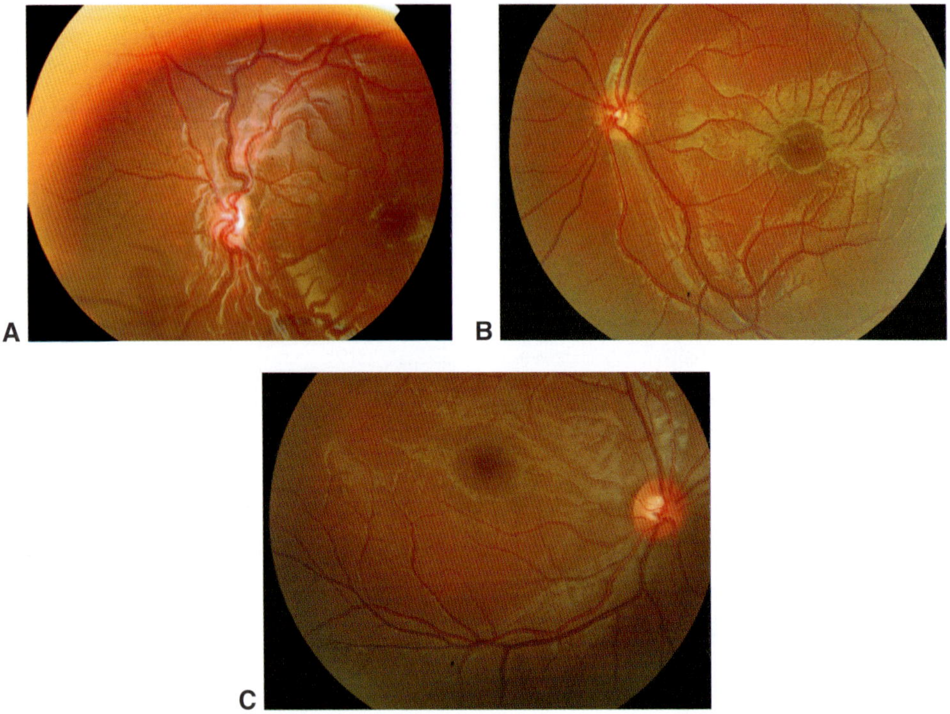

Figure 23-1 Optic nerve hypoplasia. **A,** Left optic nerve hypoplasia. Note the small, pale optic nerve head (ONH) with vascular tortuosity. The ONH-to-fovea/ONH diameter ratio is higher than 3. **B,** Left optic nerve hypoplasia with the double ring sign. When viewed quickly, the hypoplastic ONH–ring complex may be mistaken for a normal-sized optic nerve. **C,** The normal right ONH of the patient shown in part B. *(Courtesy of Arif O. Khan, MD.)*

including growth hormone deficiency, hypothyroidism, hyperprolactinemia, hypocortisolism, panhypopituitarism, and diabetes insipidus. A history of neonatal jaundice suggests hypothyroidism; neonatal hypoglycemia or seizures indicate possible panhypopituitarism. Patients with ON hypoplasia and hypocortisolism, especially those with diabetes insipidus, may have problems with thermal regulation, and dehydration and must be monitored carefully during febrile illnesses.

ON hypoplasia with agenesis of the corpus callosum and an absent septum pellucidum is called *septo-optic dysplasia* (Figs 23-2, 23-3). As isolated abnormalities, the neuroimaging findings are not associated with neurodevelopmental or endocrinologic problems. Cerebral hemisphere abnormalities such as schizencephaly, periventricular leukomalacia, and encephalomalacia occur in approximately 45% of patients with ON hypoplasia and are associated with neurodevelopmental defects.

Children with periventricular leukomalacia can have a large cup and a normal-sized ONH with or without static visual field defects. This may be mistaken for glaucomatous cupping and is not associated with endocrine abnormalities.

Garcia-Filion P, Borchert M. Optic nerve hypoplasia syndrome: a review of the epidemiology and clinical associations. *Curr Treat Options Neurol.* 2013;15(1):78–89.

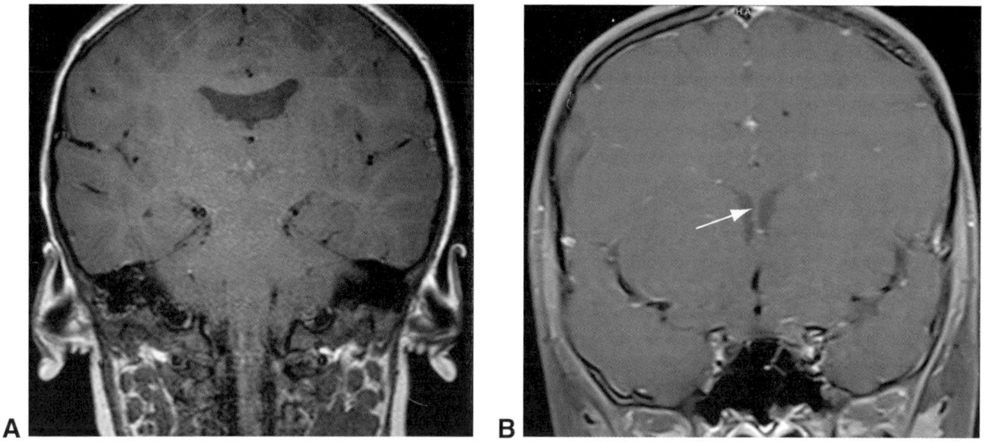

Figure 23-2 Magnetic resonance imaging (MRI) focusing on the septum pellucidum. **A,** Coronal T1-weighted MRI scan of the lateral ventricles: the septum pellucidum (interventricular septum) is absent. **B,** Normal septum pellucidum for comparison *(arrow)*. *(Part A courtesy of Jane L. Weissman, MD; part B courtesy of Mays El-Dairi, MD.)*

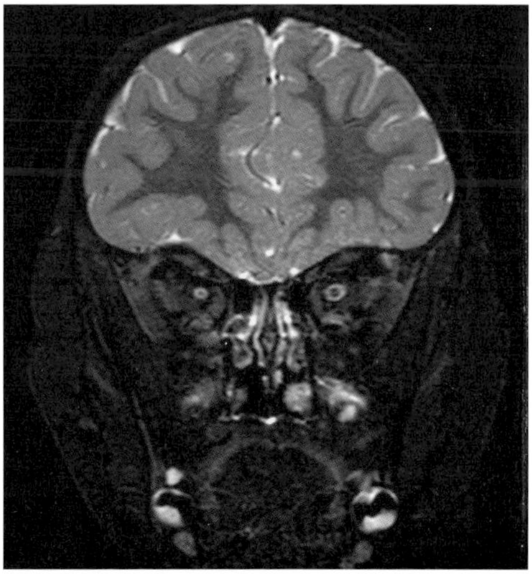

Figure 23-3 Coronal T2-weighted MRI scan of the orbits: the right optic nerve is smaller and more T2 hyperintense than the left optic nerve. *(Courtesy of Jane L. Weissman, MD.)*

Morning Glory Disc Anomaly

Morning glory disc anomaly (MGDA) is the result of abnormal development of the distal optic stalk at its junction with the primitive optic vesicle. The anomaly is typically unilateral and is more common in girls. Serous retinal detachments occur in one-third of cases. Choroidal neovascular membranes may develop. MGDA has been associated with basal encephalocele in patients with midline abnormalities, PHACE syndrome (*p*osterior fossa malformations, *h*emangiomas, *a*rterial lesions, *c*ardiac and *e*ye anomalies), and carotid circulation abnormalities (including moyamoya disease).

MGDA typically appears as a funnel-shaped excavation of the posterior fundus that incorporates an enlarged ONH with elevated surrounding retinal pigment epithelium and an increased number of blood vessels looping at the edges of the ONH (Fig 23-4). A core of white glial tissue occupies the normal position of the optic cup. This tissue may have contractile elements, as the optic cup can sometimes be seen to open and close periodically.

Visual acuity ranges from 20/20 to no light perception, but it is usually 20/100 to 20/200. Because of the potential for associated CNS abnormalities, MRI and MR angiography should be considered.

Optic Nerve Coloboma

Optic nerve coloboma results from incomplete closure of the embryonic fissure. It can be associated with iris coloboma and adjacent or peripheral chorioretinal coloboma. Optic nerve coloboma can be unilateral or bilateral and is often asymmetric.

Typically, there is an inferonasal excavation of the ONH that, when mild, may be confused with glaucomatous damage. More extensive defects appear as an enlargement of the peripapillary area with a deep central excavation lined by a glistening white tissue; blood vessels overlie this deep cavity (Fig 23-5). When chorioretinal coloboma is present, there is a risk for retinal detachment. Visual acuity is related to involvement of the papillomacular or foveal region and is difficult to predict.

Ocular colobomas may be associated with multiple systemic abnormalities and a number of syndromes, such as the CHARGE syndrome (*c*oloboma, *h*eart defects, choanal *a*tresia, mental *r*etardation, *g*enitourinary abnormalities, and *e*ar abnormalities). A careful evaluation by primary pediatrician or geneticist is recommended.

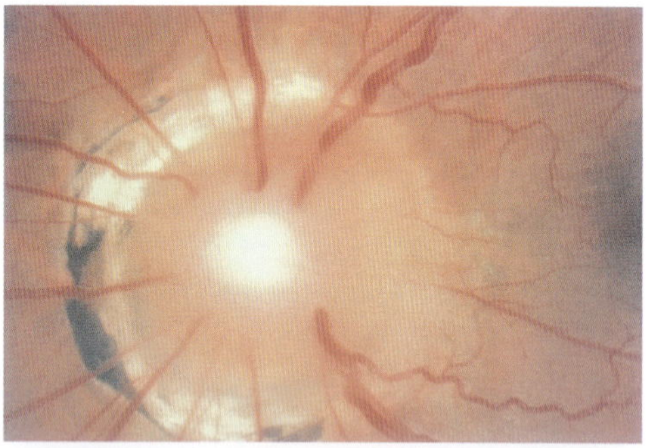

Figure 23-4 Morning glory disc anomaly, left eye. Salient features include an enlarged ONH within an excavation, a pigmented border, and radiating vasculature with a central glial tuft.

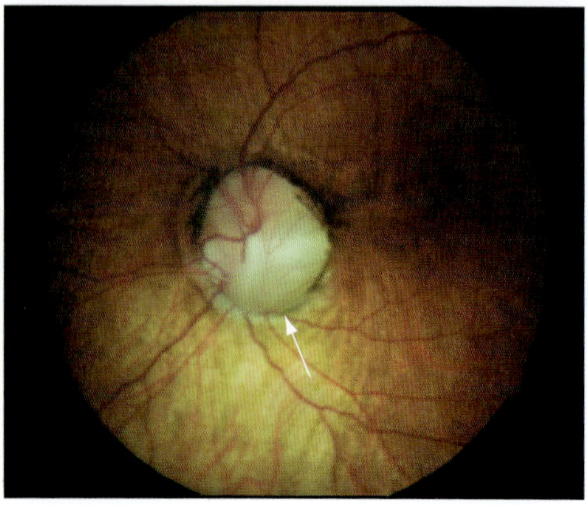

Figure 23-5 Optic nerve coloboma, left eye. Note the inferonasal location of the coloboma corresponding to the failed closure of the embryonic fissure *(arrow)*. *(Courtesy of Mays El-Dairi, MD.)*

Optic Nerve Pit

Optic nerve pit (optic hole) represents herniation of dysplastic retina into a collagen-lined pocket extending posteriorly, often into the subarachnoid space, through a defect in the lamina cribrosa. It is typically unilateral. It is associated with localized nerve fiber layer defects and serous macular detachments, typically in the second or third decade of life.

The typical appearance is a round or oval, gray, white, or yellowish depression in the inferotemporal quadrant or central portion of the ONH, often covered with a gray veil of tissue and emerging cilioretinal vessels (Fig 23-6).

Some have considered this entity to be a variant of coloboma, but it is distinct and there is no association with iris or chorioretinal coloboma.

Myelinated Retinal Nerve Fiber Layer

Myelination of the optic nerve normally stops at the lamina cribrosa. Inappropriate myelination anterior to the lamina cribrosa causes scotomata or central vision loss. Particularly when the macula is involved, myelinated retinal nerve fibers are associated with ipsilateral high myopia and resultant anisometropic amblyopia. In some cases, the fovea is hypoplastic.

Clinically, myelinated nerve fibers appear as a white superficial retinal area, the frayed and feathered edges of which tend to follow the same orientation as that of the normal retinal nerve fibers (Fig 23-7). Retinal vessels that pass within the superficial layer of the

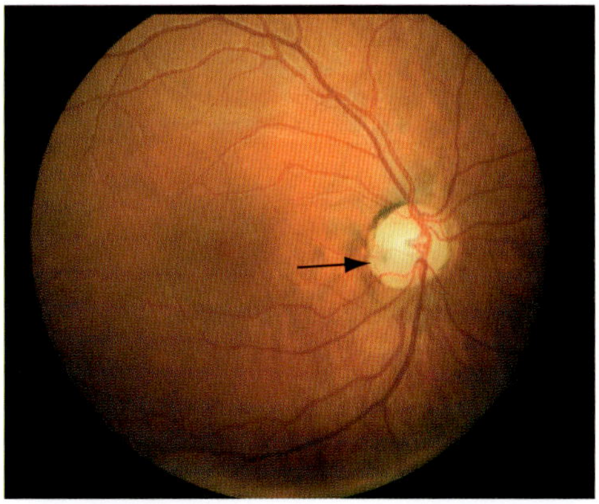

Figure 23-6 Right optic nerve with a temporal optic nerve pit *(arrow)*. Cilioretinal vessels can be seen emanating from the optic nerve pit. Serous detachments may lead to acquired vision loss; these may need to be surgically managed. *(Courtesy of Mays El-Dairi, MD.)*

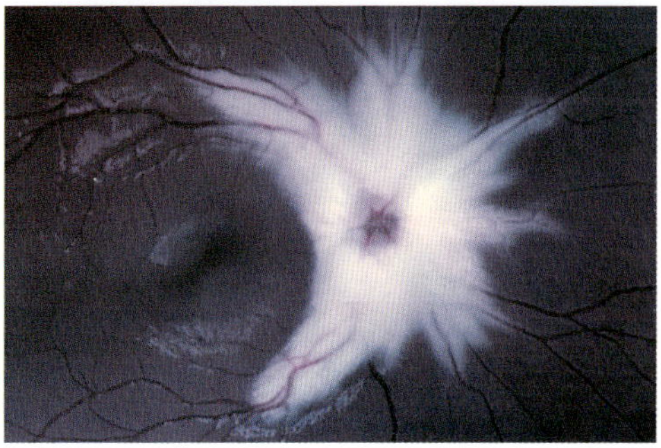

Figure 23-7 Myelinated nerve fibers of the optic nerve and retina, right eye. *(Courtesy of Arif O. Khan, MD.)*

nerve fibers are obscured. The myelinated fibers may occur as a single spot or as several noncontiguous patches. The most common location is along the ONH margin.

Tilted Optic Nerve Head

In a patient with a tilted ONH, often the superior pole of the ONH appears elevated, with posterior displacement of the inferior nasal ONH. Alternatively, the ONH is tilted horizontally, resulting in an oval ONH with an oblique long axis (Fig 23-8). Tilted ONH is often associated with a scleral crescent located inferiorly or inferonasally, situs inversus, posterior ectasia of the inferior nasal fundus, myopia, and astigmatism that is often in the axis of the ONH tilt.

Patients may demonstrate superotemporal visual field defects, which may resolve with refractive correction. Tilted optic nerve heads, myopic astigmatism, bilateral decreased vision, and visual difficulty at night are suggestive of congenital stationary night blindness (see Chapter 24 and BCSC Section 12, *Retina and Vitreous*). Acquired tilted ONH and peripapillary crescent formation have been documented in children with myopic progression.

Kim TW, Kim M, Weinreb RN, Woo SJ, Park KH, Hwang JM. Optic disc change with incipient myopia of childhood. *Ophthalmology.* 2012;119(1):21–26.

Bergmeister Papilla

A form of persistent fetal vasculature, Bergmeister papilla is a benign prepapillary glial remnant of the hyaloid artery, which is normally resorbed before birth. In some cases, a hyaloid artery remnant extends from the ONH to the lens (typically inferonasally) and may contain blood.

Megalopapilla

Megalopapilla is an abnormally large ONH (area >2.5 mm^2). The commonly associated large cup can be mistaken for glaucomatous damage.

Peripapillary Staphyloma

Peripapillary staphyloma is a posterior bulging of the sclera encompassing the ONH. White sclera encircling the ONH is often visible. Vision is usually poor. The condition is usually unilateral and rarely bilateral.

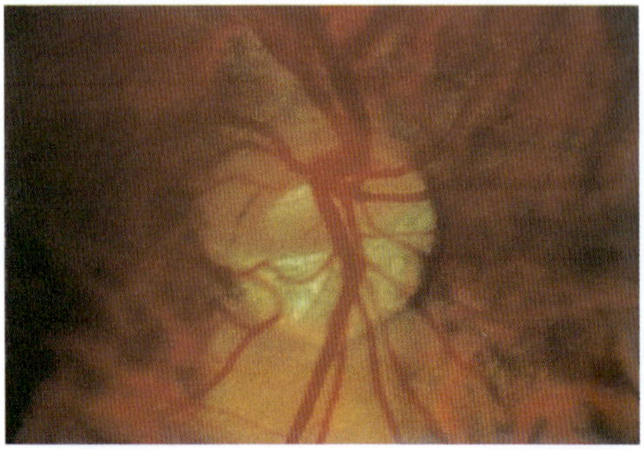

Figure 23-8 Tilted ONH, right eye.

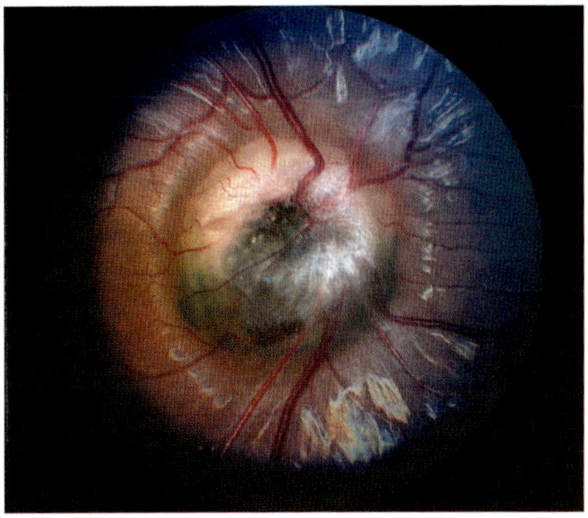

Figure 23-9 Melanocytoma of the ONH and adjacent retina. *(Courtesy of Scott Lambert, MD.)*

Optic Nerve Aplasia

Optic nerve aplasia, a lack of optic nerve axons and retinal blood vessels, is very rare. The choroidal pattern is clearly visible. When bilateral, optic nerve aplasia is usually associated with other CNS malformations; when unilateral, it can occur with normal brain development.

Melanocytoma of the Optic Nerve Head

Melanocytoma is a darkly pigmented tumor with little or no growth potential. It usually involves the ONH and adjacent retina (Fig 23-9).

Optic Atrophy

Optic atrophy in children can be secondary to anterior visual pathway disease such as perinatal hypoxic–ischemic injury, hydrocephalus, optic nerve or chiasmal tumors, nutritional deficiencies, or inflammation (optic neuritis), or it can be inherited (autosomal dominant, autosomal recessive, X-linked, or mitochondrial). A differential diagnosis for optic neuropathy is given in Table 23-1. Neuroimaging should be considered for all patients with optic atrophy of undetermined etiology. Specific underlying gene defects may be inferred from coexisting systemic features (eg, Wolfram syndrome or Behr syndrome). See BCSC Section 5, *Neuro-Ophthalmology,* for further discussion of acquired optic neuropathies.

Inherited Optic Atrophies

Dominant optic atrophy, Kjer type

Dominant optic atrophy is characterized by bilateral slow loss of central vision, usually before 10 years of age. It is caused by heterozygous mutations in *OPA1*. Visual acuity ranges from 20/40 to 20/100, with visual acuity rarely worse than 20/200. Visual field tests show central or cecocentral scotomata with normal peripheral isopters. Color vision testing reveals a blue dyschromatopsia. The ONH shows a characteristic temporal wedge of pallor, often with triangular excavation (Fig 23-10). Some patients experience hearing loss.

Table 23-1 Differential Diagnosis of Optic Neuropathies in Children

Etiology	Possible Disease Entities	Early Optic Nerve Appearance
Metabolic/toxic	B_{12}, folate, vitamin A, zinc, or copper deficiency Heavy metal toxicity Alcohol, ethambutol, or linezolid toxicity	Vitamin deficiency: normal or pale Heavy metal or medication toxicity: normal or mild swelling
Increased intracranial pressure	Obstructive hydrocephalus, craniosynostosis, venous sinus thrombosis, reaction to medication (vitamin A, estrogen, tetracyclines, growth hormone, lithium), malignant hypertension, meningitis, idiopathic intracranial hypertension	Papilledema: swelling
Traumatic	Traumatic optic neuropathy: severe trauma to eye/head	Normal or swelling; possible retinal findings
Infectious	Neuroretinitis Retrobulbar infectious optic neuropathy	Neuroretinitis: swollen with macular exudates in a stellate pattern Retrobulbar: normal or swelling; retinal changes or vitreous inflammation may also be present
Demyelinating	Neuromyelitis optica spectrum (anti-AQP4 antibodies or anti-MOG antibodies) ADEM; often associated with MOG MS Isolated	Normal or mild swelling MOG: mild to severe edema; occasional neuroretinitis-like picture
Inflammatory	Idiopathic orbital inflammatory syndrome Sarcoidosis Granulomatosis with polyangiitis Systemic lupus erythematosus Behçet disease	Normal or swelling; possible retinal findings
Neoplastic/ compressive	Optic pathway glioma Schwannomas Optic nerve sheath meningioma Craniopharyngioma Pituitary tumor Lymphoma Leukemia Aneurysm	Normal Swelling or pallor Infiltrative pathologies: retinal/ vitreous findings
Hereditary	LHON Dominant optic atrophy Wolfram and Behr syndromes	LHON: pseudoedema, peripapillary telangiectasias Dominant optic atrophy and Wolfram syndrome: temporal pallor with excavation of cup

ADEM = acute demyelinating encephalomyelopathy; AQP4 = aquaporin-4; LHON = Leber hereditary optic neuropathy; MOG = myelin oligodendrocyte glycoprotein; MS = multiple sclerosis.

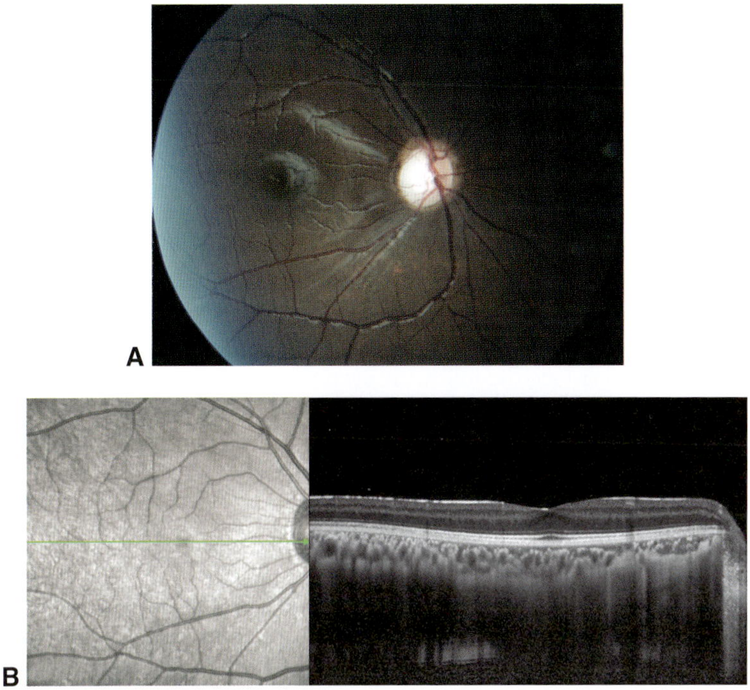

Figure 23-10 Dominant optic atrophy in a boy with confirmed heterozygous *OPA1* mutation. **A,** The ONH, right eye, shows temporal pallor. The left eye was similar. **B,** Corresponding optical coherence tomography (OCT) image shows a lack of nerve fiber and ganglion cell layers (left eye was similar). *(Courtesy of Arif O. Khan, MD.)*

Recessive optic atrophy

Recessive optic atrophy is characterized by severe bilateral vision loss before 5 years of age, often associated with nystagmus. Wolfram syndrome (also called DIDMOAD: diabetes insipidus, diabetes mellitus, optic atrophy, and deafness) is optic atrophy caused by biallelic mutations in *WFS1,* with variable expressivity of hearing loss and diabetes mellitus. Wolfram syndrome should be suspected in children with diabetes who have optic atrophy. Behr syndrome is caused by biallelic mutations in *OPA1,* with variable expressivity of neurologic findings such as ataxia, pyramidal signs, spasticity, bladder dysfunction, and intellectual disability.

Leber hereditary optic neuropathy

Leber hereditary optic neuropathy is a maternally inherited (mitochondrial) disease characterized by acute or subacute bilateral loss of central vision, ONH edema in the acute phase, acquired red-green dyschromatopsia, and central or cecocentral scotomata in otherwise healthy patients (usually men) in their second to fourth decade of life.

Optic Neuritis

Optic neuritis presents differently in children than it does in adults: it is more often bilateral, associated with ONH edema and vision loss, and can be severe. Over one-half of affected children have systemic symptoms, including headache, nausea, vomiting, lethargy, or malaise. In children, optic neuritis can occur as an isolated neurologic deficit or as a component of more generalized neurologic disease. See BCSC Section 5, *Neuro-Ophthalmology,* for further discussion of optic neuritis.

Optic Neuritis and Myelin Oligodendrocyte Glycoprotein

Patients with myelin oligodendrocyte glycoprotein (MOG) autoimmunity may present with optic neuritis. They may also present with multiple neurologic abnormalities, including transverse myelitis, acute demyelinating encephalomyelitis, and brainstem encephalitis. Patients with neuromyelitis optica may meet diagnostic criteria for neuromyelitis optica spectrum disorders (see the following section). MOG appears to be more common in children than in adults and can be recurrent. Clinically, optic neuritis associated with MOG is more likely to present with optic nerve head swelling, peripapillary hemorrhages, and retinal findings such as neuroretinitis.

Optic Neuritis and Neuromyelitis Optica Spectrum Disorders

Neuromyelitis optica (NMO) is characterized by optic neuritis (unilateral or bilateral, frequently severe) and transverse myelitis (usually spanning 3 or more vertebral segments). Seropositive NMO is associated with antibody to aquaporin 4 (NMO-IgG or AQP4-IgG). Recognizing NMO is crucial since treatment delay can cause severe visual and neurologic disability. Other manifestations of NMO can include intractable nausea and vomiting (area postrema syndrome), acute brainstem syndrome, and narcolepsy. NMO IgG testing is 99% specific and 75% sensitive.

Optic Neuritis and Multiple Sclerosis

The relationship between optic neuritis and the later development of multiple sclerosis, which is common in adults, is less clear in children. In a small subset of children with optic neuritis, signs and symptoms consistent with multiple sclerosis develop. Older age and MRI findings extrinsic to the visual system are associated with increased risk of multiple sclerosis.

Treatment of an isolated optic neuritis in children is controversial. If MOG or NMO is suspected, treatment is strongly recommended. In children with NMO, vision loss may be severe and response to corticosteroids is typically poor. Escalation of the treatment to intravenous immunoglobulins or even plasmapheresis might be indicated.

Neuroretinitis denotes inflammatory ONH edema associated with a stellate pattern of exudates in the macula (macular star; Fig 23-11). Common etiologies differ by region. In North America, a common etiology is *Bartonella henselae* infection (cat-scratch disease). Other infectious etiologies include mumps, toxocariasis, tuberculosis, and syphilis. Patients with neuroretinitis are not at risk for development of multiple sclerosis. Children initially suspected to have optic neuritis should be reevaluated for potential emergence of macular edema, which would reclassify the diagnosis as neuroretinitis. Neuroretinitis may also be a manifestation of an autoimmune disorder, such as MOG, sarcoidosis, or microvasculitis.

Chen JJ, Pittock SJ, Flanagan EP, Lennon VA, Bhatti MT. Optic neuritis in the era of biomarkers. *Surv Ophthalmol.* 2020;65(1):12–17.

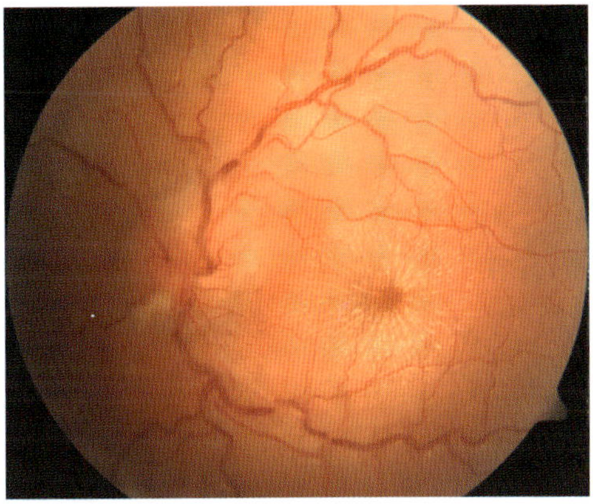

Figure 23-11 Neuroretinitis. Inflammatory ONH edema with a macular star. *(Courtesy of Paul Phillips, MD.)*

Papilledema

Papilledema refers to ONH edema that is secondary to elevated intracranial pressure (ICP) (Fig 23-12). It is typically bilateral. Initially, visual acuity, color vision, and pupillary reactions are normal. However, vision dysfunction may occur as a result of high-grade papilledema. Signs of high-grade papilledema include obscuration of vessels at the ONH or its margins, retinal peripapillary hemorrhages, and exudates.

In children, a number of conditions (eg, hydrocephalus, intracranial mass lesions, meningitis, idiopathic intracranial hypertension) can cause increased ICP and thus ONH swelling. A full evaluation, including neuroimaging possibly followed by lumbar puncture, is indicated in patients with papilledema. In infants, increased ICP results in firmness and distention of the open fontanelles. Significantly elevated pressure is usually accompanied by nausea, vomiting, and headaches. Older children may describe transient visual obscurations as transient dimming of vision, often upon sitting or standing up. Cranial nerve (CN) VI palsy may be a sign of elevated ICP.

See BCSC Section 5, *Neuro-Ophthalmology,* for further discussion of papilledema.

A

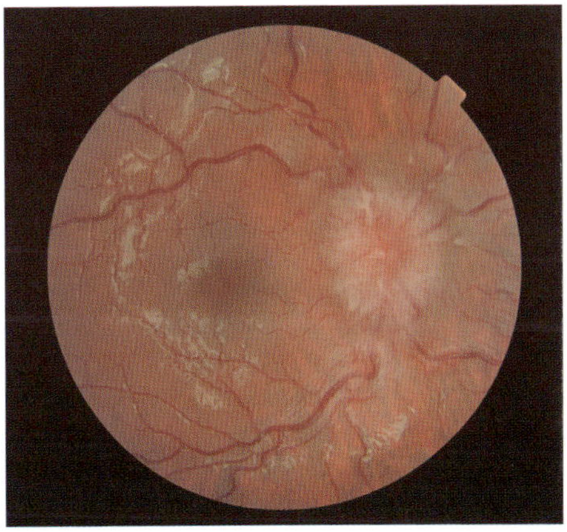

B

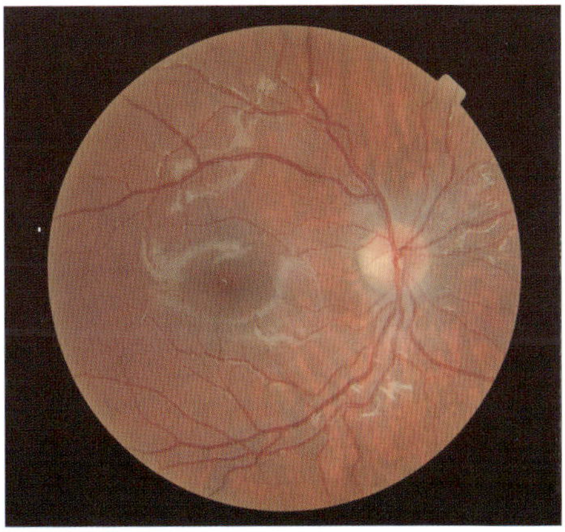

Figure 23-12 Papilledema in the right eye of a child with idiopathic intracranial hypertension before treatment **(A)** and 3 months after treatment with oral acetazolamide **(B).** Resolution in the left eye was similar. *(Courtesy of Robert W. Hered, MD.)*

Idiopathic Intracranial Hypertension

Idiopathic intracranial hypertension (IIH), or *pseudotumor cerebri,* is characterized by increased ICP in patients with normal-sized or small ventricles on neuroimaging, and normal cerebrospinal fluid composition. Although IIH is uncommon in children, it can occur at any age. It may be associated with viral infections, excessive intake of vitamin A, and certain drugs (eg, tetracyclines, corticosteroids, nalidixic acid, thyroid medications, estrogen, testosterone, and growth hormone). Although MRI in patients with IIH does not reveal a cause of increased ICP, it frequently shows other signs of elevated ICP, including a partially empty sella, flattening of the posterior poles, and distension of the optic nerve sheaths. Magnetic resonance venography is recommended to rule out cerebral venous sinus thrombosis as opposed to IIH and frequently shows venous sinus stenosis in IIH.

In *prepubescent* children with IIH, the incidence of obesity is lower compared with that in adult IIH patients, and the male-to-female ratio is approximately equal. *Postpubescent* children with IIH have a clinical profile similar to that of adult IIH patients, with a higher incidence of obesity and female preponderance.

Common presenting symptoms are headache, vision loss, transient visual obscurations, and diplopia. Papilledema may be noted on routine examination of an asymptomatic child. Examination frequently reveals excellent visual acuity with bilateral papilledema. Unilateral or bilateral CN VI palsy may be present. The patient should be monitored closely for decreased visual acuity, visual field loss, and worsening headaches. Although visual field tests can be difficult to interpret in children, they should be performed when possible. Structural imaging (fundus photos, optical coherence tomography [OCT]) is highly valuable in monitoring disease progression.

Treatment of IIH begins with discontinuation of any causative medications and weight management, if indicated. Medical treatment includes acetazolamide or topiramate (see Fig 23-12). If medical treatment is unsuccessful, surgical treatment options include optic nerve sheath fenestration or shunting procedures (lumbar or ventriculoperitoneal), both of which can reduce the incidence of vision loss. Shunting procedures are preferred for patients with vision loss or risk of vision loss and those with severe headaches unresponsive to medical management. With treatment, the vision prognosis is excellent for most patients, although vision loss can occur secondary to high-grade untreated papilledema. In most cases, spontaneous resolution occurs within 12–18 months of initial treatment.

Pseudopapilledema

Pseudopapilledema refers to any elevated anomaly of the ONH that resembles papilledema. In children, conditions that are frequently confused with papilledema include ONH drusen, hyperopic ONHs, and prominent ONH glial tissue. Pseudopapilledema can be very difficult to differentiate from true low-grade papilledema (nerve elevation with no vessel obscuration). Anomalous branching of the large peripapillary retinal vessels is often seen in eyes with pseudopapilledema (Fig 23-13).

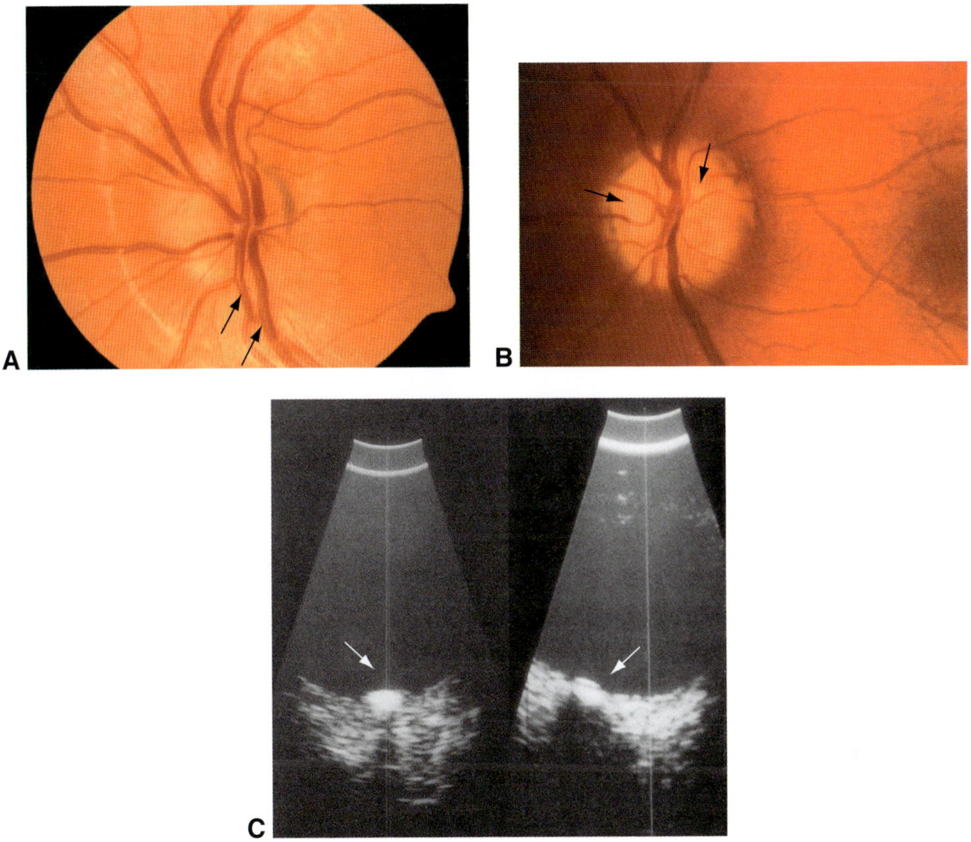

Figure 23-13 Pseudopapilledema. **A,** Note anomalous branching *(arrows)* of the large retinal vessels without ONH hyperemia, retinal hemorrhages, or exudates. **B,** ONH drusen seen as refractile opacities on the ONH surface *(arrows).* **C,** Ultrasonographic image shows a bright spot in the ONH *(arrows),* consistent with drusen. *(Parts A and B courtesy of Paul Phillips, MD; part C courtesy of Edward G. Buckley, MD.)*

Although most children with pseudopapilledema do not have other related ophthalmic or systemic abnormalities, pseudopapilledema can occur in patients with retinal dystrophy, pseudoxanthoma elasticum, Down syndrome, and Alagille syndrome. Down and Alagille syndromes are also associated with IIH; thus, close monitoring and/or workup is recommended.

Optic Nerve Head Drusen

Intrapapillary drusen, the most common cause of pseudopapilledema in children, can appear within the first or second decade of life (Fig 23-14; see also Fig 23-13B). Drusen are frequently inherited (autosomal dominant); thus, examination of the parents is helpful when drusen are suspected in children.

Clinically, the elevated ONH does not obscure the retinal arterioles lying anteriorly; it often has an irregular border, suggesting the presence of drusen beneath the surface.

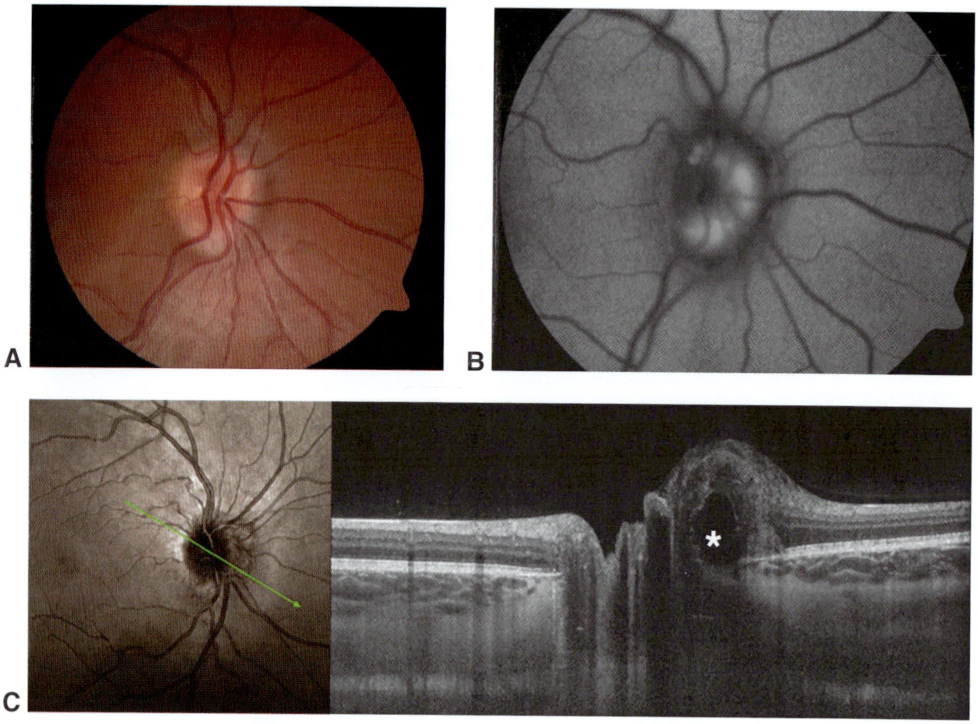

Figure 23-14 ONH drusen. **A,** Superficial ONH drusen, right eye. **B,** Appearance with autofluorescence. **C,** OCT image from a different child with drusen reveals a hyperreflective cap over a hyporeflective core *(asterisk)*. *(Courtesy of Wayne T. Cornblath, MD.)*

There is no dilatation of the papillary network, and superficial retinal hemorrhages and exudates are absent. Peripapillary subretinal hemorrhages and subretinal neovascular membranes occur only in rare cases. When drusen are not buried, they appear as shiny refractile bodies visible on the ONH surface, with a gray-yellow translucent appearance. Visual field defects are frequently associated with drusen; inferior nasal field defects are common. Concentric narrowing, an arcuate scotoma, and central defects may also occur. These defects may be slowly progressive. Visual acuity is rarely affected.

In some patients, fundus evaluation can be sufficient to enable the clinician to identify drusen as the cause of the swollen ONH appearance. In others, B-scan ultrasonography is helpful in visualizing bright calcific reflections at the ONH that remain visible after the gain is decreased (see Fig 23-13C). Autofluorescence imaging and OCT may also be useful (see Fig 23-14).

Most children with ONH drusen do not have other related ophthalmic or systemic abnormalities. However, the incidence of ONH drusen is increased in children with high hyperopia, retinal dystrophy, or pseudoxanthoma elasticum.

CHAPTER 24

Disorders of the Retina and Vitreous

This chapter includes related videos. Go to www.aao.org/bcscvideo_section06 or scan the QR codes in the text to access this content.

This chapter includes a related activity. Go to www.aao.org/bcscactivity_section06 or scan the QR code in the text to access this content.

Highlights

- While most retinopathy of prematurity spontaneously involutes, specific criteria indicate high risk for vision loss from abnormal vascularization and the need for treatment.
- Inherited retinal disorders are genotypically and phenotypically heterogeneous; genetic counseling is a component of care.
- Genetic testing and pathophysiologic understanding have led to novel treatment approaches for previously untreatable conditions.
- Retinoblastoma is the most common intraocular malignancy afflicting children; early recognition and prompt referral improve survival and visual outcomes.

Introduction

This chapter focuses on retinal diseases that are most often diagnosed in the first 2 decades of life, including acquired and inherited vascular disorders, vitreoretinopathies, retinal dystrophies, and retinoblastoma. Many of the topics covered in this chapter are also discussed in BCSC Section 12, *Retina and Vitreous.* See BCSC Section 4, *Ophthalmic Pathology and Intraocular Tumors,* for a detailed discussion of tumors.

Vascular Disorders of the Retina

Persistent Fetal Vasculature

Persistent fetal vasculature is covered in BCSC Section 11, *Lens and Cataract,* and Section 12, *Retina and Vitreous.*

Coats Disease

See BCSC 12, *Retina and Vitreous,* and the section Retinoblastoma later in this chapter.

Retinopathy of Prematurity

Retinopathy of prematurity (ROP) is a vasoproliferative retinal disorder unique to prematurely born infants. First described in the 1940s, ROP is a leading cause of childhood blindness in the United States, second only to cerebral visual impairment. See BCSC Section 12, *Retina and Vitreous,* for more on ROP.

Pathophysiology

Retinal vascularization begins during week 16 of gestation. Mesenchymal tissue, the source of retinal blood vessels, grows centrifugally from the optic nerve head (ONH; also called *optic disc*), reaching the nasal ora serrata by 36 weeks' gestation and the temporal ora serrata by 40 weeks' gestation. ROP results from abnormal growth of these retinal vessels in prematurely born infants, owing to complex interactions among environmental factors—such as oxygen levels, oxidative stress, and light—as well as endogenous factors—such as vascular endothelial growth factor (VEGF), insulin-like growth factor 1 (IGF-1), growth hormone, and neuronal signaling molecules. For a further discussion of this topic, see BCSC Section 12, *Retina and Vitreous.*

Risk factors for development of ROP

Premature birth (≤30 weeks' gestational age) and low birth weight (≤1500 g) are the most significant risk factors for development of ROP, but risk also is stratified by ethnoracial group and geographic region. Additional risk factors include oxygen (supplementation or fluctuation), slow postnatal growth, increased altitude, and day length in early gestation.

Binenbaum G, Tomlinson LA, de Alba Campomanes AG, et al. Validation of the Postnatal Growth and Retinopathy of Prematurity Screening Criteria. *JAMA Ophthalmol.* 2020;138(1): 31–37.

Reem RE, Nguyen T, Yu Y, Ying G-S, Tomlinson L, Binenbaum G. Effects of altitude on retinopathy of prematurity. *Invest Ophthalmol Vis Sci.* 2020;61:2190. [abstract]

Yang MB, Rao S, Copenhagen DR, Lang RA. Length of day during early gestation as a predictor of risk for severe retinopathy of prematurity. *Ophthalmology.* 2013;120(12): 2706–2713.

Classification

Worldwide ROP experts devised the International Classification of Retinopathy of Prematurity (ICROP). The recently published third edition (ICROP3) reflects the refined understanding of this disease and its progression, as well as advanced imaging characteristics, regional variation, and evolving treatment paradigms. Disease is classified by location (zone), severity (stage), extent, and characteristics of vessels in the posterior pole (spectrum of "plus" disease) (Table 24-1; Figs 24-1 and 24-2). Higher stage numbers, lower zone numbers, and the presence of plus disease indicate more severe ROP.

Table 24-1 International Classification of Retinopathy of Prematurity, 3rd Edition

Location: zones II and III are based on convention rather than strict anatomy (see Fig 24-1)

Zone I (posterior pole): a circle centered on the optic disc, with a radius equal to twice the distance from the center of the disc to the center of the macula

Zone II: the area extending from and anterior to zone I extending to a circle centered on the optic disc, with a radius equal to the distance from the center of the optic disc to the nasal ora serrata

Posterior zone II: the area that begins at the margin between zone I and zone II and extends into zone II for 2 disc diameters

Notch terminology: incursion of an ROP lesion 1–2 clock-hours along the horizontal meridian that is more posterior than the remainder of disease

Zone III: residual crescent anterior to zone II

Extent: defined as 12 sectors in using clock-hour designation

Stages of acute disease[a]

Stage 0: immature vascularization, no ROP

Stage 1: presence of a demarcation line between vascularized retina posteriorly and avascular retina anteriorly (see Fig 24-2A)

Stage 2: presence of a ridge with height and width, with or without small tufts of fibrovascular proliferation ("popcorn") (see Fig 24-2B)

Stage 3: ridge with extraretinal fibrovascular proliferation or flat neovascularization (see Fig 24-2C)

Stages of retinal detachment

Stage 4: subtotal retinal detachment

A. extrafoveal retinal detachment (see Fig 24-2D)

B. retinal detachment including fovea (see Fig 24-2E)

Stage 5: total retinal detachment; open or closed funnel (see Fig 24-2F)[b]

A. optic disc visible by ophthalmoscopy, suggesting open-funnel detachment

B. optic disc not visible due to retrolental fibrovascular tissue or closed-funnel detachment

C. stage 5B, plus anterior segment changes (eg, marked anterior chamber shallowing, iridocorneolenticular adhesions, corneal opacification), suggesting closed-funnel configuration

Pre–plus and plus disease

Pre–plus disease is defined by abnormal vascular dilation and/or tortuosity insufficient for plus disease (see Fig 24-4); plus disease is defined by the appearance of dilation and tortuosity of retinal vessels (see Fig 24-3):

- pre–plus to plus disease represents a continuous spectrum
- vessels should be assessed within zone I (not by quadrants)
- plus symbol (+) added to ROP stage denotes presence of plus disease (eg, stage 3 + ROP)

Aggressive ROP (A-ROP): severe, rapidly progressive form of ROP, usually located in posterior zone I or zone II; may also occur outside the posterior retina (see Fig 24-5A)

Regression: definition of ROP regression and its sequelae, whether spontaneous or following laser or anti-VEGF treatment. Can be complete or incomplete. Location and extent of PAR should be documented

Reactivation: definition and description of nomenclature representing ROP reactivation following treatment; may include new ROP lesions and vascular changes. When reactivation of ROP stages occurs, the modifier "reactivated" (eg, "reactivated stage 2") is recommended

Long-term sequelae: late retinal detachments, PAR, macular anomalies, retinal vascular changes, and glaucoma

PAR = persistent avascular retina; ROP = retinopathy of prematurity; VEGF = vascular endothelial growth factor.

[a] If more than 1 ROP stage is present in the same eye, the eye is classified by the most severe stage.

[b] Additional descriptors of funnel configuration (eg, open–closed) may be applied if clinically useful.

Information from Chiang MF, Quinn GE, Fielder AR, et al. International Classification of Retinopathy of Prematurity, 3rd ed. *Ophthalmology.* 2021;128(10):e51–e68.

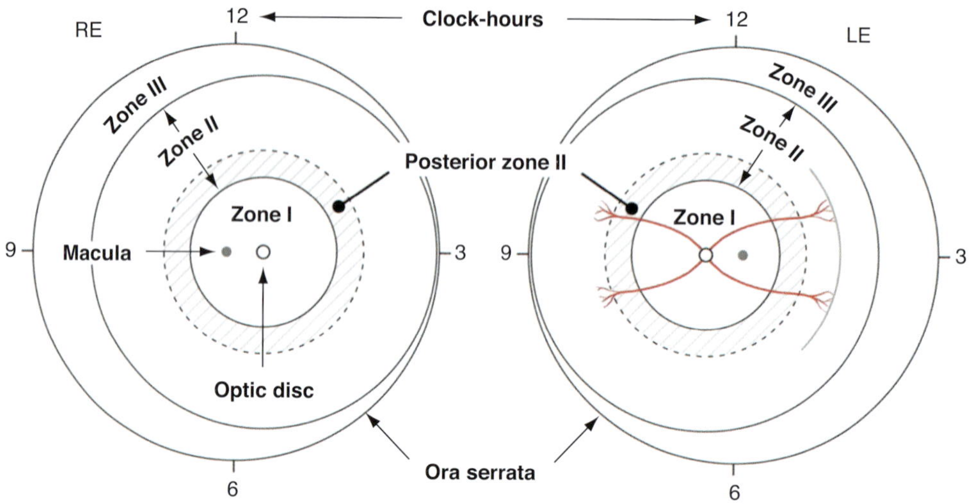

Figure 24-1 Schematic of the retina of the right eye (RE) and left eye (LE), showing zone borders and clock-hour sectors used to describe the location of vascularization and extent of retinopathy. Solid circles represent borders of zones I–III, and dashed circles represent borders of posterior zone II (2 disc diameters beyond zone I). The LE illustration shows a hypothetical example of examination findings, representing approximately 3 clock-hours of stage 1 disease in zone II (the single line documents the presence of stage 1 disease). *(Courtesy of Chiang MF, Quinn GE, Fielder AR, et al. International Classification of Retinopathy of Prematurity, 3rd ed.* Ophthalmology. *2021;128(10):e51–e68. With permission from Elsevier.)*

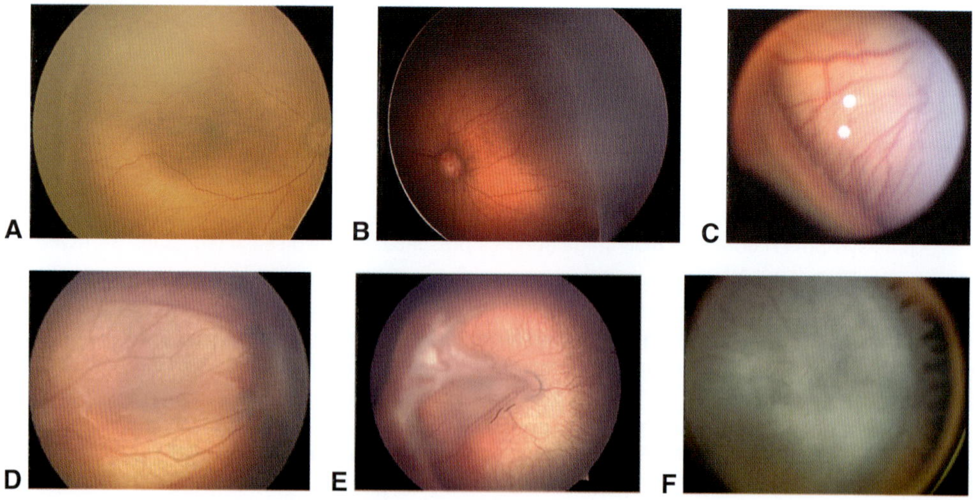

Figure 24-2 Staging of retinopathy of prematurity (ROP). **A,** Stage 1 ROP. The demarcation line has no height. **B,** Stage 2 ROP. The demarcation line has height and width, creating a ridge. **C,** Stage 3 ROP. Ridge with extraretinal fibrovascular proliferation. **D,** Stage 4A ROP. Partial detachment of the retina not involving the fovea. **E,** Stage 4B ROP. Partial detachment of the retina involving the fovea. **F,** Stage 5 ROP. Total retinal detachment. *(Part A courtesy of Daniel Weaver, MD; part B courtesy of Andrea Molinari, MD; part C reproduced with permission from Lueder GT.* Pediatric Practice Ophthalmology. *McGraw-Hill Medical; 2011:232. Permission conveyed through Copyright Clearance Center, Inc.; parts D–F courtesy of R.V. Paul Chan, MD, and Michael F. Chiang, MD.)*

CLINICAL PEARL

Clinically, the temporal edge of zone I is visible with a 25.00 D or 28.00 D lens, with the other edge of the field of view on the nasal optic nerve head margin.

Plus disease (Fig 24-3) and *pre–plus disease* (Fig 24-4) are a continuum of marked arteriolar tortuosity and venous dilation of retinal vessels as assessed in zone I (see Table 24-1).

The term *aggressive posterior ROP (AP-ROP)* was previously used to describe a severe, rapidly progressive form of ROP in posterior zone I and posterior zone II. However, because this aggressive form of ROP can occur outside the posterior zones and in larger preterm infants, particularly in countries with limited resources, the ICROP3's new preferred term is *aggressive ROP (A-ROP),* which reflects the varied location of disease. A-ROP is associated with plus disease out of proportion to the stage of ROP present. In addition, A-ROP does not progress in the typical fashion (ie, through stages 1, 2, then 3), and stage

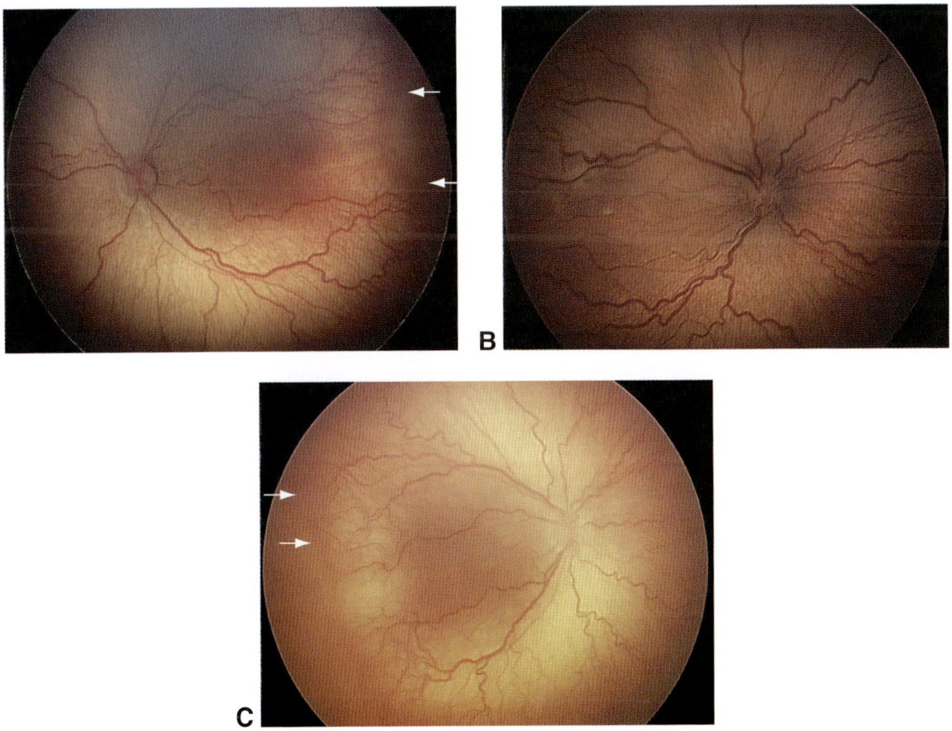

A B C

Figure 24-3 Wide-angle fundus photos demonstrating the spectrum of plus disease as defined by the International Classification of Retinopathy of Prematurity, 3rd edition (ICROP3). The vascular abnormalities are assessed in the central retina within the region of zone I. **A,** Plus disease with notable venous dilation and arterial tortuosity. The plus disease is out of proportion to visible peripheral findings, suggesting flat neovascularization (stage 3, *arrows*). **B,** Severe plus disease, with dilation and tortuosity of both arteries and veins. **C,** Severe plus disease. Note the presence of ill-defined posterior flat stage 3 *(arrows),* which, combined with severe plus disease, is typical of aggressive ROP (A-ROP). *(Courtesy of Chiang MF, Quinn GE, Fielder AR, et al. International Classification of Retinopathy of Prematurity, 3rd ed.* Ophthalmology. *2021;128(10):e51–e68. With permission from Elsevier.)*

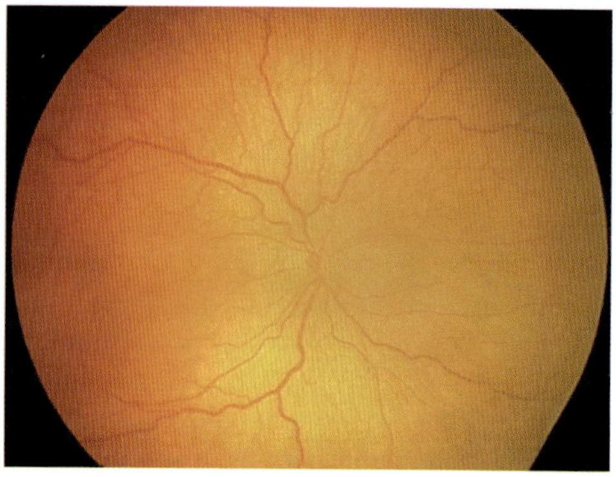

Figure 24-4 Pre–plus disease. Pre–plus disease is defined as abnormal dilation and tortuosity of the posterior pole vessels, but insufficiently severe for the diagnosis of plus disease. Pre–plus is part of a continuum of vascular abnormality from normal to plus disease. *(Courtesy of Daniel Weaver, MD.)*

3 often presents as flat neovascularization. Without treatment, A-ROP proceeds quickly to stage 5 ROP (Fig 24-5).

CLINICAL PEARL

Each eye should be classified by (1) zone, (2) presence or absence of plus disease, (3) stage, and (4) extent of disease, noting A-ROP if present.

Activity 24-1 is an interactive, case-based retinopathy of prematurity training module.

ACTIVITY 24-1 Case-based training: retinopathy of prematurity.
Courtesy of R.V. Paul Chan, MD; Michael F. Chiang, MD; and Karyn Jonas, RN.

Chiang MF, Quinn GE, Fielder AR, et al. International Classification of Retinopathy of Prematurity, 3rd ed. *Ophthalmology.* 2021;128(10):e51–e68.

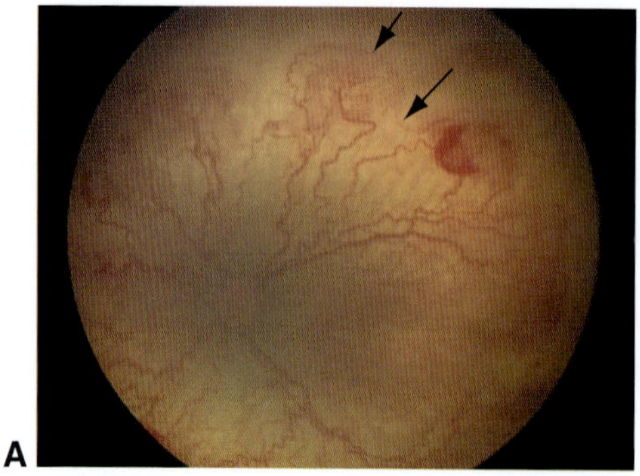

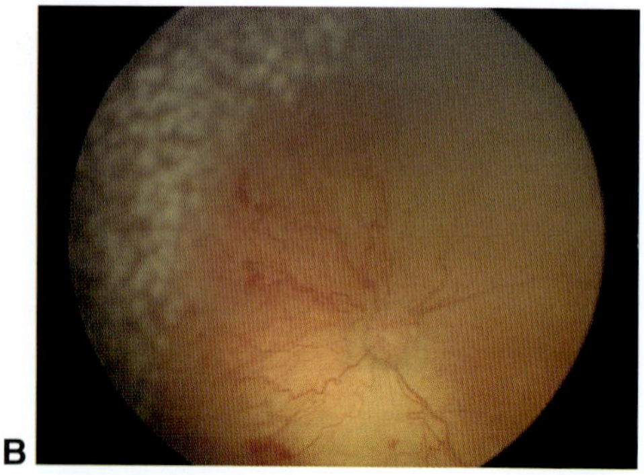

Figure 24-5 Aggressive ROP (A-ROP) before and after treatment. **A,** Tortuosity and dilation of arterioles and veins in all 4 quadrants, out of proportion to peripheral retinopathy. *Arrows* demonstrate neovascularization at the demarcation between avascular and vascular retinal tissue. **B,** Appearance of the retina shortly after laser treatment. Note vascular dilation has improved, but tortuosity still exists. *(Courtesy of Robert W. Hered, MD.)*

Screening and diagnosis

In the United States, it is recommended that infants with the following characteristics be screened for ROP:

- gestational age of 30 weeks or less
- birth weight of 1500 g or less
- complicated clinical course

For ROP examination in infants, sterile instruments are used, and pupil dilation typically is achieved with a combination of cyclopentolate (0.2%) and phenylephrine (1%). Infants receiving care in the neonatal intensive care unit may have apnea or bradycardia during the examination, so it is recommended that a nurse be present to provide support as needed. If the patient's condition requires postponement of the examination, this is documented in the medical record. Suggested intervals for follow-up examinations of patients with ROP without plus disease are given in Table 24-2; discontinuation of screening examinations is summarized in Table 24-3. Most ROP regresses spontaneously via involution. Access to screening may be expanded by implementing digital retinal photography and telemedicine.

Fierson WM; American Academy of Pediatrics Section on Ophthalmology; American Academy of Ophthalmology; American Association for Pediatric Ophthalmology and Strabismus; American Association of Certified Orthoptists. Screening examination of premature infants for retinopathy of prematurity. *Pediatrics.* 2018;142(6):e20183061.

Treatment

Approximately 10% of infants examined for ROP require treatment. Several multicenter ROP trials have been influential in guiding treatment of the disease. Treatment recommendations initially were based on findings of the Cryotherapy for Retinopathy of Prematurity

Table 24-2 Recommended Intervals of Follow-Up Eye Examinations for ROP Without Plus Disease

Follow-Up Interval	Disease Condition
1 week or less	Zone I: immature vascularization, no ROP Zone I: stage 1 or 2 ROP Posterior zone II: immature retina on the boundary between zones I and II Suspected presence of aggressive ROP (A-ROP) Stage 3 ROP, zone I requires treatment, not observation
1 to 2 weeks	Posterior zone II: immature vascularization Zone II: stage 2 Zone I: unequivocally regressing ROP
2 weeks	Zone II: stage 1 ROP Zone II: no ROP, immature vascularization Zone II: unequivocally regressing ROP
2 to 3 weeks	Zone III: stage 1 or 2 ROP Zone III: regressing ROP

ROP = retinopathy of prematurity.

Information from Fierson WM; American Academy of Pediatrics Section on Ophthalmology; American Academy of Ophthalmology; American Association for Pediatric Ophthalmology and Strabismus; American Association of Certified Orthoptists. Screening examination of premature infants for retinopathy of prematurity. *Pediatrics.* 2018;142(6):e20183061.

Table 24-3 Criteria for Discontinuation of ROP Screening Examinations[a]

Fully vascularized retina in close proximity to the ora serrata[b]
Zone III vascularization without previous zone I or II ROP
Lack of type 1 ROP[c] or worse ROP by postmenstrual age of 45 weeks
Postmenstrual age of 45 weeks and no type 1 ROP (previously called "prethreshold") disease (defined as stage 3 ROP in zone II, any ROP in zone I) or worse ROP is present
Postmenstrual age of at least 65 weeks in children treated with anti-VEGF agents[d]
Regression of ROP without abnormal vascular tissue capable of reactivation in zone II or III

ROP = retinopathy of prematurity; VEGF = vascular endothelial growth factor.
[a]Anti-VEGF agents change the natural history of disease; therefore, the retina must be fully vascularized or screening continue to at least 65 weeks to detect late occurrences.
[b]This criterion should be applied to any child treated with anti-VEGF medications.
[c]Type 1 ROP was previously called prethreshold ROP, defined as stage 3 ROP in zone II or any ROP in zone I.
[d]This criterion addresses the high risk of reactivation at 45–55 weeks.

Information from Fierson WM; American Academy of Pediatrics Section on Ophthalmology; American Academy of Ophthalmology; American Association for Pediatric Ophthalmology and Strabismus; American Association of Certified Orthoptists. Screening examination of premature infants for retinopathy of prematurity. *Pediatrics.* 2018;142(6):e20183061.

(CRYO-ROP) study; cryotherapy was recommended when the disease reached a certain severity threshold. This threshold was defined as 5 contiguous or 8 total clock-hours of stage 3 ROP in zone I or II in the presence of plus disease (see Table 24-1). However, results of the Early Treatment for Retinopathy of Prematurity (ETROP) study demonstrated that treatment of prethreshold disease yielded better structural and functional outcomes than did the threshold approach. Prethreshold disease is defined as all zone I and zone II ROP changes that do not meet threshold treatment criteria. These changes are further divided into type 1 and type 2 disease to delineate which infants would benefit from treatment. Table 24-4 details the definitions of clinically important ROP.

Current recommendations advocate performing confluent/semi-confluent panretinal laser photocoagulation of the peripheral retina (see Fig 24-5B) and administering

Table 24-4 Definitions of Clinically Important ROP

Severe ROP	Diagnosis	Zone	Stage	Plus Disease
a. Threshold	Clinical examination	I or II	Stage 3 (5 contiguous or 8 total clock-hours)	Yes
b. Type 1	Clinical examination	I	Any ROP with plus disease	Yes
		I	Stage 3 ROP without plus disease	Yes or no
		II	Stage 2 or 3 ROP with plus disease	Yes
Photographic imaging: referral-warranted ROP (in either eye)	Contact imaging	I	Any stage	
		I or II	Stage 3 ROP	
		I or II		Yes

ROP = retinopathy of prematurity.

Modified from Hartnett ME. Advances in understanding and management of retinopathy of prematurity. *Surv Ophthalmol.* 2017;62(3):257–276.

anti-VEGF treatment in select cases (Video 24-1). Once type 1 ROP develops, treatment within 72 hours is recommended. Eyes with type 2 ROP are monitored closely for progression. Videos 24-2 through 24-5 show ROP progression and response to laser treatment.

VIDEO 24-1 Intravitreal injection at bedside.
Courtesy of Audina M. Berrocal, MD.

VIDEO 24-2 Stage 3 retinopathy of prematurity.
Courtesy of Leslie D. MacKeen, BSc, and Anna L. Ells, MD. Dynamic documentation of the evolution of retinopathy of prematurity in video format. J AAPOS. *2008;12(4):349–351. With permission from Elsevier.*

VIDEO 24-3 Aggressive posterior retinopathy of prematurity with laser treatment.
Courtesy of Leslie D. MacKeen, BSc, and Anna L. Ells, MD. Dynamic documentation of the evolution of retinopathy of prematurity in video format. J AAPOS. *2008;12(4):349–351. With permission from Elsevier.*

VIDEO 24-4 Retinopathy of prematurity—the movie, 2.
Courtesy of Anna L. Ells, MD, and Leslie D. MacKeen, BSc. Retinopathy of prematurity—the movie. J AAPOS. *2004;8(4):389. With permission from Elsevier.*

VIDEO 24-5 Retinopathy of prematurity—the movie, 7.
Courtesy of Anna L. Ells, MD, and Leslie D. MacKeen, BSc. Retinopathy of prematurity—the movie. J AAPOS. *2004;8(4):389. With permission from Elsevier.*

Panretinal photocoagulation Panretinal laser photocoagulation is the mainstay of treatment for ROP. Adequate anesthesia and analgesia are needed with systemic monitoring and consultation with the neonatal intensive care unit physician.

KEY POINTS 24-1

Panretinal laser photocoagulation Panretinal photocoagulation involves less treatment-related morbidity than does cryoablation and is the preferred treatment unless media opacities obstruct visualization for the laser. The following are important tips for performing this treatment:

- A confluent or semi-confluent pattern is preferred to ablate the peripheral avascular retina.
- The laser is placed anterior to the ridge (not on the ridge) and extended 360° to the ora serrata.
- A lighter pattern is made in the horizontal meridian to avoid damaging the nerves or long ciliary vessels, which could result in anterior ischemic syndrome.

After treatment, weekly monitoring is recommended. If ROP regression is inadequate, additional laser treatment can be applied to the skip regions (see Fig 24-5B).

Shulman JP, Hobbs R, Hartnett ME. Retinopathy of prematurity: evolving concepts in diagnosis and management. *Focal Points: Clinical Modules for Ophthalmologists.* American Academy of Ophthalmology; 2015, module 1.

Anti-VEGF agents The most recent treatment option for type 1 ROP (and A-ROP) is an intravitreal injection of anti-VEGF agents (ie, bevacizumab and ranibizumab). The initial study of anti-VEGF agents for treatment of ROP was Bevacizumab Eliminates the Angiogenic Threat of Retinopathy of Prematurity (BEAT-ROP); investigators found a reduced rate of recurrence of neovascularization in eyes with stage 3, zone I that received intravitreal bevacizumab monotherapy compared with those treated with laser. In contrast, the outcomes of these treatment modalities were similar in eyes with zone II ROP. It has since been demonstrated that ROP may recur months after treatment with anti-VEGF agents; therefore, long-term surveillance is recommended, and re-treatment may be necessary. Because of this recurrence risk, anti-VEGF agents are not advised for infants who have an unstable social situation and are at risk for nonadherence to frequent follow-up examinations.

There is concern that antiangiogenic drugs may affect the developing vasculature in other areas of the body and lead to adverse developmental outcomes. To ascertain the minimum effective dose of bevacizumab, the Pediatric Eye Disease Investigator Group (PEDIG) evaluated a de-escalating dose regimen (0.25, 0.125, 0.063, 0.031 mg, all in 10 mL), defining success as improvement in plus disease or zone I, stage 3 ROP by 5 days after the injection and no recurrence of type 1 ROP or severe neovascularization requiring more treatment by 4 weeks. PEDIG's criteria for success were met at the lowest dose; however, 41% of the 61 treated eyes received additional treatment. Ranibizumab treatment and dosing have also been studied in randomized clinical trials and, unlike bevacizumab, do not alter plasma levels of VEGF.

Lepore D, Quinn GE, Molle F, et al. Intravitreal bevacizumab versus laser treatment in type 1 retinopathy of prematurity: report on fluorescein angiographic findings. *Ophthalmology.* 2014;121(11):2212–2219.

Stahl A, Lepore D, Fielder A, et al. Ranibizumab versus laser therapy for the treatment of very low birthweight infants with retinopathy of prematurity (RAINBOW): an open-label randomized controlled trial. *Lancet.* 2019;394(10208):1551–1559.

Wallace DK, Dean TW, Hartnett ME. A dosing study of bevacizumab for retinopathy of prematurity: late recurrences and additional treatments. *Ophthalmology.* 2018;125(12): 1961–1966.

Sequelae and complications

Children with ROP, especially those who have had laser treatment, are at risk of developing high myopia. Other concerns in this patient population include glaucoma—owing to crowding of the anterior chamber angle—as well as lattice-like degenerative disease, failure of peripheral vascularization, and tortuous vessels. These children also are at risk of macular dragging, yielding pseudoexotropia as a result of a large positive angle kappa (Fig 24-6; also see Chapter 6). Treated eyes are at risk of delayed retinal detachment at the border between treated and untreated retinal tissue. Late changes associated with stage 5 ROP include cataract, glaucoma, and phthisis bulbi.

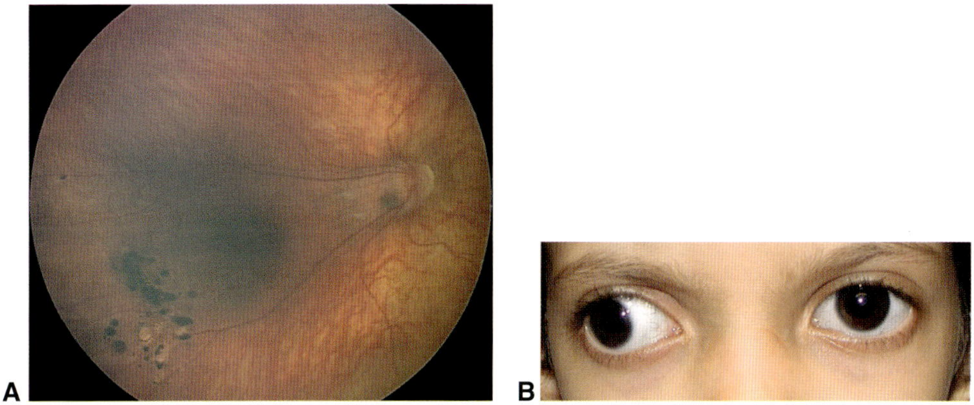

Figure 24-6 Macular dragging. **A,** Posterior pole traction and dragging of the macula (right eye), a sequela of ROP. **B,** Pseudoexotropia in a fixating right eye that has macular dragging from ROP. The temporal macular dragging in the right eye results in a large positive angle kappa in that eye. *(Part A courtesy of Robert W. Hered, MD; part B courtesy of Arif O. Khan, MD.)*

When laser treatment, cryotherapy, or intravitreal bevacizumab monotherapy has not prevented the progression of ROP to stage 4 or 5 (retinal detachment), scleral buckling and vitrectomy may be indicated. Anatomical success varies, but visual acuity results have been disappointing, particularly in eyes with stage 5 ROP.

Unfortunately, even with current recommendations for screening and treatment, approximately 400–600 babies become legally blind due to ROP each year in the United States. Poor ROP outcomes may be perceived as medical malpractice and therefore pose a risk for litigation by patients or their families. The Ophthalmic Mutual Insurance Company (www.omic.com/retinopathy-of-prematurity-requires-diligent-follow-up-care) offers tools to help ophthalmologists limit their liability risk.

Inherited Retinal Vascular Disorders

The Wnt signaling pathway plays a pivotal role in retinal angiogenesis. Pathogenic variations in genes encoding proteins in this cascade lead to a spectrum of inherited vascular disorders. Depending on the specific variant and signaling protein involved, the phenotype can range from severe retinal dysplasia (pseudoglioma) as seen in Norrie disease to subtle infantile-onset avascular peripheral retina in an asymptomatic adult. The retinal findings may be similar to those in a child with ROP but no history of prematurity. The ocular phenotype can occur in isolation (eg, familial exudative vitreoretinopathy, FEVR) or as part of a syndrome. Goals of treatment are to prevent neovascularization and retinal detachment (see BCSC Section 12, *Retina and Vitreous*). A combination of planned preterm delivery, early prophylactic laser, and anti-VEGF agents can prevent the development of severe Norrie disease in the affected sibling of a proband (Fig 24-7).

Sisk RA, Hufnagel RB, Bandi S, Polzin WJ, Ahmed ZM. Planned preterm delivery and treatment of retinal neovascularization in Norrie disease. *Ophthalmology.* 2014;121(6):1312–1313.

Wang Z, Liu CH, Huang S, Chen J. Wnt signaling in vascular eye diseases. *Prog Retin Eye Res.* 2019;70:110–133.

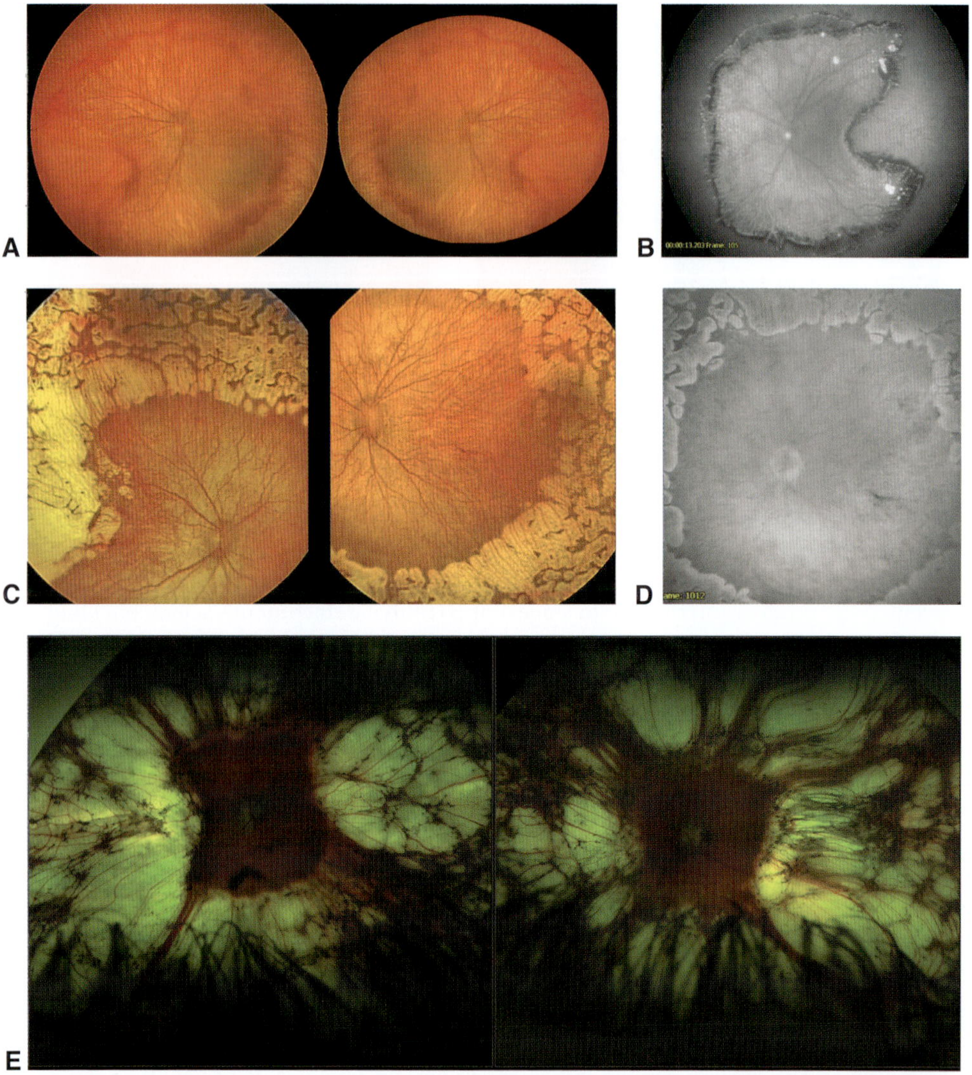

Figure 24-7 An infant with Norrie disease underwent planned preterm delivery at 34 weeks for treatment of retinopathy. The patient's affected older brother was born at 38 weeks with bilateral retinal detachments and no light perception vision, as was a maternal uncle. **A,** Note the butterfly-shaped pattern of incomplete retinal vasculogenesis resembling zone I aggressive retinopathy of prematurity (A-ROP) with plus disease. Both eyes had incomplete foveal vascularization, terminal vascular remodeling, retinal neovascularization, and a hemorrhagic border. **B,** Fluorescein angiography (FA) findings of the left eye in the arteriovenous phase demonstrate encircling, telangiectasia, a "brush-border" appearance at the leading edge of arrested vasculogenesis, and focal areas of retinal neovascularization. **C,** At 16 weeks post-treatment, note near-confluent chorioretinal scarring, reduced vascular caliber, and resolution of neovascularization. **D,** Recirculation-phase FA results show resolution of hyperfluorescence in the left eye. **E,** Wide-field images of both eyes of the patient at 8 years of age. Note extensive chorioretinal scarring. The patient is highly myopic (–10.00 D) and has retained best-corrected visual acuity of 20/250 in the right eye and 20/125 in the left eye. *(Parts A–D courtesy of Sisk RA, Hufnagel RB, Bandi S, Polzin WJ, Ahmed ZM. Planned preterm delivery and treatment of retinal neovascularization in Norrie disease.* Ophthalmology. *2014;121(6):1312–1313; with permission from Elsevier. Part E courtesy of Robert A. Sisk, MD.)*

Retinopathy Associated With Hemoglobinopathies

Refer to BCSC Section 12, *Retina and Vitreous.*

Selected Early-Onset Inherited Retinal Disorders

Inherited retinal disorders (IRDs) are genotypically and phenotypically heterogeneous (see BCSC Section 12, *Retina and Vitreous*). In early-onset IRDs, the retina may appear normal, so it is important for the presenting signs and symptoms to be recognized; nystagmus is 1 of the most common and typically occurs between 8 and 12 weeks of age (see Chapter 12). Other presenting signs and symptoms include poor vision, nyctalopia, photodysphoria, eye-poking (oculodigital sign), paradoxical pupil (see Chapter 12), and high refractive error. Table 24-5 highlights elements of the workup for suspected retinal dystrophy (also see BCSC Section 12, *Retina and Vitreous*).

IRDs may occur as part of a syndrome (eg, ciliopathy; see Chapter 27) or may be nonsyndromic; the term for severe, early-onset nonsyndromic IRD is Leber congenital amaurosis. Electroretinography (ERG) can help confirm the diagnosis or inform prognosis; genetic

Table 24-5 Evaluation of an Infant or Child With a Suspected Retinal Dystrophy[a]

History	Birth history Past medical history Ocular history Family history with pedigree
Comprehensive eye examination[b]	Eye examination including color vision
Imaging	Color photos Spectral-domain optical coherence tomography Fundus autofluorescence[c]
Visual field testing	Static perimetry Kinetic Goldmann perimetry
Electroretinography	Full-field ERG Multifocal ERG (if applicable) Pattern ERG (if applicable)
Psychophysical measurement of rod and cone thresholds	Dark adaptation testing (if applicable) Full-field threshold stimulus testing (if applicable)
Low vision[d]	Refer for early intervention, vision rehabilitation, and orientation and mobility training
Genetic testing	Provide pre- and post-test counseling
Comprehensive evaluation with medical geneticist	Consider if systemic concerns, developmental delay, dysmorphic features

ERG = electroretinography.

[a] Test selection may depend on patient's age and ability to participate in a meaningful assessment, and the modalities available.

[b] See Chapter 1 for description of a comprehensive examination.

[c] Short-wavelength, reduced illumination is advised to prevent phototoxicity.

[d] Criteria for services vary by state.

Modified from Duncan JL, Bernstein PS, Birch DG, et al. Approved by American Academy of Ophthalmology, Quality of Care Secretariat, Hoskins Center for Quality Eye Care. *Clinical Statement. Recommendations on Clinical Assessment of Patients With Inherited Retinal Degenerations.* American Academy of Ophthalmology; 2016. www.aao.org/clinical-statement/recommendations-on-clinical-assessment-of-patients testing and counseling are recommended (see BCSC Section 2, *Fundamentals and Principles of Ophthalmology*). Genetic diagnosis determines eligibility for clinical trials and available treatments (see the following section for *RPE65*-related retinal dystrophy gene therapy), and genetic counseling informs family planning. All infants and children benefit from early referral for supportive services and vision rehabilitation (see Chapter 28). IRDs with onset later in childhood are similar to those that occur in adulthood and are covered in BCSC Section 12, *Retina and Vitreous*.

> **CLINICAL PEARL**
>
> Children with IRDs often have concurrent ophthalmic issues that need to be considered, such as high refractive error, amblyopia, and strabismus. Untreated amblyopia further limits best-corrected vision. Because hypoaccommodation occurs in children with low vision, high hypermetropic refractive error should be fully corrected.

Leber Congenital Amaurosis

Leber congenital amaurosis (LCA) is a group of hereditary (usually autosomal-recessive) retinal dystrophies that affect both rod and cone photoreceptors. LCA is characterized by severe vision loss in infancy, nystagmus, poorly reactive pupils, and an extinguished ERG response. Visual acuity typically ranges from 20/200 to bare light perception but may be better in some patients.

Ophthalmoscopic appearance varies greatly, depending on the genotype (see eFig 24-1 at www.aao.org/bcscsupplement_section06 for images). It ranges from a normal appearance, particularly in infancy; to pigment clumping in the retinal pigment epithelium (RPE); to resemblance of classic retinitis pigmentosa, with bone spicules, attenuation of arterioles, and ONH pallor. Other reported but less common fundus findings include extensive chorioretinal atrophy, macular coloboma, white dots (similar to those seen in retinitis punctata albescens), and a marbleized retinal appearance. Histologic examination shows diffuse absence of photoreceptors.

> **CLINICAL PEARL**
>
> If the fundus appears normal in a child with nystagmus and poor visual response, look carefully for retinal vasculature attenuation, a potential sign of retinal dystrophy.

Additional ocular manifestations include the oculodigital reflex (rubbing or poking the eye), photoaversion, nyctalopia, cataracts, keratoconus, and keratoglobus. High refractive errors, often high hyperopia, are common. (See eTable 24-1 at www.aao.org/bcscsupplement_section06 for more information on IRDs in children.)

LCA-like phenotypes can be found in a number of systemic diseases, including peroxisomal disorders and the ciliopathies. The ciliopathies are a group of multisystemic genetic disorders in which the structure and function of the cilia are affected. Clinical findings may include retinal degeneration, renal disease, central nervous system (CNS) anomalies, skeletal anomalies, and obesity. Retinal involvement is common because the junction between the inner and outer segments of the photoreceptor cell is modified nonmotile cilium (see Chapter 27). Thus, ophthalmologists should be aware that an LCA-like phenotype may be the first sign of an undiagnosed systemic disease.

Treatment

In 2017, the US Food and Drug Administration (FDA) approved gene therapy for patients with biallelic pathogenic variants in *RPE65*. Younger children tend to have more viable retina and thus tend to have a better treatment prognosis; therefore, early identification of affected patients is important. See Figure 24-8 and Clinical Trial 24-1. (See eFig 24-2 at www.aao.org/bcscsupplement_section06 for an additional image.)

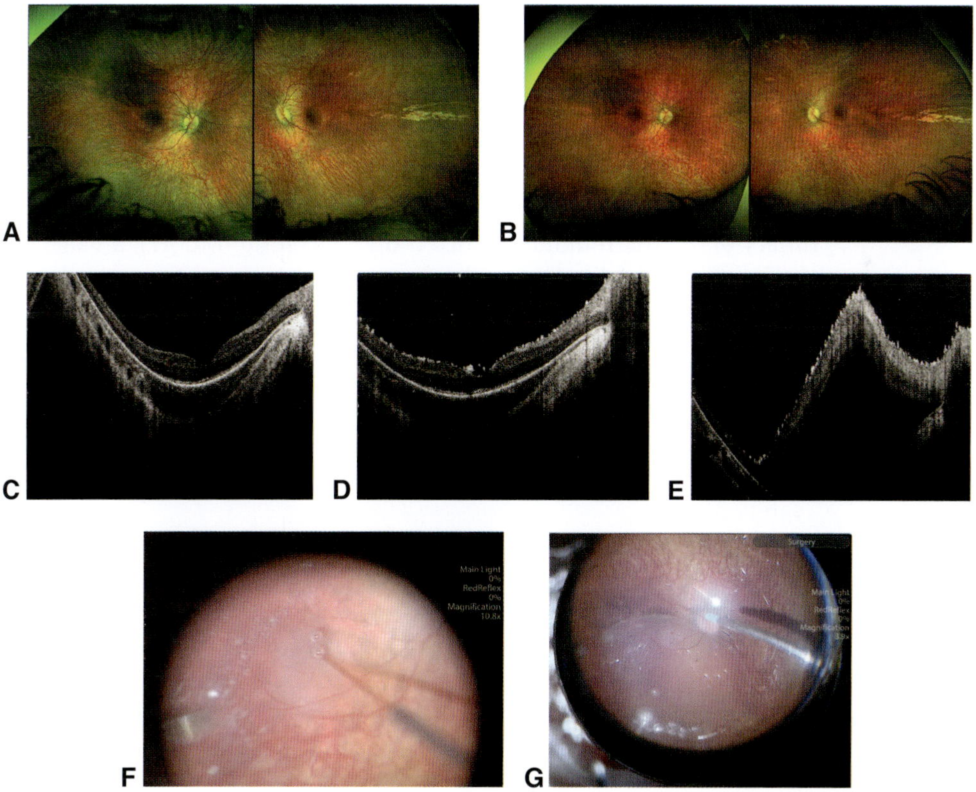

Figure 24-8 An 8-year-old child with biallelic pathogenic variants in *RPE65* who underwent subretinal gene injection of voretigene neparvovec-rzyl (VN). The patient was also highly myopic (–10.00 D). Preoperative **(A)** and postoperative **(B)** wide-field images demonstrate vascular attenuation, diffuse pigmentary mottling of the retina that relatively spares the macula, and radial hypopigmented streaks along the horizontal raphe. No major ophthalmoscopic postsurgical changes are noted. **C,** Intraoperative optical coherence tomography (OCT) preinjection. **D,** After injection of triamcinolone acetonide (hyperreflective granules on the retinal surface). **E,** At the inferior border of the bleb after subretinal injection of VN. **F,** Intraoperative color image during bleb formation. Note air bubbles at retinotomy. **G,** The completed bleb after fluid–air exchange. *(Courtesy of Robert A. Sisk, MD.)*

CLINICAL TRIAL 24-1

Phase 3 Trial Results of Voretigene Neparvovec-rzyl in *RPE65* Biallelic Pathogenic Variant–Associated Inherited Retinal Dystrophy

Study question: Does bilateral subretinal delivery of gene therapy with voretigene neparvovec-rzyl (VN) improve functional vision and visual function in patients with biallelic *RPE65* pathogenic variant–associated inherited retinal disease?

Enrollment: 31 patients ≥3 years of age with biallelic pathogenic variants in *RPE65*, best-corrected visual acuity (BCVA) worse than 20/60, and/or visual field constriction to <20 degrees from fixation.

Study groups:

- Randomized in a 2:1 fashion to receive bilateral treatment 18 days apart or to serve in the control group completing the same studies over the course of the year.
- Control group eligible for treatment at the end of year 1 if they still met enrollment criteria.

Outcome variables:

- Primary endpoint: multiluminance mobility testing (MLMT), a validated testing modality that evaluates an individual's ability to navigate a marked path while avoiding obstacles by relying solely on vision in varying luminance levels.
- Additional endpoints:
  - full-field light sensitivity threshold testing (FST)
  - BCVA, both eyes
  - Goldmann visual field (GVF; III4e isopter)
  - safety profile

Results:

- All 20 intervention participants had significant improvements in MLMT, FST thresholds, and GVF as compared to the control group (delayed intervention).
- Similar gains were seen in the delayed intervention group and the original participants.
- There was no statistically significant treatment-related change in BCVA.
- The safety profile was consistent with those of vitrectomy and subretinal injection; there were no complications related to the immune response to the injection/vector.

Conclusion: Subretinal VN injection led to sustained improvements in functional vision in patients with a previously untreatable condition.

Russell S, Bennett J, Wellman JA, et al. Efficacy and safety of voretigene neparvovec (AAV2-hRPE65v2) in patients with *RPE65*-mediated inherited retinal dystrophy: a randomised, controlled, open-label, phase 3 trial. *Lancet.* 2017;390(10097):849–860. Erratum in: *Lancet.* 2017;390(10097):848.

McGuire AM, Russell S, Wellman JA, et al. Efficacy, safety, and durability of voretigine neparvovec-rzyl in *RPE65* mutation-associated inherited retinal dystrophy: results of phase 1 and 3 trials. *Ophthalmology.* 2019;126(9):1273–1285.

Achromatopsia

Complete achromatopsia, also known as *rod monochromatism,* is an autosomal-recessive congenital disorder of the cone photoreceptors. Patients typically present in early infancy with nystagmus, photophobia, and reduced central visual response. Additional clinical features include reduced visual acuity (20/120–20/200), absent color discrimination, and absent cone ERG responses with normal rod function. Dark adaptometry shows no cone plateau and no cone–rod break. Fundus examination findings are usually normal, although the fovea may demonstrate reduced reflex and variable RPE disturbance. Optical coherence tomography (OCT) findings may include normal lamination, variable degrees of disruption of the hyperreflective photoreceptor bands (inner segment/outer segment junction), an optically empty cavity, or outer segment loss (see eTable 24-1). Pathogenic variations in several recessive genes have been identified as the cause of achromatopsia, including mutations in *CNGA3, CNGB3* (most common), *GNAT2, PDE6C,* and *PDE6H.*

Other cone dystrophies that cause early-onset visual impairment and nystagmus include *incomplete achromatopsia,* which is an autosomal-recessive condition, and *blue-cone monochromatism,* which is an X-linked disorder. In both disorders, patients usually have better vision than do those with complete achromatopsia. In incomplete achromatopsia, some residual cone function is observed on ERG testing. In blue-cone monochromatism, the blue (short-wavelength) cones show normal function on specialized ERG testing, but the photopic response is usually extinguished.

Treatment

Glasses with dark lenses or red lenses that exclude short wavelengths may help, in addition to other vision rehabilitation services. Gene therapy with *AAV* gene replacement has been successful in murine and canine models. Phase I/II clinical trials in humans are ongoing for achromatopsia related to pathogenic variants in *CNGA3* and *CNGB3.*

Congenital Stationary Night Blindness

Congenital stationary night blindness (CSNB) comprises a group of nonprogressive retinal disorders characterized predominantly by abnormal function of rod photoreceptors or with photoreceptor–bipolar synapses. The condition may be X-linked, autosomal recessive, or autosomal dominant, and is further classified into complete and incomplete CSNB according to ERG characteristics.

Children with complete CSNB, especially the autosomal-recessive and X-linked forms, may present in early infancy with nystagmus or strabismus accompanied by pre–school-age myopia. Visual acuity can range from 20/20 to 20/200. Nyctalopia may not be apparent in young children. The retina usually appears normal, but the optic nerve may show myopic tilt and temporal pallor.

An ERG is diagnostic for CSNB, demonstrating an electronegative waveform (a large a-wave and a reduced-amplitude [negative] b-wave) on the dark-adapted ERG 3 (combined rod–cone standard flash response). In individuals with CSNB, a negative b-wave occurs because of synaptic dysfunction between the photoreceptors and bipolar cells, leading to reduced inner retinal signaling. Dark adaptation testing and full-field threshold stimulus testing results are abnormal (see eTable 24-1).

Treatment

Refractive errors should be corrected in individuals with CSNB. Bright illumination should be used for visual tasks; carrying a flashlight or cell phone with flashlight may be helpful for these patients.

Miraldi Utz V, Pfeifer W, Longmuir SQ, Olson RJ, Wang K, Drack AV. Presentation of *TRPM1*-associated congenital stationary night blindness in children. *JAMA Ophthalmol.* 2018;136(4):389–398.

Zeitz C, Robson AG, Audo I. Congenital stationary night blindness: an analysis and update of genotype-phenotype correlations and pathogenic mechanisms. *Prog Retin Eye Res.* 2015;45:58–110.

Hereditary Macular Dystrophies

Macular abnormalities are seen in a number of hereditary disorders. The abnormality can be associated with a hereditary systemic disease (eg, the cherry-red spot in GM_2 gangliosidosis type I) or can reflect a primary retinal disorder. See BCSC Section 12, *Retina and Vitreous.*

Stargardt disease

Stargardt disease (juvenile macular degeneration) is the most common hereditary macular dystrophy. Inheritance is usually autosomal recessive; in rare cases, it is autosomal dominant. Most cases are caused by pathogenic variants in the retina-specific adenosine triphosphate–binding transporter gene *(ABCA4).* Children with Stargardt disease usually present between ages 8 and 15 years with a decrease in vision, photophobia, or color vision abnormalities. The condition is bilateral, symmetric, and progressive; visual acuity levels off at approximately 20/50–20/200.

Initially, the fundus appears normal even when vision is decreased, and the condition may be misdiagnosed as nonorganic vision loss. The first ophthalmoscopic changes observed are loss of foveal reflex and a peculiar light-reflecting quality called "beaten bronze" appearance, followed by development of a characteristic macular bull's-eye atrophy surrounded by round or pisciform yellowish flecks, which develop in the posterior pole at the level of the RPE (Fig 24-9). Approximately 30% of children may not have characteristic flecks.

CLINICAL PEARL

In a child with vision loss, subnormal visual acuity, and a normal-appearing fundus, the clinician should consider obtaining OCT and fundus autofluorescence imaging to evaluate for Stargardt disease. Vision loss typically precedes ophthalmoscopic changes in these patients.

The "dark choroid" sign on fluorescein angiography is distinctive but is not present in all patients. This phenomenon is due to the accumulation of lipofuscin within the RPE,

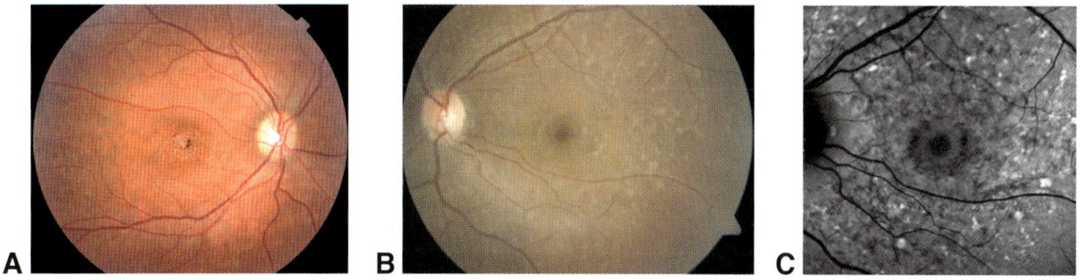

Figure 24-9 Varied clinical phenotype in 2 different patients with Stargardt disease. **A,** Macular atrophy is noted with pisciform yellow-white flecks and a beaten-bronze appearance. Note the peripapillary sparing of retina. **B,** Classic pisciform yellow-white flecks throughout the macula, with mottling of the central retinal pigment epithelium (RPE). **C,** Fundus autofluorescence (FAF) images from the same patient as in part B reveal mottled hypo- and hyperautofluorescence with hyperautofluorescent flecks (corresponding to the pisciform flecks) and a bull's-eye maculopathy. *(Courtesy of Marc T. Mathias, MD.)*

which blocks the choroidal fluorescence. Fluorescein angiography has been largely replaced by fundus autofluorescence (FAF) testing for the confirmation of Stargardt disease. FAF reveals both increased autofluorescence due to lipofuscin accumulation in the RPE and reduced autofluorescence in areas of RPE atrophy and photoreceptor loss (see Fig 24-9C). OCT imaging of the macula can reveal lipofuscin accumulation in the RPE and photoreceptor loss.

Results of visual field testing may be normal in the early stages of the disease. Disease progression will result in a central scotoma. ERG results are often normal in the early stages. A more aggressive form of *ABCA4*-related retinopathy is a progressive cone–rod dystrophy that can lead to a nonrecordable ERG.

Treatment Several approaches to the treatment of Stargardt disease that address various aspects of pathophysiology of disease are in human clinical trials. These treatments include medications that reduce the accumulation of the toxic metabolic product A2E, complement inhibitors, stem-cell replacement therapies, and gene replacement of *ABCA4*. (Updated lists of these clinical trials, with age and eligibility requirements, can be found at www.clinicaltrials.gov.)

Excessive vitamin A intake may hasten lipofuscin accumulation; therefore, such supplements are not recommended in these individuals. Excessive bright light may also be detrimental; the patient may find wearing a wide-brimmed hat and sunglasses helpful.

Rahman N, Georgiou M, Khan KN, Michaelides M. Macular dystrophies: clinical and imaging features, molecular genetics and therapeutic options. *Br J Ophthalmol.* 2020;104(4):451–460.

Best disease and other bestrophinopathies

Bestrophinopathies constitute a heterogeneous group of phenotypes related to pathogenic variation in the *BEST1* gene. The most common phenotype is autosomal-dominant Best vitelliform macular dystrophy. Children with Best disease may present with mildly decreased visual acuity (20/30–20/60) and a yellow, egg yolk–like (vitelliform) lesion in the macula. Stages and ophthalmoscopic appearance are described in Figure 24-10 and eTable 24-1. The

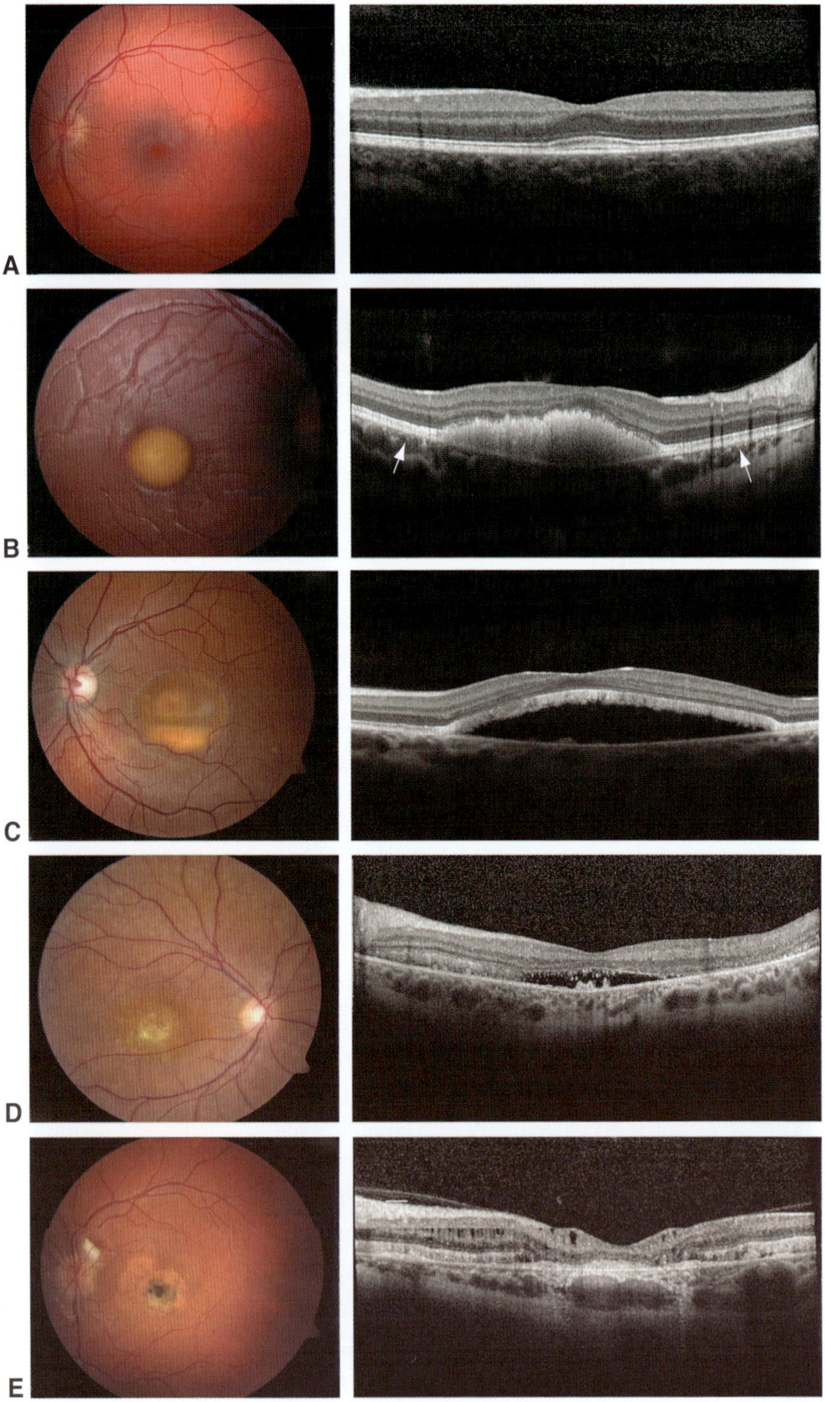

Figure 24-10 Stages of Best vitelliform dystrophy. Images from different patients demonstrating clinical stages of Best disease on fundus photography *(left)* compared with simultaneous OCT *(right)*. **A**, Previtelliform lesion with slight thickening of the interdigitation zone. **B**, Vitelliform lesion ("egg yolk") with early disintegration of the overlying ellipsoid zone. Note the thickening of the area of the interdigitation zone outside of the lesion *(white arrows)*. **C**, Pseudohypopyon lesion, cut through the superior liquefied level, with more solid area inferiorly. **D**, Vitelleruptive lesion "scrambled egg" with further disintegration of the lesion material and surrounding structures, RPE, ellipsoid, and photoreceptors. **E**, Atrophic lesion with loss of outer retina, fibrotic changes, and cystic changes within the retina. The RPE pump is nonfunctional, and the fluid accumulates within the retina. *(Courtesy of Qian CX, Charran D, Strong CR, Steffens TJ, Jayasundera T, Heckenlively JR. Optical coherence tomography examination of the retinal pigment epithelium in Best vitelliform macular dystrophy.* Ophthalmology. *2017;124(4):456–463. With permission from Elsevier.)*

ERG results are typically normal, and the electro-oculogram (EOG) Arden ratio is almost always abnormal, even in seemingly unaffected patients. A rarer phenotype is autosomal-dominant vitreoretinochoroidopathy.

Characteristics of autosomal-recessive *BEST1*-associated disease may include hyperopia, shallow anterior chamber, multifocal macular lesions, macular edema and subretinal fluid, reduced ERG scotopic and photopic responses, and severely reduced EOG light rise. Visual acuity typically decreases very slowly.

Patients with both autosomal-dominant and autosomal-recessive forms should be monitored for the development of choroidal neovascularization, which may further accelerate vision loss if left untreated (see eFig 24-3 at www.aao.org/bcscsupplement_section06 for additional images of Best disease).

Inherited Vitreoretinopathies

Hereditary vitreoretinopathies include a broad range of disease entities that may be isolated to the eye or part of a syndrome. X-linked retinoschisis is an example of a vitreous–inner retina interface disorder. Patients may present with reduced vision (failed vision screening) and moderate to high hyperopia. The fundus examination reveals small cystoid spaces and fine radial striae in the central macula (Fig 24-11); 50% of these patients may have peripheral schisis (see BCSC Section 12, *Retina and Vitreous,* and eTable 24-1).

Stickler syndrome and related disorders should be considered in the differential diagnosis of any young child who presents with high myopia. Characteristic posterior segment findings include vitreous liquefaction (optically empty vitreous) and perivascular lattice degeneration (Fig 24-12). Extraocular features can include sensorineural hearing loss, Pierre Robin sequence, micrognathia (small jaw or chin), cleft palate, and glossoptosis (tongue is further back and may cause airway obstruction), joint hyperextensibility,

A

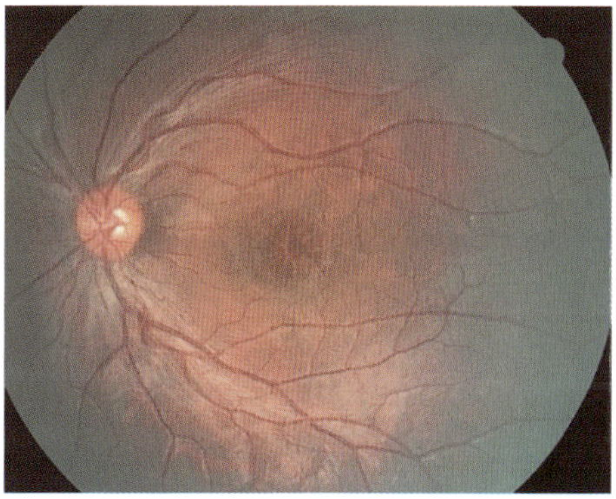

B

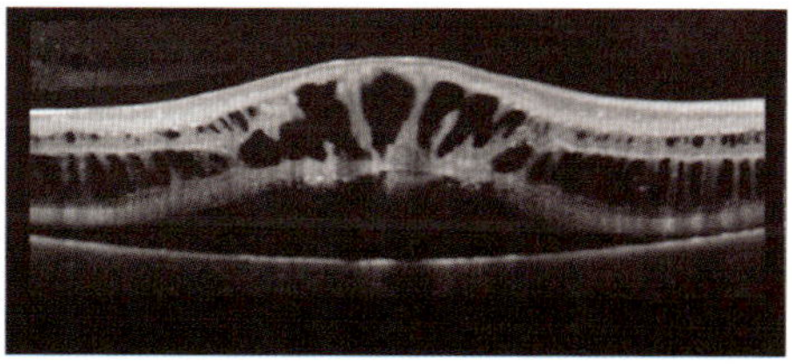

Figure 24-11 Juvenile retinoschisis. **A,** Fundus image demonstrates foveal microcystic changes in a child with X-linked retinoschisis. **B,** OCT shows foveal retinoschisis. *(Part A ©2021 American Academy of Ophthalmology; part B courtesy of Lee BA, van Kuijk E, Seely KR, et al.* X-Linked Retinoschisis. *American Academy of Ophthalmology; 2020. https://eyewiki.aao.org/X-linked_Retinoschisis)*

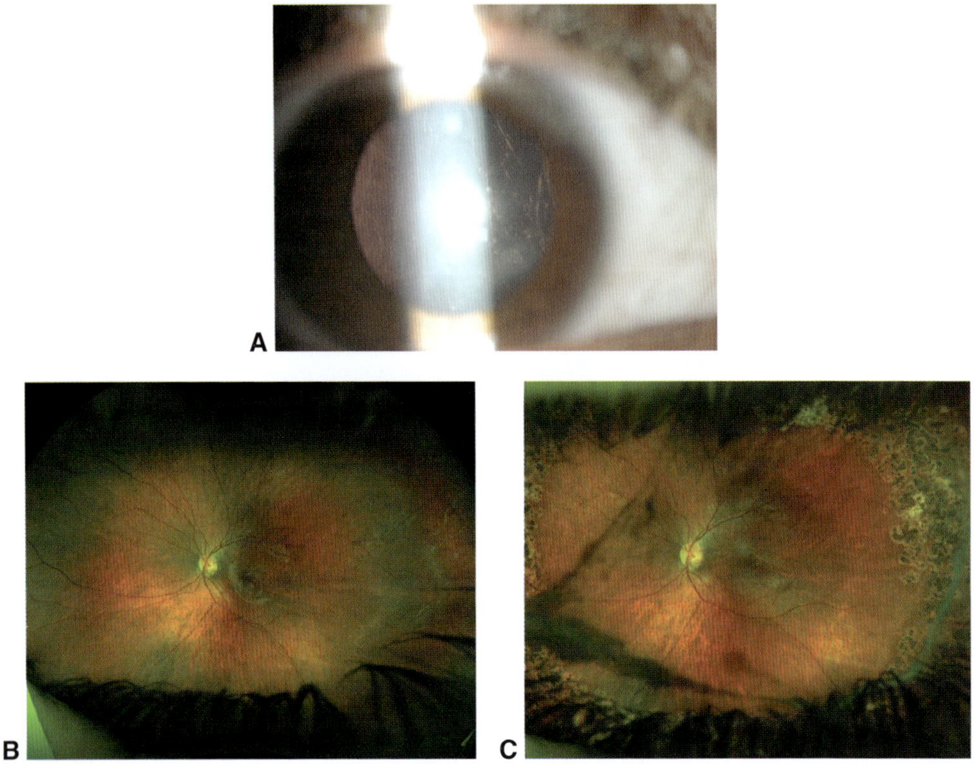

Figure 24-12 Stickler syndrome. **A,** Beaded vitreous condensations in a patient with type II Stickler syndrome. **B,** Classic perivascular lattice in a child with Stickler syndrome. Because the patient's father and sibling had a history of retinal detachment, the family elected for barricade laser to be performed. **C,** At 5-year follow-up, dense vitreous condensations are noted. *(Part A courtesy of Michael Shapiro, MD; parts B and C courtesy of Robert A Sisk, MD.)*

or skeletal malformations (see eFig 24-4 at www.aao.org/bcscsupplement_section06). Stickler syndrome is often autosomal dominant and related to pathogenic variation in *COL2A1*. However, other autosomal-dominant and -recessive collagen genes can be associated with the phenotype. Affected patients may require more frequent ophthalmic examinations to monitor for retinal detachment, and some may be treated prophylactically with barrier laser. (See BCSC Section 12, *Retina and Vitreous.*)

Another syndrome associated with pediatric high myopia is Knobloch syndrome, which is characterized by a distinct fundus appearance with macular atrophic lesions. Affected patients often have an occipital scalp defect (see eTable 24-1 and eFig 24-5 at www.aao.org/bcscsupplement_section06 for more on Knobloch syndrome).

Toxic Retinopathies

Recommendations have recently been published for monitoring children with rheumatologic disorders who are on hydroxychloroquine. Because of variability in testing

Table 24-6 American Academy of Pediatrics Ophthalmic Screening Examinations for Children on Hydroxychloroquine

Age	Baseline and Annual Ophthalmic Examination	Additional Ophthalmic Studies
<7 years	BCVA Complete ophthalmic examination, evaluating for any retinal abnormalities SD-OCT macula[a]	Fundus autofluorescence[b]
≥7 years	BCVA Complete ophthalmic examination, evaluating for any retinal abnormalities SD-OCT macula[a] Visual field testing[c]	Fundus autofluorescence[b] mfERG

BCVA = best-corrected visual acuity, mfERG = multifocal electroretinogram, SD-OCT = spectral-domain optical coherence tomography.

[a] At least a single line raster scan through the central fovea (center of the macula) should be obtained. Vertical as well as horizontal scans add information.

[b] Fundus autofluorescence may also be helpful in monitoring nonparafoveal disease, such as seen in patients of Asian descent.

[c] Humphrey Visual Field Analyzer, program 10-2 or similar study; consider wider visual field for children of Asian descent.

Courtesy of Virginia Miraldi Utz, MD; ©2022 American Academy of Ophthalmology.

performance, age-appropriate studies are completed at baseline and then yearly (Table 24-6). Also see BCSC Section 12, *Retina and Vitreous,* for further discussion of toxic retinopathies.

Infectious Diseases

Congenital and acquired infectious diseases that involve the retina include toxoplasmosis, toxocariasis, Zika virus, lymphocytic choriomeningitis, rubella, cytomegalovirus, herpes simplex virus, varicella zoster virus, and *Bartonella.* Toxoplasmosis and toxocariasis are covered in Chapter 25. The other entities are covered extensively in BCSC Section 9, *Uveitis and Ocular Inflammation,* and Section 12, *Retina and Vitreous.*

Human Immunodeficiency Virus

Since the introduction of potent antiretroviral therapy, ocular complications of HIV infection in childhood have been reported only in rare cases. Such complications typically occur only in children with advanced HIV infection who are severely immunocompromised. For more information, see BCSC Section 9, *Uveitis and Ocular Inflammation,* and Section 12, *Retina and Vitreous.*

Tumors

Choroidal and Retinal Pigment Epithelial Lesions

A pigmented fundus lesion in a child is usually benign. Flat choroidal nevi are common and are not a cause for concern; malignant melanoma of the choroid is extremely rare in children. Choroidal osteoma is a benign bony tumor of the uveal tract that may occur in childhood and usually presents as decreased vision. Diffuse hemangioma of the choroid associated with encephalofacial angiomatosis (Sturge-Weber syndrome) is discussed in Chapter 27. Patients with neurofibromatosis type 1 often have flat, hyperpigmented spots in the choroid that may be visible only with near-infrared imaging (see Chapter 27).

Congenital hypertrophy of the retinal pigment epithelium (CHRPE) is a sharply demarcated, flat, hyperpigmented lesion that may be isolated or multifocal (Fig 24-13). Such lesions are sometimes grouped, in which case they are also called *bear tracks.*

Pigmented lesions similar to CHRPE have been associated with Gardner syndrome, an autosomal-dominant condition caused by pathogenic variants in the *APC* gene, located at 5q22.2. Patients with Gardner syndrome have many polyps of the colon, and the polyps pose a high risk of malignant transformation. Affected individuals often require a colectomy in early adulthood to prevent cancer. They may also have skeletal hamartomas and various other soft-tissue tumors.

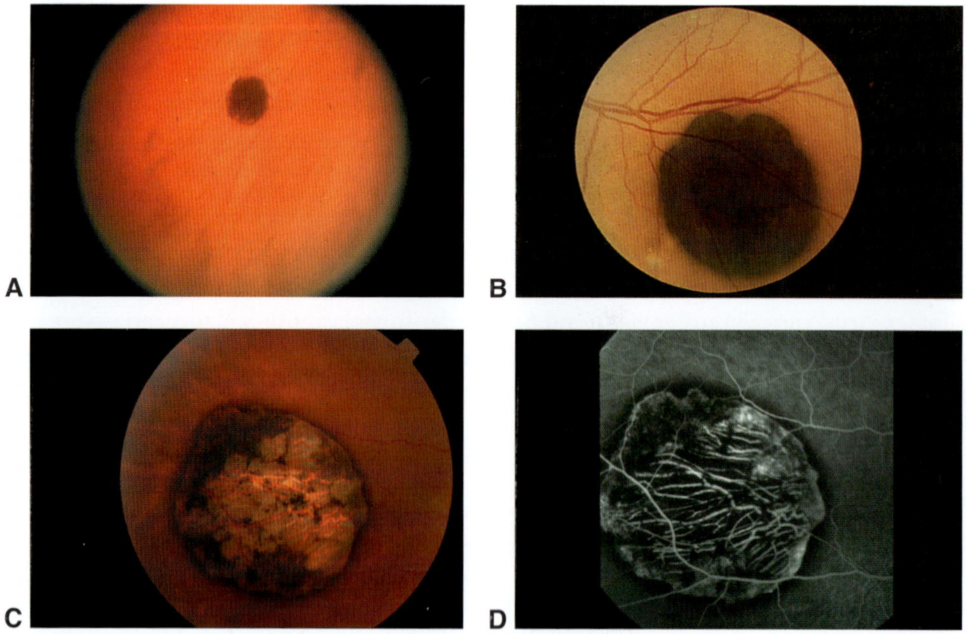

Figure 24-13 Congenital hypertrophy of the RPE (CHRPE). Examples of varying clinical appearances. **A,** Small lesion. **B,** Medium-sized lesion; note the homogeneous black color and well-defined margins of this nummular lesion. **C,** Color fundus photograph of a large lesion. **D,** Corresponding fluorescein angiogram of the large lesion. Note the loss of RPE architecture and highlighted choroidal vasculature. *(Parts A, C, and D courtesy of Timothy G. Murray, MD.)*

KEY POINTS 24-2

Differentiating Gardner syndrome lesions from CHRPE Certain features of pigmented fundus lesions in Gardner syndrome can help rule out CHRPE in the differential diagnosis:

- hyperplasia as opposed to hypertrophy
- lesions that are multiple, bilateral, and dispersed
- often a surrounding halo and tail of depigmentation that is oriented radially and directed toward the optic nerve (Fig 24-14)

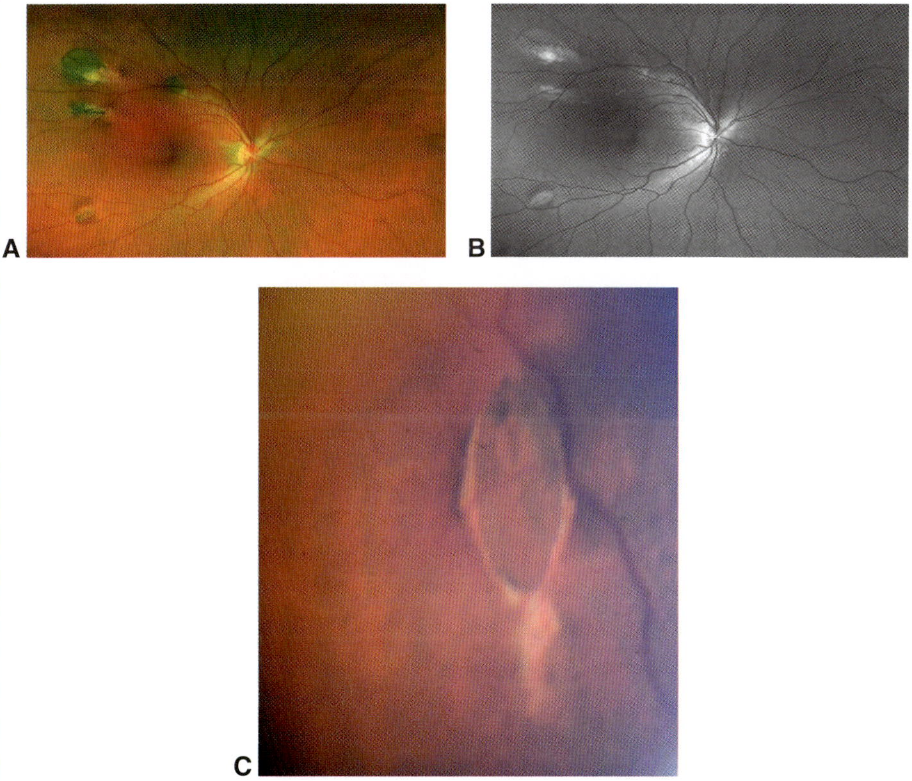

Figure 24-14 Gardner syndrome. **A,** Wide-angle fundus photograph shows multiple pigmented retinal lesions with areas of depigmentation oriented radially to the optic nerve. **B,** FAF reveals areas of hypo- and hyperautofluorescence within pigmented lesions. **C,** Retinal lesion with a "fishtail" configuration. *(Parts A and B courtesy of Cara E. Capitena, MD; part C courtesy of Robert W. Hered, MD.)*

Combined hamartoma of the retina and RPE is an ill-defined, variably pigmented tumor that may be juxtapapillary or located in the retinal periphery. The tumor is often minimally elevated, and retinal traction and tortuous retinal vessels usually are present. In peripheral tumors, dragging of the retinal vessels is a prominent feature. These tumors have a variable composition of glial tissue and RPE.

Combined hamartoma of the retina and RPE may occur in neurofibromatosis (type 1 or 2), incontinentia pigmenti, X-linked retinoschisis, and facial hemangiomas. The presence of bilateral lesions in a child is suggestive of neurofibromatosis type 2.

Traboulsi EI. Pigmented and depigmented lesions of the ocular fundus. *Curr Opin Ophthalmol.* 2012;23(5):337–343.

Retinoblastoma

Retinoblastoma (RB) is the most common malignant intraocular tumor of childhood and 1 of the most common pediatric solid tumors, with an incidence of 1:14,000–1:20,000 live births, leading to approximately 9000 new cases annually worldwide. For details, see BCSC Section 4, *Ophthalmic Pathology and Intraocular Tumors.*

KEY POINTS 24-3

Retinoblastoma epidemiology

- Males = females
- 30%–40% of cases are bilateral
- Familial/bilateral cases: diagnosed in the first year of life
- Sporadic cases: between 1 and 3 years of age (90% diagnosed by 3 years)
- Diffuse infiltrating subtype has a later presentation; 5–6 years, male predominance, uveitis masquerade

The most common initial sign is leukocoria (white pupillary reflex), which is usually first noticed by the family and described as a glow, glint, or cat's-eye appearance (Fig 24-15). The differential diagnosis of leukocoria is presented in Table 24-7. Approximately 25% of cases present with strabismus (esotropia or exotropia). Less common presentations include vitreous hemorrhage, hyphema, ocular or periocular inflammation, glaucoma, proptosis, and pseudohypopyon.

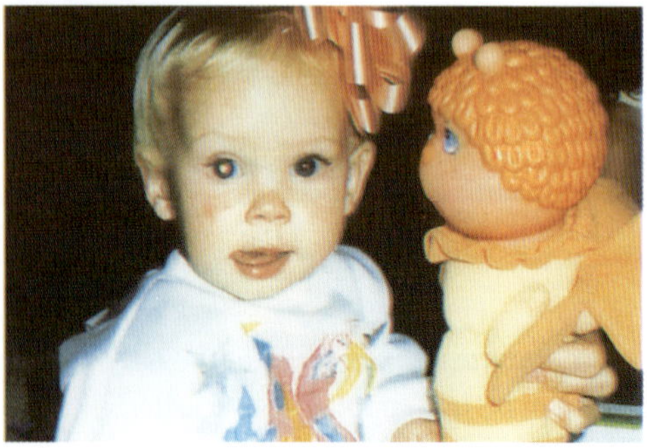

Figure 24-15 Leukocoria of the right eye, which is visible in this family photograph of a 1-year-old girl with retinoblastoma. *(Courtesy of A. Linn Murphree, MD.)*

Table 24-7 Differential Diagnosis of Leukocoria

Retinoblastoma
Coats disease
Coloboma of choroid or optic nerve head
Congenital retinal fold
Corneal opacity
Cataract
Familial exudative vitreoretinopathy/Norrie disease
High myopia or anisometropia
Myelinated nerve fibers
Organizing vitreous hemorrhage
Persistent fetal vasculature
Photographic artifact[a]
Retinal detachment
Astrocytic hamartoma
Retinal dysplasia
Retinopathy of prematurity
Toxocariasis
Uveitis

[a]The red reflex may manifest differently in the 2 eyes if the image is taken at an angle, or the image may be capturing the Brückner test phenomenon.

KEY POINTS 24-4

Coats disease It is particularly important not to mistake retinoblastoma for Coats disease; certain clinical characteristics are helpful in distinguishing the 2 conditions:

- disorder involving retinal vascular abnormalities; genetic basis unknown
- findings: telangiectasias, aneurysmal dilatations, retinal capillary nonperfusion and leakage on fluorescein angiography, exudative retinal detachment, and lipoidal exudates (Fig 24-16)
- usually unilateral, primarily affects males, onset 6–8 years
- typically, absence of calcifications, xanthocoria; if in doubt, consult ocular oncology

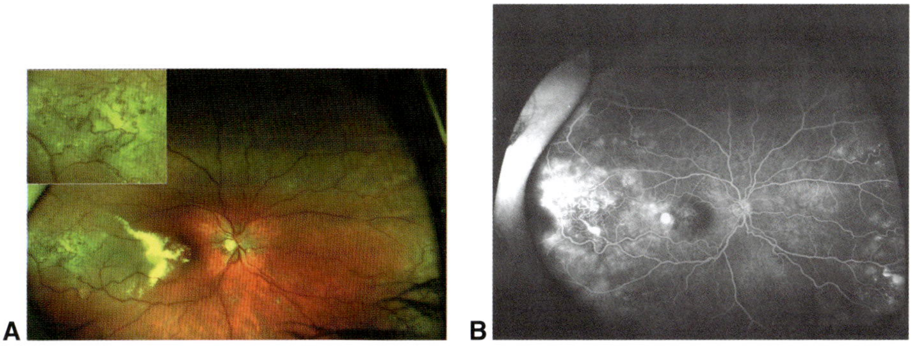

Figure 24-16 Coats disease. **A,** Wide-angle color photograph reveals foveal exudation with temporal macroaneurysms and telangiectasias. *Inset* shows magnification of macroaneurysms and telangiectasias. Subtle nasal telangiectasias are also present. **B,** Image obtained with oral fluorescein angiography shows extensive leakage from temporal macroaneurysms, mild leakage from temporal and nasal telangiectasias, and macular leakage with some staining. *(Courtesy of Scott C. Oliver, MD.)*

Diagnosis

In suspected retinoblastoma, prompt referral to an ocular oncology center is advised. Computed tomography is discouraged in this patient population because of the risk of secondary tumors due to radiation exposure.

Tumor growth patterns

Diagnosis of retinoblastoma usually is based on its ophthalmoscopic appearance and on ultrasonographic findings. See BCSC Section 4, *Ophthalmic Pathology and Intraocular Tumors,* for discussion of growth patterns and histopathology.

Genetics

Genetic counseling for families of retinoblastoma patients is complex (Table 24-8). Key points include:

- Retinoblastoma is *recessive* at the *cellular level.* Both alleles have to be affected for RB or other tumor to develop; however, because the retina undergoes so many somatic cell divisions, a spontaneous pathogenic change in one of the *RB1* genes may occur by chance alone.
- Retinoblastoma acts as a *dominant trait* at the *individual level* because the chance of an additional spontaneous pathogenic change in the developing retina is high.
- Penetrance is high (80%–90%).
- Most (but not all) unifocal cases are new somatic pathogenic variants that are not heritable.

Visit www.aao.org/bcscsupplement_section06 for supplemental Clinical Examples about genetics.

It is recommended for parents and all siblings be examined. In approximately 1% of cases, a parent will have an unsuspected fundus lesion that represents a spontaneously regressed retinoblastoma (ie, retinocytoma).

Genetic testing for retinoblastoma is useful for estimating the risk of subsequent cancers (both retinoblastoma and other primary neoplasms) in the affected child and the risk (or lack of risk) of retinoblastoma in other family members. The probability of detecting the *RB1* gene pathogenic variation depends on many factors, including the capabilities of the molecular diagnostic laboratory, the presence of tumor tissue, and the ability to test family members.

Preimplantation genetic testing can be performed, and in vitro fertilization techniques have been used successfully to select embryos that are free from a germline *RB1* pathogenic variant.

Treatment

Management of retinoblastoma is evolving and is best done in referral ocular oncology centers. Many specialists are involved, including ocular oncologists, pediatric ophthalmologists, geneticists, genetic counselors, pediatric oncologists, and radiation oncologists. The primary goal of RB treatment is to preserve life, followed by globe preservation and protection and maximalization of useful vision. The treatment regimen depends on several factors, including germline molecular status, globe classification, laterality, anticipated visual function, and risks of metastatic disease. Modalities for treating RB include chemotherapy (systemic, intra-arterial, intravitreal,

Table 24-8 Genetic Counseling for Retinoblastoma

If Parent:	Has Bilateral Retinoblastoma				Has Unilateral Retinoblastoma				Is Unaffected			
Chance of offspring having retinoblastoma	45% affected			55% unaffected	7%–15% affected			85%–93% unaffected	<1% affected			99% unaffected
Laterality	85% bilateral	15% unilateral		0%	85% bilateral	15% unilateral		0%	33% bilateral	67% unilateral		0%
Focality	100% multifocal	96% multifocal	4% unifocal	0%	100% multifocal	96% multifocal	4% unifocal	0%	100% multifocal	15% multifocal	85% unifocal	0%
Chance of next sibling having retinoblastoma	45%	45%	45%	45%	45%	45%	45%	7%–15%	5%[a]	<1%[a]	<1%[a]	<1%

[a]If parent is a carrier, then 45%

Table created by David H. Abramson, MD.

or intracameral; Fig 24-17) and focal therapies (laser photocoagulation, cryotherapy, plaque therapy, and enucleation). Chemotherapy typically is given in combination with local therapy. External beam radiotherapy is rarely used to treat retinoblastoma because it is associated with development of craniofacial deformity and secondary tumors in the field of radiation.

Regressed, treated retinoblastoma may have the following appearances:

- Type 1: calcified mass (ie, cottage cheese pattern)
- Type 2: translucent, noncalcified, grayish lesion (ie, fish flesh pattern); may be difficult to distinguish from active tumor
- Type 3: elements of types 1 and 2
- Type 4: flat, atrophic scar

After treatment, children with retinoblastoma continue to be monitored closely for new or recurrent tumor formation; typically, this follow-up involves examinations under anesthesia.

Extraocular retinoblastoma is uncommon in the United States but remains a problem in resource-limited countries, primarily because of delays in diagnosis. Extraocular retinoblastoma occurs in 4 major types:

1. optic nerve involvement
2. orbital invasion
3. CNS involvement
4. distant metastasis

Treatment of extraocular retinoblastoma includes intensive multimodality chemotherapy, autologous hematopoietic stem cell rescue, and external-beam radiotherapy. Long-term disease-free survival is possible if the central nervous system is not involved; otherwise, the prognosis is usually poor.

In patients with trilateral retinoblastoma, a primitive neuroectodermal tumor (PNET) of the pineal gland or parasellar region occurs in addition to retinoblastoma. For patients with unilateral retinoblastoma, the risk of trilateral retinoblastoma is <0.5%; for those with bilateral retinoblastoma, risk estimates range from <5% to 15%. The risk of trilateral retinoblastoma appears to be lower in patients who undergo chemoreduction. Treatment usually involves a multimodal approach, and the prognosis is poor.

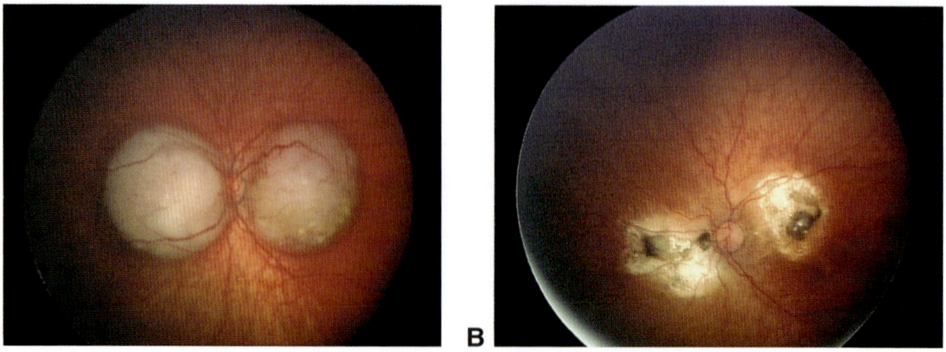

A B

Figure 24-17 Retinoblastoma. **A,** Left eye of an infant with bilateral retinoblastoma; 2 tumors straddle the optic nerve. **B,** After chemoreduction and laser consolidation, the tumors are nonviable. The child's visual acuity was 20/25 at age 5 years.

Shields CL, Alset AE, Say EA, Caywood E, Jabbour P, Shields JA. Retinoblastoma control with primary intra-arterial chemotherapy: outcomes before and during the intravitreal chemotherapy era. *J Pediatr Ophthalmol Strabismus*. 2016;53(5):275–284.

Monitoring Knowing a patient's *RB1* molecular status helps the clinician decide how frequently to monitor that individual. Patients with unilateral tumors in the context of somatic variants are not at risk of additional tumor development (ocular or systemic). Patients who undergo globe salvage require frequent examinations to monitor for tumor recurrence. In these patients, examinations under anesthesia are typically performed every 4–8 weeks until age 3 years. Recurrence of retinoblastoma is common and can occur years after treatment. In patients with germline variants, periodic magnetic resonance imaging of the brain is performed to screen for CNS metastases and PNET.

Results of genetic testing in siblings also is helpful for determining monitoring frequency. If genetic testing is not available, surveillance recommendations have been developed for children at risk of having retinoblastoma, including those with a parent, sibling, or first- or second-degree relative with the disease. Surveillance is based on pre-test probability of the mutant allele, with screening becoming less frequent after the age of 7 years.

Because of the risk of secondary malignancies, patients with germline pathogenic variants require long-term follow-up by oncologists and ophthalmologists. Nonocular tumors are common in these patients; the estimated incidence rate is 1% per year of life (ie, 10% prevalence by age 10 years, 30% by age 30 years). This incidence is higher for patients treated with external-beam radiation before 1 year of age. The most common secondary tumors (and the mean age at diagnosis) are PNET (2.7 years), sarcoma (13 years), melanoma (27 years), and carcinoma (29 years). For patients with secondary nonocular tumors, the risk of additional malignant tumors is even greater.

Correa ZM, Berry JL. Review of retinoblastoma. Knights Templar Eye Foundation Pediatric Ophthalmology Education Center. American Academy of Ophthalmology; 2016. www.aao.org/disease-review/review-of-retinoblastoma

Tomar AS, Finger PT, Gallie B, et al. A multicenter, international collaborative study for American Joint Committee on Cancer Staging of Retinoblastoma: part I: metastasis-associated mortality. *Ophthalmology*. 2020;127(12):1719–1732.

Woo KI, Harbour JW. Review of 676 second primary tumors in patients with retinoblastoma: association between age at onset and tumor type. *Arch Ophthalmol*. 2010;128(7): 865–870.

Miscellaneous Retinal Disorders

Foveal Hypoplasia

Foveal hypoplasia, or incomplete development of the fovea, often presents as nystagmus in early infancy. Although this condition is usually associated with albinism or aniridia, it may also be isolated or familial and may be related to a defect in the *PAX6* gene. Patients with achromatopsia, Stickler syndrome, ROP, and FEVR can also have foveal hypoplasia.

Diagnosis Fundus examination shows a poor or dull foveal reflex. OCT is useful and may have predictive prognostic value. (See BCSC Section 12, *Retina and Vitreous*, and Chapter 12.)

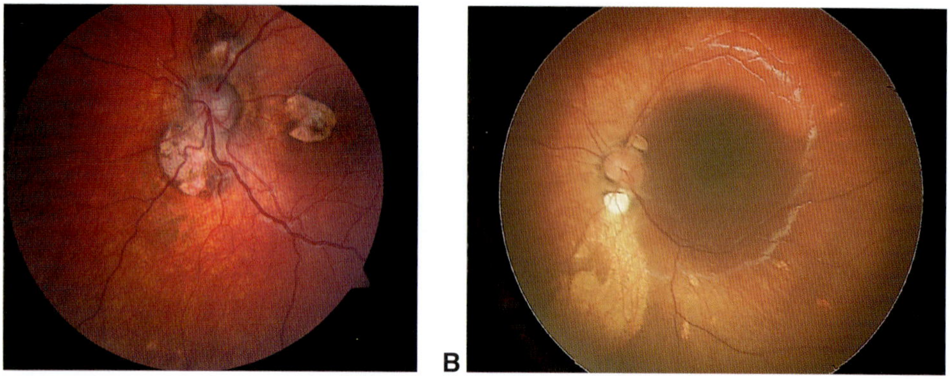

Figure 24-18 Aicardi syndrome. **A,** Fundus photograph demonstrating chorioretinal lacunae circumferential to the optic nerve. **B,** Fundus photograph with chorioretinal lacunae adjacent to the optic nerve with large and small areas of hypopigmentation resulting from chorioretinal atrophy. *(Courtesy of Elias I. Traboulsi, MD, MEd.)*

Treatment No treatment is currently available.

Rufai SR, Thomas MG, Purohit R, et al. Can structural grading of foveal hypoplasia predict future vision in infantile nystagmus? A longitudinal study. *Ophthalmology.* 2020;127(4):492–500.

Aicardi Syndrome

Aicardi syndrome is an X-linked autosomal-dominant disorder characterized by the clinical triad of widespread round or oval depigmented chorioretinal lacunae (Fig 24-18), infantile spasms, and agenesis of the corpus callosum. Chorioretinal lacunae have been shown to occur in 88% of patients; optic nerve abnormalities in 81%. Colobomas, persistent pupillary membranes, and microphthalmia may also occur. Aicardi syndrome is typically lethal in males; however, postzygotic mosaicism or aneuploidy of the X chromosome may lead to disease presentation in males.

Fruhman G, Eble TN, Gambhir N, Sutton VR, Van den Veyver IB, Lewis RA. Ophthalmologic findings in Aicardi syndrome. *J AAPOS.* 2012;16(3):238–241.

Diagnosis The disorder is diagnosed by clinical findings.

Treatment Patients with Aicardi syndrome benefit from management of seizures, physical and occupational therapy, and rehabilitation of low vision and cerebral visual impairment.

CHAPTER 25

Pediatric Uveitis

This chapter includes a related video. Go to www.aao.org/bcscvideo_section06 or scan the QR code in the text to access this content.

This chapter includes a related activity. Go to www.aao.org/bcscactivity_section06 or scan the QR code in the text to access this content.

This chapter includes case studies. Go to www.aao.org/bcsccasestudy_section06 or scan the QR codes in the text to access this content.

Highlights

- Most cases of uveitis in children are noninfectious; however, it is important to rule out and appropriately treat infection and masquerade syndromes.
- Juvenile idiopathic arthritis, the most common systemic disease association, has recommendations for screening, monitoring, and treatment of uveitis.
- Challenges and considerations for pediatric uveitis management include commonly asymptomatic presentation, difficulty of examinations, risk of amblyopia, disease chronicity, psychosocial health, and quality of life.

Introduction

Uveitis is broadly defined as inflammation of the uvea, including the iris, ciliary body, and choroid. See BCSC Section 9, *Uveitis and Ocular Inflammation,* for a more detailed description of the clinical features and inflammatory mechanisms of the conditions discussed in this chapter.

Epidemiology

Pediatric uveitis represents about 10% of all uveitis cases. The mean age at diagnosis is 8–9 years, and 75%–87% of patients have bilateral disease. Three-quarters of all pediatric uveitis cases are noninfectious and anterior, but certain geographic areas have disproportionately higher prevalences of region-specific infectious disease. The most common systemic association is juvenile idiopathic arthritis (JIA), which comprises 21%–35% of cases. Human leukocyte antigen (HLA) associations have been established for some subtypes, but most cases of uveitis are not monogenic.

Smith JA, Mackensen F, Sen HN, et al. Epidemiology and course of disease in childhood uveitis. *Ophthalmology.* 2009;116(8):1544–1551.e1.
Thorne JE, Suhler E, Skup M, et al. Prevalence of noninfectious uveitis in the United States: a claims-based analysis. *JAMA Ophthalmol.* 2016;134(11):1237–1245.

Classification

In the Standardization of Uveitis Nomenclature (SUN), pediatric uveitis is classified based on the location of the inflammation and on descriptors such as onset, course, and duration (see BCSC Section 9, *Uveitis and Ocular Inflammation*). Etiologies are broadly divided into infectious and noninfectious categories (Table 25-1).

Table 25-1 Differential Diagnosis of Uveitis in Children

Anterior	Intermediate	Posterior/Panuveitis
Infectious causes based on anatomic location		
Herpes (HSV, VZV, CMV)	Lyme disease	Herpes (HSV, VZV, CMV)
Bartonella[a]	*Bartonella*[a]	*Bartonella*[a]
Rubella	Toxocariasis	Toxocariasis
Syphilis	Toxoplasmosis	Toxoplasmosis
Tuberculosis	Syphilis	Syphilis
	Tuberculosis	Tuberculosis
		Candida albicans
		Rubella and rubeola (measles)
		HTLV-1 (common in Japan)
		TORCH, Zika virus, LCMV
		Diffuse unilateral subacute neuroretinitis
Noninfectious causes based on anatomic location		
JIA[b]	Sarcoidosis	Sarcoidosis
HLA-B27	TINU (rare)	TINU
TINU	Multiple sclerosis	VKH syndrome (Harada disease)
Sarcoidosis	Pars planitis (idiopathic)	Behçet disease
Idiopathic orbital inflammation		ANCA-associated
IBD-associated		*NOD2*-spectrum disorder (Blau syndrome)
Drug-induced		Sympathetic ophthalmia
Trauma		Systemic lupus erythematosus
Kawasaki disease		Autoinflammatory immunodeficiency syndromes
Idiopathic		Chronic granulomatous disease
		Idiopathic

ANCA = antineutrophil cytoplastic antibodies; CMV = cytomegalovirus; HLA-B27 = human leukocyte antigen B27; HSV = herpes simplex virus; HTLV-1 = human T-cell leukemia virus 1; IBD = inflammatory bowel disease; JIA = juvenile idiopathic arthritis; LCMV = lymphocytic choriomeningitis virus; TINU = tubulointerstitial nephritis and uveitis; TORCH = toxoplasmosis, other agents, rubella, cytomegalovirus, herpes simplex; VKH = Vogt-Koyanagi-Harada; VZV = varicella-zoster virus.

[a] May include anterior/intermediate uveitis but usually with concomitant posterior-segment findings (neuroretinitis, retinal infiltrates, vasculitis).

[b] May involve all compartments of the eye, but chronic anterior uveitis is the most common phenotype.

CLINICAL PEARL

Cytomegalovirus (CMV) in the anterior segment occurs in immunocompetent patients and can be acute or chronic. CMV retinitis can be congenital or acquired. Acquired cases of CMV retinitis usually occur in patients with severe immunodeficiency.

Evaluation of Pediatric Uveitis

A detailed history (see BCSC Section 9, *Uveitis and Ocular Inflammation*), a thorough ophthalmic examination (see Chapter 1), and phenotype-driven ancillary testing all are crucial steps in making an accurate diagnosis.

KEY POINTS 25-1

Considerations for examining children at risk for or diagnosed with uveitis

- Lenticular changes, vitritis, and cystoid macular edema are common causes of nonrefractive changes in vision.
- A myopic shift can result from lenticular changes or from axial elongation related to glaucoma.
- Conventional slit-lamp biomicroscopy is used to visualize anterior-segment cells. With patience and care, a quality slit-lamp examination is possible in most pediatric cases (Video 25-1). If a first attempt is unsuccessful, a second examination 2–3 weeks later is advised before resorting to examination under anesthesia (EUA) to obtain a slit-lamp examination.
- If posterior segment findings are suspected or present in a young or uncooperative child, EUA with scleral depression, optical coherence tomography, fundus photography, and fluorescein angiography may be considered.

VIDEO 25-1 Approach to slit-lamp examination in a young child.
Courtesy of Virginia Miraldi Utz, MD.

CLINICAL PEARL

Asking about immunization status is recommended. Some families choose not to vaccinate their children, and certain geographic regions have limited vaccine access.

Diagnostic Considerations

Ophthalmic Imaging and Functional Testing

Most of the modalities used to monitor disease in adults may be applied to children (see BCSC Section 12, *Retina and Vitreous*, and Section 9, *Uveitis and Ocular Inflammation*).

These include photography of the anterior segment (for keratopathy, lens opacities, and synechiae) and wide-field imaging of the posterior segment (for chorioretinal lesions) as well as optical coherence tomography (for cystoid macular edema), fluorescein angiography (for edema and vascular inflammation), and ultrasound (for media opacities and structural abnormalities of the angle or ciliary body). To adapt these modalities for use in children, decreased acquisition times and oral (rather than intravenous) fluorescein can be considered.

Ancillary Laboratory Testing and Imaging

Phenotype-driven testing is better than "shotgun" approaches (see Chapter 5, Diagnostic Considerations in Uveitis, in BCSC Section 9, *Uveitis and Ocular Inflammation*). Additional considerations for laboratory testing and imaging are summarized in eTable 25-1 at www.aao.org/bcscsupplement_section06. See Activity 25-1 for a decision-tree algorithm.

ACTIVITY 25-1 Uveitis patient evaluation flowchart.
Activity developed by Thellea K. Leveque, MD, MPH.

Case Studies 25-1 through 25-4 provide case examples, differential diagnosis, and phenotype-driven evaluation.

CASE STUDY 25-1 Phenotype-driven evaluation and testing.
Courtesy of Virginia Miraldi Utz, MD.

CASE STUDY 25-2 Phenotype-driven evaluation and testing.
Courtesy of Virginia Miraldi Utz, MD.

CASE STUDY 25-3 Phenotype-driven evaluation and testing.
Courtesy of Virginia Miraldi Utz, MD.

CASE STUDY 25-4 Phenotype-driven evaluation and testing.
Courtesy of Virginia Miraldi Utz, MD.

General Approach to Treatment of Pediatric Uveitis

Once infectious diseases and masquerading causes (addressed later in this chapter) are ruled out, the approach to managing noninfectious uveitis can be conceptualized as a stepladder, with goals of controlling ocular and systemic disease, preventing new ocular complications, and minimizing treatment side effects (Figs 25-1, 25-2).

Initial treatment of anterior-segment inflammation is with mydriatic/cycloplegic agents and topical corticosteroids. Long-term corticosteroids are usually avoided in the pediatric population because of the potential for significant ocular and systemic adverse effects (see BCSC Section 2, *Fundamentals and Principles of Ophthalmology*), including cataract,

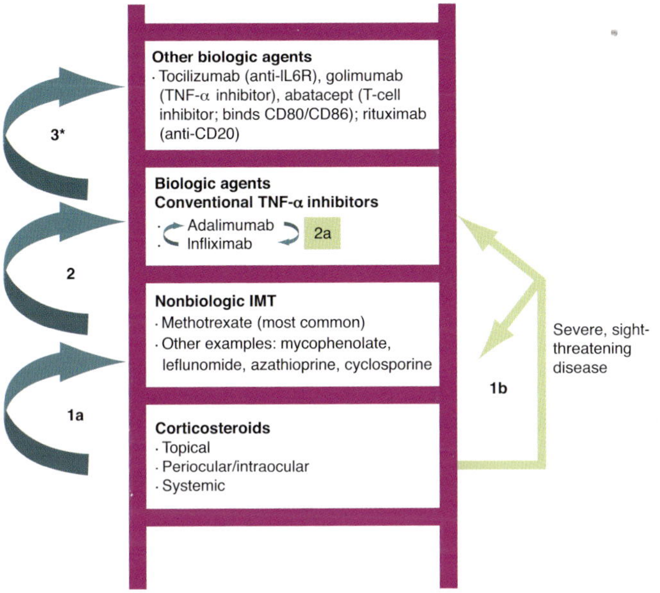

Figure 25-1 The stepladder approach to treating noninfectious uveitis. Corticosteroids are the initial treatment; selection depends on anatomic location and extent of inflammation. Systemic disease, if present, may drive the therapeutic choice. **1a,** Initial corticosteroid-sparing immunomodulatory treatment (IMT). **1b,** To control severe, vision-threatening disease, an antimetabolite may be started simultaneously with a tumor necrosis factor-alpha (TNF-α) inhibitor. **2,** Adalimumab or infliximab may be added if the treatment response is insufficient. The nonbiologic IMT should be continued as long as it is tolerated; it may prevent antibodies to the TNF-α inhibitor and work synergistically with the biologic to control disease. Prior to switching biologic therapy, dosage and frequency should be maximized. **2a,** Different TNF-α inhibitors may be tried before stepping up the ladder. **3,** Other biologic agents can be considered after failure of 2 TNF-α inhibitors. *Note:* Biologic agents are listed, but nonbiologic agents may be considered (eg, cyclosporine, mycophenolate, leflunomide). CD = clusters of differentiation; CTLA = cytotoxic T-lymphocyte–associated; IgG = immunoglobulin G; IL = interleukin. *(Courtesy of Virginia Miraldi Utz, MD.)*

glaucoma, adrenal suppression, and exogenous Cushing syndrome. Prednisolone acetate 1% or weaker corticosteroid is preferred over difluprednate. Vision-threatening disease may warrant oral corticosteroids as a bridge to definitive management with nonsteroidal immunomodulatory therapy (IMT).

Treatment escalation is considered if a patient requires ≥1–2 drops of prednisolone acetate 1% (or equivalent per day) at 3 months or if new ocular complications develop (see Fig 25-2) from inflammation or are induced by corticosteroids. Systemic IMT is best undertaken in cooperation with a pediatric specialist familiar with the use of immunosuppressive treatments and IMT. It is recommended that care be established with a pediatric rheumatologist early in the disease course.

Methotrexate is the first-line antimetabolite IMT for treatment of arthritis and uveitis in children. Approximately 70% of children have a treatment response. Subcutaneous injections are preferred because they enable more predictable dosing and bioavailability. Gastrointestinal disturbances, such as nausea, emesis, oral ulcers, and fatigue, are the most common adverse effects. Hepatic toxicity, interstitial pneumonitis,

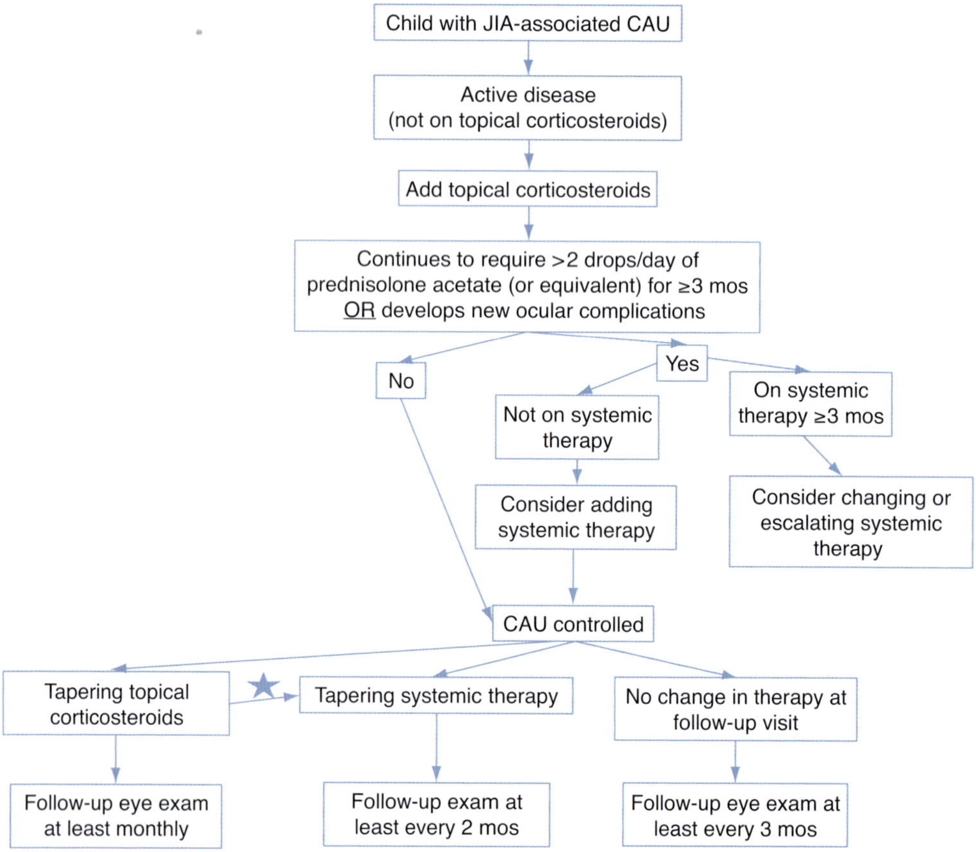

Figure 25-2 Treatment escalation algorithm in a child with noninfectious chronic anterior uveitis (CAU). *Star* indicates that topical corticosteroids should be preferentially tapered prior to systemic therapy. JIA = juvenile idiopathic arthritis. *(Created by Virginia Miraldi Utz, MD, with data from Angeles-Han ST, Ringold S, Beukelman T, et al. 2019 American College of Rheumatology/Arthritis Foundation guideline for the screening, monitoring, and treatment of juvenile idiopathic arthritis-associated uveitis.* Arthritis Care Res (Hoboken). *2019;71(6):703–716.)*

and cytopenia are rare but serious side effects. If disease is not fully controlled with methotrexate, treatment escalation is with biologics (see Figs 25-1, 25-2). Tapering of systemic therapy may be considered after at least 2 years of inactive disease, preferably with the patient also off topical corticosteroids. For more about specific IMT agents, see BCSC Section 9, *Uveitis and Ocular Inflammation.*

Angeles-Han ST, Ringold S, Beukelman T, et al. 2019 American College of Rheumatology/Arthritis Foundation Guideline for the Screening, Monitoring, and Treatment of Juvenile Idiopathic Arthritis-Associated Uveitis. *Arthritis Care Res (Hoboken).* 2019;71(6): 703–716.

Quartier P, Baptiste A, Despert V, et al. ADJUVITE: a double-blind, randomised, placebo-controlled trial of adalimumab in early onset, chronic, juvenile idiopathic arthritis-associated anterior uveitis. *Ann Rheum Dis.* 2018;77(7):1003–1011.

Ramanan AV, Dick AD, Jones AP, et al. Adalimumab plus methotrexate for uveitis in juvenile idiopathic arthritis. *N Engl J Med.* 2017;376(17):1637–1646.

Anterior Uveitis

The anterior chamber is the primary site of inflammation in patients with anterior uveitis; the uveal structures involved include the iris (iritis) and ciliary body (cyclitis).

CLINICAL PEARL

When the anterior chamber is the primary site of inflammation, the term *iritis* is used; when inflammation is also observed in the anterior vitreous and ciliary body, it is termed *iridocyclitis*.

Noninfectious Anterior Uveitis

Juvenile idiopathic arthritis

Juvenile idiopathic arthritis (JIA) is the most common identifiable etiology of childhood anterior uveitis in North America. JIA is defined as arthritis for at least 6 weeks without an identifiable cause in children younger than 16 years. The International League of Associations for Rheumatology recognizes 7 subtypes of JIA based on the number of joints involved, extra-articular manifestations, and laboratory markers of antinuclear antibody (ANA) and HLA-B27 seropositivity (Table 25-2).

Table 25-2 International League of Associations of Rheumatology Classification System of Juvenile Idiopathic Arthritis

Category	Joint Involvement	Select Extra-articular/ Serologic Manifestations	Uveitis Frequency and Phenotype
Oligoarticular arthritis	≥4 joints	Uveitis	~30%; chronic anterior uveitis
RF-negative, polyarticular arthritis	>4 joints	RF-negative	~10%; chronic anterior uveitis
RF-positive, polyarticular arthritis	>4 joints	RF-positive (similar to adult RA); +/− anti-CCP	Uveitis is rare
Psoriatic arthritis	Arthritis	Psoriasis rash	~10%; chronic anterior uveitis[a]
Enthesitis-related arthritis	Arthritis may involve spine, SI joints	Enthesitis[b] +/− HLA-B27	~10%; acute anterior uveitis
Systemic arthritis	Arthritis	Fever, evanescent rash, hepatosplenomegaly, serositis	Rare
Undifferentiated	Fits into >1 category	Any of the above	Unknown

CCP = citrullinated peptide; HLA-B27 = human leukocyte antigen B27; RA = rheumatoid arthritis; RF = rheumatoid factor; SI = sacroiliac.

[a]Occasionally acute presentation, especially in those with HLA-B27 positivity.

[b]Enthesitis is inflammation where the tendons or ligaments insert into the bone.

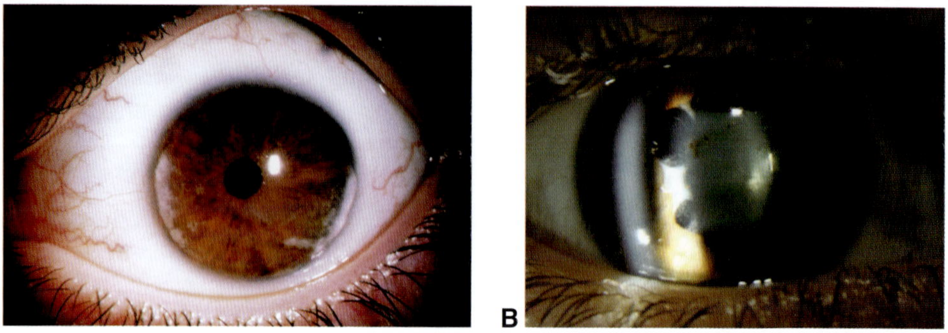

Figure 25-3 Slit-lamp photographs from 2 patients with uveitis associated with juvenile idiopathic arthritis (JIA). **A,** As is typical in oligoarticular or rheumatoid factor (RF)-negative polyarticular JIA, the conjunctiva is "white." Band keratopathy is present. **B,** Asymptomatic patient with extensive synechiae, pigmentary deposition on the lens, and posterior subcapsular cataract. *(Part A courtesy of Amy Hutchinson, MD; part B courtesy of Virginia MIraldi Utz, MD.)*

Clinical presentation of JIA-associated uveitis Uveitis, the most common extra-articular manifestation of JIA, is predominantly anterior and may be chronic or acute. Patients with oligoarticular, rheumatoid factor (RF)–negative polyarticular, and psoriatic JIA subtypes generally develop asymptomatic, bilateral chronic anterior uveitis (CAU). In contrast, enthesitis-related arthritis is associated with a symptomatic, acute, unilateral presentation.

Chronic inflammation can cause band keratopathy (Fig 25-3A), posterior synechiae (Fig 25-3B), ciliary body membrane formation, hypotony, cataract, glaucoma, and phthisis. Vitritis and macular edema occur infrequently.

Screening for uveitis in children with JIA It is recommended that a patient with JIA be screened regularly for early asymptomatic uveitis; 90% of uveitis cases occur within 4 years of the JIA diagnosis. The goal is to prevent severe ocular complications. There are 4 major risk factors for uveitis development: JIA subtype (oligoarticular, RF-negative, polyarticular, psoriatic, and undifferentiated), disease duration (≤4 years), ANA positivity, and young age (≤6 years) (Fig 25-4).

CLINICAL PEARL

In children with JIA at high risk of uveitis, monitoring at 3-month intervals is advised after discontinuation of systemic IMT because IMT can mask the presentation of uveitis.

Risk factors in JIA associated with poor visual prognosis Risk factors associated with poor visual prognosis include male gender; African American, non-Hispanic race; a short interval between arthritis onset and uveitis; uveitis before or at onset of joint symptoms; and complications (see the section "Clinical presentation of JIA-associated uveitis") and vision loss at presentation. Hypotony and posterior synechiae are predictive of ongoing uveitis after age 16.

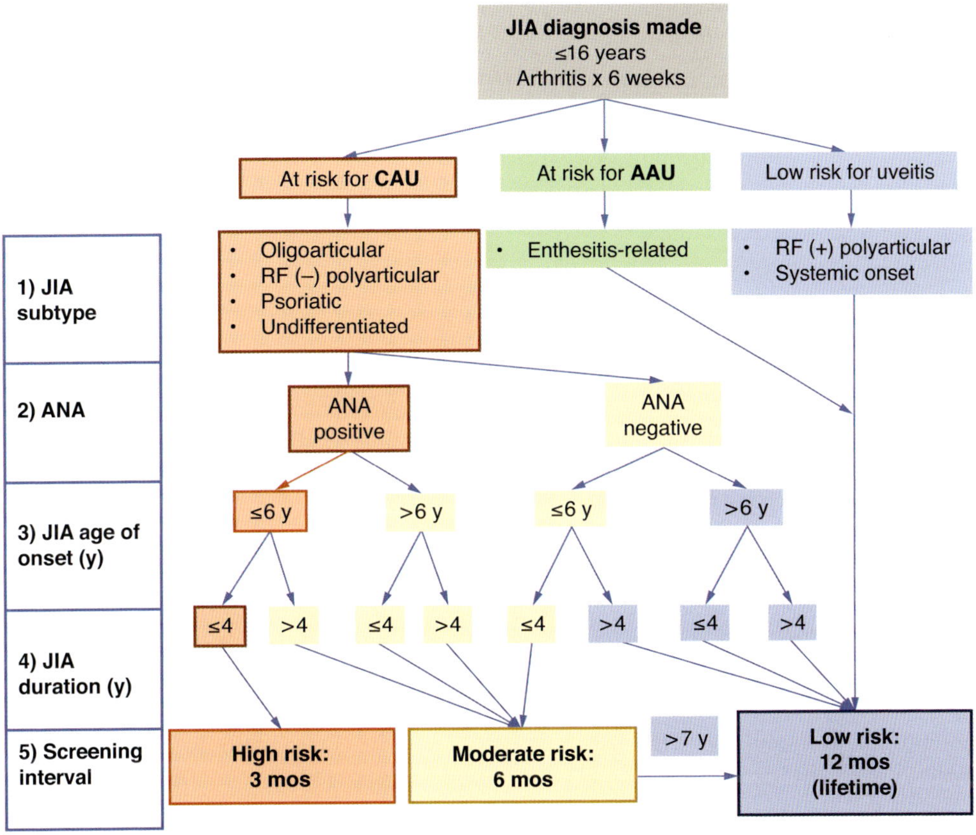

Figure 25-4 Screening intervals are determined by 4 major risk factors: JIA subtype, antinuclear antibody (ANA) status, age of JIA onset, and JIA duration. If uveitis is absent after 7 years of disease, screening should still occur yearly because there is still a lifetime risk. AAU = acute anterior uveitis. *(Courtesy of Virginia Miraldi Utz, MD; © 2022 American Academy of Ophthalmology.)*

Angeles-Han ST, Pelajo CF, Vogler LB, et al. Risk markers of juvenile idiopathic arthritis-associated uveitis in the Childhood Arthritis and Rheumatology Research Alliance (CARRA) Registry. *J Rheumatol.* 2013;40(12):2088–2096.

Monitoring and treatment of JIA-associated uveitis The guidelines of the American College of Rheumatology specify monitoring frequency of stable cases, especially after changes to treatment (see the section General Approach to Treatment of Pediatric Uveitis as well as Figs 25-1, 25-2).

CLINICAL PEARL

Most children with JIA-associated CAU experience improvement when given prednisolone acetate (1%) 4–6 times per day as initial treatment. Advise the family to shake the medication 50 times to ensure reconstitution.

Inflammatory bowel disease in children

Children with Crohn disease and ulcerative colitis are at risk for uveitis, although the prevalence is lower than in adults—less than 2%. The signs and risk factors are similar to those of children with enthesitis-related JIA; children with inflammatory bowel disease usually present with acute anterior uveitis, especially in HLA-B27–positive disease. However, several studies have reported an asymptomatic chronic anterior uveitis presentation. Routine ophthalmic screening is not recommended.

Ottaviano G, Salvatore S, Salvatoni A, et al. Ocular manifestations of paediatric inflammatory bowel disease: a systematic review and meta-analysis. *J Crohns Colitis.* 2018;12(7):870–879.

Tubulointerstitial nephritis and uveitis syndrome

Tubulointerstitial nephritis and uveitis (TINU) syndrome is a form of kidney disease associated with chronic or recurrent nongranulomatous anterior uveitis in adolescents, especially adolescent girls. Occasionally, the posterior segment is involved. TINU often presents as systemic illness characterized by fatigue, weight loss, and low-grade fever. Urinalysis findings include elevated urinary β2-microglobulin level, proteinuria, white blood cell casts, and eosinophilia. Additionally, serum creatinine levels may be elevated, and glomerular filtration rate may be decreased, indicating renal dysfunction. Renal biopsy may be needed to confirm the diagnosis and exclude other causes.

The prognosis of TINU is generally good, but long-term follow-up is required because inflammation may recur. Early treatment with systemic corticosteroids usually is necessary; chronic uveitis may require corticosteroid-sparing IMT.

Other noninfectious causes of anterior uveitis

Kawasaki disease Kawasaki disease, also known as *mucocutaneous lymph node syndrome,* is a primary vasculitis affecting children younger than 5 years. Signs include fever, conjunctival injection, mucous membrane changes, rash, and cervical lymphadenopathy. After conjunctivitis, the second most common ocular finding in the acute phase of illness is a generally self-limited anterior uveitis, which occurs in approximately 10% of cases. The most significant complication of Kawasaki disease is coronary artery aneurysm, which occurs in 15%–25% of untreated children. Treatment with aspirin and intravenous immunoglobulin G (IgG) reduces the risk of coronary artery aneurysm formation.

Behçet disease Behçet disease is a rare cause of acute anterior uveitis in children. Pediatric Behçet disease predominantly affects boys and does not necessarily involve oral and genital ulcers. It is important to rule out posterior-segment disease, which requires aggressive immunosuppressive treatment. See Chapter 9 in BCSC Section 9, *Uveitis and Ocular Inflammation.*

Idiopathic uveitis Although most cases of anterior uveitis are idiopathic, potential alternative causes to consider are masquerade syndromes (see the section Masquerade Syndromes later in this chapter), infections (see Table 25-1), medication effects (see BCSC Section 9, *Uveitis and Ocular Inflammation*), and trauma.

Infectious Anterior Uveitis

Herpesviruses (herpes simplex virus, cytomegalovirus, and varicella-zoster virus) are important infectious etiologies to consider in the differential diagnosis of anterior uveitis, especially in cases of unilateral disease with ocular hypertension and without synechiae. Other common signs include keratitis and iris atrophy.

If herpetic disease is suspected, a trial of acyclovir or valacyclovir plus topical corticosteroids may be considered. Anterior-chamber paracentesis may be performed to enable viral identification by polymerase chain reaction (PCR). (See BCSC Section 8, *External Disease and Cornea,* and Section 9, *Uveitis and Ocular Inflammation.*)

Intermediate Uveitis

The SUN Working Group defines intermediate uveitis as primary inflammation of the vitreous body, the vitreous base overlying the ciliary body, the pars plana, and the peripheral retina (Fig 25-5). Intermediate uveitis accounts for 12%–28% of pediatric uveitis cases. Noninfectious and infectious causes are listed in Table 25-1.

Pars planitis is an idiopathic form of intermediate uveitis involving the pars plana. It is a diagnosis of exclusion, accounting for 85%–90% of intermediate uveitis cases. Typical signs include

- condensations of white blood cells ("snowballs")
- peripheral exudation ("snowbanking")
- peripheral vasculitis

CLINICAL PEARL

The differential diagnosis of intermediate uveitis includes Coats disease and inherited retinal dystrophies.

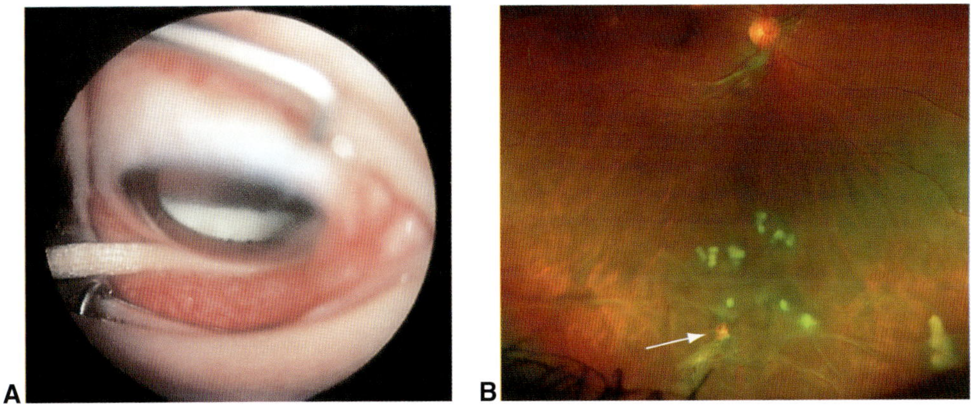

Figure 25-5 Examples of intermediate uveitis. **A,** Intermediate uveitis with inferior "snowbank" formation (inflammatory exudative accumulation on the inferior pars plana), right eye. **B,** Active intermediate uveitis with fibrosis and neovascularization *(arrow)* and "snowballs" (condensations of white blood cells). *(Part B courtesy of Virginia Miraldi Utz, MD.)*

Periocular or systemic corticosteroids may be used as initial treatment for active disease while waiting for the full effectiveness of corticosteroid-sparing IMT to be reached (see Fig 25-1). Laser photocoagulation or cryotherapy can be applied to manage peripheral exudation or neovascularization. Potential complications of intermediate uveitis include papillitis, macular edema, and peripheral neovascularization. Peripheral neovascularization may lead to tractional retinal detachment.

Posterior Uveitis

Posterior uveitis is defined as intraocular inflammation primarily involving the choroid; often, the retina is also involved. Posterior uveitis can be infectious or noninfectious. Two important pediatric infectious causes are toxoplasmosis and toxocariasis.

Toxoplasmosis

Toxoplasmosis is the most common cause of infectious posterior uveitis in children (see BCSC Section 9, *Uveitis and Ocular Inflammation*). Systemic infection with the obligate intracellular parasite *Toxoplasma gondii* is common in humans and usually goes undiagnosed; felines are the definitive host. Signs and symptoms include fever, lymphadenopathy, and sore throat. In the United States, approximately 11% of children older than 6 years have been infected by the parasite. Seropositivity increases with age and can exceed 60% in certain countries. Transplacental infection occurs. Congenital toxoplasmosis is bilateral in 85% of cases and has a predilection to the posterior pole (Fig 25-6A). The classic presentation is white retinochoroiditis with overlying vitreous inflammation ("headlight in the fog") adjacent to a pigmented retinochoroidal scar (Fig 25-6B, C). Evidence suggests this presentation can represent postnatal infection. For lesions that threaten vision, systemic treatment is with 1 or more antimicrobial drugs with or without oral corticosteroids.

> **CLINICAL PEARL**
>
> The Sabin tetrad for congenital toxoplasmosis is (1) retinochoroiditis (bilateral, predilection for posterior pole and macula), (2) hydrocephalus or microcephaly, (3) intracranial calcifications, and (4) cognitive impairment.

Toxocariasis

Ocular toxocariasis (OT) is caused by the nematode larvae of common intestinal parasites of dogs *(Toxocara canis)* and cats *(Toxocara cati)*. The disease primarily affects children and is contracted by ingestion of ascarid ova in soil contaminated with dog or cat feces. *Visceral toxocariasis (VT)* is an acute systemic infection produced by these organisms that usually affects children younger than 3 years. Symptoms include fever, cough, rash, hepatomegaly, pneumonia, malaise, anorexia, and meningoencephalitis.

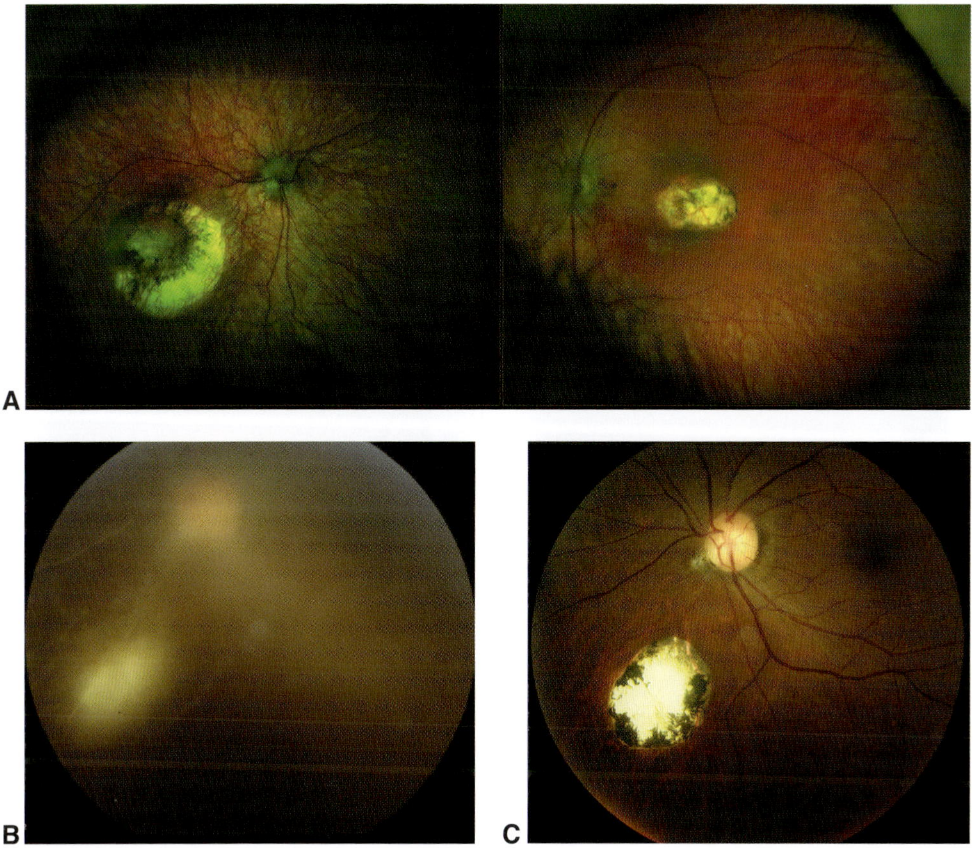

Figure 25-6 Examples of toxoplasmosis in children. **A,** Wide-field images of the right and left eyes of a 4-month-old child with bilateral toxoplasmosis–associated chorioretinal scars. The optic nerve is hypoplastic in the right eye and pale in the left eye. The patient presented with poor visual response and nystagmus (right > left). **B,** Eye with classic "headlight in the fog" appearance on presentation. **C,** Patient in **(B)** after treatment, with a chorioretinal scar. *(Part A courtesy of Virginia Miraldi Utz, MD; parts B and C courtesy of E. Mitchel Opremcak, MD.)*

Laboratory test results reveal eosinophilia. For unknown reasons, VT and OT seldom occur in the same patient.

Ocular toxocariasis is usually unilateral and is not associated with systemic illness or systemic eosinophilia. In the United States, the average age of presentation is 8 years. Specific ocular presentations correspond to the following age ranges:

- *2–9 years:* chronic endophthalmitis; chronic unilateral uveitis
- *6–11 years:* localized granuloma; present in macula or peripapillary region (Fig 25-7A, B)
- *6–40 years:* peripheral granuloma; peripheral hemispheric masses with dense connective tissue strands (Fig 25-7C, D)

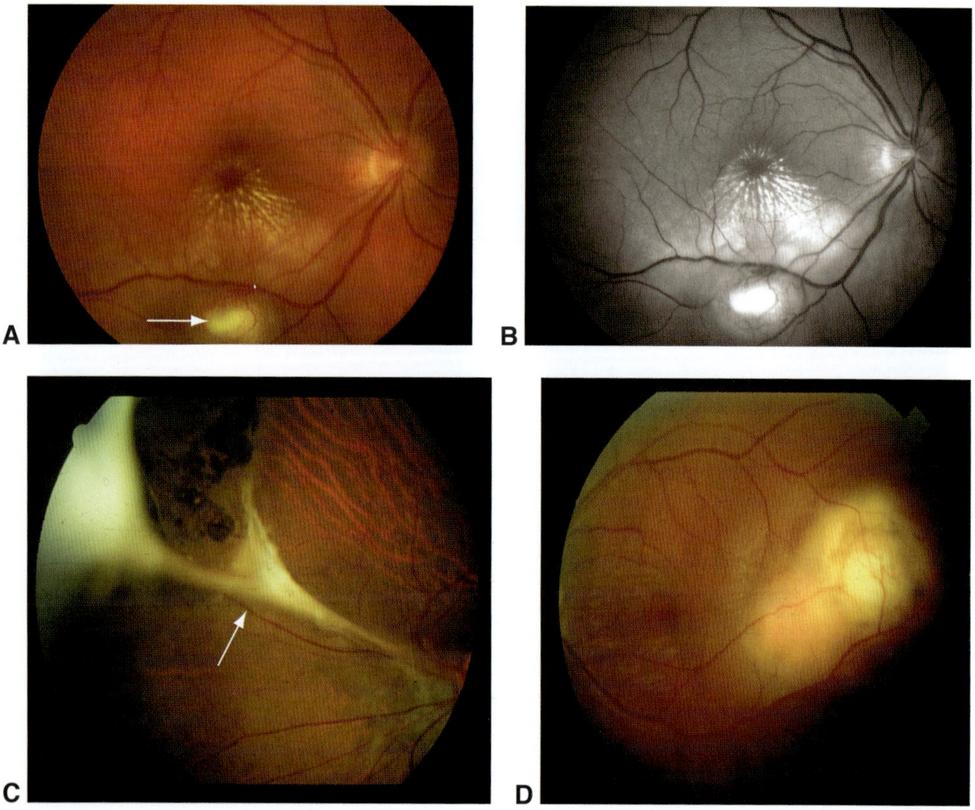

Figure 25-7 Toxocariasis. **A** and **B,** Peripheral granuloma *(arrow)* associated with a macular star. **C,** Falciform fold *(arrow)* associated with a peripheral granuloma. **D,** Fundus photograph of peripheral granuloma causing macular striations and vascular distortion. *(Courtesy of E. Mitchel Opremcak, MD.)*

Treatment includes observation, steroids for posterior lesions and endophthalmitis, or surgical intervention to address retinal traction, cataract, glaucoma, or cyclitic membranes. Treatment of OT with systemic anthelmintics is discouraged because the organisms may already be dead, or their deaths may elicit a significant host inflammatory response. See BCSC Section 9, *Uveitis and Ocular Inflammation.*

Woodhall D, Starr MC, Montgomery SP, et al. Ocular toxocariasis: epidemiologic, anatomic, and therapeutic variations based on a survey of ophthalmic subspecialists. *Ophthalmology.* 2012;119(6):1211–1217.

Other Causes of Posterior Uveitis

Other causes of posterior uveitis are listed in Table 25-1.

Panuveitis

In panuveitis, the inflammation is diffuse, occurring in the anterior chamber, vitreous, and choroid without a predominant site.

Sarcoidosis

Sarcoidosis comprises 2 distinct presentations in children. Early-onset sarcoidosis—occurring in children younger than 5 years—entails arthritis, rash, and uveitis but includes pulmonary disease only in rare cases. Features of early-onset ocular sarcoidosis overlap with those of JIA and Blau syndrome (the latter is discussed in the next section). In older children (8–15 years), the presentation of sarcoidosis is similar to that in the adult form of the disease, with pulmonary and lymph node abnormalities and increased risk of uveitis. Although the most common manifestation of ocular sarcoidosis is acute or chronic granulomatous anterior uveitis, classically with "mutton fat" keratic precipitates, the spectrum of disease includes posterior-segment manifestations such as multifocal choroiditis, optic nerve head edema, segmental periphlebitis with characteristic "candle wax drippings," and panuveitis (Fig 25-8).

Sarcoidosis is diagnosed and treated similarly in adults and children. (See BCSC Section 9, *Uveitis and Ocular Inflammation*.) However, serum angiotensin-converting enzyme levels, which may be abnormally elevated in patients with sarcoidosis, are normally higher in healthy children than in adults and thus can be misleading. Definitive diagnosis is made from results of a biopsy specimen analysis (see Case Study 25-3).

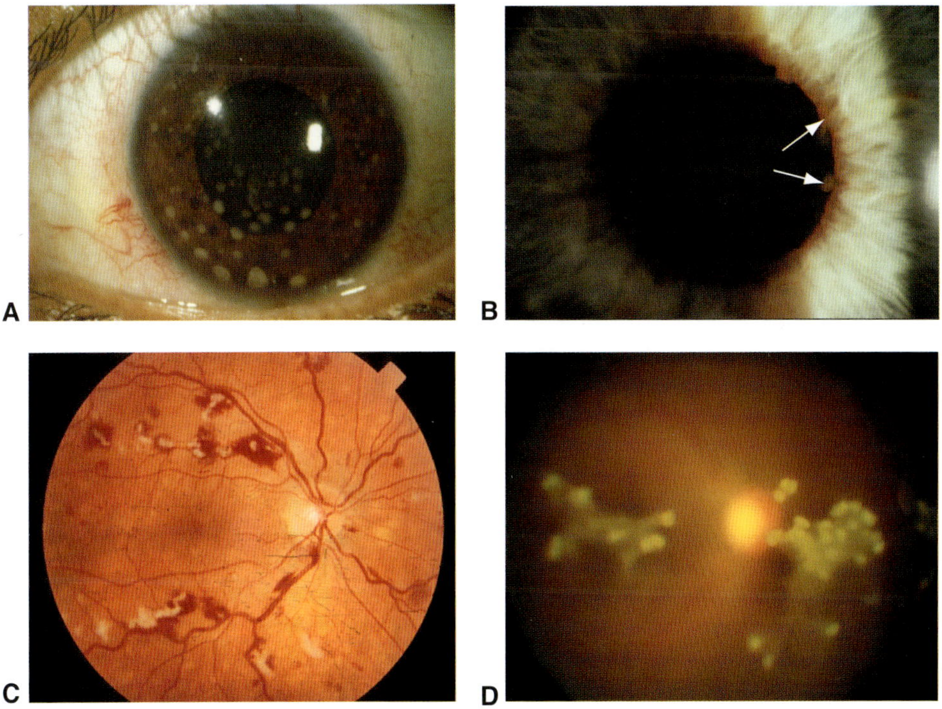

Figure 25-8 Select ophthalmic manifestations of ocular sarcoidosis. **A,** Classic "mutton fat" granulomatous keratic precipitates. **B,** Iris nodules (*arrows* indicate Koeppe nodules). **C,** Periphlebitis with irregular perivascular granulomas ("candle wax drippings"). **D,** Snowballs in sarcoid uveitis. If in a linear array, this is called a "string of pearls." *(Courtesy of E. Mitchel Opremcak, MD.)*

Familial Juvenile Systemic Granulomatosis

Early-onset sarcoidosis and Blau syndrome are the sporadic and familial forms, respectively, of granulomatous autoinflammatory disease that is inherited in an autosomal dominant disorder secondary to a pathogenic variant in *NOD2* on chromosome 16. *NOD2* encodes the nucleotide-binding oligomerization domain–containing 2 protein. Although different disease manifestations can emerge simultaneously, the median age of dermatitis onset is at 1 year; arthritis, 2 years; and ocular disease, 4.4 years. Ocular involvement can occur as early as 6 months and as late as 22 years of age. Pulmonary involvement and lymphadenopathy are usually absent. Progressive panuveitis with multifocal choroiditis is the most common ocular presentation. Inflammatory ocular complications are common.

Sarens IL. Blau syndrome-associated uveitis: preliminary results from an international prospective interventional case series. *Am J Ophthalmol.* 2018;187:158–166.

Vogt-Koyanagi-Harada Syndrome

Vogt-Koyanagi-Harada (VKH) syndrome is a chronic, progressive bilateral panuveitis associated with exudative retinal detachments that may be accompanied by meningeal irritation, auditory disturbances, and skin changes. VKH syndrome occurs in children only in rare instances, but in those affected, ocular complications (eg, cataracts and glaucoma) occur at a higher rate and the visual prognosis is poorer, compared with affected adults. For further discussion, see BCSC Section 9, *Uveitis and Ocular Inflammation.*

Other Causes of Panuveitis

Other causes of panuveitis are listed in Table 25-1.

Masquerade Syndromes

Various conditions can simulate pediatric uveitis. Table 25-3 lists some masquerade syndromes and their diagnostic features (see BCSC Section 9, *Uveitis and Ocular Inflammation*). The possibility of diffuse infiltrating retinoblastoma is particularly important to recognize. Presentation may involve a unilateral, "uveitic-like" syndrome, with tumor cells in the anterior chamber and pseudohypopyon (Fig 25-9). When diffuse infiltrating retinoblastoma is suspected, prompt referral of the patient to an experienced ocular oncologist is crucial.

Traine PG, Schedler KJ, Rodrigues EB. Clinical presentation and genetic paradigm of diffuse infiltrating retinoblastoma: a review. *Ocul Oncol Pathol.* 2016;2(3):128–132.

Psychosocial Concerns and Adherence

Vision loss, fear of blindness, burden of medical examinations, treatment regimens, medication side effects, and chronicity of disease impact both the child and the family. The Effects of Youngsters' Eyesight on Quality of Life (EYE-Q) questionnaire is a validated

Table 25-3 Uveitis Masquerade Syndromes in Children

Disease or Condition	Age (Years)	Signs of Inflammation	Examination/Diagnostic Studies
Anterior segment			
Diffuse infiltrating retinoblastoma	Average, 5.7 (M > F)	Flare, cells, pseudohypopyon	Aqueous paracentesis by an experienced ocular oncologist; genetic counseling and testing; occasionally patients can have a combined presentation
Leukemia	<15	Flare, cells, hypopyon, iris heterochromia, hyphema	Bone marrow biopsy, peripheral blood smear
Intraocular foreign body	Any	Flare, cells	X-ray, CT, ultrasonography
Malignant melanoma	Any	Flare, cells	Fluorescein angiography, ultrasonography, OCT
Juvenile xanthogranuloma	<15	Flare, cells, "spontaneous" hyphema, iris lesions	Examination of skin, iris biopsy
Peripheral retinal detachment	Any	Flare, cells (usually pigmented); IOP may be elevated in Schwartz Matsuo syndrome	Ophthalmoscopy, wide-field imaging, ultrasonography
Posterior segment			
Inherited retinal disease	Any	Cells in vitreous, waxy ONH pallor, bone-spicule pigmentary changes in the midperiphery	Nyctalopia; ERG, Goldmann visual fields, OCT, FAF; genetic counseling and testing
Systemic lymphoma	≥15	Retinal hemorrhage or exudates, vitreous cells	Lymph node biopsy, bone marrow biopsy, physical examination
Retinoblastoma	<15	Vitreous cells, retinal exudates	Ultrasonography, MRI
Malignant melanoma	≥15	Vitreous cells, choroidal pigmentary lesion	Fluorescein angiography, b-scan ultrasonography, OCT, FAF

CT = computed tomography; ERG = electroretinography; FAF = fundus autofluorescence; IOP = intraocular pressure; MRI = magnetic resonance imaging; OCT = optical coherence tomography; ONH = optic nerve head.

instrument used to assess child- and parent-reported visual function and vision-related quality of life in children aged 5–18. To address academic concerns, an educational plan (https://aapos.org/patients/patient-resources/pediatric-uveitis) can be implemented.

Follow-up and treatment adherence present unique challenges in the pediatric population. A parent or guardian must manage scheduling and transport for the child's appointments and infusions and must administer at-home medications. In teens and young adults, treatment may be a shared responsibility, further complicating adherence. For disorders like JIA-associated uveitis, the disease may be asymptomatic, and the effects of indolent, uncontrolled inflammation may not be realized until complications have occurred. Despite advances in treatment, children with incomplete adherence to follow-up or treatment are 10 times more likely to have active disease at any given visit, resulting in further morbidity. Understanding family dynamics and barriers to care may help to

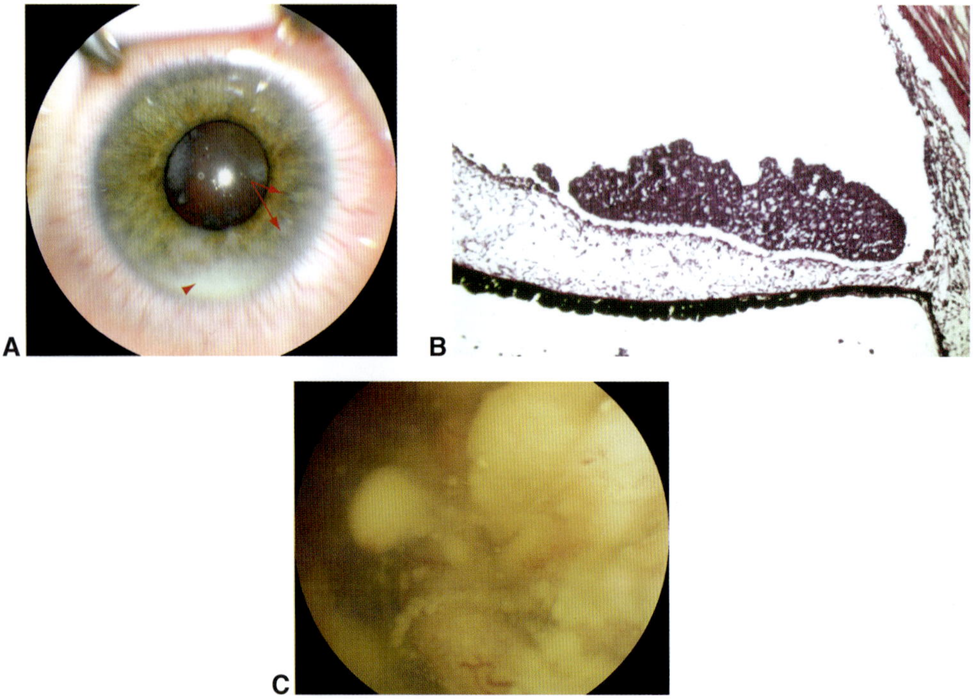

Figure 25-9 Diffuse infiltrating retinoblastoma: a crucial diagnosis. **A,** Whitish pseudohypopyon *(arrowhead)* is present along with small white nodules of tumor on the iris *(arrows).* Retroillumination reveals media opacities, likely tumor cells on the posterior surface of the lens. **B,** Histopathologic section demonstrating nodules of retinoblastoma adherent to the iris and infiltrating the angle. **C,** Posterior segment indicating diffuse vitritis. *(Courtesy of James J. Augsburger, MD.)*

promote adherence and disease control. A social worker or psychologist can help address barriers to care and adjustment to illness and may promote well-being. See Chapter 28, Pediatric Chronic Eye Care and Low Vision Rehabilitation.

McDonald J, Cassedy C, Altaye M, et al. Comprehensive assessment of quality of life, functioning and mental health in children with juvenile idiopathic arthritis and non-infectious uveitis [epub ahead of print January 9, 2021]. *Arthritis Care Res (Hoboken).* doi: 10.1002/acr.24551.

Miraldi Utz V, Bulas S, Lopper S, et al. Effectiveness of long-term infliximab use and impact of treatment adherence on disease control in refractory, non-infectious pediatric uveitis. *Pediatr Rheumatol Online J.* 2019;17(1):79.

Surgical Treatment of Complications of Uveitis

Complications of uveitis include band keratopathy, cataract, and glaucoma. Band keratopathy can be treated by removal of the corneal epithelium and calcium chelation with EDTA. Treatment may have to be repeated. Phototherapeutic keratectomy has also been used to treat band keratopathy.

Cataract surgery for patients with uveitis can be complicated by hypotony, glaucoma, synechiae formation, cystoid macular edema, and retinal detachment. Controlling the uveitis preoperatively, perioperatively, and postoperatively is necessary for a successful outcome. The use of intraocular lenses (IOLs) in these patients is controversial. Long-term well-controlled disease is important before consideration of IOL implantation, as are judicious use of perioperative corticosteroids, meticulous technique, and frequent postoperative follow-up to detect complications early. See BCSC Section 9, *Uveitis and Ocular Inflammation.*

Glaucoma surgery is necessary in certain cases of pediatric uveitis. Many techniques have been used, and long-term success rates vary. Standard trabeculectomy is associated with a high rate of failure due to scarring. Goniotomy or trabeculotomy is often effective in children and is an appropriate initial surgery if the anterior-chamber angle is visible and the uveitis is well-controlled. Tube shunts can be used when goniotomy fails or when the angle is closed. Control of inflammation with systemic IMT is advised prior to surgical intervention for glaucoma whenever possible.

Bohnsack BL, Freedman SF. Surgical outcomes in childhood uveitic glaucoma. *Am J Ophthalmol.* 2013;155(1):134–142.

CHAPTER 26

Ocular Trauma in Childhood

This chapter includes a related video. Go to www.aao.org/bcscvideo_section06 or scan the QR code in the text to access this content.

Highlights

- A low threshold for examination under anesthesia is acceptable if significant ocular trauma and an open globe injury are suspected.
- Cataract surgery often is not performed at the same time as the primary globe repair, even if the lens capsule is breached.
- Nonaccidental injury should always be considered if the circumstances and clinical features of an ocular injury are suspicious.

Introduction

Trauma is one of the most prevalent causes of ocular morbidity in childhood. In younger children, most accidental ocular trauma occurs during casual play with other children. Older children and adolescents are most likely to be injured while participating in sports. Although fireworks, pellets from BB guns, and various other projectiles are less frequent causes of pediatric ocular trauma, when they are causes, they are likely to cause severe injuries. The incidence of severe eye injury is particularly high in children aged 11–15 years compared with the incidence in other age groups. Injured boys outnumber injured girls by a factor of 4 to 1.

Most serious childhood eye injuries could, in principle, be prevented by appropriate adult supervision and by regular use of protective eyewear during sports activities and play involving projectiles. These measures are particularly important for children who already have monocular vision loss.

Special Considerations in the Management of Pediatric Ocular Trauma

Many aspects of ocular trauma are similar in both adults and children, including classification of the trauma into closed globe injury (CGI) and open globe injury (OGI) as well as the principles of trauma management. An OGI is defined by a full-thickness break in the "eye wall" (ie, the cornea and sclera), whereas in eyes with CGI, the eye wall has no full-thickness defect.

A comprehensive discussion of all aspects of trauma is beyond the scope of this chapter. However, pediatric eye trauma requires special consideration of issues common in or unique to this patient population:

- **Trauma is often unwitnessed, or an accurate history is not available or reliable.** Important factors such as the mechanism of injury (eg, force, trajectory, speed) as well as the type of causative agent (eg, sharp or blunt, contaminated, chemical) may not be known.
- **If the patient is unable to cooperate, the clinician may not be able to perform a detailed examination.** Using force to open a child's eye risks exacerbating preexisting damage in an eye with OGI. Examination under anesthesia (EUA) may be warranted if there was significant ocular trauma and signs that suggest an OGI (eg, blood or pink tears with no obvious cause).
- **Children younger than 5–7 years have a high risk of developing amblyopia.** Any unilateral media opacity (eg, traumatic cataract, corneal scar, vitreous hemorrhage) can cause severe amblyopia. Restoration of medial clarity and initiation of amblyopia treatment are thus a high priority.
- **The possibility of nonaccidental trauma should always be considered** (see the section Nonaccidental Trauma).

CLINICAL PEARL

An anesthetic eyedrop followed by waiting a few minutes for parents to calm the child may allow enough assessment for the clinician to distinguish an ocular surface pain (abrasion or foreign body) from a more severe injury.

Closed Globe Injury

Corneal Abrasion

Corneal abrasion is one of the most common ocular injuries. Disruption of the corneal epithelium is usually associated with immediate pain, foreign-body sensation, tearing, and discomfort with blinking. Topical cycloplegic eyedrops and antibiotic ointment may help reduce discomfort and the risk of infection, respectively. In healthy children, most epithelial defects heal within 1–2 days. A pressure patch to keep the eyelids closed is generally unnecessary; it does not reduce the time required for the abrasion to heal, and many children find patches uncomfortable.

Corneal Foreign Body

Corneal foreign bodies in children can sometimes be dislodged with a forceful stream of irrigating solution. Alternatively, after topical anesthetic is applied, a cotton swab or blunt spatula can be used to remove the foreign body, with or without a slit lamp. Use of sharp instruments should be avoided in young children. If these methods are unsuccessful, sedation or general anesthesia may be required.

Thermal Injury

Cigarette burns of the cornea are the most common thermal injuries to the ocular surface in childhood and are often accidental. The burns usually result from the child running into a cigarette held at eye level by an adult. Despite the alarming initial white appearance of coagulated corneal epithelium, cigarette burns typically heal in a few days and without scarring. Treatment is the same as treatment of corneal abrasions (discussed in a previous section).

Hot drinks pulled down from a table are a common cause of facial and eyelid burns in toddlers. It is rare for ocular surface burns to occur due to the protective effect of the blink reflex. Furthermore, cicatricial ectropion from severe skin burns are also rare in these patients.

Chemical Injury

Chemical burns in childhood are generally caused by organic solvents, detergent pods, or household cleaning agents. Acid and alkali burns in children, as in adults, can be very serious. The initial and most important steps in management of all chemical injuries are immediate copious irrigation and meticulous removal of any particulate matter from the conjunctival fornices. Even burns involving almost total loss of corneal epithelium are likely to heal in a week or less. See BCSC Section 8, *External Disease and Cornea.*

Blunt (Contusional) Injury

As in adults, blunt trauma to a child's eye causes a sudden deformation of the globe. The compression and expansion of the relatively rigid eye wall against the attached internal structures result in typical patterns of contusional injury (eg, hyphema, iridodialysis, zonular dialysis, vitreous hemorrhage). The management of blunt trauma and its complications in children is similar to management in adults, bearing in mind the special considerations for pediatric patients, mentioned earlier in this chapter.

Because of the potential complications of cataract, retinal detachment, and glaucoma, all children who have experienced a blunt injury should be monitored closely. To assess long-term glaucoma risk, gonioscopy should be performed in children with suspected angle damage after the eye has healed and the child is able to cooperate with the examination.

Hyphema

Other than trauma, the differential diagnosis of hyphema includes rare spontaneous causes that should be considered and investigated as appropriate (eg, retinoblastoma, juvenile xanthogranuloma of the iris, and bleeding diathesis from leukemia or other blood dyscrasia). If the fundus cannot be adequately examined, ultrasonography should be performed to rule out intraocular pathology.

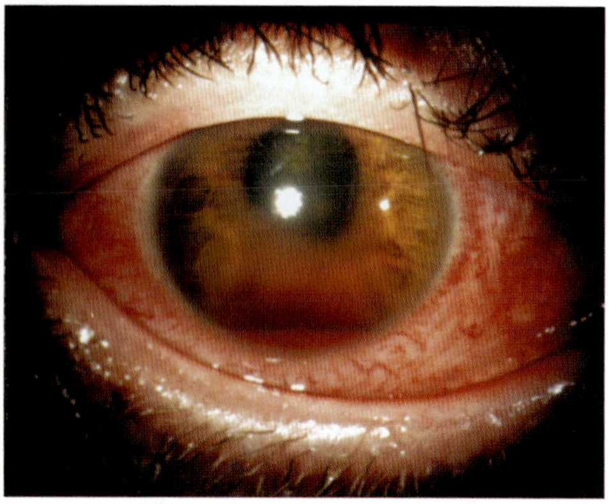

Figure 26-1 Small hyphema. Note the layering of blood inferiorly. *(Courtesy of Edward L. Raab, MD.)*

Medical management of hyphema in children remains controversial. Care must be taken to minimize the risk of rebleeding, which usually occurs between 3 and 7 days postinjury as a result of clot lysis and retraction. Outpatient management with activity restriction and close follow-up is generally accepted. However, if parental cooperation is questionable or if the patient has sickle cell trait, hospitalization for several days after injury may be warranted. Many ophthalmologists routinely use cycloplegic and corticosteroid eyedrops to improve comfort, facilitate fundus examination, and reduce the risk of inflammatory complications and rebleeding. The value of these topical agents as well as other treatments is unproven, and some clinicians prefer to use them selectively or to avoid them altogether, to minimize manipulation of the eye. Small hyphemas (Fig 26-1) generally resolve quickly. See BCSC Section 8, *External Disease and Cornea*. Aspirin-containing compounds and nonsteroidal anti-inflammatory drugs can increase the risk of rebleeding and should be avoided.

Intraocular pressure (IOP), an important factor in therapeutic planning for patients with traumatic hyphema, may be difficult to monitor acutely in the pediatric patient. With a total hyphema, especially if it persists beyond 4–5 days, the risk of corneal blood staining and severe deprivation amblyopia increases in patients with high IOP. A lower threshold for evacuation of the clot may be considered if IOP assessment is not possible in these patients. In children with sickle cell trait or disease, sickling may develop in the anterior chamber, elevating IOP and retarding resorption of blood; due to the risk for optic nerve infarction, it may be necessary to perform clot evacuation sooner and at lower IOP thresholds. Sickle cell screening is recommended for all African American children with traumatic hyphema.

Open Globe Injury

OGI may be caused by sharp trauma or by blunt trauma in which the compression force on the globe (hence deformation) is so great that it "ruptures" the eye wall. By definition, a "globe rupture" is the result of blunt force, but this term is often used incorrectly to describe all OGIs. Because the damage to the internal structures of the eye is so great, a globe rupture usually has a very poor prognosis. A sharp object or small high-velocity projectile can cause a penetration injury (eg, a laceration) or a perforation (ie, with separate entry and exit wounds); either may result in an intraocular foreign body. Because a sharp injury may only cause damage at the entry site, the prognosis for this type of injury is usually better than that of globe rupture, with over 50% of cases achieving a visual acuity of 20/40 or better.

In pediatric patients who have experienced injury due to trauma, the anterior segment and fundus must be thoroughly inspected if an OGI is suspected. An EUA may be necessary. An area of subconjunctival hemorrhage or chemosis or a small break in the skin of the eyelid may be the only surface manifestation of scleral perforation by a sharp object, such as a pencil or scissors blade (Fig 26-2). Distortion of the pupil may be the most evident sign of a small corneal or limbal perforation. Imaging should be considered if there is any reason to suspect the presence of an intraocular or orbital foreign body.

Corneoscleral lacerations in children are repaired using the same principles employed for these repairs in adults (Video 26-1; also see BCSC Section 8, *External Disease and Cornea*). Corneal wounds should be closed with 10/0 nylon sutures and limbal and scleral

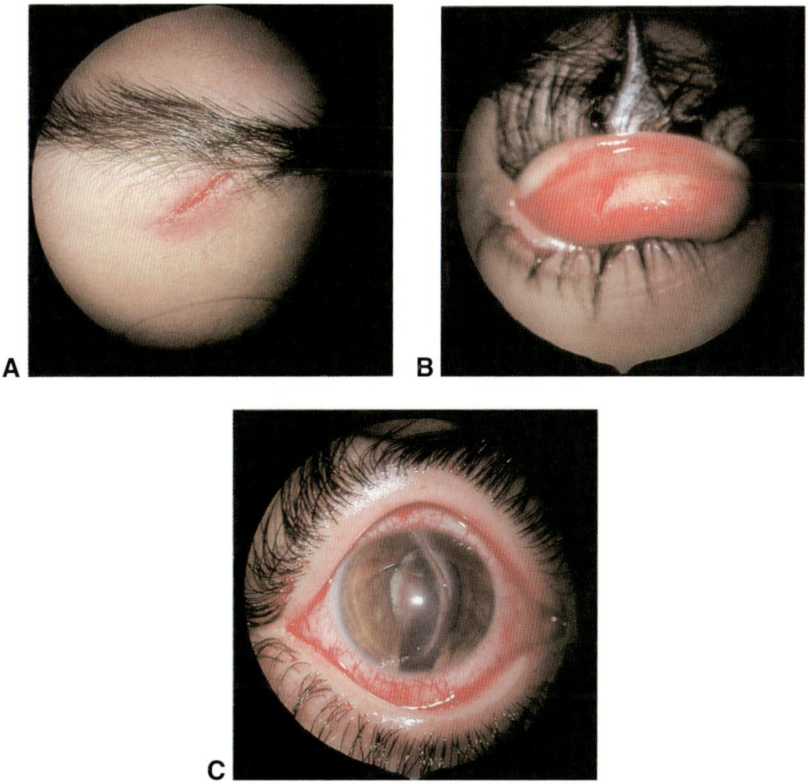

Figure 26-2 Open globe injury. **A,** Small skin entry wound, right brow region, in a 7-year-old boy. The wound was created by a thrown dart. **B,** Conjunctival exit wound indicates complete perforation of the eyelid. **C,** Extensive injury to the anterior segment of the same eye.

wounds with 9/0 nylon sutures. Absorbable sutures should be avoided because they have progressively less strength over a few weeks, especially considering the risk of eye rubbing in children (Fig 26-3). The sutures should be buried and can be removed when adequate healing has occurred, when they become loose, or when they attract vascularization. Generally, corneal wounds heal adequately within 3–4 months.

VIDEO 26-1 Basic principles of open globe injury repair.
Courtesy of Kamiar Mireskandari, MBChB, PhD.

After an OGI, fibrin clots may form quickly in the anterior chamber of a child's eye; these clots can simulate the appearance of fluffy cataractous lens cortex. To avoid rendering the eye aphakic unnecessarily (and thereby compromising vision rehabilitation), the clinician should not remove the lens as part of primary wound repair. Even if the lens capsule is breached, postponing cataract surgery for 1–2 weeks, until severe posttraumatic inflammation has resolved, may result in a smoother postoperative recovery and reduced risk of complications without compromising the vision prognosis. Furthermore, taking the time to plan the cataract surgery may allow better biometry calculation, intraocular lens placement, and vitreous management. However, in very young children, delaying cataract removal beyond a few weeks increases the risk of deprivation amblyopia. See also BCSC Section 11, *Lens and Cataract.*

Bunting H, Stephens D, Mireskandari K. Prediction of visual outcomes after open globe injury in children: a 17-year Canadian experience. *J AAPOS.* 2013;17(1):43–48.

Yardley AM, Ali A, Najm-Tehrani N, Mireskandari K. Refractive and visual outcomes after surgery for pediatric traumatic cataract. *J Cataract Refract Surg.* 2018;44(1):85–90.

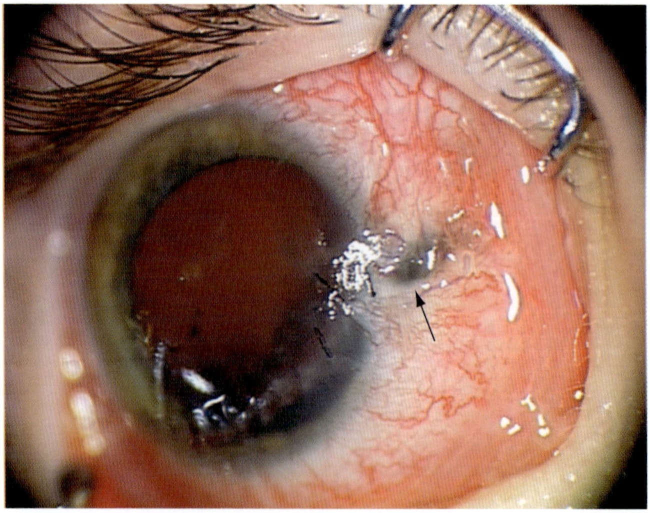

Figure 26-3 Corneoscleral laceration in an 8-year-old boy. Scleral wound dehiscence with uveal prolapse *(arrow)* occurred 3 weeks after primary repair of the sclera with polyglactin sutures (absorbable sutures lost their tensile strength). *(Courtesy of Kamiar Mireskandari, MBChB, PhD.)*

Adnexal and Orbital Trauma

For all trauma that involves the ocular adnexa, the possibility of an underlying CGI or OGI should be considered (see Fig 26-2). Full-thickness eyelid lacerations, especially those involving the eyelid margin and/or a canaliculus, should be repaired meticulously. Sedation or general anesthesia is usually required, even in older children. Working near the eyes with sharp instruments and draping the face to create a sterile field are likely to frighten an awake child and add to the difficulty of the repair. Principles of repair in children are similar to those in adults (see BCSC Section 7, *Oculofacial Plastic and Orbital Surgery*).

Orbital Fractures

The term *blowout fracture* is used when the orbital rim remains intact. Such orbital wall fractures may result from an acute increase in intraorbital pressure, which occurs when a direct impact occludes the orbital entrance; or from compression of the rim, which results in buckling of the orbital wall. Fractures may be part of more extensive fractures of the orbit and midface.

Wei LA, Durairaj VD. Pediatric orbital floor fractures. *J AAPOS*. 2011;15(2):173–180.

Orbital floor fractures

Blunt facial trauma is the usual cause of orbital floor fractures. Periorbital ecchymosis and diplopia are common in the immediate posttrauma period. Injury to the inferior rectus muscle or to its nerve, with resultant weakness, may be caused by hemorrhage or ischemia. In addition, entrapment of the inferior rectus or associated connective tissue in the fracture may occur with restricted upgaze. Bradycardia, heart block, nausea, or syncope can occur as a vagal response to entrapment. When the entrapment involves the more anterior portion of the orbital floor or when there is associated injury to the inferior rectus muscle or its nerve, there can also be limited depression. Reduced saccadic velocity and force generation on attempted downgaze suggest weak muscle action. In a patient with limited elevation, a positive forced duction test indicates the presence of restriction. Hypoesthesia in the cutaneous distribution of the infraorbital nerve can also occur. Orbital computed tomography and high-resolution, multipositional magnetic resonance imaging are useful for revealing the presence and extent of the injury.

A *white-eyed blowout fracture* is characterized by marked restriction in elevation and depression of the eye despite minimal signs of soft-tissue injury. This restriction is due to entrapment of the inferior rectus muscle or orbital tissue either beneath a trapdoor fracture or in a linear opening caused by flexion deformity of the floor. The latter condition is unique to children, and in these cases early surgery, rather than observation, is required in order to minimize permanent muscle and nerve damage.

Management There are diverse approaches to the management of orbital floor fractures. Diplopia immediately after the injury is common and is not necessarily an indication for urgent intervention, except in patients with a white-eyed blowout fracture (described earlier). Many surgeons recommend waiting up to 2 weeks after the injury to allow periorbital swelling to subside before considering floor fracture repair in patients with residual

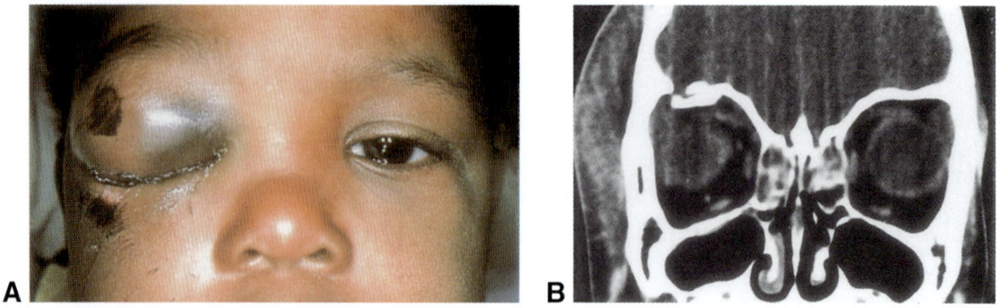

Figure 26-4 Orbital roof fracture in a child, resulting from direct impact to the brow region in a fall. **A,** Marked right upper eyelid swelling from a hematoma originating in the superior orbit, adjacent to a linear fracture. **B,** Coronal computed tomography shows a bone fragment displaced into the right orbit.

restriction and unresolved diplopia in primary position. Some clinicians advocate surgical treatment for large bony defects, even without evidence of entrapment, because progressive herniation of orbital contents into the adjacent maxillary sinus may result in disfiguring enophthalmos. For further discussion of diagnosis and management of orbital trauma, see BCSC Section 7, *Oculofacial Plastic and Orbital Surgery.* Management of persistent diplopia is covered in Chapter 10.

Orbital roof fractures

Orbital roof fractures are more common in children younger than 10 years than in adults. Isolated roof fractures typically result from impact to the brow region during a fall, often from a height of only a few feet. The principal external manifestation is upper eyelid hematoma (Fig 26-4). These fractures often heal without treatment.

Traumatic Optic Neuropathy

The optic nerve may be damaged by trauma to the head, orbit, or globe. Vision loss is usually immediate and severe, and a relative afferent pupillary defect is typically present. Initially, the optic nerve appears normal, but it becomes atrophic within 1–2 months of injury. Treatment with high-dose intravenous corticosteroids is controversial and may even be harmful in patients with an associated head injury.

For further discussion of diagnosis and management of traumatic optic neuropathy, see BCSC Section 5, *Neuro-Ophthalmology.*

Nonaccidental Trauma

Although most eye injuries in childhood are accidental or innocently caused by other children, a significant minority result from physical abuse by adults. The terms used for intentional physical abuse of a child include *nonaccidental trauma* and *child abuse.* Child abuse includes emotional abuse, sexual abuse, and neglect as well as physical abuse. It is a pervasive problem, with an estimated 750,000 cases per year in the United States.

A reliable history is often difficult to obtain when nonaccidental trauma has occurred. Nonaccidental trauma should be suspected when repeated accounts of the circumstances of injury or histories obtained from different individuals are inconsistent or when the events described do not correlate with the injuries (eg, bruises on multiple aspects of the head after "a fall") or with the child's developmental level (eg, a 1-month-old "rolling off a bed" or a 4-month-old "climbing out of a high chair").

Any physician who suspects child abuse is required by law in every US state and Canadian province to report the incident to a designated governmental agency. Once this obligation has been discharged, full investigation of the situation by appropriate specialists and authorities is usually performed. Physicians should be familiar with the regulations in their own country. If possible, ocular abnormalities should be documented photographically or with a detailed drawing to use as evidence in court.

Abusive Head Trauma

A unique complex of ocular, intracranial, and sometimes other injuries occurs in infants who have been abused by violent shaking. It is important to recognize this as a manifestation of child abuse. Although the term *shaken baby syndrome* is still occasionally used, it has largely been replaced with the terms *abusive head trauma (AHT)* and *inflicted childhood neurotrauma* because these infants may sustain impact injury as well as shaking injury involving the head.

Patients with AHT are usually younger than 5 years and most often younger than 12 months. When a reliable history is available, it typically involves a parent or other caregiver who shook an inconsolable crying baby in anger or frustration. Often, however, the only information provided is that the child's mental status deteriorated or that a seizure or respiratory difficulty developed. The involved caregiver may relate that an episode of relatively minor trauma occurred, such as a fall from a bed.

Intracranial injury in AHT frequently includes subdural hematoma (typically bilateral over the cerebral convexities or in the interhemispheric fissure) and subarachnoid hemorrhage. These findings are thought to result from repetitive, abrupt acceleration-deceleration of the child's head as it whiplashes back and forth during the shaking episode. Displacement of the brain in relation to the skull and dura mater ruptures bridging vessels, and compression against the cranial bones produces further damage. Neuroimaging may also reveal intracranial edema, ischemia, or contusion in the acute stage and atrophy in later stages. Some authorities, citing the frequency with which patients with AHT also show evidence of having received blows to the head, think that impact may be an essential component, although in many cases no sign of impact is found.

A notable feature of AHT is the typical lack of external evidence of trauma. Occasionally, the patient's trunk or extremities may show bruises representing the imprint of the perpetrator's hands. In some cases, broken ribs or metaphyseal fractures of the long bones result from forces generated during shaking. It must be kept in mind, however, that these patients may have been subjected to other forms of abuse (eg, neglect).

Ocular involvement

The most common ocular manifestation of AHT, present in approximately 80% of cases, is retinal hemorrhage. The ocular adnexa and anterior segment usually appear entirely normal. Retinal hemorrhages can occur in all layers of the retina and may be unilateral or bilateral.

They are found most commonly in the posterior pole but often extend to the periphery (Fig 26-5). Vitreous hemorrhage may also occur and may be caused primarily by the trauma or secondary to migration of blood from a preretinal hemorrhage into the vitreous. Occasionally, the vitreous hemorrhage can be dense. Retinal hemorrhages in shaken infants cannot be dated with precision and usually resolve over a period of weeks to months. Vitrectomy should be considered if there is a risk of amblyopia due to persistent vitreous hemorrhage.

Some eyes show evidence of retinal tissue disruption in addition to hemorrhage. Full-thickness perimacular folds in the neurosensory retina, typically with circumferential orientation around the macula, are highly characteristic. Splitting of the retina (traumatic retinoschisis), either deep to the nerve fiber layer or superficial (involving only the internal limiting membrane), may create cavities of considerable extent that are partially filled with blood, also usually in the macular region (Fig 26-6). Full-thickness retinal breaks and detachment are rare. Retinal folds usually flatten out within a few weeks of injury, but schisis cavities can persist indefinitely.

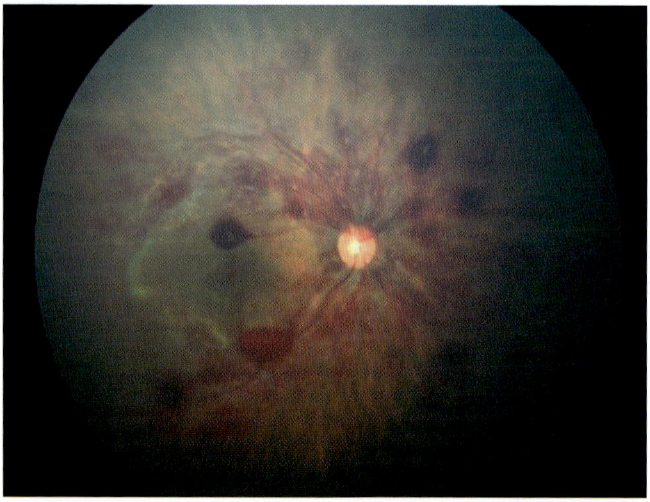

Figure 26-5 Extensive retinal hemorrhages in a 4-month-old infant suspected to have been violently shaken. *(Courtesy of Sophia Ying Fang, MD.)*

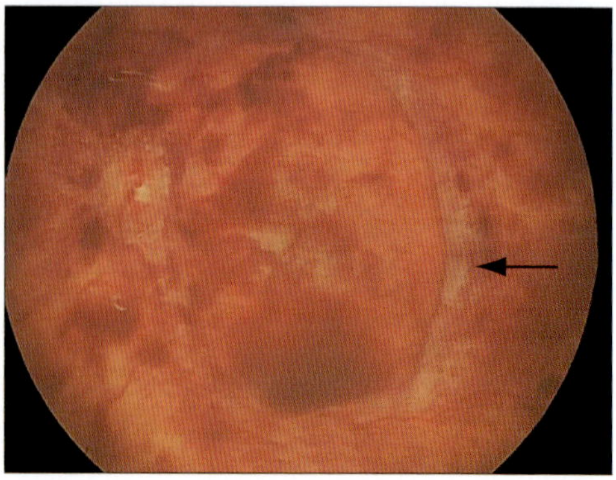

Figure 26-6 Traumatic retinoschisis with perimacular folds *(arrow)*. *(Courtesy of Ken K. Nischal, MD.)*

Diagnostic considerations

Severe accidental head trauma (eg, trauma sustained in a fall from a second-story level or in a motor vehicle collision) is not frequently accompanied by retinal hemorrhage, and when it is present, the hemorrhage is not extensive. Retinal hemorrhage is rare and has never been documented to be extensive following cardiopulmonary resuscitation by trained personnel. Severe, fatal, acute head-crush injury rarely causes hemorrhagic retinopathy with perimacular folds, which can nonetheless be differentiated from AHT by the associated injuries.

Extensive retinal hemorrhage without other ocular findings strongly suggests that associated intracranial injury has been caused by AHT, but alternative possibilities such as a coagulation disorder must be considered as well. Retinal hemorrhages resulting from birth trauma are common in newborns, but they seldom persist beyond the age of 1 month. Other possible causes of retinal hemorrhage in children include anemia, hypertension, acutely increased intracranial pressure, leukemia, meningitis, glutaricaciduria, and retinopathy of prematurity; however, the quantity and distribution of hemorrhages seen in patients with these conditions are often different from the patterns typically seen in those with AHT.

The diagnosis of AHT is not made on the basis of ophthalmic findings in isolation. When extensive retinal hemorrhage accompanied by perimacular folds and schisis cavities is found in association with intracranial hemorrhage or other evidence of trauma to the brain in an infant, the diagnosis of AHT can be made with confidence by a multidisciplinary team upon review of all clinical findings. It must be remembered, however, that the timing and circumstances of injury and the identity of the perpetrator often cannot be inferred from medical evidence alone.

Levin AV, Alexander R, Binenbaum G, Forbes B, Jenny C. Revised and endorsed by the American Academy of Ophthalmology, Quality of Care Secretariat, Hoskins Center for Quality Eye Care. Clinical Statement. *Abusive Head Trauma/Shaken Baby Syndrome—2015.* American Academy of Ophthalmology; 2015. www.aao.org/clinical-statement/abusive-head-traumashaken-baby-syndrome

Maguire SA, Watts PO, Shaw AD, et al. Retinal haemorrhages and related findings in abusive and nonabusive head trauma: a systematic review. *Eye (Lond).* 2013;27(1):28–36.

Narang SK, Fingarson A, Lukefahr J; Council on Child Abuse and Neglect. Abusive head trauma in infants and children. *Pediatrics.* 2020;145(4):e20200203.

Prognosis

In 1 large study, 29% of children with AHT died of their injuries. Poor visual and pupillary responses were correlated with a higher risk of mortality. Survivors often had permanent impairment ranging from mild learning disability and motor disturbances to severe cognitive impairment and quadriparesis. The most common cause of vision loss is cortical injury followed by optic atrophy. Dense vitreous hemorrhage, which is usually associated with deep traumatic retinoschisis, carries a poor prognosis for both vision and life.

Kivlin JD, Simons KB, Lazoritz S, Ruttum MS. Shaken baby syndrome. *Ophthalmology.* 2000;107(7):1246–1254.

Other Ocular Injury Secondary to Nonaccidental Trauma

The presenting sign of child abuse involves the eye in approximately 5% of cases. Blunt trauma inflicted with fingers, fists, or implements such as belts or straps is the most common mechanism of nonaccidental injury to the ocular adnexa or anterior segment. Periorbital ecchymosis, subconjunctival hemorrhage, and hyphema should raise suspicion of recent abuse if the explanation provided is implausible. Cataract and lens dislocation may be a sign of repeated injury or of previously inflicted trauma. Child abuse should also be suspected when rhegmatogenous retinal detachment occurs in a child without a history of injury or an apparent predisposing factor, such as high myopia.

CHAPTER 27

Ocular Manifestations of Systemic Disease

Highlights

- Systemic disease may be first recognized by an ophthalmologist on the basis of its ophthalmic signs.
- Earlier diagnosis of systemic diseases can help to decrease morbidity and mortality.
- Multidisciplinary teams often are needed for optimal care of a child with ocular manifestations of systemic disease.

Introduction

This chapter addresses systemic disorders with multiple types of ocular involvement. Systemic disorders characterized by a single ocular abnormality are discussed in other chapters in this volume.

Chromosomal Abnormalities

Abnormalities in chromosome number (aneuploidy; eg, trisomy or monosomy), structure (duplications, deletions, translocations, inversions, or rings), or type (autosomal or sex chromosome) occur in approximately 1 in 150 live births. Table 27-1 lists select chromosomal abnormalities commonly associated with ocular findings. Also see BCSC Section 2, *Fundamentals and Principles of Ophthalmology,* Chapter 6.

Inborn Errors of Metabolism

Inborn errors of metabolism occur in approximately 1 in 1400 births, often as a result of biallelic pathogenic variants, and can produce ocular findings through toxicity of metabolic products or deficiencies in synthetic pathways or energy production.

Certain ocular manifestations are suggestive of systemic disorders, as listed below, and can emerge at various ages (Table 27-2; also see Chapter 20 in this volume):

- corneal clouding, corneal deposits: certain mucopolysaccharidoses (Fig 27-1), cystinosis (Fig 27-2), Schnyder corneal dystrophy (Fig 27-3)
- corneal pseudodendritic ulcerations: tyrosinemia

Table 27-1 Common Chromosomal Abnormalities With Ocular Findings

Chromosomal Abnormality	Incidence in Newborns	Common Associated Ocular Findings	Uncommon Associated Ocular Findings
Trisomy 13, Patau syndrome	1/16,000	Microphthalmia, coloboma, retinal dysplasia with frequent islands of intraocular cartilage	Cataract, corneal opacification, cyclopia, persistent fetal vasculature, shallow supraorbital ridges, upward-slanting palpebral fissures, absent eyebrows, hypotelorism, hypertelorism, anophthalmia, glaucoma
Trisomy 18, Edwards syndrome	1/6000–8000[a]	Short palpebral fissure, hypertelorism, epicanthus, hypoplastic supraorbital ridge	Cataract, microcornea, corneal opacification, congenital glaucoma, retinal depigmentation, colobomatous microphthalmia, cyclopia
Trisomy 21, Down syndrome (most common trisomy)	1/1400	Epicanthus with upward-slanting palpebral fissures, blepharitis, Brushfield spots, congenital or acquired cataract, refractive error, congenital nasolacrimal duct obstruction and difficulty with probing, ectropion, strabismus, hypoaccommodation	Infantile glaucoma, keratoconus, nystagmus, additional vessels at the margin of the optic nerve head
Deletion 4p, Wolf-Hirschhorn syndrome	1/50,000	Colobomatous microphthalmia, epicanthus, downward-slanting palpebral fissures, hypertelorism, strabismus, ptosis, corneal opacification (Peters anomaly)	Anterior segment anomalies, cataract
Deletion 5p, cri-du-chat syndrome	1/20,000–50,000	Upward- or downward-slanting palpebral fissures, hypotelorism or hypertelorism, epicanthus, strabismus	Ptosis, decreased tear production, myopia, cataract, glaucoma, tortuous retinal vessels, foveal hypoplasia, optic atrophy, colobomatous microphthalmia
Deletion 18p	1/50,000	Hypertelorism, ptosis, epicanthus, strabismus	Cataracts, retinal dysplasia, colobomatous microphthalmia, synophthalmia/cyclopia
Deletion 18q	1/55,000	Epicanthus, hypertelorism, downward-slanting palpebral fissures, strabismus, dysplastic or atrophic optic nerve, nystagmus	Corneal abnormalities, cataracts, blue sclera, myopia, colobomatous microphthalmia
Monosomy X, Turner syndrome	1/2000–2500 females	Strabismus, ptosis	Cataracts, refractive errors, corneal scars, blue sclera, incidence of color blindness similar to that in males

[a] Those with mosaic disease are more likely to survive.

Table 27-2 Select Metabolic Disorders With Ophthalmic Manifestations[a]

Metabolic Category	Select Examples	Anterior Segment	Posterior Segment	Motility Findings
Carbohydrate synthesis	Classic galactosemia Enzyme: Gal-1PO_4 uridyltransferase (GALT)	Cataract (infantile onset)		
	Galactokinase or epimerase deficiency	Cataract (developmental)		
Amino acid metabolism	*CBS*-related homocystinuria Enzyme: cystathionine β-synthetase (*CBS* gene)	Subluxation/luxation Cataract	Optic atrophy (23%)	
Peroxisomal disorders	Zellweger spectrum disorders (cerebrohepatorenal syndrome)	Corneal clouding Bilateral cataracts	Optic atrophy Rod–cone degeneration	Poor pursuit movements
	Mucopolysaccharidosis (MPS)[b]			
Lysosomal storage disorders	MPS I (severe and attenuated)	+ corneal haze and +++ corneal haze	Mild (+) to moderate (++) retinopathy	
	MPS II (Hunter) → X-linked		++ retinopathy	
	MPS III (Sanfilippo A, B, C, D)	+ corneal haze	+++ retinopathy	
	MPS IV (Morquio A, B)	+ corneal haze	++ retinopathy	
	MPS VI (Maroteaux-Lamy)	+++ corneal haze		
	MPS VII (Sly)	++ corneal haze		
	MPS IX (Natowicz)			

(Continued)

Table 27-2 *(continued)*

Metabolic Category	Select Examples	Anterior Segment	Posterior Segment	Motility Findings
	Sphingolipidosis[c]			
	Generalized gangliosidosis (GM_1 gangliosidosis)	Corneal haze	Optic atrophy	
			Tortuous vessels, cherry-red spot	
	Tay-Sachs disease (GM_2 gangliosidosis) Enzyme: hexosaminidase A (HEXA)		Cherry-red spot	
	Sandhoff disease (GM_2) Enzyme: hexosaminidase A&B (HEXB)		Cherry-red spot	
	Niemann-Pick disease Enzyme: sphingomyelinase (*SPMD1, NPC1/NPC2* genes)	Opacified cornea (type A, *SPMD1* gene)	Optic atrophy (type C, *NPC1/NPC2* genes) Cherry-red spot	Supranuclear gaze palsy (type C, *NPC1/NPC2* genes)
	Metachromatic leukodystrophy Enzyme: arylsulfatase A (ARSA)		Cherry-red spot (rare)	
	Gaucher disease Enzyme: β-glucocerebrosidase		Preretinal white spots, vitreous opacities, retinal vascular anomalies	Supranuclear gaze palsy, ocular motor apraxia, paralytic strabismus
	Fabry disease Enzyme: α-galactosidase A (X-linked)	Cornea verticillata (vortex keratopathy, whorl keratopathy)		
	Cystinosis (*CTNS* encoding lysosomal carrier protein)	Corneal crystals	Pigment epithelial mottling, intraretinal crystals, diminished scotopic and photopic responses	
	Neuronal ceroid lipofuscinosis (NCL)			
	CLN1 (infantile, 6–12 months)		Minimal pigmentary changes, early extinction of ERG	
	CLN2 (late infantile–onset, 2–4 years)		Optic atrophy Early bull's-eye maculopathy	

Metabolic Category	Select Examples	Anterior Segment	Posterior Segment	Motility Findings
	CLN3 (juvenile-onset, 4–8 years)		Early-onset rapid retinal dystrophy, bull's-eye maculopathy; early ERG results are electronegative and later become nonrecordable	
	CLN4–8; CNL10–14	Overlapping features; several of the childhood forms demonstrate ophthalmic findings (retinal dystrophy, optic atrophy, etc.). Adult-onset forms (*CLN4* and *CLN13*) lack retinal findings.		
Lipoprotein	Abetalipoproteinemia (Bassen-Kornzweig syndrome) Gene: *MTP*, microsomal triglyceride transfer protein		Retinal degeneration (nyctalopia → atypical retinopathy with vision loss → pigmentary retinopathy, perivascular deposits)	

ERG = electroretinography.

[a] It is important to diagnosis metabolic disorders early and provide patients access to the latest relevant treatment or treatment trials.

[b] Optic atrophy and papilledema have been reported for MPS; craniosynostosis can lead to increased intracranial pressure, except in MPS IV.

[c] Many sphingolipidoses are characterized by neurologic degeneration (eg, loss of milestones, progressive neurologic signs).

Plus (+) signs indicate the relative likelihood of occurrence of ocular findings in these systemic disorders. Inheritance is autosomal recessive unless otherwise stated.

Note: Please refer to BCSC Section 2, *Fundamentals and Principles of Ophthalmology*, Chapter 6, Clinical Genetics, for more information about genetic counseling and treatment options.

Data from Adam MP, Ardinger HH, Pagon RA, Wallace SE, eds. *GeneReviews* [Internet]. University of Washington, Seattle; 1993–2021. Accessed February 15, 2022. www.ncbi.nlm.nih.gov/books/NBK1116/

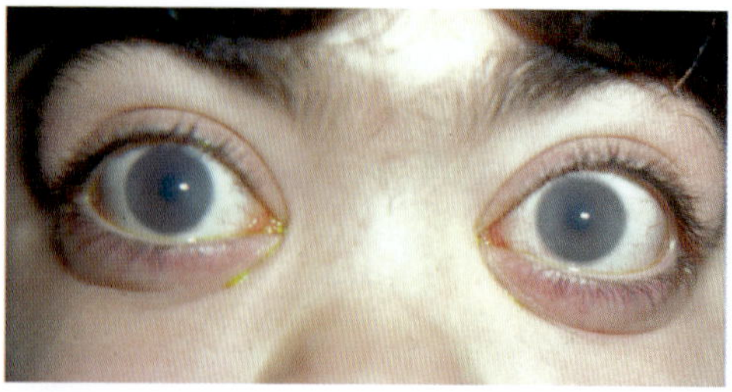

Figure 27-1 Bilateral corneal clouding in mucopolysaccharidosis VI. *(Courtesy of Edward L. Raab, MD.)*

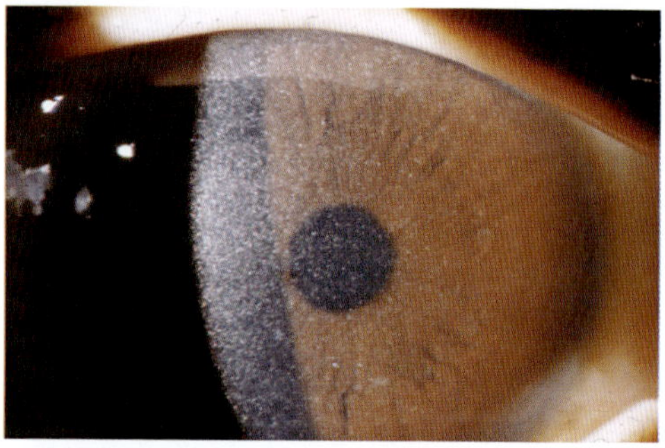

Figure 27-2 Cystinosis with corneal involvement. *(Courtesy of Gregg T. Lueder, MD.)*

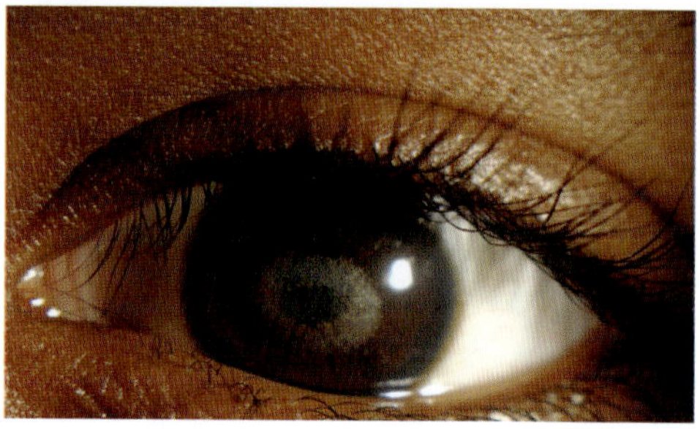

Figure 27-3 Corneal crystals in a girl with Schnyder corneal dystrophy. *(Courtesy of Arif O. Khan, MD.)*

- cataracts: diabetes, galactosemia, Smith-Lemli-Opitz syndrome, cerebrotendinous xanthomatosis (Fig 27-4)
- lens luxation or subluxation: homocystinuria (Fig 27-5)
- retinal degeneration: peroxisomal disorders (Zellweger spectrum disorders), lysosomal disorders (eg, neuronal ceroid lipofuscinosis), mitochondrial disorders (eg, Kearns-Sayre syndrome [Fig 27-6])
- central macular cherry-red spot: GM_2 gangliosidosis type I (Tay-Sachs disease) and type II (Sandhoff disease), Niemann-Pick disease

CLINICAL PEARL

The central macular cherry-red spot disappears over time as intumescent ganglion cells die and optic atrophy develops. Thus, the absence of a cherry-red spot should not exclude a diagnosis that includes cherry-red spot, especially in older children.

CLINICAL PEARL

In patients with *CBS*-related homocystinuria, lens subluxation is classically inferonasal from broken zonules (as opposed to Marfan syndrome, for which lens subluxation is classically temporal from stretched zonules). Patients can have Marfanoid body habitus and osteoporosis. Early dietary modification can prevent intellectual disability. There is an increased risk of mortality from thromboembolic events, and this needs to be considered if general anesthesia is needed for ocular surgery.

CLINICAL PEARL

The age of presentation in patients with juvenile-onset NCL *(CLN3)* overlaps with that of childhood-onset Stargardt disease. Vision problems may precede neurologic signs by 1–2 years. Clues to distinguish juvenile-onset NCL from childhood-onset Stargardt disease include

- withdrawn/inattentive behavior and sleep problems
- optic atrophy and bull's-eye maculopathy
- rapidly progressive retinal dystrophy (faster than expected for Stargardt disease)
- an electronegative ERG waveform early in the disease process

CLINICAL PEARL

Inherited causes of early-onset hearing loss and pigmentary retinopathy include

- Usher syndrome type I
- peroxisomal disease
- mitochondrial disease
- ciliopathies
- Alport syndrome
- MPS I

CLINICAL PEARL

The differential diagnosis of bull's-eye maculopathy in infancy and childhood includes

- NCL
- spinocerebellar ataxia VII
- Leber congenital amaurosis
- cone dystrophy
- cone–rod dystrophy
- Stargardt disease and other macular dystrophies
- Cohen syndrome
- ciliopathies

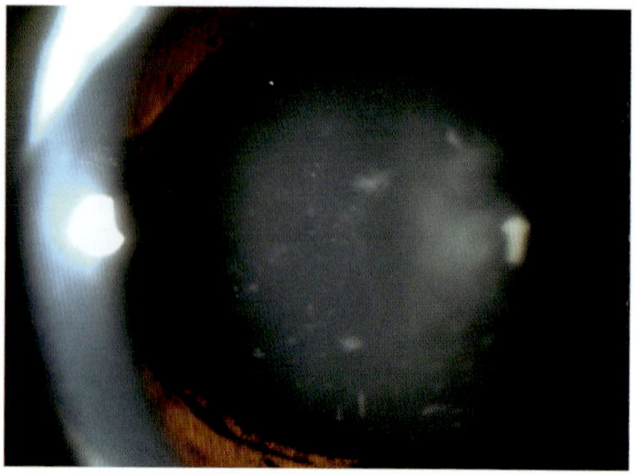

Figure 27-4 Fleck opacities and posterior capsular cataract secondary to cerebrotendinous xanthomatosis in the right eye of a boy. The patient had a history of intractable infantile diarrhea. *(Modified with permission from Khan AO, Al-dahmesh MA, Mohamed JY, Alkuraya FS. Juvenile cataract morphology in 3 siblings not yet diagnosed with cerebrotendinous xanthomatosis.* Ophthalmology. *2013;120(5):956–960. Copyright 2013, with permission from Elsevier.)*

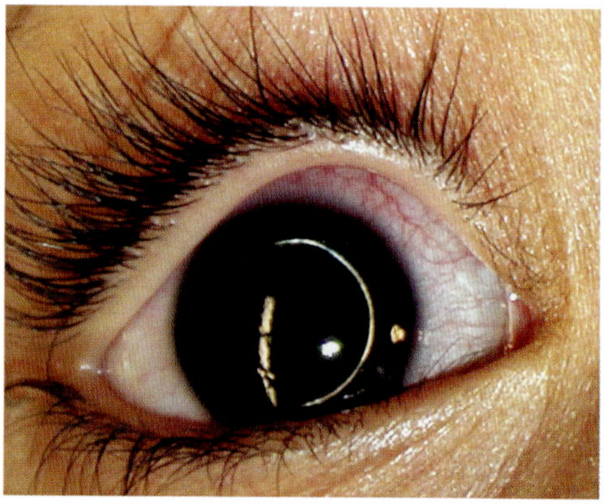

Figure 27-5 Total lens dislocation into the anterior chamber and acute glaucoma as the presenting sign of homocystinuria in a boy. *(Courtesy of Arif O. Khan, MD.)*

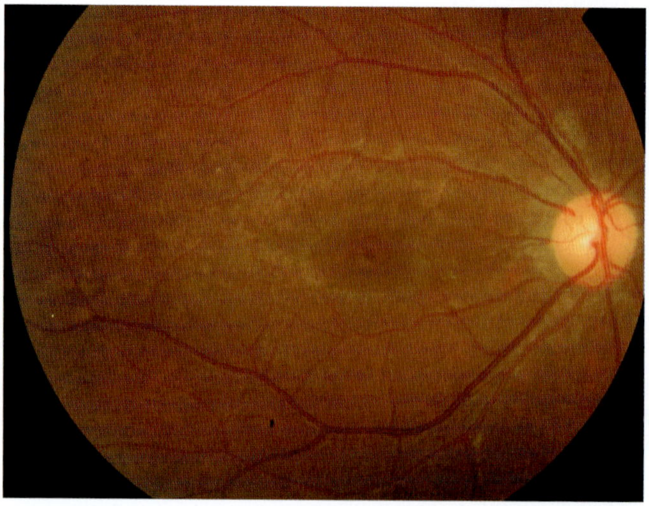

Figure 27-6 Juvenile retinal dystrophy in a boy with recent slow development of ptosis and ophthalmoplegia, which led to the diagnosis of Kearns-Sayre syndrome. *(Courtesy of Arif O. Khan, MD.)*

Early identification and control of metabolic disease can greatly lower the risk of ocular and systemic sequelae. The ophthalmologist often is the first to suspect a metabolic disorder, based on the presence of ophthalmic signs, such as galactosemia, classic homocystinuria (see Chapter 22), cystinosis (see Chapter 20), certain mucopolysaccharidoses, and cerebrotendinous xanthomatosis (see Chapter 22). Prompt referral to a geneticist is essential.

Familial Oculorenal Syndromes

Alport Syndrome

Alport syndrome is X-linked in two-thirds of patients and involves abnormalities in collagen type IV, a key component of basement membranes. Ocular findings include anterior lenticonus, posterior polymorphous corneal dystrophy, fleck maculopathy, and recurrent erosion syndrome and may be accompanied by progressive renal disease, progressive sensorineural hearing loss, and risk of thoracic or abdominal aortic aneurysm.

Ciliopathies

Ciliopathies are functional disorders of organ-specific or systemic cilia. Nonmotile cilia have roles in cell signaling, detection of chemical gradients, and intracellular transport. Ciliopathies commonly have retinal involvement because the junction between the inner and outer segments of the photoreceptor cell is a modified nonmotile cilium. A child with retinopathy secondary to a systemic ciliopathy is at risk of concurrent or later renal dysfunction. For any child with early-onset retinal dystrophy, consideration of systemic ciliopathy and referral to a genetic counselor and medical geneticist are advised.

Systemic ciliopathies involving the retina and kidney include the following:

- Senior-Løken syndrome: retinopathy, renal dysfunction
- Bardet-Biedl syndrome: retinopathy, polydactyly (Fig 27-7), obesity, renal dysfunction
- Alström syndrome: retinopathy, cardiomyopathy, obesity, renal dysfunction
- Joubert syndrome: retinopathy, ocular motor apraxia, developmental delay, characteristic magnetic resonance imaging (MRI) findings (Fig 27-8), renal dysfunction

Lowe (oculocerebrorenal) syndrome is an X-linked ciliopathy (hemizygous *OCRL* mutation) characterized by congenital cataracts at birth, glaucoma in 50% of cases, and corneal or conjunctival keloids in 25%. Mothers who are carriers for this trait commonly have radially oriented punctate snowflake opacities (Fig 27-9). In individuals with this syndrome, the pupils are typically miotic, and the lenses are small, thick, and may exhibit posterior lenticonus. Systemic findings include congenital hypotonia, central nervous system (CNS) anomalies, cognitive impairment, and infantile proximal renal tubulopathy (Fanconi type) with resultant aminoaciduria, metabolic acidosis, proteinuria, and rickets.

Chen HY, Kelley RA, Li T, Swaroop A. Primary cilia biogenesis and associated retinal ciliopathies. *Semin Cell Dev Biol.* 2021;110:70–88.

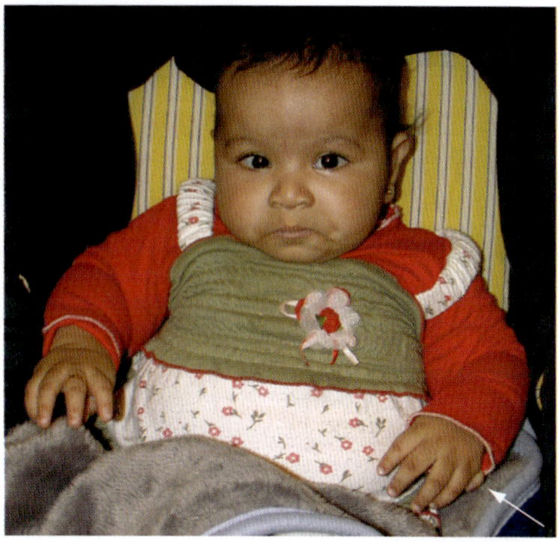

Figure 27-7 This infant with nystagmus related to retinal dystrophy also had polydactyly *(arrow)*, which led to the diagnosis of Bardet-Biedl syndrome. Systemic features, such as renal impairment, may not emerge until later childhood. *(Courtesy of Arif O. Khan, MD.)*

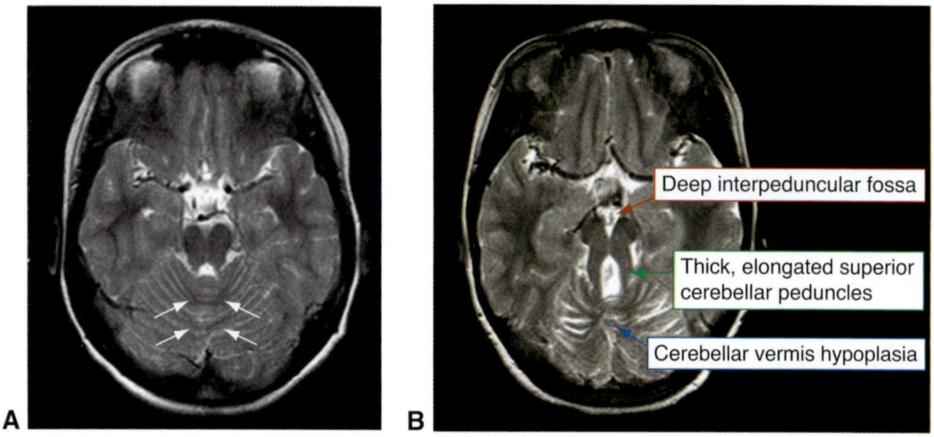

Figure 27-8 Molar tooth sign in Joubert syndrome. **A,** Axial magnetic resonance imaging (MRI) through the cerebellum and brainstem of an unaffected individual showing intact cerebellar vermis (outlined by *arrows*). **B,** Axial MRI through the cerebellum and brainstem of a child with Joubert syndrome. *Arrows* indicate the 3 key components of the molar tooth sign: deep interpeduncular fossa; thick, elongated superior cerebellar peduncles; and cerebellar vermis hypoplasia. *(Reprinted with permission from Parisi M, Glass I. Joubert syndrome. In: Adam MP, Ardinger HH, Pagon RA, Wallace SE, eds.* GeneReviews *[Internet]. University of Washington, Seattle; 1993–2020: Figure 1. www.ncbi.nlm.nih.gov/books/NBK1325.)*

Neuro-Oculocutaneous Syndromes

Neuro-oculocutaneous syndromes (phakomatoses) are a heterogeneous group of congenital syndromes characterized by systemic hamartomas of the eye, CNS, and skin. Diagnosis is clinical, but most cases have a molecular etiology involving loss of a tumor suppressor gene, autosomal recessive inheritance, or somatic mosaicism. Recognition of the common ocular manifestations of these disorders allows for expeditious systemic evaluation and surveillance for vision- and life-threatening manifestations. An overview of these conditions is provided in Table 27-3.

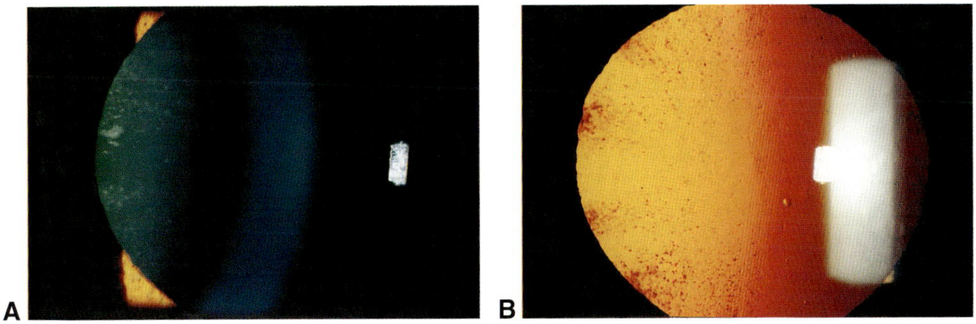

Figure 27-9 Slit-lamp images of the lens of an adult Lowe syndrome carrier. **A,** Equatorial and anterior cortical clusters of smooth, off-white opacities of various sizes and shapes distributed in radial clusters. **B,** The same opacities are seen in retroillumination to emphasize the wedges of clustered opacities. *(Reprinted from Lin T, Lewis RA, Nussbaum, RL. Molecular confirmation of carriers for Lowe syndrome.* Ophthalmology. *1999;106(1):119–122. Copyright 1999, with permission from Elsevier.)*

Neurofibromatosis Type 1

Neurofibromatosis type 1 (NF1) is characterized by melanocytic and neuroglial lesions, including *café-au-lait spots*—uniformly hyperpigmented macules of varying size (Fig 27-10). Three or fewer café-au-lait spots may be observed in unaffected individuals, but the presence of more than 6 spots and larger spots is suggestive of NF1. Clinical diagnosis is by consensus criteria. See Table 27-3 for common features.

Ocular melanocytic lesions

Lisch nodules are small (usually <1 mm), sharply demarcated, dome-shaped excrescences of the iris (Fig 27-11). Lisch nodules most often develop between ages 5 and 10 years and are present in nearly all adults with NF1. *Melanocytic* lesions of the choroid also are common in patients with NF1 but typically are not observable on fundus examination; near-infrared reflectance imaging has a high sensitivity for detection (Fig 27-12). Neither lesion affects vision.

Neuroglial lesions

Nodular cutaneous and *subcutaneous neurofibromas,* or *fibroma molluscum,* are by far the most common lesions of neuroglial origin. They typically develop in late childhood.

Plexiform neurofibromas occur in approximately 30% of cases and are observed as extensive, soft, poorly demarcated subcutaneous swellings, with hyperpigmentation or hypertrichosis of the overlying skin. Often, hypertrophy of the underlying soft tissue and bone (regional gigantism) is also present. Plexiform neurofibromas develop earlier than nodular lesions, are frequently evident in infancy or childhood, and may cause severe disfigurement and functional impairment. Approximately 10% of plexiform neurofibromas involve the face, commonly the upper eyelid and orbit (Fig 27-13). Greater involvement of the upper eyelid's temporal portion results in an S-shaped configuration that patients often describe as feeling like a "bag of worms." Orbital neurofibromas can be amblyogenic and may cause vision loss by deprivation (due to tumor bulk), anisometropia, and strabismus. Glaucoma in the ipsilateral eye is found in up to 50% of cases.

Table 27-3 Overview and Select Features of Neurocutaneous Syndromes

Disease	Gene Symbol/ Chromosome Location	Inheritance Pattern	Ocular Features	Cutaneous Features	CNS and Other Systemic Features	Incidence and Comments
Neurofibromatosis type 1 (von Recklinghausen disease) (OMIM 162200 [a])	*NF1* (17q11.2); tumor suppressor	AD	Orbital or eyelid neurofibroma, glaucoma, prominent corneal nerves, Lisch nodules, iris ectropion, retinal and choroidal hamartomas, optic pathway glioma, refractive error	Café-au-lait spots, neurofibromas, freckling of the axillary or inguinal regions	Sphenoid dysplasia, optic pathway glioma	1/3500 New pathogenic variants common; variable expressivity common; patients with genetic mosaicism should follow same screening guidelines as those with germline mutations
Neurofibromatosis type 2 (OMIM 101000)	*NF2* (22q12); tumor suppressor	AD	Cataract (PSC most common), combined hamartoma of the RPE and retina, epiretinal membrane, optic nerve sheath meningiomas	Café-au-lait spots	Bilateral acoustic neuromas, spinal cord tumors, meningiomas, cranial nerve palsies	1/33,000 New pathogenic variants common
Tuberous sclerosis complex (Bourneville disease) (OMIM 191100 and 613254)	*TSC1* (9q34), *TSC2* (16p13.3); tumor suppressor	AD	Retinal astrocytic hamartomas, peripheral depigmented or hypopigmented lesions	Angiofibromas, hypopigmented macules, subungual fibromas, shagreen patch	Infantile spasms/seizures, cognitive impairment, SEGA, subependymal nodules, cardiac rhabdomyoma, lymphangiomyomatosis, renal angiomyolipoma	1/10,000 New pathogenic variants very common

Disease	Gene Symbol/ Chromosome Location	Inheritance Pattern	Ocular Features	Cutaneous Features	CNS and Other Systemic Features	Incidence and Comments
Retinocerebral angiomatosis (von Hippel–Lindau disease; VHL) (OMIM 193300)	*VHL* (3p26-p25); tumor suppressor	AD	Retinal capillary hemangioblastoma	Café-au-lait spots, vascular nevi, rare cutaneous manifestations (<5%)	Hemangioblastoma, renal cell carcinoma, pheochromocytoma	1/36,000, de novo in 70%–80% High penetrance; benign and malignant tumors
Encephalofacial angiomatosis (Sturge-Weber syndrome) (OMIM 185300)	*GNAQ* (9q21)	Somatic mosaicism	Diffuse choroidal cavernous angioma, glaucoma	Nevus flammeus	Meningeal angiomas, seizures/infantile spasms	1/50,000 Nevus flammeus alone not pathognomonic
Ataxia-telangiectasia (Louis-Bar syndrome) (OMIM 208900)	*ATM* (11q22.3)	AR	Saccadic initiation failure, conjunctival telangiectasias	Telangiectasias	Cerebellar dysfunction, immunodeficiency, malignancy	1/40,000 *ATM* is regulator of tumor-suppressor genes and DNA repair
Incontinentia pigmenti (Bloch-Sulzberger syndrome) (OMIM 308300)	*IKBKG* (Xq28)	X-linked dominant	Retinal vasculopathy	Vesicles with evolution to hyperpigmented lesions	Seizures, cognitive impairment	Evolution of skin lesions can occur in utero
Racemose angioma (Wyburn-Mason syndrome)	Nonhereditary	Sporadic	Retinal racemose angioma	Facial lesions (if present)	Intracranial AVMs with bleeding as sequelae	Isolated finding more common than syndrome
Klippel-Trénaunay-Weber syndrome *PIK3CA*-related overgrowth spectrum (PROS)	*PIK3CA* gene	Mosaic	Glaucoma	Nevus flammeus similar to that in encephalofacial angiomatosis; hyperpigmented nevi and streak	Limb anomalies (asymmetric limb hypertrophy, poly-/syn-/oligodactyly), seizures, Kasabach-Merritt syndrome	Capillary and venous malformations with limb overgrowth with or without lymphatic malformation

AD = autosomal dominant; AR = autosomal recessive; AVM = arteriovenous malformation; CNS = central nervous system; PSC = posterior subcapsular cataract; RPE = retinal pigment epithelium; SEGA = subependymal giant cell astrocytoma.

[a] OMIM = Online Mendelian Inheritance in Man; database is online at www.omim.org.

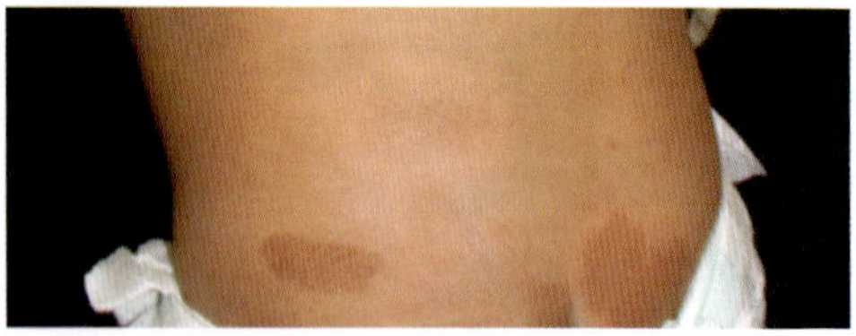

Figure 27-10 Multiple café-au-lait spots on the lower back of an infant with unilateral glaucoma; neurofibromatosis type 1 (NF1) was ultimately diagnosed. *(Courtesy of Arif O. Khan, MD.)*

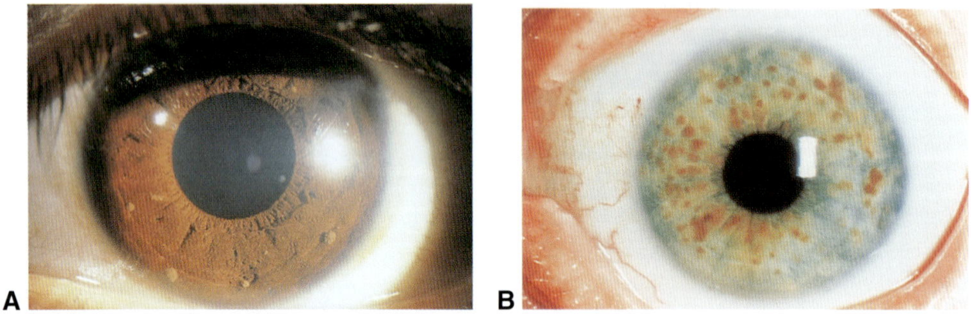

Figure 27-11 Lisch nodules of the iris in 2 patients with NF1. The brown iris has lighter-colored Lisch nodules **(A),** whereas the blue iris has darker-colored nodules **(B).**

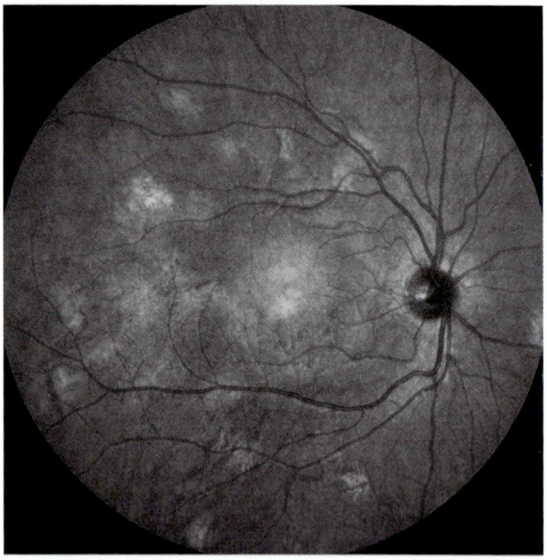

Figure 27-12 Near-infrared imaging of the right eye of an 11-year-old boy with NF1 and 20/20 visual acuity. Both eyes had a normal retinal appearance. However, imaging revealed choroidal melanocytic lesions in both eyes. *(Courtesy of Arif O. Khan, MD.)*

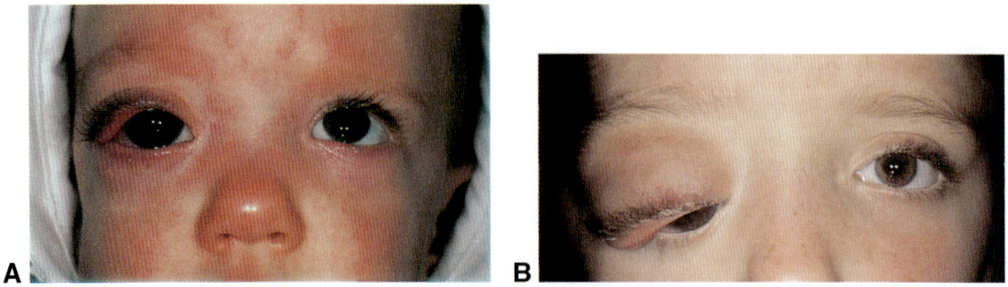

Figure 27-13 Plexiform neurofibroma involving the right upper eyelid, associated with ipsilateral buphthalmos, in a girl with NF1. **A,** Age 8 months. **B,** Age 8 years.

Complete excision of a plexiform neurofibroma of the eyelid is generally not possible. Instead, the aim of treatment is to relieve symptoms. Surgical debulking and suspension of the frontalis can reduce ptosis enough to allow binocular vision. Selumetinib, an inhibitor of mitogen-activated protein kinase (MAPK) kinase 1/2 (MEK1/2), was approved by the US Food and Drug Administration (FDA) in April 2020 to treat inoperable plexiform neurofibromas in children older than 2 years. In clinical trials, sustained tumor shrinkage occurred in 70% of patients.

Optic pathway glioma (OPG) is a low-grade pilocytic astrocytoma involving the optic nerve, chiasm, or both. It is present in approximately 15% of affected patients and is symptomatic in 1%–5% (almost always before age 10 years, after a brief period of rapid enlargement). The efficacy of treatment (ie, chemotherapy) is unclear because of the condition's highly variable natural history, including relative stability after rapid growth and spontaneous improvement in a few cases. MRI findings usually show cylindrical or fusiform enlargement (Fig 27-14), often with exaggerated sinuousness or kinking, creating an appearance of discontinuity or localized constriction on axial images. In addition to causing bilateral vision loss, tumors of the chiasm produce significant morbidity, including hydrocephalus and hypothalamic dysfunction. Patients with NF1 in whom OPGs develop have a better prognosis than do patients without NF1 in whom OPGs occur spontaneously.

Less common neuroglial abnormalities include spinal and gastrointestinal neurofibromas, pheochromocytomas, prominence of corneal nerves (≤20%), and localized orbital neurofibromas (see Table 27-3).

Gross AM, Wolters PL, Dombi E, et al. Selumetinib in children with inoperable plexiform neurofibromas. *N Engl J Med.* 2020;382(15):1430–1442.

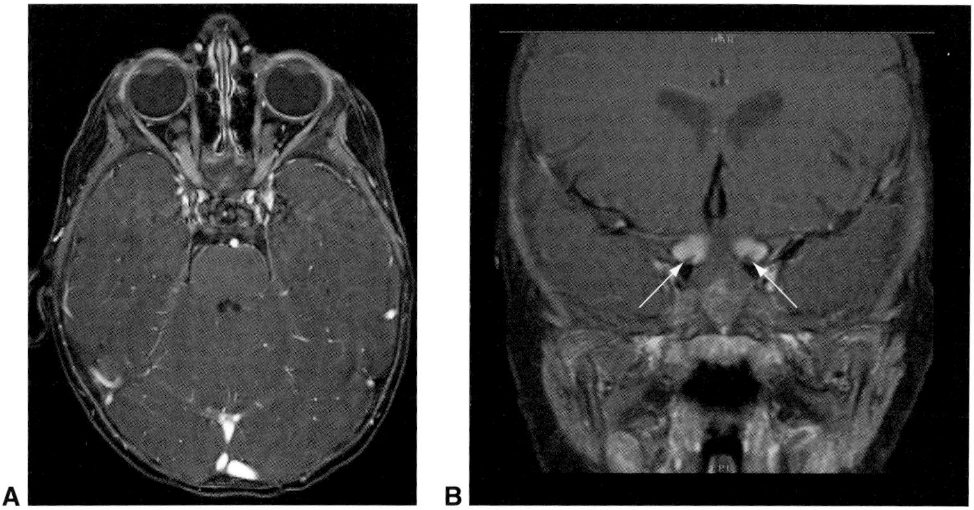

Figure 27-14 Bilateral optic pathway gliomas in a child with NF1. **A,** T2-weighted MRI axial section demonstrates fusiform enlargement and kinking of both right and left optic nerves. **B,** Coronal MRI demonstrates bilateral hyperintense signal of the optic tracks *(arrows)*. *(Courtesy of Mays El-Dairi, MD.)*

Other manifestations

Additional manifestations of NF1 include benign tumors of the skin or eye (eg, juvenile xanthogranuloma, retinal capillary hemangioma), several forms of malignancy (leukemia, rhabdomyosarcoma, pheochromocytoma, Wilms tumor), and bony defects such as scoliosis, pseudarthrosis of the tibia, and hypoplasia of the sphenoid bone (which may cause ocular pulsation). Sphenoid dysplasia may be associated with neurofibromas in the ipsilateral superficial temporal fossa as well as in the deep orbit. Several ill-defined abnormalities of the CNS (macrocephaly, aqueductal stenosis, seizures, and developmental delay) also are seen with greater frequency in patients with NF1. NF1 is a diagnosis to consider in any child who presents with unilateral glaucoma.

In otherwise uncomplicated NF1, an appropriate interval for pediatric ophthalmic reassessment is 1–2 years. In patients with known or suspected OGPs, screening is recommended every 6–12 months, especially in those younger than 6 years.

Fisher MJ, Loguidice M, Gutmann DH, et al. Visual outcomes in children with neurofibromatosis type 1–associated optic pathway glioma following chemotherapy: a multicenter retrospective analysis. *Neuro Oncol.* 2012;14(6):790–797.

Miller DT, Freedenberg D, Schorry E, et al; Council on Genetics, American College of Medical Genetics and Genomics. Health supervision for children with neurofibromatosis type 1. *Pediatrics.* 2019;143(5):e20190660.

Neurofibromatosis Type 2

Neurofibromatosis type 2 (NF2) is characterized by either bilateral cranial nerve (CN) VIII tumors (acoustic neuromas) or by any of the following in a patient with a first-degree relative with NF2: unilateral CN VIII tumors, neurofibroma, meningioma, schwannoma, glioma, or early-onset posterior subcapsular cataract. Patients typically present in their teens or early adulthood with signs or symptoms of CN VIII tumors, including decreased hearing or tinnitus. The most characteristic ocular finding in NF2 is lens opacity, especially posterior subcapsular cataract or wedge-shaped cortical cataracts. Up to 80% of patients have epiretinal membranes or combined hamartomas of the retina and retinal pigment epithelium (RPE). Lisch nodules of the iris can occur in NF2 but are infrequent. Salient features are summarized in Table 27-3.

Tuberous Sclerosis Complex

Tuberous sclerosis complex (TSC) is characterized by benign tumor growth in multiple organs, predominantly the skin, brain, heart, kidney, and eye. Prominent extraocular features are summarized in Table 27-4, and examples are shown in Figures 27-15 and 27-16. The classic *Vogt triad* of clinical findings is cognitive impairment, seizures, and facial angiofibromas. The facial angiofibromas are not usually present in young children, but hypomelanotic macules ("ash-leaf spots") are.

The ocular hallmark of TSC is retinal astrocytic hamartoma (retinal phakoma) (Fig 27-17). Pathologically, this growth arises from the innermost layer of the retina and is composed of nerve fibers and relatively undifferentiated cells that appear to be of glial origin. Astrocyctic hamartomas are usually found near the posterior pole and involve the retina, the

Table 27-4 Extraocular Features in Tuberous Sclerosis Complex

Feature	Characteristic
Ash-leaf spot	Sharply demarcated, hypopigmented skin lesion Visibility increased by ultraviolet light Onset during infancy
Adenoma sebaceum	Facial angiofibromas Occurrence in three-quarters of patients Can be mistaken for acne Onset during childhood
Subungual fibroma	Most common but can be periungual
Shagreen patch	Typically located in lumbosacral area Onset after puberty
Seizures	Periventricular or basal ganglia calcification (representing benign astrocytomas) Tuberous malformations of the cortex Cognitive impairment in 50% of patients
Other tumors	Cardiac rhabdomyomas Bone and kidney lesions

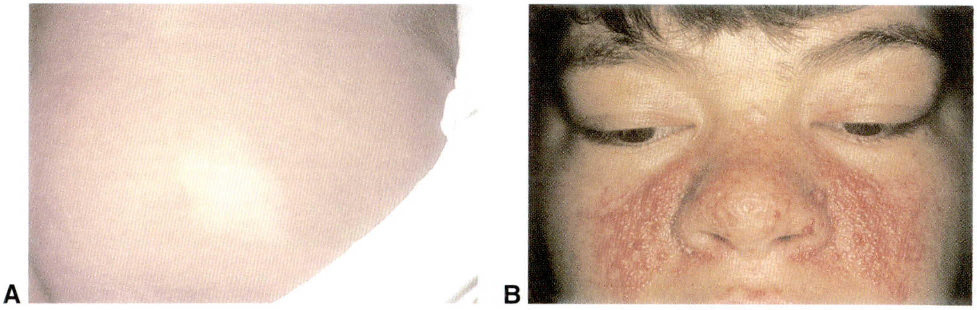

Figure 27-15 Cutaneous lesions of tuberous sclerosis complex (TSC). **A,** Hypomelanotic macule (ash-leaf spot). **B,** Adenoma sebaceum of the face.

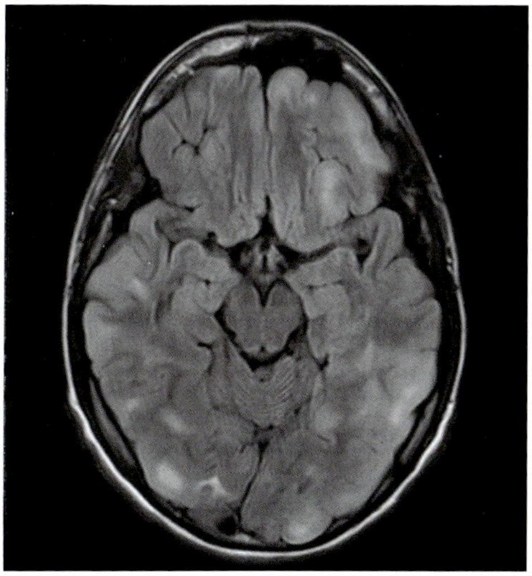

Figure 27-16 Brain lesions in a patient with TSC. Axial flair image demonstrates tuberous malformations (hyperintense lesions throughout white matter). *(Courtesy of Mays El-Dairi, MD.)*

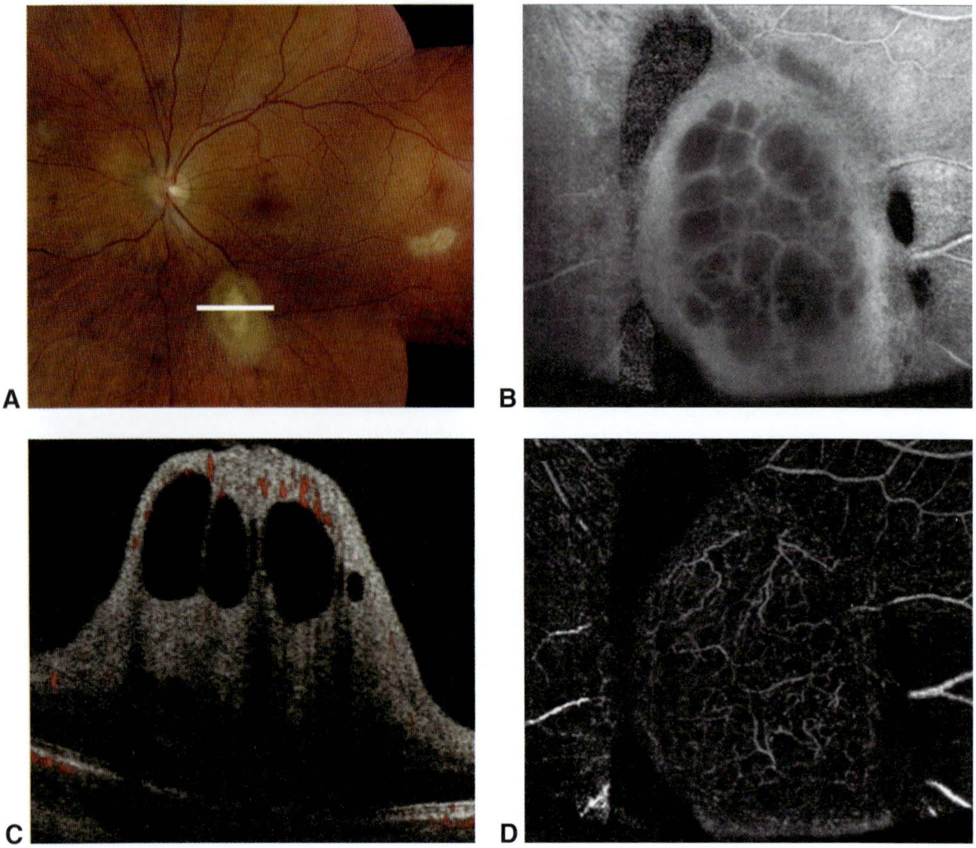

Figure 27-17 Retinal astrocytic hamartoma (retinal phakoma) in TSC. **A,** Multiple white globular elevated lesions bilaterally in a 23-year-old male with TSC. *White line* demonstrates a calcific, elevated astrocytoma that is shown in parts B–D. **B,** En face optical coherence tomography (OCT) infrared scan highlights the clear cystic spaces. Angiographic flow **(C)** and en face OCT angiography **(D)** demonstrate a plexus of capillary vessels in the apex of the hamartoma. The lesions of TSC can vary considerably in their opaqueness and visibility. *(Reprinted from Peng MY, Agarwal A, McDonald HR. Multimodal imaging findings in a retinal astrocytic hamartoma.* Ophthalmology. *2021;128(1):99. Copyright 2021, with permission from Elsevier.)*

optic nerve head, or both. They vary in size from approximately one-half to double the diameter of the optic nerve head. Vision is rarely affected.

Retinal astrocytic hamartomas have 3 distinct appearances:

1. relatively flat with a smooth, gray-white surface and indistinct margins, making detection difficult; typically found in very young children
2. sharply demarcated, calcified, raised, and irregular yellow-white surface, akin to a mulberry; often found in older patients, on or adjacent to the optic nerve head
3. transitional lesion combining features of types 1 and 2

Astrocytic hamartomas are present in 30%–50% of patients with TSC. One or more hamartomas may be found in a single eye, and 40% of cases are bilateral. There is no evidence that the number of lesions increases with age, but individual tumors have been documented to grow over time. Astrocyctic hamartomas are not pathognomonic of TSC; they may occur in people with or without TSC. Retinal lesions are more common in individuals with mutations in the *TSC2* gene. Hypopigmented lesions analogous to ash-leaf spots are occasionally seen in the iris or choroid.

Ophthalmic care of patients with TSC includes monitoring for changes in visual function and ocular lesions. For seizure control, vigabatrin can be used; up to 95% of patients with TSC and intractable seizures had significant reduction in seizure frequency on vigabatrin. Vigabatrin has been reported to cause peripheral visual field loss from retinal toxicity in a dose-dependent manner, and monitoring with visual field testing and electroretinography is recommended by some centers.

Aronow ME, Nakagawa JA, Gupta A, Traboulsi EI, Singh AD. Tuberous sclerosis complex: genotype/phenotype correlation of retinal findings. *Ophthalmology.* 2012;119(9): 1917–1923.

Retinocerebral Angiomatosis

Retinocerebral angiomatosis (also known as von Hippel–Lindau disease) is an autosomal dominant, highly penetrant systemic disorder characterized by hemangioblastomas of the brain, spinal cord, and retina. The systemic findings are summarized in Table 27-5. Capillary hemangioblastomas of the retina are found in up to 85% of patients with the *VHL* mutation and may be the first clinical sign of retinocerebral angiomatosis, becoming visible ophthalmoscopically between ages 10 and 35 years, with an average age at onset of 25 years. Tumors occur unilaterally in approximately one-third of cases; in up to one-half of cases, the tumors affect both eyes. Tumors typically occur in the peripheral fundus, but lesions adjacent to the optic nerve head have been described.

The hallmark of the mature tumor is a pair of markedly dilated vessels (artery and vein) running between the lesion and the optic nerve head, indicating significant arteriovenous shunting (Fig 27-18). Characteristic paired or twin retinal vessels of normal caliber may be evident before the tumor becomes visible.

Histologically, retinal capillary hemangioblastomas consist of relatively well-formed capillaries; however, fluorescein angiography findings indicate that these vessels are leaky.

Table 27-5 Extraocular Features in Retinocerebral Angiomatosis

Feature	Characteristic
Brain hemangioblastomas	Usually located in cerebellum Exudation from thin tumor vessel walls causes significant fluid accumulations
Cysts and tumors	Potential for cyst or tumor development in kidneys (renal cell carcinoma, clear cell subtype), pancreas, endolymphatic sac tumors, neuroendocrine tumors, liver, epididymis, and adrenal glands (pheochromocytoma)
Rare skin lesions	Café-au-lait spots and port-wine birthmarks (nevus flammeus) seen occasionally (5%)

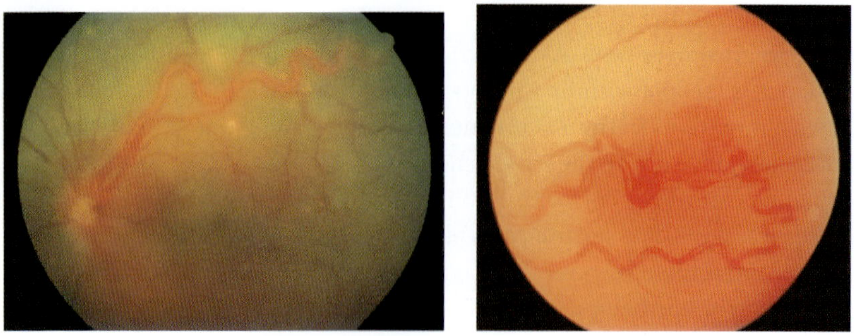

Figure 27-18 Retinal angiomatosis, left eye.

Transudation of fluid into the subretinal space causes lipid accumulation, retinal detachment, and consequent vision loss.

In about two-thirds of cases, particularly those with small lesions, treatment with cryotherapy or laser photocoagulation is effective. Antiangiogenic therapy and oral propranolol may also be considered. Early diagnosis increases the likelihood of successful treatment. The ocular lesions of retinocerebral angiomatosis are asymptomatic prior to retinal detachment. Therefore, periodic ophthalmic monitoring of young children at risk for the disease is advised.

Early diagnosis also is crucial to reduce morbidity and mortality from extraocular tumors in retinocerebral angiomatosis. Prompt referral to a geneticist for a systemic workup is recommended for any patient with an early-onset retinal capillary hemangioblastoma.

Karimi S, Arabi A, Shahraki T, et al. Von Hippel–Lindau disease and the eye. *J Ophthalmic Vis Res.* 2020;15(1):78–94.

Toy BC, Agrón E, Nigam D, Chew EY, Wong WT. Longitudinal analysis of retinal hemangioblastomatosis and visual function in ocular von Hippel–Lindau disease. *Ophthalmology.* 2012;119(12):2622–2630.

Encephalofacial Angiomatosis

Encephalofacial angiomatosis (also called Sturge-Weber syndrome) presents as a facial cutaneous vascular malformation (port-wine birthmark) with an ipsilateral leptomeningeal vascular malformation. Extraocular features are summarized in Table 27-6, with examples shown in Figures 27-19 and 27-20.

Table 27-6 Extraocular Features in Encephalofacial Angiomatosis

Feature	Characteristics
Port-wine birthmark	Congenital facial cutaneous vascular malformation (dilatation of the deep dermal plexus) Hemifacial lesion, typically unilateral
Leptomeningeal vascular malformation	Ipsilateral to port-wine birthmark Potentially associated with cerebral calcification (occipital, parietal, temporal, and occasionally frontal lobe), seizures, focal neurologic defect, and highly variable cognitive impairment

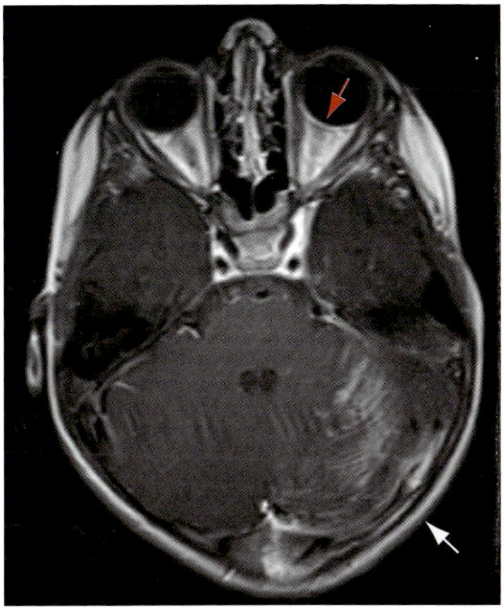

Figure 27-19 Axial gadolinium-enhanced T2-weighted MRI of the brain and orbits demonstrates enhancement of the choroid of the left eye *(red arrow)* and vascular malformation of the left lobe *(white arrow)* of the cerebellum at the level of the superior cerebellar peduncle in a patient with encephalofacial angiomatosis. *(Courtesy of Mays El-Dairi, MD.)*

A

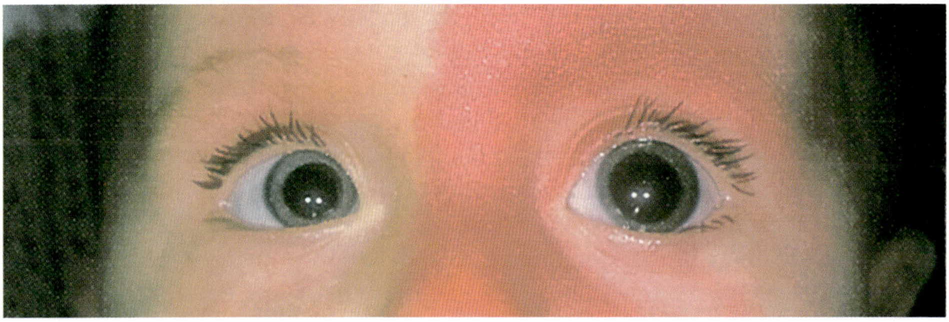

B

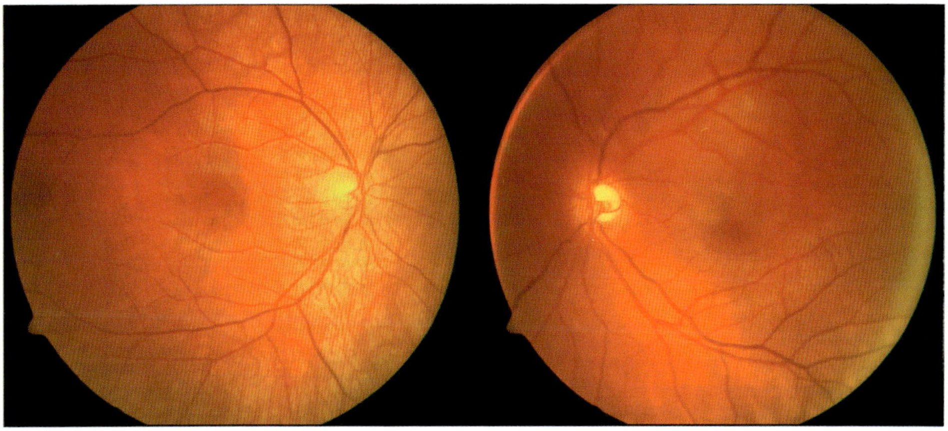

Figure 27-20 Encephalofacial angiomatosis. **A,** Facial port-wine birthmark involving the left eyelids, associated with ipsilateral buphthalmia, in an infant girl with encephalofacial angiomatosis and glaucoma. **B,** Fundus appearance in a child with encephalofacial angiomatosis. Note the glaucomatous cupping of the left optic nerve associated with a diffuse choroidal hemangioma (ie, "ketchup fundus") compared with the right, healthy fellow eye. *(Part B courtesy of Mays El-Dairi, MD.)*

Any portion of the ocular circulation may be anomalous in encephalofacial angiomatosis. When the skin lesion involves the eyelids, increased conjunctival vascularity commonly produces a pinkish discoloration. An abnormal plexus of episcleral vessels often is present.

Retinal findings in encephalofacial angiomatosis may include tortuous vessels, arteriovenous communications, and most significantly, choroidal hemangioma with well-formed choroidal vessels that cause the fundus to appear dark red (see Fig 27-20B). Either the posterior pole alone or the entire fundus may be affected. Choroidal hemangiomas usually are asymptomatic in childhood. During adolescence or adulthood, the choroid may substantially thicken, with subsequent degeneration or detachment of the overlying retina. No treatment has been proven to prevent or reverse such deterioration, but scattered application of laser photocoagulation may help.

Glaucoma is the most common and most serious ocular complication of encephalofacial angiomatosis, occurring in up to 70% of patients. Increased intraocular pressure (IOP) may result from elevated episcleral venous pressure, hyperemia of the ciliary body with hypersecretion of aqueous, or a developmental anomaly of the anterior chamber angle. Glaucoma in encephalofacial angiomatosis may occur at birth or later in childhood and is more likely in cases with involvement of the skin of the upper and lower eyelids, choroidal hemangioma, iris heterochromia, or episcleral hemangioma.

Glaucoma management in patients with encephalofacial angiomatosis is challenging. Eyedrops can be effective—especially in later-onset cases—but surgery typically is indicated in early-onset cases and when medical treatment is inadequate. Long-term control of IOP generally requires multiple operations, which pose risks of intraoperative or postoperative exudation or hemorrhage owing to rapid ocular decompression in patients with anomalous choroidal vessels. Extreme care is needed during glaucoma tube shunt surgery to avoid early postoperative hypotony. Postsurgical accumulation of choroidal or subretinal fluid may be dramatic, but resorption usually occurs spontaneously within 1–2 weeks.

In some patients with encephalofacial angiomatosis, angle surgery (goniotomy and trabeculotomy) has been effective, and treatment of affected skin with a pulsed-dye laser can reduce vascularity, improving appearance without much damage to dermal tissue.

Khaier A, Nischal KK, Espinosa M, Manoj B. Periocular port wine stain: the Great Ormond Street Hospital experience. *Ophthalmology.* 2011;118(11):2274–2278.e1.

Ataxia-Telangiectasia

Ataxia-telangiectasia (AT; Louis-Bar syndrome) affects the cerebellum, ocular surface, skin, and immune system. Extraocular features are summarized in Table 27-7.

Ocular motor abnormalities are found in many patients with AT and are among the earliest disease manifestations. Poor initiation of saccades with preservation of vestibular-ocular movements is common, similar to congenital ocular motor apraxia. Head thrusts are used to compensate for saccades. Strabismus and nystagmus also may be present.

Telangiectasia of the conjunctiva occurs in 91% of patients and develops between the ages of 3 and 5 years. Initially, involvement is interpalpebral and away from the limbus (Fig 27-21), but involvement eventually becomes generalized. Similar vessel changes may occur in the eyelids and other sun-exposed skin.

Table 27-7 Extraocular Features in Ataxia-Telangiectasia

Feature	Characteristics
Neurologic findings	Truncal ataxia usually noted during second year of life Subsequent development of dysarthria, dystonia, and choreoathetosis Progressive deterioration of motor function, leading to serious disability by age 10 years Intellectual disability and microcephaly in some patients
Immunologic findings	Defective T-cell function is usually associated with hypoplasia of the thymus and decreased levels of circulating immunoglobulin Recurrent respiratory tract infections (frequent cause of mortality) Increased susceptibility to malignancy (frequent cause of mortality)
Oncologic findings	Greatly increased sensitivity to the tissue-damaging adverse effects of therapeutic radiation and many chemotherapeutic agents Increased risk of malignancy and radiation damage can also occur in heterozygous carriers

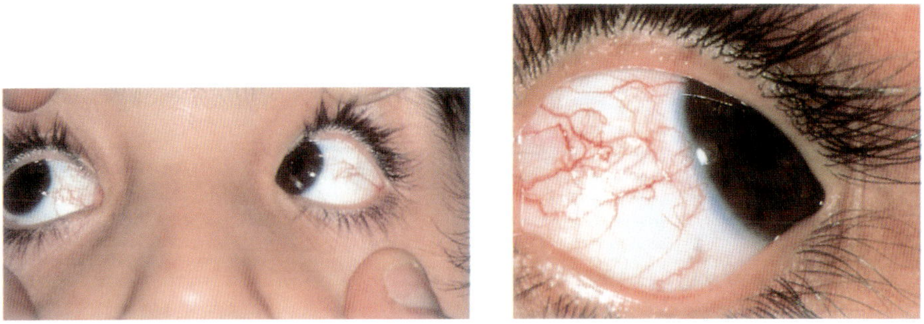

Figure 27-21 Abnormally dilated and tortuous interpalpebral conjunctival vessels in a child with ataxia-telangiectasia, seen only in the interpalpebral fissure.

Individuals with AT are highly sensitive to the tissue-damaging adverse effects of chemotherapy and radiation. Defective T-cell function in patients with AT usually is associated with hypoplasia of the thymus and decreased levels of circulating immunoglobulin. Respiratory tract infections and malignant tumors are frequent causes of mortality in this population.

Incontinentia Pigmenti

Incontinentia pigmenti (IP; also called Bloch-Sulzberger syndrome) affects the skin, brain, and eyes. Extraocular features are summarized in Table 27-8, with examples of skin lesions shown in Figure 27-22. The condition has an X-linked dominant inheritance pattern, with presumed fetal lethality in hemizygous males.

Approximately 35%–77% of patients with IP have ocular involvement, characterized by proliferative retinal vasculopathy that closely resembles retinopathy of prematurity. The presentation typically is unilateral or very asymmetric. At birth, incomplete peripheral retinal vascularization may be the only recognized defect, but abnormal arteriovenous connections, microvascular anomalies, and neovascular membranes develop at or near the junction of

Table 27-8 Extraocular Features in Incontinentia Pigmenti

Feature	Characteristics
Dermatologic findings	Usually normal skin appearance at birth Development of erythema and bullae during the first few days of life, usually on the extremities (see Fig 27-22A) Persistence of lesions for weeks to months When healed, appearance of lesions as clusters of small, hyperpigmented macules in a characteristic "splashed paint" distribution (see Fig 27-22B), most prominently on the trunk
Neurologic findings	Microcephaly, hydrocephalus, seizures, and varying degrees of cognitive impairment in one-third of patients
Dental findings	Missing and malformed teeth in roughly two-thirds of cases
Other findings	Scoliosis, skull deformities, cleft palate, and dwarfism, among other findings, occur less commonly

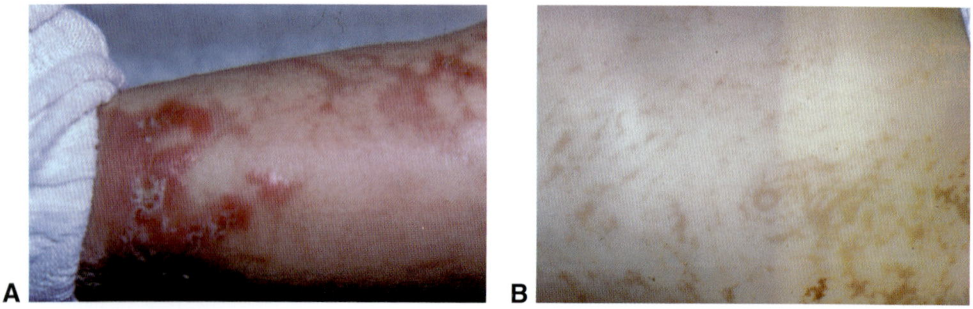

Figure 27-22 Pigmented skin lesions in a patient with incontinentia pigmenti (IP). **A,** Bullous lesions. **B,** Hyperpigmented macules. *(Courtesy of Edward L. Raab, MD.)*

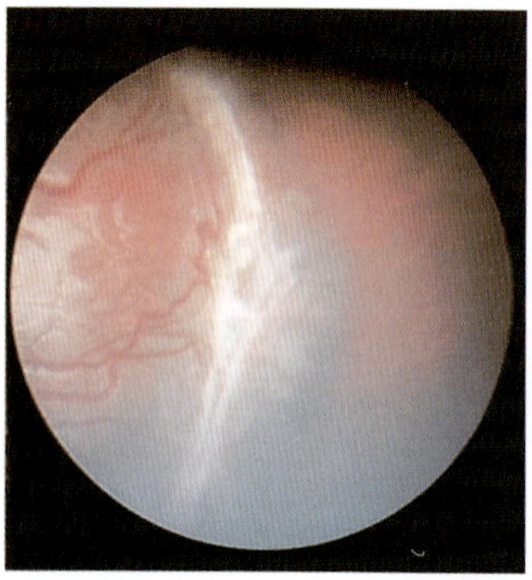

Figure 27-23 Vascular abnormalities of the temporal retina, in the right eye of a 2-year-old with IP. Note the avascularity peripheral to the circumferential white vasoproliferative lesion, which showed profuse leakage on fluorescein angiography.

the vascular and avascular retina (Fig 27-23). Rapid progression sometimes leads to total retinal detachment and retrolental membrane formation within the first few months of life. Microphthalmia, cataract, glaucoma, optic atrophy, strabismus, and nystagmus may occur, usually secondary to end-stage retinopathy.

Serial retinal monitoring for the first 1–2 years of life is necessary to identify patients who require ophthalmic treatment. The retinopathy of IP responds to photocoagulation or cryotherapy with varying degrees of success. Treatment primarily targets the avascular peripheral retina, as in management of retinopathy of prematurity or other early-onset familial exudative vitreoretinopathies.

O'Doherty M, Mc Creery K, Green AJ, Tuwir I, Brosnahan D. Incontinentia pigmenti—ophthalmological observation of a series of cases and review of the literature. *Br J Ophthalmol.* 2011;95(1):11–16.

Racemose Angioma

Racemose angioma (also called Wyburn-Mason syndrome) is a nonhereditary arteriovenous malformation of the eye and brain. Extraocular features are summarized in Table 27-9.

Ocular manifestations are unilateral and congenital, and they may progress during childhood. The typical lesion consists of markedly dilated and tortuous vessels that shunt blood directly from the arteries to the veins (Fig 27-24). Unlike in retinocerebral angiomatosis–associated hemangioblastomas, the abnormal vessels in racemose angioma do not leak fluid. Intraocular hemorrhage and secondary neovascular glaucoma are possible complications. Some patients with racemose angioma have normal vision, but approximately half of affected eyes are blind, and an additional one-quarter are severely impaired.

No treatment is indicated for primary lesions. Treatment may be considered for associated complications, such as scatter photocoagulation for ischemic venous occlusive disease, vitrectomy for nonclearing vitreous hemorrhage, and cyclodestructive therapy for neovascular glaucoma.

Table 27-9 Extraocular Features in Racemose Angioma

Feature	Characteristics
Dermatologic findings	Maxillofacial or cutaneous facial AVM
Neurologic findings	AVM, especially in midbrain
	Frequent source of hemorrhage
	May result in seizures, mental changes, hemiparesis, and papilledema
	Mandibular AVMs can lead to bleeding with dental extraction

AVM = arteriovenous malformation.

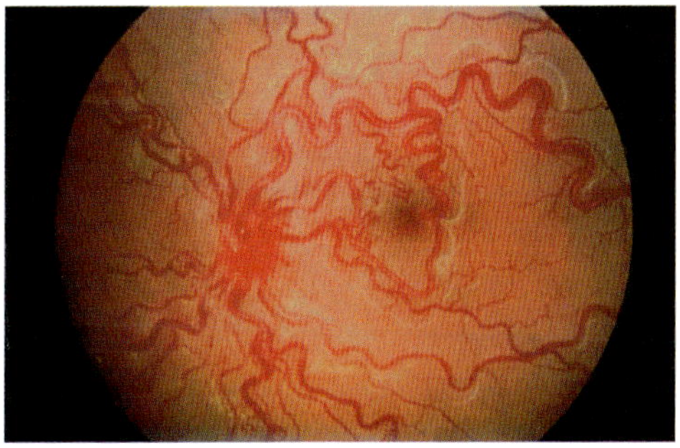

Figure 27-24 Racemose angioma of the retina, left eye.

Klippel-Trénaunay-Weber Syndrome

Klippel-Trénaunay-Weber syndrome (KTWS) is a neuro-oculocutaneous disorder consisting of a vascular nevus involving an extremity, varicosities of that extremity, and hypertrophy of the underlying bone and soft tissue. KTWS is a *PIK3CA*-related overgrowth spectrum (PROS) disorder, in which mosaic activating mutations in *PIK3CA* lead to vascular and hypertrophic manifestations. Thromboembolic events may complicate the clinical course and treatment. Ophthalmic findings include vascular anomalies of the orbit, iris, retina, choroid, and optic nerve, as well as optic nerve and chiasmal gliomas. Patients with KTWS are at increased risk of glaucoma.

KTWS is a complex syndrome that requires individualized treatment.

Hughes M, Hao M, Luu M. PIK3CA vascular overgrowth syndromes: an update. *Curr Opin Pediatr.* 2020;32(4):539–546.

Albinism

Albinism comprises conditions affecting melanin synthesis in the skin and eye *(oculocutaneous albinism [OCA])* or in the eye alone *(ocular albinism [OA])*. OCA is inherited in an autosomal-recessive manner. Pathogenic variants in *TYR, OCA2, TYRP1, SLC45A2, SLC24A5*, and *LRMDA* lead to OCA1, OCA2, OCA3, OCA4, OCA6, and OCA7, respectively, and are characterized by various degrees of skin and hair pigmentation (Fig 27-25A). The OCA5 locus candidate region is at 4q24, but the causative gene has not been identified.

Hermansky-Pudlak syndrome is characterized by pulmonary interstitial fibrosis, bleeding abnormalities, immunodeficiency, and granulomatous colitis. It is caused by bialleic mutations in several *HPS* genes. *Chédiak-Higashi syndrome* is a rare condition involving increased susceptibility to bacterial infections that results from biallelic *LYST* mutations.

> **CLINICAL PEARL**
>
> When a child is diagnosed with albinism, it is recommended that the clinician inquire whether the patient has bleeding or bruising tendencies or frequent infections.

OA is an X-linked recessive disorder caused by a hemizygous pathogenic variant in *GPR143* that affects melanosome number and size. Carrier females may demonstrate mosaic pigmentary changes and mild transillumination defects but are asymptomatic otherwise.

Ocular Features

Major ophthalmic findings of albinism include

- iris transillumination from decreased pigmentation
- foveal aplasia or hypoplasia
- retinal pigmentary deficit, especially peripheral to the posterior pole (Fig 27-25B, C)
- nystagmus, photophobia, and reduced central visual acuity

A B C

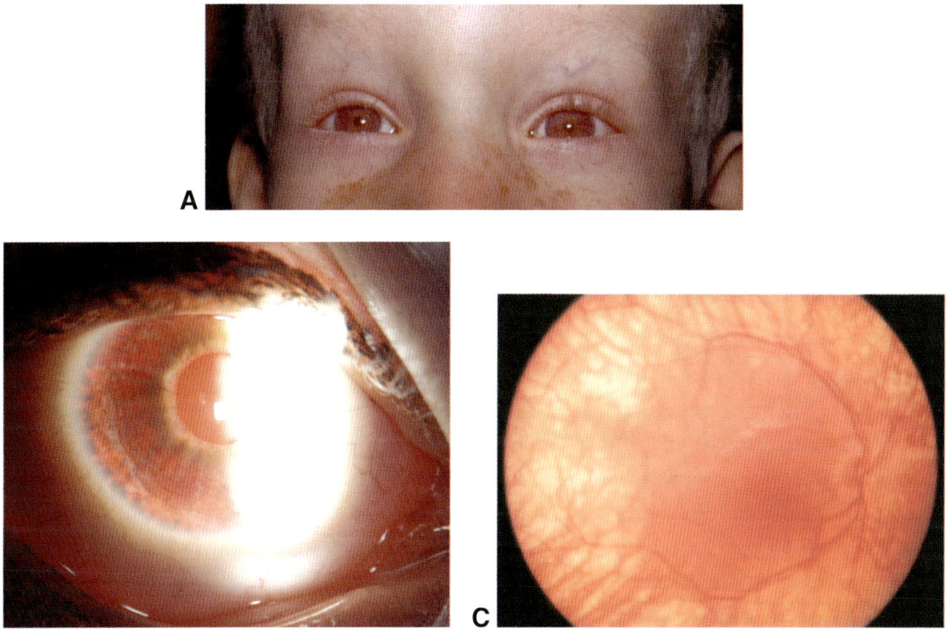

Figure 27-25 Ophthalmic findings in albinism. **A,** Child with oculocutaneous albinism type 2. Note the white hair, eyebrows, and lashes and the light-colored irides and freckles. **B,** Transillumination of the iris in albinism, right eye. **C,** Fundus in albinism, right eye, demonstrating complete lack of pigment and foveal hypoplasia. *(Parts A and B courtesy of Edward L. Raab, MD.)*

Although some patients with albinism have good vision, visual acuity usually ranges from 20/80 to worse than 20/400, and high refractive error is common, particularly with-the-rule astigmatism. In an infant with foveal hypoplasia, nystagmus typically begins at 2–3 months of age and dampens in the first year of life. The severity of the visual impairment tends to be proportional to the grade of foveal hypoplasia by optical coherence tomography, although variations in visual acuity are present within each grade. Visual acuity also seems to be inversely related to the amplitude of nystagmus. A multitude of crossed fibers appears in the optic chiasm of patients with albinism and preclinical models; this structural anomaly precludes stereopsis and often induces strabismus. Asymmetric visually evoked potentials often are seen in affected patients and may be helpful in diagnosis.

Ocular findings in albinism vary; an absence of transillumination defects or of foveal hypoplasia does not exclude the diagnosis.

Management

Genetic counseling and testing are offered to patients with albinism and their families. Patients with OCA are advised to wear protective clothing, avoid sunlight, and use sunscreen because of the increased risk for skin cancer.

Ophthalmic management of these cases is correction of high refractive error and use of glasses or contact lenses with ultraviolet (UV) protection and tinting to protect the retina and alleviate photodysphoria. Eye muscle surgery may be considered for strabismus and torticollis associated with a null position. Early intervention with vision rehabilitation and orientation/mobility training is crucial in children with albinism and low vision (see Chapter 28, Pediatric Chronic Eye Care and Low Vision Rehabilitation).

Khan AO, Tamimi M, Lenzner S, Bolz HJ. Hermansky-Pudlak syndrome genes are frequently mutated in patients with albinism from the Arabian Peninsula. *Clin Genet.* 2016;90(1):96–98.

Schidlowski L, Liebert F, Iankilevich PG, et al. Non-syndromic oculocutaneous albinism: novel genetic variants and clinical follow up of a Brazilian pediatric cohort. *Front Genet.* 2020;11:397.

Thomas MG, Kumar A, Mohammad S, et al. Structural grading of foveal hypoplasia using spectral-domain optical coherence tomography: a predictor of visual acuity? *Ophthalmology.* 2011;118(8):1653–1660.

Diabetes

In type 1, or insulin-dependent, diabetes (T1D; formerly called *juvenile-onset diabetes*), the prevalence of retinopathy is directly proportional to the duration of poorly controlled disease after puberty. Poor glucose control also can cause cataract. Retinopathy rarely occurs less than 15 years after the onset of diabetes; as such, proliferative diabetic retinopathy is rare in pediatric cases.

Type 2, or insulin-resistant, diabetes (T2D) is becoming increasingly common in pediatric patients. Testing for rare genetic causes of diabetes is useful because positive findings could lead to screening and treatment of family members with the trait. See BCSC Section 1, *Update on General Medicine.*

The American Academy of Ophthalmology recommends screening for diabetic retinopathy beginning 5 years from the onset of T1D or on presentation of T2D and continuing annually thereafter. However, results of a recent observational study of patients with T1D or T2D demonstrated diabetic retinopathy in 20% and 7.2%, respectively, by year 3 of follow-up. Additionally, for every 1-point increase in hemoglobin A1c (a proxy for glycemic control), the hazard ratio increased by 20% for T1D and by 30% for T2D. Therefore, screening prior to 5 years of disease is likely warranted, especially in cases of poor glycemic control. Telemedicine using nonmydriatic photographs is a promising approach to increase access to diabetic retinopathy screening.

See BCSC Section 12, *Retina and Vitreous.*

American Academy of Ophthalmology Retina/Vitreous Panel. Preferred Practice Pattern Guidelines. *Diabetic Retinopathy.* American Academy of Ophthalmology; 2019. www.aao.org/ppp

Intrauterine or Perinatal Infection

Congenital infections may harm the eye through numerous pathologic mechanisms:

- direct tissue damage from the infecting agent
- teratogenic effects, resulting in malformations
- delayed reactivation of the agent after birth by direct action or inflammation, and associated tissue damage

Most perinatal disorders involve a spectrum of clinical presentations, ranging from silent disease to life-threatening tissue and organ damage. The classical series of congenital infections are represented by the mnemonic *TORCH: to*xoplasmosis, *o*ther (Zika, lymphocytic choriomeningitis (LCMV), *r*ubella, *c*ytomegalovirus, and *h*erpesviruses.

Toxoplasmosis

See Chapter 25 in this volume and BCSC Section 9, *Uveitis and Ocular Inflammation,* for discussion of toxoplasmosis.

Rubella

Congenital rubella (German measles) syndrome involves well-defined ocular, otologic, and cardiac abnormalities, accompanied by microcephaly and variable developmental delay. The incidence of congenital rubella has decreased markedly in North America since widespread vaccination of children was instituted in the late 1960s; however, this condition remains a cause of infant morbidity and mortality in less-developed countries.

Ocular abnormalities include a characteristic nuclear cataract (that may be observed floating in a liquefied lens cortex), glaucoma, microphthalmia, and retinal abnormalities that vary from subtle salt-and-pepper retinopathy (most common finding; Fig 27-26) to pseudoretinitis pigmentosa. Diagnosis is based on these clinical findings as well as serologic testing. The virus can be isolated from pharyngeal swab specimens and from the lens contents at time of cataract surgery.

Lensectomy is usually required for management of cataracts in children with rubella. Pregnant staff should not participate in the surgical procedure due to the risk of contagion. After the operation, infected eyes are prone to inflammation and formation of a secondary membrane. These outcomes are managed with high doses of topical corticosteroids and mydriatics. In adults, rubella virus infection is associated with Fuchs heterochromic uveitis.

Cytomegalovirus

Infection with the ubiquitous herpesvirus cytomegalovirus (CMV) produces host responses ranging from asymptomatic (in immunocompetent individuals) to severe (in newborns and immunocompromised patients). Over 80% of adults in developed countries have antibodies to the virus.

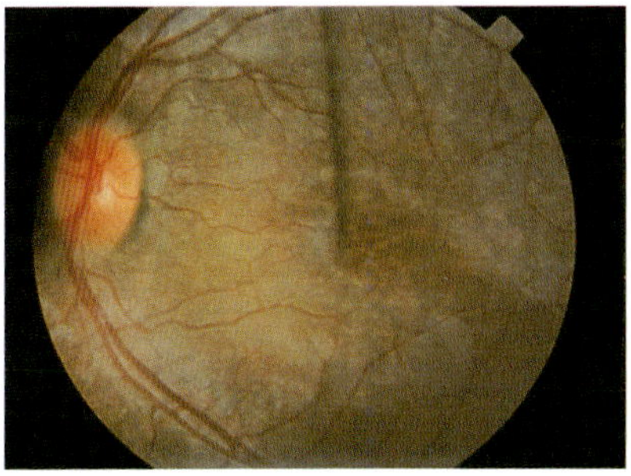

Figure 27-26 Fundus photograph from a 6-year-old patient with rubella syndrome (electroretinography results were normal).

CMV is the most common etiology of congenital infection, affecting approximately 1% of infants. Clinically apparent disease is present in 10%–15% of infected neonates, and 20%–30% of these cases are fatal. Vertical transmission to the fetus or newborn can occur transplacentally, from contact with an infected birth canal during delivery, or from ingestion of infected breast milk or maternal secretions. Congenital CMV disease is characterized by fever, jaundice, hematologic abnormalities, deafness, microcephaly, and periventricular calcifications.

The following are ophthalmic manifestations of congenital CMV infection; these occur primarily in infants with systemic symptoms:

- retinochoroiditis (Fig 27-27)
- optic nerve anomalies
- microphthalmia
- cataract
- uveitis

The retinochoroiditis entails bilateral focal involvement with areas of RPE atrophy and whitish opacities mixed with retinal hemorrhages. CMV retinitis can be acquired in children who are immunocompromised; this is most frequently associated with HIV infection or AIDS, organ transplantation, or chemotherapy. A diffuse retinal necrosis is observed, with areas of retinal thickening and whitening, hemorrhages, and venous sheathing. The retinitis can be progressive, or it may masquerade as toxoplasmosis by presenting as a quiescent retinochoroidal scar. Vitritis may also be present.

In acquired CMV, diagnosis is based on the clinical presentation; in congenital CMV, diagnosis is supplemented by serologic testing. In infected infants, the virus can be recovered from bodily secretions.

Infants with systemic or ocular disease are usually treated with ganciclovir or its prodrug, valganciclovir.

Herpes Simplex Virus

Congenital infection with herpes simplex virus (HSV1 or HSV2) occurs in 1 in 3000 to 1 in 20,000 births and typically involves infection with HSV2 during passage through the

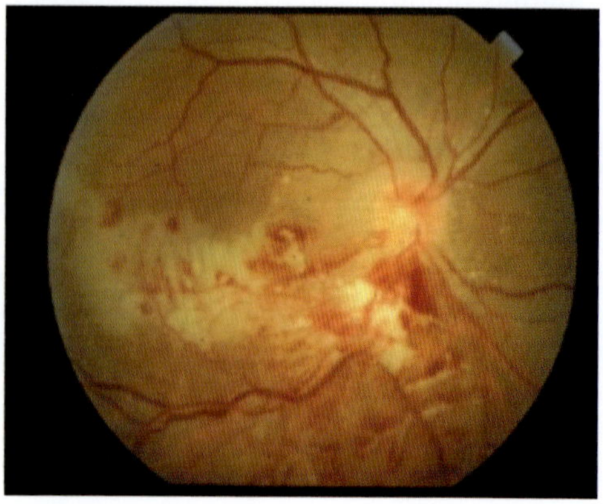

Figure 27-27 Retinochoroiditis associated with active cytomegalovirus infection in a pediatric bone-marrow transplant recipient with immunosuppression. Note the retinal whitening, hemorrhage, and venous sheathing, giving the classic "ketchup and cottage cheese" appearance. *(Courtesy of E. Mitchel Opremcak, MD.)*

birth canal. The neonatal infection is confined to the CNS, skin, oral cavity, and eyes in one-third of cases. Disseminated disease occurs in two-thirds of cases and can involve the liver, adrenal glands, and lungs. Eye involvement in congenital HSV infection can include conjunctivitis, keratitis, retinochoroiditis, and cataracts. Keratitis can be epithelial or stromal. Retinal involvement can be severe and may include massive exudates and retinal necrosis.

Affected infants are treated with systemic acyclovir. The mortality rate from disseminated disease is significant, and survivors usually have permanent ocular and CNS impairment.

Marquez L, Levy ML, Munoz FM, Palazzi DL. A report of three cases and review of intrauterine herpes simplex virus infection. *Pediatr Infect Dis J.* 2011;30(2):153–157.

Syphilis

Syphilis is caused by the spirochete *Treponema pallidum;* transmission is through sexual contact. Fetal infection follows from maternal spirochetemia, but the longer the mother has had syphilis, the lower the risk of vertical transmission. If a mother has primary or secondary disease, approximately half of her offspring will be infected. In untreated late maternal syphilis, approximately 30% of infants have congenital infection. The incidence of congenital syphilis in the United States is 23.7 cases per 100,000 live births, with the highest rates among Black and Hispanic women.

Signs and symptoms of congenital syphilis include unexplained premature birth, large placenta, persistent rhinitis, intractable rash, unexplained jaundice, hepatosplenomegaly, pneumonia, anemia, generalized lymphadenopathy, and metaphyseal abnormalities or periostitis on radiographs. Congenital infection can lead to neonatal death.

Early eye involvement in congenital syphilis is rare. In some infants, chorioretinitis appears as a salt-and-pepper granularity of the fundus. Pseudoretinitis pigmentosa may follow. In rare cases, anterior uveitis, glaucoma, or both develop. Certain signs and symptoms of congenital syphilis may not appear until late childhood or adolescence, such as widely spaced peg-shaped teeth, sensorineural hearing loss, saddle nose, short maxilla, and linear scars around the body orifices. Bilateral interstitial keratitis, the classic ophthalmic finding in older children and adults, occurs in approximately 10% of patients.

CLINICAL PEARL

Late-presenting signs of congenital syphilis include those of the Hutchinson triad:

- widely spaced, peg-shaped teeth
- sensorineural hearing loss
- interstitial keratitis

A diagnosis of congenital syphilis is confirmed by identification of *T pallidum* by dark-field microscopy or fluorescent antibody testing. The detection of specific immunoglobulin M is the most sensitive serologic method.

Congenital syphilis in neonates is treated with intravenous aqueous crystalline penicillin G. Serologic analyses are repeated at 2 to 4, 6, and 12 months after conclusion of treatment—or until antibody reactivity can no longer be detected or the titer decreases fourfold. Persistent positive titers or a positive result of the cerebrospinal fluid VDRL test at 6 months indicate need for retreatment.

Also see BCSC Section 9, *Uveitis and Ocular Inflammation.*

Centers for Disease Control and Prevention. Sexually transmitted infections treatment guidelines, 2021: syphilis. US Department of Health and Human Services; 2021. Accessed February 15, 2022. www.cdc.gov/std/treatment-guidelines/syphilis.htm

Lymphocytic Choriomeningitis

Lymphocytic choriomeningitis virus (LCMV) is an arenavirus that is acquired by exposure to infected rodents (including house and laboratory mice and pet hamsters) and can be transmitted vertically. Infants with congenital LCMV infection present with CNS abnormalities including hydrocephaly, microcephaly, intracranial calcifications, and cognitive impairment. Chorioretinal scars may occur without neurologic abnormalities and may involve the entire macula. These scars are similar to those associated with toxoplasmosis, CMV infection, and Aicardi syndrome. A diagnosis of LCMV infection is considered in infants with chorioretinal scars when results of tests for these more common etiologies are negative. Elevated LCMV antibody titers establish the diagnosis. No specific treatment is available apart from exposure prevention.

Zika Virus

Zika virus is a flavivirus transmitted by the *Aedes aegypti* mosquito. Zika virus infection historically was thought to produce only nonspecific viral symptoms but recently was found to be associated with congenital microcephaly, chorioretinal lesions, and cerebral visual impairment. In a series of 29 infants in Brazil with presumed intrauterine Zika virus infection, 10 infants (35%) had ocular abnormalities, and 7 of these infants were affected bilaterally. Specifically, clumps of pigment in the posterior pole and circumscribed areas of chorioretinal atrophy were observed. One infant had iris colobomas and lens subluxation.

de Paula Freitas B, de Oliveira Dias JR, Prazeres J, et al. Ocular findings in infants with microcephaly associated with presumed Zika virus congenital infection in Salvador, Brazil. *JAMA Ophthalmol.* 2016;134(5):529–535.

Malignant Disease

Leukemia

Leukemia in childhood is acute in 95% of cases and is more often lymphocytic than myelocytic. Acute lymphoblastic leukemia is the most common malignant disease of childhood and is responsible for 30% of all pediatric cancer cases; there are 4000 new cases per year in the United States. Although the most common ocular manifestation of leukemia is leukemic retinopathy, any ocular structure can be affected. Ocular involvement is highly correlated with CNS involvement.

Leukemic infiltrates in the anterior segment may lead to heterochromia iridis, architectural changes in the iris, frank iris infiltrates, spontaneous hyphemas, leukemic cells in the anterior chamber, or pseudohypopyon. Keratic precipitates may occur, and glaucoma may develop from tumor cells clogging the trabecular meshwork. Results of anterior-chamber paracentesis for cytologic studies may be diagnostic in cases involving the anterior segment. To manage these anterior-segment complications, systemic chemotherapy, local radiation therapy, and topical steroids may be given. Leukemic involvement of the iris may masquerade as juvenile xanthogranuloma.

The most common ocular findings of leukemia are retinal hemorrhages, especially flame-shaped lesions in the nerve fiber layer. The hemorrhages may have white centers. They involve the posterior fundus and correlate with other aspects of the disease, including anemia, thrombocytopenia, and coagulation abnormalities. Retinal hemorrhages in leukemia can resemble those associated with abusive head trauma (see Chapter 26) and may be the first manifestation of leukemia. Other signs of leukemic retinal involvement are localized perivascular infiltrations, microinfarction, and discrete tumor infiltrations. Histologically, the choroid is the most frequently affected ocular tissue, but choroidal involvement usually is not apparent clinically.

Optic nerve involvement occurs if the nerve head has been infiltrated by leukemic cells (Fig 27-28); this may cause loss of central vision. Translucent swelling of the optic nerve head obscures the normal landmarks; with florid involvement, only a white mass is visible in the region of the nerve head. An afferent pupillary defect may be present, and there may be reductions in visual acuity and color discrimination.

CLINICAL PEARL

The presence of edema of the optic nerve head and loss of central vision in a child with leukemia is a medical emergency because of the risk for blindness if not treated promptly.

In suspected leukemic infiltration of the optic nerve, urgent neuroimaging and consultation with oncology and radiation oncology are needed. Treatment is usually multidisciplinary and may include intrathecal chemotherapy and orbital radiation.

Myers KA, Nikolic A, Romanchuk K, et al. Optic neuropathy in the context of leukemia or lymphoma: diagnostic approach to a neuro-oncologic emergency. *Neurooncol Pract.* 2017;4(1):60–66.

Neuroblastoma

Neuroblastoma is one of the most common childhood cancers and is the most frequent source of childhood orbital metastasis (89% of cases). Neuroblastoma usually originates in the adrenal gland or in the sympathetic ganglion chain of the retroperitoneum or

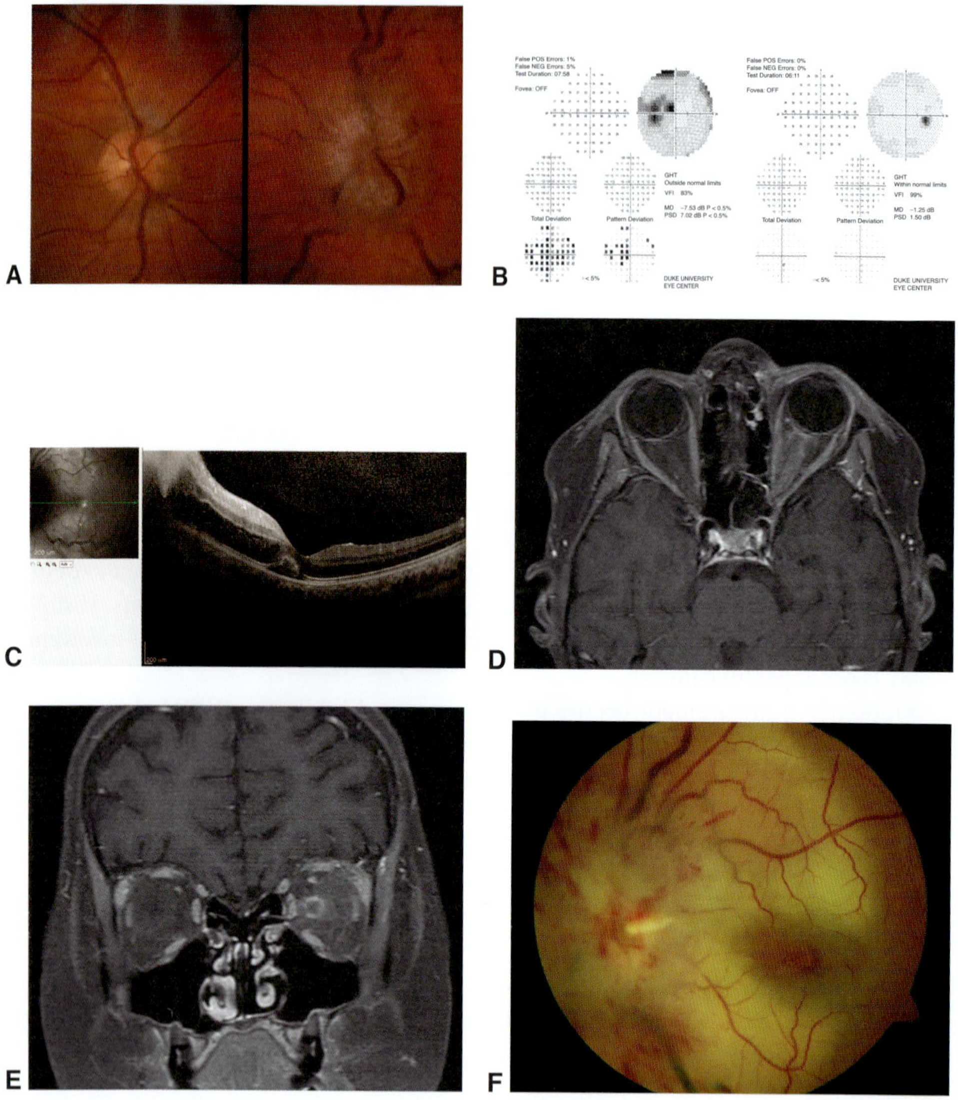

Figure 27-28 Child with leukemic infiltration of the left optic nerve from central nervous system involvement of acute lymphocytic leukemia at presentation **(A–E)** and 4 weeks later **(F). A,** Leukemic infiltration of the left optic nerve. **B,** Visual field demonstrates a left cecocentral scotoma. **C,** Subretinal foveal infiltration. **D,** Axial T1 MRI demonstrates enhancement and enlargement of the intraorbital portion of the optic nerve. **E,** Coronal T1 MRI shows enhancement of the left optic nerve from leukemic infiltration. **F,** Progression of optic nerve infiltration, subretinal leukemic infiltration, and secondary retinal ischemia. *(Courtesy of Mays El-Dairi, MD.)*

mediastinum. Approximately 20% of patients with neuroblastoma have clinically evident orbital involvement; this is sometimes the initial manifestation of the tumor.

The mean patient age at diagnosis of metastatic orbital neuroblastoma is approximately 2 years; 90% are diagnosed by 5 years of age. Unilateral or bilateral proptosis and eyelid ecchymosis are the classic presentations (Fig 27-29). Systemic signs and symptoms

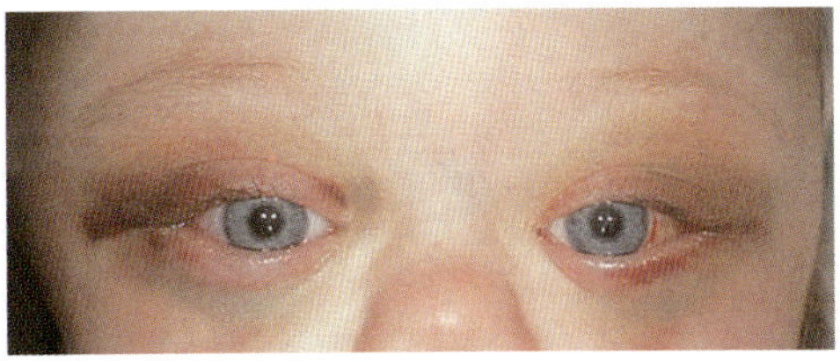

Figure 27-29 Bilateral orbital metastasis from neuroblastoma in a 2-year-old girl, presenting with periorbital ecchymosis.

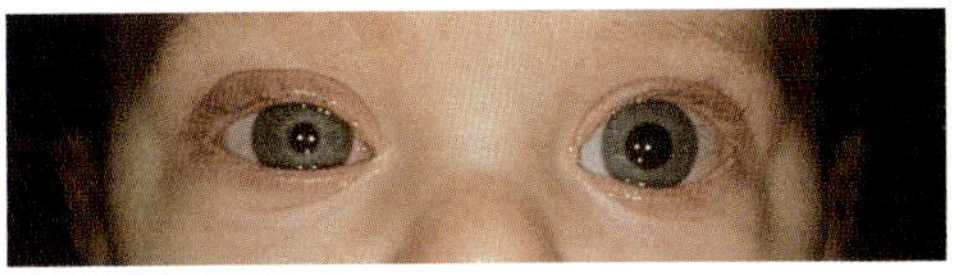

Figure 27-30 Right Horner syndrome, the presenting sign of localized intrathoracic neuroblastoma in a 6-month-old boy.

include abdominal fullness and pain, venous obstruction and edema, hypertension caused by renal vascular compromise, and bone pain. Urinalysis for catecholamines yields positive results in 90%–95% of cases.

Opsoclonus is a paraneoplastic syndrome characterized by rapid, multidirectional saccadic eye movements. It is associated with neuroblastoma but is not related to orbital involvement. Opsoclonus is associated with a good prognosis for survival, but neurologic deficits may persist. Primary cervical or apical thoracic neuroblastoma that involves the sympathetic chain may result in Horner syndrome (Fig 27-30).

Treatment modalities for neuroblastoma include surgery, chemotherapy, autologous stem cell transplant, immunotherapy, and radiation. Advances in multimodal treatments and supportive care have improved survival in children with neuroblastoma.

See BCSC Section 7, *Oculofacial Plastic and Orbital Surgery,* for additional information.

Coughlan D, Gianferante M, Lynch CF, Stevens JL, Harlan LC. Treatment and survival of childhood neuroblastoma: evidence from a population-based study in the United States. *Pediatr Hematol Oncol.* 2017;34(5):320–330.

CHAPTER 28

Pediatric Chronic Eye Care and Low Vision Rehabilitation

Highlights

- Successful management of pediatric chronic eye disease involves the child as a whole and accounts for potential barriers to treatment, including social determinants of health.
- Low vision rehabilitation in childhood can maximize the patient's ability to learn, thereby improving quality of life in the long term.

Pediatric Chronic Eye Care

For ophthalmologists who provide care to children with chronic eye disorders, there are 2 essential factors to address: (1) the child as a whole and (2) all potential barriers to treatment adherence (also see Chapter 25), including social determinants of health (SDOH).

If the eye disorder co-occurs with systemic disease (see Chapter 27), it is crucial that the manifestations of the disease and the possible adverse effects of its treatment be considered in the child's ophthalmic management plan. For instance, systemic therapies given in childhood may impact growth and development, and some can affect monocular and binocular reflexes crucial to the eye movements involved in reading (eg, convergence, accommodation, and saccades). Pediatric patients recovering from traumatic brain injury also may experience these deficits in visual function.

Visual impairment is more impactful when it occurs in childhood than in adulthood because of the effects on learning and development. Disorders as common as simple amblyopia have been associated with reading and hand–eye coordination difficulties. A team approach is crucial for comprehensive low vision rehabilitation in the pediatric population.

In caring for the whole child, addressing the psychological impact of the disease also is advised. Children may have fears about the visual impairment (eg, of it worsening) or may feel different from other children because of the disability or its appearance.

SDOH are conditions in the environment in which people grow, live, learn, work, and age that affect health outcomes. Over the past few decades, increasing evidence has suggested that complex social, physical, and economic conditions have a greater impact than medical care on health outcomes and life expectancy. Recognizing the social, economic, and physical conditions that different populations experience because of their environments is fundamental to understanding and addressing SDOH, which can be grouped into 5 domains:

- health care access and quality (eg, insurance, physician availability, communication)
- economic stability (eg, employment, income, housing, food security)
- education access and quality (eg, education, literacy, language skills)
- neighborhood and built environment (eg, transportation, safety, geography, parks)
- social and community context (eg, community engagement, social cohesion, incarceration rates)

The caregivers of children with chronic eye disorders face financial and time burdens and may have difficulties accessing and understanding the health care system. Adherence to the child's care plan may be compromised by barriers related to language, transportation, housing, employment, education, and other socioeconomic factors. Certain family dynamics also can disrupt continuity of care, including divorce, relocation, death, and adoption. Adolescence is a particularly vulnerable stage when patients begin to assume agency and responsibility over management of their chronic condition.

It is vital to recognize these barriers while striving to provide excellent care, regardless of gender, age, culture, race, religion, disability, national origin, socioeconomic status, or sexual orientation. Ophthalmologists can play an important role in addressing SDOH in vulnerable patient populations. Various strategies can be used:

- Assess the impact of SDOH in patients' lives as part of every patient encounter.
- Address biases in your practice.
- Provide patient-centered care based on the principles of empathy, curiosity, and respect.
- Integrate patient social support structures into your practice.
- Improve access to care and quality of care.

See Chapter 17 in BCSC Section 1, *Update on General Medicine,* for further discussion of social determinants of health.

Sokol R, Austin A, Chandler C, et al. Screening children for social determinants of health: a systematic review. *Pediatrics.* 2019;144(4):e20191622.

Pediatric Low Vision Rehabilitation

Vision is measured not only as visual acuity in the clinic, but also as visual perception and processing under a variety of real-world circumstances and environments. Vision rehabilitation and supportive care are advised for any visual impairment that affects the child's ability to access the visual environment, including best-corrected visual acuity worse than 20/40 in the better-seeing eye, decreased visual field, central field loss, reduced contrast sensitivity, nyctalopia, or impaired visual processing. From diagnosis onward, the ophthalmologist plays an important role in recommending that children with low vision receive comprehensive vision rehabilitation.

For children with acquired visual impairment, early referral is associated with better adjustment to the vision loss, optimal visual performance, improved access to instruction and learning, and achievement of safe and independent mobility. Even though preschool-aged children with impaired vision can function reasonably well without low vision aids, they ultimately have poorer school performance compared with visually impaired children who had received early intervention in preschool.

In pediatric vision rehabilitation, the care team may comprise the parents or caregivers, pediatric ophthalmologists, vision rehabilitation clinicians, teachers of the visually impaired (TVI), occupational therapists, other teachers, orientation and mobility specialists, technology experts, state societies, and other professionals and organizations.

In the United States, approaches for educating children with visual impairment vary regionally and include the following:

- state-funded residential schools for the visually impaired
- district-level clustering of students with visual impairment into the same school
- cooperation of schools with itinerant TVI at the neighborhood level (most common)

An individualized education plan (IEP) outlines the needs of an individual child in the school setting; a 504 plan can be implemented for those children with an isolated visual disability. The child's needs at home and in other nonacademic settings generally are considered independently from these plans.

Many children with partial sight can function well with low vision aids; others benefit from braille literacy, which is most easily acquired in childhood. Most children have large accommodative amplitudes, enabling them to hold an object closer than normal to enlarge its retinal image. Thus, magnification may not be necessary for very young patients with low vision. However, accommodative amplitudes decrease with age, and visual demands increase as students are faced with smaller print size. For these reasons, holding objects close to the eyes becomes an unsustainable strategy in older children.

For older children with visual impairment engaged in near work, printed material can be enlarged, and dome-type magnifiers may be utilized. Video magnification can be employed for near- or distance-vision tasks, and handheld monocular telescopes can assist with viewing at a distance. An array of tablets, smartphones, e-textbooks, and text-to-speech conversion software is available to meet the needs of visually impaired children; these technologies also have the advantage of being socially acceptable among peers. See also BCSC Section 3, *Clinical Optics and Vision Rehabilitation,* for a detailed discussion of low vision aids.

The American Academy of Ophthalmology's Preferred Practice Pattern guidelines on vision rehabilitation outline the rehabilitation process from early childhood to young adulthood. The availability of rehabilitation resources varies across communities, but the following online resources, which can be searched by location, may be helpful for clinicians and families seeking services in their community:

- American Foundation for the Blind: www.afb.org
- Texas School for the Blind and Visually Impaired resources home page: www.tsbvi.edu/tagged-resources

To learn about the Academy's Initiative in Vision Rehabilitation, visit the Low Vision and Vision Rehabilitation page, which also offers a patient handout, on the ONE Network at www.aao.org/low-vision-and-vision-rehab. Table 28-1 lists additional sources of information on low vision.

Table 28-1 Sources of Information on Low Vision

Websites

American Council of the Blind; www.acb.org
American Foundation for the Blind; www.afb.org
American Printing House for the Blind, Inc; www.aph.org
 Large-print and braille books, tapes, talking computer software, and low vision aids
Family Support America; www.familysupportamerica.org
 Parent support groups in the United States
Learning Ally; www.learningally.org
 Audiobooks for blind or dyslexic individuals
Lighthouse Guild; www.lighthouseguild.org
National Federation of the Blind; www.nfb.org
National Library Service for the Blind and Print Disabled, Library of Congress; www.loc.gov/nls
 Free library program of braille and audio materials, including books and magazines
National Organization for Albinism and Hypopigmentation; www.albinism.org
Prevent Blindness; www.preventblindness.org
Royal National Institute of Blind People (RNIB); www.rnib.org.uk

National toll-free numbers

American Council of the Blind; (800) 424-8666
New York Times Large-Print Weekly; (800) 631-2580
Reader's Digest Large Print; (877) 732-4438

American Academy of Ophthalmology Vision Rehabilitation Committee. Preferred Practice Pattern Guidelines. *Vision Rehabilitation.* American Academy of Ophthalmology; 2013. www.aao.org/ppp

APPENDIX

Strabismus Terminology

Definitions

The term *strabismus* is derived from the Greek word *strabismos*—"to squint, to look obliquely or askance"—and means ocular misalignment.

Orthophoria is the ideal condition of perfect ocular alignment, even during monocular viewing. In practice, orthophoria is seldom encountered, because a small heterophoria can be found in most people. *Orthotropia* is the term used more commonly, denoting correct ocular alignment under binocular conditions. Both terms describe eyes without manifest strabismus.

Heterophoria is an ocular deviation kept latent by the fusional mechanism (latent strabismus). *Heterotropia* is a deviation that is present when both eyes are open and used for viewing (manifest strabismus).

It is sometimes helpful to specify the deviating eye, particularly when vertical deviations or restrictive or paretic strabismus is being measured, or when amblyopia is present in a preverbal child.

Prefixes and Suffixes

A detailed nomenclature has evolved to describe the various types of ocular deviations. In this vocabulary, the prefix used indicates the relative position of the visual axes of the 2 eyes, or the direction of deviation.

Prefixes

Eso- The eye is rotated so that the visual axis is deviated nasally. Because the visual axes align at a point closer than the fixation target, this state is also known as *convergent strabismus,* a form of horizontal strabismus.

Exo- The eye is rotated so that the visual axis is deviated temporally. Because the visual axis of the deviated eye diverges from the fixation target, this state is also known as *divergent strabismus,* another form of horizontal strabismus.

Hyper- The eye is rotated so that the visual axis is deviated superiorly; this describes a form of *vertical strabismus.*

Hypo- The eye is rotated so that the visual axis is deviated inferiorly; this describes another form of *vertical strabismus.*

Incyclo- The eye is rotated so that the superior pole of the vertical meridian is rotated nasally. This state is known as *intorsion.*

Excyclo- The eye is rotated so that the superior pole of the vertical meridian is rotated temporally. This state is known as *extorsion.*

Suffixes

-phoria A latent deviation (eg, esophoria, exophoria, right hyperphoria, left hyperphoria); the deviation is controlled by the fusional mechanism so that the eyes remain aligned under binocular conditions.

-tropia A manifest deviation (eg, esotropia, exotropia, right hypertropia, left hypertropia); the deviation exceeds the control of the fusional mechanism so that the eyes are misaligned even under binocular conditions. Heterotropias can be constant or intermittent.

Strabismus Classification Terms

No classification system is perfect or all-inclusive. This section presents commonly used terms.

Onset

Infantile A deviation documented at or before age 6 months, presumably related to a defect present at birth. The term *congenital* is sometimes used, but that term may be less accurate because the deviation is usually not present at birth.

Acquired A deviation with onset after 6 months of age, following a period of presumably normal ocular alignment.

Consecutive A deviation that is in the direction opposite that of a previous strabismus. For example, consecutive exotropia is an exotropia that follows an esotropia (eg, as a result of overcorrection from surgery for esotropia).

Fixation

Alternating Spontaneous alternation of fixation from 1 eye to the other.

Monocular Fixation with 1 eye only.

Variation of the deviation with gaze position

Comitant (concomitant) The size of the deviation does not vary by more than a few prism diopters in different positions of gaze.

Incomitant (noncomitant) The deviation varies in size in different positions of gaze. Examples of incomitant deviations are cranial nerve VI palsy (deviation larger in the gaze direction ipsilateral to the palsy than the gaze direction contralateral to the palsy) and pattern strabismus (deviation different in upgaze and downgaze).

Primary deviation In patients with incomitant strabismus due to paresis or palsy, this is the deviation that occurs when the unaffected eye is in primary position and prism is held over the paretic eye.

Secondary deviation In patients with incomitant strabismus due to paresis or palsy, this is the deviation that occurs when the paretic eye is in primary position and prism is held over the unaffected eye. In individuals with paretic strabismus, the secondary deviation is larger than the primary deviation.

Miscellaneous terms

Overelevation in adduction and overdepression in adduction These motility anomalies—also sometimes termed *inferior oblique overaction* and *superior oblique overaction,* respectively—can be caused by overaction of the oblique muscles, as well as by other mechanisms (see Chapter 10).

Underelevation in adduction and underdepression in adduction These motility anomalies—also sometimes termed *inferior oblique underaction* and *superior oblique underaction,* respectively—can be caused by underaction of the oblique muscles, as well as by other mechanisms (see Chapter 10).

Dissociated strabismus complex This includes dissociated vertical deviation (DVD) (elevation of the nonfixating eye), dissociated horizontal deviation (typically abduction of the nonfixating eye), and dissociated torsional deviation (extorsion of the nonfixating eye). The term *dissociated* indicates that the characteristics of the relative misalignment of the eyes depend on which eye is fixating. In DVD, when the right eye is fixating, the nonfixating left eye elevates; the vertical deviation is a *left* hyperdeviation. However, when the left eye is fixating, the nonfixating right eye elevates; the vertical deviation is a *right* hyperdeviation. No other type of strabismus varies like this according to which eye is fixating.

Abbreviations for Notation of Strabismus

Addition of the prime symbol (′) to any of the following indicates that measurement of ocular alignment is made at near fixation (eg, E′ indicates esophoria at near).

E, X, RH, LH Esophoria, exophoria, right hyperphoria, left hyperphoria at distance fixation, respectively.

ET, XT, RHT, LHT Constant esotropia, exotropia, right hypertropia, left hypertropia at distance fixation, respectively.

E(T), X(T), RH(T), LH(T) Intermittent esotropia, exotropia, right hypertropia, left hypertropia at distance fixation, respectively. The addition of parentheses around the *T* indicates an intermittent tropia.

RHoT, LHoT Right hypotropia, left hypotropia at distance fixation, respectively.

OEAd or IOOA Overelevation in adduction or inferior oblique overaction, respectively.

ODAd or SOOA Overdepression in adduction or superior oblique overaction, respectively.

UDAd or SOUA Underdepression in adduction or superior oblique underaction, respectively.

UEAd or IOUA Underelevation in adduction or inferior oblique underaction, respectively.

DSC Dissociated strabismus complex.

DHD, DTD, DVD Dissociated horizontal deviation, dissociated torsional deviation, dissociated vertical deviation, respectively.

Additional Materials and Resources

Related Academy Materials

The American Academy of Ophthalmology is dedicated to providing a wealth of high-quality clinical education resources for ophthalmologists.

Print Publications and Electronic Products

For a complete listing of Academy products related to topics covered in this BCSC Section, visit our online store at:

https://store.aao.org/clinical-education/topic/pediatric-ophth-strabismus.html

Or call Customer Service at 866.561.8558 (toll free, US only) or +1 415.561.8540, Monday through Friday, between 8:00 AM and 5:00 PM (PST).

Online Resources

Visit the Ophthalmic News and Education (ONE®) Network at https://www.aao.org/pediatric-ophthalmology-strabismus to find relevant videos, online courses, journal articles, practice guidelines, self-assessment quizzes, images, and more. The ONE Network is a free Academy-member benefit.

Access free, trusted articles and content with the Academy's collaborative online encyclopedia, EyeWiki, at aao.org/eyewiki.

Get mobile access to the *Wills Eye Manual,* watch the latest 1-minute videos, and set up alerts for clinical updates relevant to you with the AAO Ophthalmic Education App. Download today: Search for "AAO Ophthalmic Education" in the Apple app store or in Google Play.

Basic Texts and Additional Resources

Brodsky MC. *Pediatric Neuro-Ophthalmology.* 3rd ed. Springer-Verlag; 2016.

Buckley EG, Freedman S, Shields MB. *Atlas of Ophthalmic Surgery, Vol III: Strabismus and Glaucoma.* Mosby-Year Book; 1995.

Buckley EG, Plager DA, Repka MX, Wilson ME. *Strabismus Surgery: Basic and Advanced Strategies.* Oxford University Press; 2005.

Coats DK, Olitsky SE. *Strabismus Surgery and Its Complications.* Springer-Verlag; 2007.

Dutton J. *Atlas of Clinical and Surgical Orbital Anatomy.* 2nd ed. Elsevier; 2011.

Hartnett ME, ed. *Pediatric Retina.* 3rd ed. Wolters Kluwer; 2020.

Helveston EM. *Surgical Management of Strabismus.* 5th ed. Wayenborgh Publishing; 2005.*

Jones KL, Jones MC, del Campo M. *Smith's Recognizable Patterns of Human Malformation.* 8th ed. Elsevier; 2021.

Katowitz JA, Katowitz WR. *Pediatric Oculoplastic Surgery.* 2nd ed. Springer; 2018.

Lambert SR, Lyons CJ, eds. *Taylor and Hoyt's Pediatric Ophthalmology and Strabismus.* 5th ed. Elsevier; 2017.

Leigh RJ, Zee DS. *The Neurology of Eye Movements.* 5th ed. Oxford University Press; 2015.

Miller NR, Newman NJ, Biousse V, Kerrison JB, eds. *Walsh and Hoyt's Clinical Neuro-Ophthalmology.* 6th ed. Lippincott Williams & Wilkins; 2005.

Nelson LB, Olitsky SE, eds. *Harley's Pediatric Ophthalmology.* 6th ed. Lippincott Williams & Wilkins; 2014.

Parks MM. *Atlas of Strabismus Surgery.* Harper & Row; 1983.

Parks MM. *Ocular Motility and Strabismus.* Harper & Row; 1975.

Pratt-Johnson JA, Tillson G. *Management of Strabismus and Amblyopia: A Practical Guide.* 2nd ed. Thieme; 2001.

Rosenbaum AL, Santiago AP, eds. *Clinical Strabismus Management: Principles and Surgical Techniques.* Saunders; 1999.

Tasman W, Jaeger EA, eds. *Duane's Ophthalmology on DVD-ROM.* Lippincott Williams & Wilkins; 2013.

Traboulsi EI. *A Compendium of Inherited Disorders and the Eye.* Oxford University Press; 2006.

von Noorden GK. *Atlas of Strabismus.* 4th ed. Mosby; 1983.

von Noorden GK, Campos EC. *Binocular Vision and Ocular Motility.* 6th ed. Mosby; 2002.*

von Noorden GK, Helveston EM. *Strabismus: A Decision Making Approach.* Mosby; 1994.*

Wilson ME, Saunders RA, Trivedi RH, eds. *Pediatric Ophthalmology: Current Thought and A Practical Guide.* Springer; 2009.

Wright KW, Strube YJ, eds. *Color Atlas of Strabismus Surgery: Strategies and Techniques.* 4th ed. Springer; 2015.

Wright KW, Strube YJ, eds. *Pediatric Ophthalmology and Strabismus.* 3rd ed. Oxford University Press; 2012.

* Available online on the Ophthalmic News and Education (ONE®) Network in the Pediatric Ophthalmology Education Center (https://www.aao.org/pediatric-ophthalmology-strabismus) and on the Cybersight website (https://cybersight.org).

Requesting Continuing Medical Education Credit

The American Academy of Ophthalmology is accredited by the Accreditation Council for Continuing Medical Education (ACCME) to provide continuing medical education for physicians.

The American Academy of Ophthalmology designates this enduring material for a maximum of 15 *AMA PRA Category 1 Credits*™. Physicians should claim only the credit commensurate with the extent of their participation in the activity.

To claim *AMA PRA Category 1 Credits*™ upon completion of this activity, learners must demonstrate appropriate knowledge and participation in the activity by taking the posttest for Section 6 and achieving a score of 80% or higher.

This activity meets the Self-Assessment CME requirements defined by the American Board of Ophthalmology (ABO). Please be advised that the ABO is not an accrediting body for purposes of any CME program. ABO does not sponsor this or any outside activity, and ABO does not endorse any particular CME activity. Complete information regarding the ABO Self-Assessment CME Maintenance of Certification requirements is available at https://abop.org/maintain-certification/cme-self-assessment/.

To take the posttest and request CME credit online:

1. Go to www.aao.org/cme-central and log in.
2. Click on "Claim CME Credit and View My CME Transcript" and then "Report AAO Credits."
3. Select the appropriate media type and then the Academy activity. You will be directed to the posttest.
4. Once you have passed the test with a score of 80% or higher, you will be directed to your transcript. *If you are not an Academy member, you will be able to print out a certificate of participation once you have passed the test.*

CME expiration date: June 1, 2025. *AMA PRA Category 1 Credits*™ may be claimed only once between June 1, 2022, and the expiration date.

For assistance, contact the Academy's Customer Service department at 866.561.8558 (US only) or +1 415.561.8540 between 8:00 AM and 5:00 PM (PST), Monday through Friday, or send an e-mail to customer_service@aao.org.

Study Questions

Please note that these questions are not part of your CME reporting process. They are provided here for your own educational use and for identification of any professional practice gaps. The required CME posttest is available online (see "Requesting Continuing Medical Education Credit"). Following the questions are answers with discussions. Although a concerted effort has been made to avoid ambiguity and redundancy in these questions, the authors recognize that differences of opinion may occur regarding the "best" answer. The discussions are provided to demonstrate the rationale used to derive the answer. They may also be helpful in confirming that your approach to the problem was correct or, if necessary, in fixing the principle in your memory. The Section 6 faculty thanks the Resident Self-Assessment Committee for developing these self-assessment questions and the discussions that follow.

1. In testing visual acuity in preliterate children, what optotype has the best calibration and reliability?
   a. HOTV
   b. Tumbling E
   c. Allen figures
   d. Lighthouse chart

2. The lateral muscular branch of the ophthalmic artery supplies which extraocular muscle (EOM)?
   a. superior rectus
   b. medial rectus
   c. inferior rectus
   d. inferior oblique

3. In right gaze, the innervation to the right lateral rectus will increase. What determines the amount of innervation to the right medial rectus in this situation?
   a. arc of contact
   b. Sherrington's law
   c. vergence amplitudes
   d. recruitment

4. What are the primary synergistic (yoke) muscles that are used for gazing up and to the right?
   a. left inferior oblique and right superior oblique
   b. left superior rectus and right inferior oblique
   c. left inferior oblique and right superior rectus
   d. left superior oblique and right superior rectus

5. In a complete cranial nerve (CN) III palsy, what action of the superior oblique muscle exacerbates the outward position of the eye?
   a. primary
   b. secondary
   c. tertiary
   d. quaternary

6. A parent brings a child to the clinic for evaluation of strabismus. What finding on examination would suggest that the strabismus is long-standing?
   a. incomitant deviation
   b. diplopia
   c. anomalous retinal correspondence (ARC)
   d. normal head position

7. What is the essential feature of monofixation syndrome?
   a. normal stereo acuity
   b. loss of peripheral sensory fusion
   c. amblyopia
   d. presence of peripheral fusion with the absence of bifoveal fusion

8. To test for a horizontal deviation using the Maddox rod, in what direction should the cylinders be placed in front of the right eye?
   a. 15° meridian
   b. 45° meridian
   c. 90° meridian
   d. 180° meridian

9. A patient has a comitant esotropia. What is the most likely diagnosis?
   a. nasal wall fracture
   b. infantile esotropia
   c. thyroid orbitopathy
   d. CN VI palsy

10. A 12-year-old boy is diagnosed with well-controlled, intermittent exotropia. What is stereopsis testing most likely to reveal?
   a. monofixation syndrome
   b. no stereopsis because of diplopia
   c. excellent stereopsis
   d. no stereopsis because of temporal hemiretinal suppression

11. A 6-year-old child presents with a 35 prism diopters (Δ) intermittent exotropia at distance and a 20Δ intermittent exotropia at near. After the patch test, measurements for this patient are 35Δ exotropia at distance and 30Δ exotropia at near. What is the most likely diagnosis?
    a. pseudodivergence excess intermittent exotropia
    b. divergence excess intermittent exotropia
    c. intermittent exotropia with a high accommodative convergence/accommodation (AC/A) ratio
    d. basic intermittent exotropia

12. What is the most appropriate surgery to perform for a V-pattern esotropia without overelevation in adduction?
    a. bilateral medial rectus recession with inferior transposition (inferoplacement)
    b. bilateral medial rectus recession with superior transposition (superoplacement)
    c. bilateral lateral rectus resection with inferior transposition (inferoplacement)
    d. unilateral medial rectus recession and lateral rectus resection with inferior transposition (inferoplacement)

13. What pattern strabismus would be most successfully addressed with bilateral weakening of the inferior oblique muscles?
    a. A pattern
    b. V pattern
    c. X pattern
    d. Y pattern

14. A patient undergoes surgery to repair an orbital floor fracture and free an entrapped inferior rectus muscle. The surgery is technically successful. Postoperatively, a hypotropia is present in that eye and persists for 6 months following the surgery. What surgery is most likely to provide benefit at this time?
    a. superior rectus resection
    b. inferior rectus recession
    c. re-exploration of the fracture
    d. transposition procedure

15. What defines type 2 Duane syndrome?
    a. poor adduction and exotropia
    b. poor abduction and esotropia
    c. poor abduction and adduction
    d. poor abduction and exotropia

16. What intracranial structural abnormality could most likely account for new-onset downbeat nystagmus in a 4-year-old girl?
    a. pinealoma
    b. chiasmal tumor
    c. craniopharyngioma
    d. Arnold-Chiari malformation

17. A 6-year-old child undergoes bilateral 5-mm medial rectus recession for 35Δ esotropia. One week after surgery, there is a measurement of 30Δ exotropia. What is the most appropriate test to perform next?
    a. test of EOM movements
    b. measurement of stereopsis
    c. measurement of vertical deviations
    d. slit-lamp examination

18. What sort of anomaly is represented by a choroidal coloboma?
    a. agenesis
    b. hypoplasia
    c. hyperplasia
    d. dysraphism

19. The results of a cycloplegic retinoscopy in an otherwise healthy, asymptomatic 3-year-old child are likely to reveal what approximate refractive error?
    a. 0.00–1.00 diopters (D) myopia
    b. 0.00–1.00 D hyperopia
    c. 2.00–3.00 D hyperopia
    d. 2.00–3.00 D myopia

20. A 4-month-old boy does not fix or follow but has an otherwise normal eye examination. The child is reexamined when he is 6 months old and is noted to have normal responses to visual stimuli. What is the most likely diagnosis?
    a. cerebral visual impairment (CVI)
    b. delayed visual maturation (DVM)
    c. intrauterine infection
    d. uncorrected high refractive error

21. For a 5-month-old child with poor visual behavior but no nystagmus, what diagnosis is likely?
    a. retinal dystrophy
    b. CVI
    c. optic nerve hypoplasia
    d. congenital cataract

22. For a child with right severe congenital ptosis and no ipsilateral levator function, what is the most appropriate method of ptosis repair?
    a. blepharoplasty
    b. levator resection
    c. frontalis suspension
    d. brow lift

23. Blepharophimosis–ptosis–epicanthus inversus syndrome is usually inherited in what manner?
    a. autosomal dominant
    b. autosomal recessive
    c. X-linked dominant
    d. X-linked recessive

24. Crouzon syndrome differs from Apert syndrome in that the latter is associated with what finding?
    a. hypertelorism
    b. proptosis
    c. significant syndactyly
    d. inferior scleral show

25. What is the most common type of strabismus associated with craniosynostosis?
    a. A-pattern esotropia
    b. V-pattern esotropia
    c. V-pattern exotropia
    d. A-pattern exotropia

26. A 4-day-old infant presents with chemosis, significant discharge, and corneal ulceration. What is the most likely diagnosis?
    a. chemical conjunctivitis
    b. herpes simplex virus conjunctivitis
    c. *Neisseria gonorrhoeae* conjunctivitis
    d. chlamydial conjunctivitis

27. What is an early ocular manifestation of Stevens-Johnson syndrome?
    a. mucopurulent conjunctivitis
    b. symblepharon
    c. corneal vascularization
    d. entropion

28. A child with new-onset ptosis should be examined for what other potentially associated finding?
    a. cataract
    b. anisocoria
    c. dacryostenosis
    d. corneal haze

29. In patients with aniridia, what is the most common cause of progressive corneal scarring?
    a. endothelial decompensation
    b. exposure keratopathy
    c. limbal stem cell deficiency
    d. herpes simplex keratitis

30. A 6-week-old boy presents with unilateral epiphora and ocular irritation. The cornea is enlarged but clear. The intraocular pressure (IOP) is 38 mm Hg. What is the preferred initial treatment?
    a. Ahmed valve placement
    b. cycloablation via diode laser
    c. trabeculectomy
    d. goniotomy

31. What is the preferred laboratory testing for a child with a unilateral congenital cataract?
    a. TORCH (*t*oxoplasmosis, *o*ther agents, *r*ubella, *c*ytomegalovirus, *h*erpes simplex) titers
    b. serum for calcium and phosphorus
    c. no testing (typically none is needed)
    d. urine for amino acids

32. Children with optic nerve hypoplasia should undergo magnetic resonance imaging (MRI) to evaluate for what finding?
    a. bifid septum pellucidum
    b. empty sella
    c. ectopic posterior pituitary bright spot
    d. chiasmal glioma

33. What growth pattern of retinoblastoma is most likely to be mistaken as childhood uveitis?
    a. diffuse infiltrating
    b. retinocytoma
    c. unilateral multifocal
    d. unilateral unifocal

34. A 6-month-old child has poor vision with nystagmus and eye-poking. The retinal appearance is normal. What is the best test to evaluate this patient?
    a. MRI
    b. fluorescein angiography
    c. A-scan ultrasonography
    d. electroretinography

35. An infant is diagnosed with type 1, prethreshold retinopathy of prematurity (ROP). What is the best step in management, according to the Early Treatment for Retinopathy of Prematurity (ETROP) study?
    a. observation
    b. cryotherapy to ablate the peripheral retina
    c. panretinal laser photocoagulation to ablate the peripheral retina
    d. intravitreal injection of steroid

36. What test is most likely to determine the etiology of anterior uveitis in a child?
    a. antinuclear antibodies
    b. rheumatoid factor
    c. human leukocyte antigen B27 (HLA-B27)
    d. Lyme serology

37. Tubulointerstitial nephritis is associated with what ocular condition?
    a. bilateral anterior uveitis
    b. cataract formation
    c. serous retinal detachment
    d. papilledema

38. Spontaneous hyphema can occur with what intraocular lesion?
    a. juvenile xanthogranuloma of the iris
    b. iris nevus
    c. iris capillary hemangioma
    d. iris cyst

39. The greatest risk of rebleeding in traumatic hyphema occurs how long after initial injury?
    a. 3–7 days
    b. 8–12 days
    c. 13–17 days
    d. 18–25 days

40. What is the most common ocular manifestation of abusive head trauma (AHT)?
    a. corneal abrasion
    b. hyphema
    c. subconjunctival hemorrhage
    d. retinal hemorrhage

41. What condition is associated with an abnormally high number of crossed fibers in the optic chiasm?
    a. ocular albinism
    b. optic nerve hypoplasia
    c. achromatopsia
    d. morning glory disc anomaly

42. A 4-year-old boy presents with salt-and-pepper fundus and cataracts in both eyes. What congenital infection did he most likely have?
    a. rubella
    b. toxoplasmosis
    c. toxocariasis
    d. syphilis

43. A child has uncontrolled glaucoma due to encephalofacial angiomatosis (also known as Sturge-Weber syndrome). If glaucoma surgery is needed, what is a particular intraoperative risk?
    a. choroidal hemorrhage
    b. hyphema
    c. exposure of tube under conjunctiva
    d. leakage from trabeculectomy flap

44. Hermansky-Pudlak albinism is associated with what systemic clinical feature?
    a. soft tissue tumors
    b. recurrent infections
    c. easy bruising
    d. immunoglobulin A deficiency

Answers

1. **a.** Various optotypes are available for recognition visual acuity testing in preliterate children. LEA symbols and the HOTV test are reliably calibrated and have high testability rates for preschool-aged children. For a shy child, testability may be improved by having the child point to match optotypes on a chart with those on a handheld card rather than verbally identify them. Several symbol charts, such as Allen figures and the Lighthouse chart, are not recommended by the World Health Organization or the National Academy of Sciences because the optotypes are considered confusing, culturally biased, or nonstandardized. The Tumbling E chart is accurate but conceptually difficult for many preschool-aged children.
2. **a.** The muscular branches of the ophthalmic artery provide the most important blood supply to the extraocular muscles (EOMs). The lateral muscular branch supplies the lateral rectus, superior rectus, superior oblique, and levator palpebrae superioris muscles; the medial muscular branch, the larger of the 2, supplies the inferior rectus, medial rectus, and inferior oblique muscles.
3. **b.** Sherrington's law of reciprocal innervation states that increased innervation of a given EOM is accompanied by a reciprocal decrease in innervation of its antagonist. As the right eye abducts, innervation of the right lateral rectus muscle increases and innervation of the right medial rectus muscle decreases. The arc of contact refers to the length of muscle in contact with the globe. Vergence amplitudes have to do with the eyes working together to converge or diverge. Recruitment is the orderly increase in the number of activated motor units, thus increasing the strength of muscle contraction.
4. **c.** The left inferior oblique and right superior rectus muscles are the prime agonists for gazing up and to the right. The superior oblique muscle is an eye depressor, and the main elevation action of the right inferior oblique is in left gaze.
5. **c.** The tertiary action of the superior oblique is abduction, and this exacerbates the outward position of the eye in a complete cranial nerve (CN) III palsy. In a complete CN III palsy, the only functioning EOMs are the lateral rectus and superior oblique.
6. **c.** Anomalous retinal correspondence (ARC) occurs when the fovea of the fixating eye has acquired a visual direction in common with a peripheral retinal element in the deviated eye. This is an adaptive mechanism that takes time to develop; therefore, a short history of esotropia would not be associated with ARC. Abnormal head position, "spread of comitance," and suppression, as opposed to diplopia, would be features suggesting a longstanding deviation.
7. **d.** Monofixation syndrome is a sensory state in strabismus where peripheral fusion is present and bifoveal fusion is absent, due to a macular scotoma. Thus, amblyopia may be present in the deviated eye, along with a reduction of stereopsis. Because of peripheral fusion and anomalous retinal correspondence, the Worth 4-dot test demonstrates suppression at distance, but fusion at near.
8. **d.** In the Maddox rod test, a series of parallel cylinders convert a point source of light into a line image perpendicular to the cylinders. To test for horizontal deviations, the Maddox rod cylinders are placed horizontally in front of the right eye (180° meridian). The patient, fixating on a point source of light, sees a vertical line with the right eye and the point source of light with the left.

9. **b.** A comitant deviation is one in which the size of the deviation does not vary by more than a few prism diopters (Δ) in different positions of gaze or with either eye used for fixating. Of the choices provided, the best answer is infantile esotropia. A restrictive orbitopathy (such as nasal wall fracture with entrapment or thyroid orbitopathy) or a paretic process (such as CN VI palsy) would lead to an incomitant deviation, in which the measurement varies significantly in different positions of gaze.

10. **c.** Intermittent exotropia is an outward deviation that becomes manifest during times of visual inattention, fatigue, or stress. In the early stages of the disorder, the deviation is usually larger for distance viewing than for near. Thus, sensory testing at near is typically excellent, including stereopsis and fusion on Worth 4-dot testing. When the eye deviates, suppression of the image typically occurs, rather than the recognition of diplopia.

11. **a.** When the exodeviation at distance is larger than the deviation at near fixation by 10Δ or more but the distance and near measurements become similar after 30–60 minutes of binocular occlusion using a patch (the patch test), pseudodivergence excess intermittent exotropia is the likely diagnosis. In true divergence excess intermittent exotropia, the distance–near discrepancy would persist after patch testing. A patient with distance–near discrepancy may have a high accommodative convergence/accommodation (AC/A) ratio, which would be defined by persistence of the distance–near discrepancy after the patch test but resolution of this discrepancy with a +3.00 add. In a patient with basic intermittent exotropia, the measurement of the deviation at distance would be within 10Δ of the deviation measurement at near without patch testing or a +3.00 add.

12. **a.** In a V-pattern esotropia, the medial rectus muscles can be recessed and moved toward the apex of the deviation, which would be inferiorly in this case. Lateral muscles should be moved away from the apex of the deviation. A useful mnemonic is MALE: *m*edial rectus muscle to the *a*pex, *l*ateral rectus muscle to the *e*mpty space. When horizontal muscle recession-resection is performed, displacement should be in opposite directions, but this could cause symptomatic torsion.

13. **b.** Inferior oblique overaction commonly causes a V pattern. A patterns are most commonly caused by superior oblique overaction. X and Y patterns result from pseudo-overaction of the inferior oblique muscles; weakening them would not collapse the pattern.

14. **b.** Despite the repair of the orbital floor and release of the entrapped muscle, restriction can persist, so re-exploration of the fracture will not be of benefit. In these cases, recession of the restricted muscle is the next step. An inferior rectus recession is indicated in this case. A superior rectus resection may be done if the inferior rectus recession results in undercorrection. A transposition could be considered for a muscle palsy, but an inferior rectus muscle palsy would result in a hypertropia, not a hypotropia.

15. **a.** Type 1, the most common form of Duane syndrome, is classically characterized by poor abduction and esotropia. A patient may adopt a head turn to establish binocular fusion, and the esotropia may be seen only in primary gaze or with a head turn to the opposite direction. Type 2 is classically characterized by limited adduction and exotropia. Type 3 is characterized by poor abduction and adduction; either esotropia or exotropia may result.

16. **d.** Acquired downbeat nystagmus can be secondary to Arnold-Chiari malformation. Pinealoma is associated with convergence-retraction nystagmus. Chiasmal tumors have been associated with spasmus nutans, a triad of nystagmus, head bobbing, and torticollis. Craniopharyngioma is associated with see-saw nystagmus.

17. **a.** The extreme overcorrection suggests that there is a slipped medial rectus muscle. This would be evident by limited adduction in either eye. In this patient, absence of stereopsis would be expected but not helpful diagnostically. Vertical measurements would not be helpful, nor would findings from a slit-lamp examination.
18. **d.** Dysraphism represents a failure to fuse. Agenesis represents developmental failure, as is found in anophthalmia, whereas hypoplasia is due to developmental arrest. Developmental excess such as that observed with distichiasis is the cause of hyperplasia.
19. **c.** A 3-year-old child is expected to have some hyperopia, approximately between 2.00 and 3.00 diopters (D). Infants are hyperopic and can become slightly more hyperopic until approximately 6–8 years of age. Then the refraction shifts toward plano until approximately age 16, during the process of emmetropization. If myopia presents before age 10 years, later high myopia (6.00 D or more) has a greater likelihood of developing. Low amounts of astigmatism, typically with the rule, are common in infants and can resolve. Large ametropias or anisometropias can be amblyogenic.
20. **b.** The term *delayed visual maturation (DVM)* describes a condition wherein normal fixation and tracking do not develop within the first 3–4 months of life, but visual behavior subsequently normalizes. Cerebral visual impairment (CVI) is caused by pathology posterior to the lateral geniculate nucleus. CVI can be congenital or acquired. Causes include structural central nervous system abnormalities, intrauterine infection, periventricular leukomalacia, hypoxia, hydrocephalus, abusive head trauma, and encephalitis. Although some improvement in vision can occur, a complete normalization of vision is uncommon. Uncorrected refractive error and intrauterine infection would not be associated with spontaneous normalization of vision.
21. **b.** When vision loss is due to pathology posterior to the lateral geniculate nucleus, nystagmus is generally not present.
22. **c.** As long as there is adequate levator function, levator resection is an appropriate option for congenital ptosis treatment; in this case, levator resection would fail. Neither blepharoplasty nor brow lift would be successful—congenital ptosis is not typically associated with dermatochalasis or brow ptosis. In this case, a frontalis suspension is the appropriate procedure. Harvesting autologous fascia lata may be difficult in very young children. Many surgeons would utilize either suture (prolene, nylon) or a silicone rod to temporarily elevate the eyelid and proceed with a fascial sling once the child is older. Some surgeons would opt for banked fascia lata.
23. **a.** Blepharophimosis–ptosis–epicanthus inversus syndrome may occur as a sporadic or autosomal-dominant disorder. It consists of blepharophimosis, congenital ptosis, telecanthus, and epicanthus inversus. Surgery may be necessary early in life.
24. **c.** Crouzon and Apert syndromes appear similar clinically. However, Apert syndrome is associated with an extreme amount of syndactyly. Both syndromes are associated with hypertelorism, proptosis, and inferior scleral show.
25. **c.** Patients with craniosynostoses can have various types of horizontal strabismus. V-pattern exotropia is the most common type.
26. **c.** Ophthalmia neonatorum caused by *Neisseria gonorrhoeae* typically presents in the first 3–4 days of life. In severe cases, it is associated with marked chemosis, significant discharge, and a risk of corneal perforation. Chemical conjunctivitis is a mild, self-limited inflammation occurring in the first 24 hours of life due to instillation of silver nitrate.

Herpes simplex virus conjunctivitis usually presents later, often in the second week of life. Chlamydial conjunctivitis usually occurs around 1 week of age and is associated with minimal to moderate discharge and possible pseudomembrane formation.

27. **a.** Stevens-Johnson syndrome is a hypersensitivity reaction that affects the skin and mucous membranes. Early ocular involvement may range from conjunctivitis to corneal perforation. Symblepharon, corneal vascularization, and eyelid anomalies such as entropion are later sequelae.

28. **b.** Horner syndrome caused by a lesion along the oculosympathetic pathway must be ruled out in a patient with new-onset ptosis. Affected patients have anisocoria that is greater in dim light and ptosis secondary to paralysis of the Müller muscle. In a child, new-onset Horner syndrome can be idiopathic or secondary to trauma, surgery, or neuroblastoma along the sympathetic chain in the chest. Cataract, dacryostenosis, and corneal haze are not associated with acute ptosis.

29. **c.** Classic aniridia is autosomal dominant, associated with a pathogenic variant in the *PAX6* gene. Large deletions of the gene are typically sporadic and can confer a risk for Wilms tumor of the kidney. Patients with congenital aniridia can develop progressive corneal scarring within the first decade of life, necessitating corneal transplantation to restore vision. Adult patients with aniridia can also develop later-onset issues with nonhealing epithelial defects and corneal neovascularization. The major underlying mechanism is related to limbal stem cell deficiency, although abnormal cell differentiation may play a role as well.

30. **d.** Congenital glaucoma can present with epiphora and ocular irritation. The initial treatment is surgical, with goniotomy or trabeculotomy preferred for the initial treatment. Primary trabeculectomy has a high failure rate and is contraindicated as primary treatment. Both Ahmed valve placement and cycloablation are reserved for secondary treatments.

31. **c.** Unilateral cataracts are not usually associated with occult systemic or metabolic disease; therefore, laboratory tests are not warranted. Note that bilateral cataracts can have significant asymmetry. In cases of bilateral cataracts, the history and physical examination guide whether and which laboratory investigations are indicated. A complete ocular evaluation is needed to rule out a secondary ocular cause.

32. **c.** Optic nerve hypoplasia is characterized by a decreased number of optic nerve axons. It is associated with absence of the septum pellucidum, not a bifid septum pellucidum; with agenesis of the corpus callosum; and with pituitary gland abnormalities. Magnetic resonance imaging (MRI) reveals an ectopic posterior pituitary bright spot at the upper infundibulum. This finding is associated with pituitary hormone deficiencies. Optic nerve hypoplasia is not associated with an empty sella on MRI. Chiasmal gliomas are associated with optic nerve elevation, not optic nerve hypoplasia.

33. **a.** Diffuse infiltrating retinoblastoma can mimic childhood uveitis. It typically presents in older children (5–6 years old). Retinocytoma is a spontaneously regressed retinoblastoma.

34. **d.** Early-onset inherited retinal disorders (IRDs) are genotypically and phenotypically heterogeneous. Because the retinal appearance is sometimes normal in early-onset IRDs, signs and symptoms are particularly important to recognize. For early-onset IRDs, nystagmus is one of the most common presenting signs, typically occurring between 8 and 12 weeks of age. In addition to poor vision, symptoms include nyctalopia, photodysphoria, and eye-poking (oculodigital sign). Signs include paradoxical pupil and high refractive error. An electroretinogram is typically used to make the diagnosis, showing extinguished waveforms.

A-scan ultrasonography, fluorescein angiography, and MRI would not be helpful in making the diagnosis.

35. **c.** Prethreshold retinopathy of prematurity (ROP) is classified into 2 types. Type 1 includes zone I, any stage ROP with plus disease; zone I, stage 3 ROP, without plus disease; and zone II, stage 2 or 3 ROP, with plus disease. The Early Treatment for Retinopathy of Prematurity (ETROP) trial found that earlier treatment at prethreshold resulted in better structural and visual outcomes when compared with conventional treatment at threshold. On the basis of ETROP, laser treatment is recommended for any eye with type 1 ROP.

36. **a.** The most common identifiable etiology of anterior uveitis in a child is juvenile idiopathic arthritis, which occurs in 15%–47% of cases. Antinuclear antibody positivity is typically present in these children; rheumatoid factor is typically negative. Although juvenile spondyloarthropathies are associated with anterior uveitis in children, they are less common; thus, human leukocyte antigen B27 (HLA-B27) testing is less likely to be beneficial. Infectious etiologies of anterior uveitis in children are less common, and results of serologic testing are less likely to reveal the etiology in these patients.

37. **a.** Tubulointerstitial nephritis and uveitis (TINU) syndrome is kidney disease associated with chronic or recurrent anterior uveitis in adolescents; the median age at onset is 15 years. The renal disease is characterized by low-grade fever, fatigue, pallor, and weight loss. The uveitis is usually bilateral and may occur before, simultaneously with, or after the renal disease. TINU nephritis is not commonly associated with cataract, serous retinal detachment, or papilledema.

38. **a.** Although trauma is the most common cause of hyphema in children, spontaneous hyphemas can occur in juvenile xanthogranuloma of the iris, retinoblastoma, leukemia, and blood dyscrasias. Iris nevus, iris capillary hemangioma, and iris cyst are not associated with spontaneous hyphema formation.

39. **a.** One of the risks of hyphema is rebleeding, with worsening symptoms. This is especially critical in children, who often do not adhere to activity restrictions. The greatest risk for rebleeding occurs within 3 to 7 days. After 7 days, the risk progressively decreases.

40. **d.** The most common ocular manifestation of abusive head trauma (AHT), present in approximately 80% of cases, is retinal hemorrhage. These hemorrhages can be seen in all layers of the retina and may be unilateral or bilateral. They are found most commonly in the posterior pole but can also be present peripherally. The anterior segment and ocular adnexa are often normal. Hyphema, corneal abrasion, and subconjunctival hemorrhages are less commonly seen in AHT.

41. **a.** Ocular albinism is associated with iris transillumination, foveal aplasia or hypoplasia, and decreased retinal pigmentation. Both human and animal studies have shown an abnormally high number of crossed fibers in the optic chiasm, which precludes stereopsis and is associated with strabismus. Optic nerve hypoplasia and morning glory disc anomaly are not associated with abnormalities in the crossed fibers of the optic chiasm. Achromatopsia is not typically associated with optic nerve abnormalities.

42. **a.** Congenital rubella syndrome is caused by rubella virus that is transmitted transplacentally to a fetus. Eye findings include a variable pigmentary retinopathy, ranging from a salt-and-pepper appearance to pseudoretinitis pigmentosa. In this case, the patient has macular pigmentary changes as well as peripheral pigmentary changes. Other eye findings

in congenital rubella syndrome include cataract, glaucoma, and microphthalmia. Rubella has also been identified as a cause of Fuchs heterochromic iridocyclitis. Extraocular manifestations include hearing loss and cardiac abnormalities.

43. **a.** Encephalofacial angiomatosis, or Sturge-Weber syndrome, is a capillary malformation of the leptomeninges with or without ocular or facial involvement. This patient has the classic manifestations of a port-wine birthmark and associated glaucoma manifesting as an enlarged cornea. Encephalofacial angiomatosis glaucoma is difficult to treat. Surgery is indicated in early-onset cases and when medical treatment is inadequate. Multiple operations are typically necessary. A particular risk of glaucoma surgery in encephalofacial angiomatosis is intraoperative or postoperative exudation or hemorrhage from anomalous choroidal vessels; this complication is caused by rapid ocular decompression. The other complications (hyphema, exposure of tube under conjunctiva, leakage from trabeculectomy flap) are not particularly higher in encephalofacial angiomatosis glaucoma.

44. **c.** Albinism can be part of a broader syndrome, such as Hermansky-Pudlak syndrome, which is associated with bleeding abnormalities and pulmonary interstitial fibrosis. This syndrome occurs with higher frequency in persons with Puerto Rican ancestry. Recurrent bacterial infections are more common in Chédiak-Higashi syndrome. Both syndromes are autosomal recessive.

Index

(*f* = figure; *t* = table)